T0092210

OXFORD MEDICAL PUBLICATIONS

Oxford Handbook of Expedition and Wilderness Medicine

Published and forthcoming Oxford Handbooks

OXFORD HANDBOOK OF

Expedition and Wilderness Medicine

Third Edition

EDITED BY

Dr Jon Dallimore

General Practitioner, Chepstow, Wales, UK; Director,
International Diploma in Expedition and Wilderness Medicine,
Royal College of Physicians and Surgeons of Glasgow, Medical
Officer, Severn Area Rescue Association, UK

Dr Sarah R. Anderson

Consultant in Public Health, UK Health Security Agency, UK

Professor Chris Imray

Professor of Vascular and Renal Transplant Surgery University
Hospital, Coventry and Warwickshire NHS Trust; Director of
NIHR Coventry Clinical Research Facility, UHCW NHS Trust,
Coventry; Professor, Warwick Medical School; Professor,
Coventry University; Professor, Exeter University, UK

Dr Chris Johnson

Retired Consultant Anaesthetist, UK

James Moore

Director, Travel Health Consultancy,
Director, International Diploma in Expedition and Wilderness
Medicine, Royal College of Physicians and Surgeons of Glasgow, UK

Shane Winser

Expeditions and Field Science Advisor, Royal Geographical
Society (with IBG), London, UK

OXFORD
UNIVERSITY PRESS

OXFORD
UNIVERSITY PRESS

Great Clarendon Street, Oxford, OX2 6DP,
United Kingdom

Oxford University Press is a department of the University of Oxford.
It furthers the University's objective of excellence in research, scholarship,
and education by publishing worldwide. Oxford is a registered trade mark of
Oxford University Press in the UK and in certain other countries

© Oxford University Press 2023

The moral rights of the authors have been asserted

First Edition published in 2008
Second Edition published in 2015
Third Edition published in 2023

Published in the United States of America by Oxford University Press
198 Madison Avenue, New York, NY 10016, United States of America

British Library Cataloguing in Publication Data
Data available

Library of Congress Control Number: 2022943952

ISBN 978–0–19–886701–2

DOI: 10.1093/med/9780198867012.001.0001

Printed and bound in Turkey by Promat

Dedication

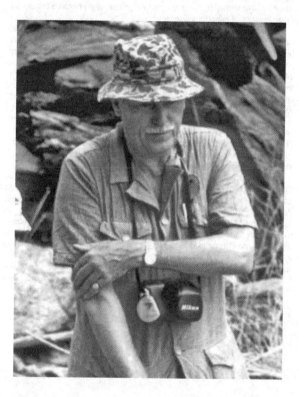

Dr Bent Einer Juel-Jensen (1922–2006)

MA, DM (Cand. Med. Copenhagen) FRCP, MRCGP, HonFRGS

This book is dedicated to the memory of our late very dear friend Bent Juel-Jensen who stimulated, encouraged, and supported us together with generations of other young explorers and expeditioners at the Royal Geographical Society and the University of Oxford. He was the archetypal and model expedition medical officer.

Born in Odense, Denmark, Bent qualified in medicine in Copenhagen in 1949 but spent the rest of his life based in Oxford with his devoted wife Mary. At New College he studied physiology and Elizabethan literature and later became a loyal Fellow of St Cross College. His medical career began at the Radcliffe Infirmary with Dr Fred Hobson and Professor George Pickering, working on hypertension. In 1960, he became hospital Medical Officer and, from 1977 to 1990, University Medical Officer. Bent took charge of infectious diseases in Oxford and pioneered the treatment of herpes zoster with antiviral drugs. Many of his protégés became consultants or professors of infectious diseases.

Bent's greatest enthusiasm was exploration and expeditions. He was passionately committed to the Oxford University Exploration Club, eventually becoming its Honorary President. Bent greatly improved the medical preparedness and training of its largely undergraduate members and was the inspiration, advisor, and friend to many budding young explorers, including the editors of this handbook. Pharmaceutical companies were pressurized into donating essential drugs for their medical kits. As founding medical advisor to the Royal Geographical Society, he created a new awareness of the medical aspects of exploration. This contribution was recognized by his election to an Honorary Fellowship. The RGS-NMK Kora Research Project (Tana River, Kenya) in 1983 had Bent as its energetic medical officer. He was friend and advisor to many famous explorers and travellers, the likes of Sir Wilfred Thesiger, Sir Vivian Fuchs, and Bruce Chatwin.

After England and Denmark, Bent's favourite country was Ethiopia. Oxford expeditions to explore the rock-hewn churches of Tigre in 1973 and 1974 resulted in his forming a close friendship with the local ruler, Prince Ras Mangashia. Bent's enthusiasm for Ethiopia stimulated him to learn Amharic and the priests' language Ge'ez, to embrace its history, literature, culture, and food. He always carried his own supply of fiery berbera to ignite tame European dishes. His great physical courage, early displayed in his resistance to the Nazis in wartime Copenhagen, was again very much to the fore as he gave medical support across the Sudanese border to the Ethiopian Democratic Union's army battling the evil despot Mengistu Haile Mariam.

Bent Juel-Jensen, what an incredible man and a marvellous friend for all seasons!

Foreword

An altered perspective

In the past, the main emphasis of publications on expedition and wilderness medicine was to encourage ambitious (even daring) travel and activities off the beaten track, while reducing the risk of associated diseases, injuries, and accidents. That emphasis has changed! Enthusiasm for adventurous exploration of remote locations, promoted by previous editions of the *Oxford Handbook of Expedition and Wilderness Medicine* (OHEWM), is now threatening to crowd-out, pollute, damage, and even destroy many of the most challenging destinations. In the face of climate change, expanding human population, and occupation of the planet leading to environmental degradation, as well as political uncertainties and pandemics, we should now recognize responsibility towards the environment as the overriding concern of expedition and wilderness medicine.

Responsible enjoyment of the environment

While encouraging participation in properly-planned travels and expeditions, the third edition of *OHEWM* emphasizes a more responsible, contributory, and sensitive approach to enjoying our natural environment. In Chapter 4, 'Ethics and professional responsibilities', under 'Environmental impact', those planning expeditions are urged to analyse and minimize the consequences of their activities. How best to travel to the site of the expedition? Reducing one's carbon footprint should, perhaps, encourage rail or sea as an alternative to flying, even though they will be slower. Once arrived, conservation of local fauna and flora and respect for indigenous people should be the priority. Collection of voucher specimens for research studies or museums should be rigorously justified and controlled.

The fragility of nature is captured beautifully by Gerard Manley Hopkins' poem 'Binsey Poplars', written in 1879.

> O if we but knew what we do
>   When we delve or hew—
>   Hack and rack the growing green!
>   Since country is so tender
>   To touch, her being so slender, …

Chapter 4 gives sound and detailed advice about mitigating environmental damage, but the hardest decision of all would be to opt for an alternative, perhaps less immediately appealing, destination, or for a less demanding scientific aim for the expedition, in the interests of preserving precious countryside and wildlife. Some of the most fragile and threatened locations will have to be closed to all visitors, to allow their return to a more serene primal state, before further incursion can be allowed.

Paul Auerbach (1951–2021)—'the father of wilderness medicine'

Let us celebrate the many contributions and achievements of my American friend Paul Auerbach, who died of a cerebral glioblastoma on 23 June 2021. He is widely regarded as being 'the father of wilderness medicine' having practically invented this subspeciality of emergency medicine. While a resident at UCLA in 1978, he began working on a landmark publication, *Management of Wilderness and Environmental Emergencies*, which evolved into *Auerbach's Wilderness Medicine* (7th edition, 2017), the most comprehensive database available in this field. He co-founded the Wilderness Medical Society in 1983. Paul strongly supported the development of expedition and wilderness medicine in the UK, notably by attending and enlivening the Oxford meeting of the Student Wilderness Medicine UK National Conference in November 2003. In choosing an appropriate and internationally recognizable title for the *OHEWM*, we were influenced by the transatlantic term 'wilderness medicine', promoted, if not coined, by Paul himself. His later espousal of the environmental imperative, as shown by his book *Enviromedics: The Impact of Climate Change on Human Health*, published in 2017, supports the contentions I have expressed above.

OHEWM's lineage of authorship

It is good to see contributions from a number of new authors and reviewers. However, in the *OHEWM*, authorship is built on previous contributions by a succession of writers and advisors, as is acknowledged on the title page of each chapter. All the chapters have been enhanced and updated over the three editions, that, in turn, were based on antecedent versions, before we were adopted by Oxford University Press in 2008.

Dr Bent Juel-Jensen remembered

The origins of this book were cyclostyled sheets, prepared by Oxford University Expedition Club's medical advisor, Dr Bent Juel-Jensen, to equip undergraduate expeditioners for their adventures. The editors of this current edition, and many of its authors, were fortunate enough to have known Bent and to have been inspired by his example. However, most of its readers will not have had that privilege, so please read the Dedication.

I warmly congratulate my successors as editors of the *OHEWM* for their achievement in publishing a magnificent new edition, and I wish the readers enjoyable, successful, but above all, environmentally responsible expeditions.

David A. Warrell
Oxford
October 2021

Preface

Expedition medicine (also known as 'wilderness medicine') is concerned with maintaining physical and psychological well-being during travel to remote and challenging places. Adventurous travel is to be encouraged and wilderness medicine attempts to minimize the risk of injury and disease by proper planning, preventive measures such as vaccinations, sensible behaviour, and acquisition of relevant medical skills.

Exploration and wilderness travel has proved distinctly dangerous in the past because of poor understanding of the environment, limited medical knowledge, and inadequate equipment. Admiral Anson circumnavigated the globe in 1741–1742, losing five of his six ships and 626 of his 961 crew. All 124 members of Sir John Franklin's ill-fated voyage to the northwest passage died. During Stanley's trans-Africa expedition from Zanzibar to the Congo 1874–1877, 114 of his original 228 expedition members died from battle, murder, smallpox, dysentery, drowning, crocodile attack, fever, execution, getting lost, or falling victim to cannibalism post starvation. This level of expedition mortality was unacceptable even in those days. It led to Stanley being branded a ruthless and irresponsible leader, exhibiting highly disrespectful behaviours associated with colonialization, a system we now recognize as deeply wrong, and that must not be repeated.

The twentieth century saw safety improve and mortality fall but many expeditioners perished in the quest for mountain summits or during polar and remote area exploration. Until the 1980s, 1% of Antarctic base members died of accident or disease, while for every ten climbers who summited Everest roughly one person died on the mountain.

The twenty-first century has seen a vast increase in the number of people visiting remote areas for research, education, and recreation. In 2019, over 400,000 UK nationals booked an adventure holiday. In 2018, 242,000 passengers visited remote destinations on expedition cruises. Visitors to Nepal increased from 460,000 in 2000 to 1.2 million in 2019 and on 19 May 2012, 234 climbers summited Everest. This desire to reach all parts of the earth means that there are now few unexplored land areas and so the aim of expeditions has shifted from discovery, sovereign possession, and scientific investigation in the nineteenth and twentieth centuries to adventure, personal development, and cultural exchange. Commercial expedition opportunities have resulted in the marketing of adventurous journeys by numerous companies, blurring the distinction between an expedition and a leisure activity, and exposing people to physical and psychological hazards for which they may be unprepared. Explicit standards such as British Standard (BS) 8848— a specification for the provision of visits, fieldwork, expeditions, and adventurous activities, outside the UK—set out good practice for organizing adventures and seek to optimize planning and risk management. The medical section of BS 8848 describes the need to consider pre-existing medical problems, disease prevention, first-aid kits, environmental illnesses, and levels of medical expertise. All of these areas are carefully considered in this book.

Many of the environmental hazards encountered by previous generations of explorers still challenge expeditions in the twenty-first century, but we are now in a much stronger position to minimize risk through careful planning based on a vast fund of medical knowledge and the development of drugs, vaccines, technology, and skills. In recent years, the advent of smartphones and tablets has altered the way we access knowledge while cellular and satellite networks link us to the internet from previously isolated locations. In the 1980s, expeditions would seldom have communication with the outside world. Modern technology now means that it is possible to track the movements of an expedition remotely and to have real-time communication with expert help when required.

Clinicians, quite rightly, expect to receive appropriate training to equip themselves for new challenges. A number of organizations have produced competency-based syllabuses for expedition and wilderness medicine. This manual has proved a useful supplement for these courses.

This handbook, now in its third edition, started as a product of the Medical Cell at the Royal Geographical Society (with the Institute of British Geographers). The Medical Cell was set up to provide medical advice to expeditions and those seeking advice from the Society. The handbook is a distillation of the experience and skills accumulated by clinicians, explorers, expeditioners, local people, researchers, and remote area travellers from all around the world. The first edition, published in 2008, was designed to be a practical and portable guide to the prevention and treatment of common medical problems and injury conditions in extreme and remote environments. The handbook format proved very popular and has been used during the course of many expeditions by doctors, nurses, paramedics, and first-aiders, as well as by non-medical expedition members. The second edition of this handbook, published in 2015, included more topics and treatment algorithms and had greater emphasis on risk management.

This edition has been fully revised and the editors are grateful for the valuable contributions from our new authors and reviewers. There are new colour plates, more treatment algorithms to guide care, and some chapters have been re-written. The work remains in its convenient rucksack-size handbook format but is also available electronically to save space and weight—both of which are at a premium on almost all expeditions. The information presented is based on the latest clinical guidelines or, where these do not exist, on best practice.

The world is a very different place since we edited the last edition. The COVID-19 pandemic delayed publication as many of our contributors have been involved with managing patients and health services during that time. We are hugely grateful to all of our contributors for devoting time to this work when so many healthcare providers have been busier than at any time in their working lives. While the pandemic caused great suffering, it also brought opportunities. Everyone has a greater awareness of the interconnected nature of human societies, animals, and the planet, the impact of global warming, and the opportunities presented through shared medical research for the common good of all humankind.

As international travel increases, we hope this handbook will encourage many people to experience and enjoy remote travel in a responsible way. Once the world begins to refocus after the pandemic, it is hoped that everyone will be more aware of the effects of burning fossil fuels and climate change. We must all play our part in reducing the damage to our fragile planet. Our original aim when creating this handbook was to highlight the need to identify and minimize avoidable risks without allowing these concerns to detract from the essential excitement and sense of achievement while exploring the wilderness. Now, we need to add that our wish for adventure travel must not be to the detriment of our shared home. We want to encourage people to enjoy remote travel in a more responsible, contributive, and sensitive manner.

Jon Dallimore
Sarah R. Anderson
Chris Imray
Chris Johnson
James Moore
Shane Winser
September 2021

Contents

Contributors

Edi Albert

Senior Lecturer in Remote and Polar Medicine, and Rural Generalist in Emergency Medicine, University of Tasmania, Hobart, Tasmania, Australia; Director, Wilderness Education Group

Sarah R. Anderson

Consultant in Health Protection, Public Health England, London, UK

Jules Blackham

Consultant Emergency Physician and HEMS Consultant, North Bristol NHS Trust and Great Western Air Ambulance, UK

Jim Bond

Specialist in Travel and Expedition Medicine, TrExMed Travel Clinic, Edinburgh, UK

Peter Bradley

Anaesthetist, Expedition, Medical and Prolonged Field Care Lead, Remote Area Risk International, UK

Spike Briggs

Consultant in Intensive Care and Anaesthesia, Poole Hospital NHS Foundation Trust; Director of Medical Support Offshore Ltd, UK

Rose Buckley

Consultant Anaesthetist, Sheffield Teaching Hospitals NHS Foundation Trust, UK

Tim Campbell-Smith

Consultant General and Colorectal Surgeon, Surrey and Sussex NHS Healthcare Trust, UK

Nicholas Chilvers

Specialty Trainee in Cardiothoracic Surgery, The James Cook University Hospital, Middlesbrough, UK; Medical Officer, Royal Army Medical Corps.

Alistair Cobb

Consultant Oral & Maxillofacial Surgeon, Southwest Regional Cleft Service, Bristol, UK

Robert Conway

Anaesthetist and Expedition Doctor, Wild Medic Ltd, Brighton, UK

Paul Cooper

Consultant Neurologist, Greater Manchester Neuroscience Centre, Salford Royal Foundation Trust, UK

Rachael Craven

Consultant Anaesthetist, University Hospitals, Bristol, UK

Dr Jon Dallimore

General Practitioner, Chepstow, Wales, UK; Director, International Diploma in Expedition and Wilderness Medicine, Royal College of Physicians and Surgeons of Glasgow; Medical Officer, Severn Area Rescue Association, UK

Matthew Davies

Solicitor-Advocate. Remote Area Legal and Travel Risk Management. Duty of Care Subject Matter Expert at Remote Area Risk International. BS:8848 & ISO: 31030 committee member

Ian Davis

General Practitioner and Polar Explorer, UK

Richard Dawood
Medical Director, Fleet Street Clinic, London, UK

Matthew Dryden
Consultant in Infection, UKOT Program and RIPL, Porton Down, UK Overseas Territories, Global Operations, UK Health Security Agency

Matthew Ellis
Honorary Senior Lecturer in Global Child Health, University of Bristol, UK

Derek Evans
Independent Travel Medicine Specialist, Newport, Wales, UK Adjunct Clinical Professor in Pharmacy Practice, Doctor of World Sciences, USA

Jonathan Ferguson
Consultant Cardiothoracic Surgeon, The James Cook University Hospital, Middlesbrough, UK

Simon Flower
General Practitioner, Bristol, UK; Medical Officer, Mendip Cave Rescue

Prof Karen Forbes
Professorial Teaching Fellow in Palliative Medicine, Programme Director, University of Bristol Medical School, UK

Prof Larry Goodyer
Professor of Pharmacy Practice, De Montfort University, Leicester, UK

Penelope B. Granger
General Dental Practitioner, BASMU, Derriford Hospital, Plymouth, UK; Norrbottens Läns Landsting, Sweden

Richard Griffiths
Consultant in Emergency Medicine, Ysbyty Gwynedd, Wales, UK; Chairman, Llanberis Mountain Rescue Team

Rebecca Harris
Freelance TV Producer, London, UK

Peter Harvey
Risk Management Specialist, Hampshire, UK

Debbie Hawker
Clinical Psychologist, InterHealth Worldwide, London, UK

Roderick Hay
Emeritus Professor of Cutaneous Infection, King's College Hospital, London, UK

Craig Holdstock
Consultant Cardiothoracic Anaesthetist, University Hospitals Plymouth NHS Trust, UK; Medical Officer, Devon Cave Rescue Organisation

Amy Hughes
Flight Doctor, Essex and Herts Air Ambulance, Research Fellow, National Institute for Health and Care Research, Barts and The Royal London;
Senior Education Fellow, Institute of Pre-hospital Care, Queen Mary University, London, UK

Chris Johnson
Retired Consultant Anaesthetist, Frenchay, Bristol, UK

Clive Johnson
Retired Polar Specialist, Buxton, UK

Stephen Jones
Operations Manager, Antarctic Logistics & Expeditions LLC, UK

Burjor K. Langdana
Honorary Clinical Professor, University of Exeter, Founder of Wilderness Expedition Dentistry (WED), Leeds, UK

Nick Lewis
Environmental Scientist and
Mountaineer;
Antarctic Logistics and Expeditions
LLC, Salt Lake City, USA

Tom Mallinson
Rural GP and Co-Director of
Prehospital Care,
BASICS Scotland, Brora, Scotland,
UK

Carey M. McClellan
Advanced Physiotherapy
Practitioner, Clinical Director,
getUBetter, Bristol, UK

Iain McIntosh
Travel Health Consultant, St
Ninian's Travel Health Research
Centre, Stirling, UK

Alastair Miller
Consultant Physician,
Deputy Medical Director,
Joint Royal Colleges of Physicians
Training Board, London, UK

Ben Molyneaux
Dental Surgeon, London, UK

James Moore
Director and Nurse Specialist,
Travel Health Consultancy, Exeter
Director, International Diploma
in Expedition and Wilderness
Medicine, Royal College of
Physicians and Surgeons of
Glasgow, UK

Paddy Morgan
Consultant in Anaesthesia and
Pre-Hospital Care, North Bristol
NHS Trust, & Emergency Medical
Retrieval and Transfer Service,
Wales, UK

Daniel S. Morris
Consultant Ophtahlmologist,
Cardiff Eye Unit, University of
Wales, UK

Harvey Pynn
Consultant in Emergency Medicine
and Pre-hospital Emergency
Medicine, Bristol, UK

Defence Consultant Advisor in Pre-
hospital Emergency Care

Paul Richards
General Practitioner, Mid and
South Essex Integrated Care
System; Member, Travel Medicine
Subcommittee, Joint Committee on
Vaccination and Immunisation

Barry Roberts
Director, Wilderness Medical
Training, Kendal, UK

Marc Shaw
Professor, College of Public Health,
Medical and Veterinary Sciences,
Division of Tropical Health and
Medicine, James Cook University,
Townsville, Australia;
Medical Director, Worldwise
Geographic Medicine, New Zealand

Julian Thompson
Consultant in Intensive Care
Medicine, Southmead Hospital,
Bristol, UK

Lesley F. Thomson
Consultant Anaesthetist
University Hospitals Plymouth NHS
Trust, Derriford Road, Plymouth,
UK

Clare Warrell
Consultant in Tropical Medicine
and Infectious Diseases, London,
UK; Clinical Fellow, London
School of Hygiene and Tropical
Medicine

Prof Sir David A. Warrell
Emeritus Professor of Tropical
Medicine, University of
Oxford, UK

Andy Watt

Consultant Physician, Ayrshire and Arran NHS, UK

Jane Wilson-Howarth

General Practitioner and Global Health Specialist, Cambridge, UK

Jeremy Windsor

Consultant in Anaesthesia and Intensive Care, Chesterfield Royal Hospital, Derbyshire, UK; Senior Lecturer in Mountain Medicine, University of Central Lancashire, UK

Shane Winser

Expeditions and Field Science Advisor, Royal Geographical Society (with IBG), London, UK

Contributors to the second edition

Dr Edi Albert

Senior Lecturer in Remote and Polar Medicine, and Rural Generalist in Emergency Medicine, University of Tasmania, Hobart, Tasmania, Australia; Director, Wilderness Education Group

Dr Sarah R. Anderson

Consultant in Health Protection, Public Health England, London, UK

Dr Kristina Birch

Consultant in Anaesthetics and Intensive Care Medicine, North Bristol NHS Trust, UK

Dr Jules Blackham

Consultant Emergency Physician and HEMS Consultant, North Bristol NHS Trust and Great Western Air Ambulance, UK

Dr Jim Bond

Specialist in Travel and Expedition Medicine, TrExMed Travel Clinic, Edinburgh, UK

Dr Spike Briggs

Consultant in Intensive Care and Anaesthesia, Poole Hospital NHS Foundation Trust; Director of Medical Support Offshore Ltd, UK

Mr Tim Campbell Smith

Consultant General and Colorectal Surgeon, Surrey and Sussex NHS Healthcare Trust, UK

Mr Alistair R. M. Cobb

Consultant Oral and Maxillofacial Surgeon, Southwest Regional Cleft Service, Bristol, UK

Dr Robert Conway

Anaesthetist and Expedition Doctor, Wild Medic Ltd, Brighton, UK

Dr Paul Cooper

Consultant Neurologist, Greater Manchester Neuroscience Centre, Salford Royal Foundation Trust, UK

Dr Rachael Craven

Consultant Anaesthetist, University Hospitals, Bristol, UK

Dr Jon Dallimore

General Practitioner and Specialty Doctor in Emergency Medicine, Bristol Royal Infirmary, UK

Dr Claire Davies

Travel Health Doctor/General Practitioner, InterHealth Worldwide, London, UK

Dr Ian Davis

General Practitioner and Polar Explorer, UK

Dr Richard Dawood

Medical Director, Fleet Street Clinic, London, UK

Dr Sundeep Dhillon

Honorary Research Fellow, Centre for Altitude, Space & Extreme Medicine (CASE), Institute of Sport, Exercise & Health, London, UK

Dr Rose Drew
Registrar in Anaesthesia and Intensive Care Medicine, Sheffield School of Anaesthesia, UK

Dr Matthew Dryden
Director of Infection, Rare and Imported Pathogens Department, Public Health England, Porton, Hampshire Hospitals NHS Foundation Trust and Southampton School of Medicine, UK

Dr Linda Dykes
Consultant in Emergency Medicine, Ysbyty Gwynedd, Bangor, UK

Mr Jonathan Ferguson
Consultant Cardiothoracic Surgeon, The James Cook University Hospital, Middlesbrough, UK

Prof Karen Forbes
Professorial Teaching Fellow and Consultant in Palliative Medicine, University of Bristol, UK

Prof Larry Goodyer
Head of the Leicester School of Pharmacy, De Montfort University, Leicester, UK

Paul F. Goodyer
CEO and Founder of Nomad Travel Stores and Travel Clinics, Enfield, UK

Penelope B. Granger
General Dental Practitioner, BASMU, Derriford Hospital, Plymouth, UK; Norrbottens Läns Landsting, Sweden

Rebecca Harris
Freelance TV Producer, London, UK

Peter Harvey
Risk Management Specialist, Hampshire, UK

Dr Debbie Hawker
Clinical Psychologist, InterHealth Worldwide, London, UK

Dr Amy Hughes
Clinical Lecturer in Emergency Response, Humanitarian and Conflict Response Institute, University of Manchester, UK

Prof Chris Imray
Consultant Vascular and Renal Transplant Surgeon, Warwick Medical School and University Hospital Coventry and Warwickshire NHS Trust, UK

Dr Chris Johnson
Consultant Anaesthetist, North Bristol NHS Trust, Westbury-on-Trym, Bristol, UK

Clive Johnson
Polarsphere, Polar Logistics, Buxton, UK

Stephen Jones
Operations Manager, Antarctic Logistics & Expeditions LLC, UK

Burjor K. Langdana
General and Expedition Dental Practitioner, Leeds, Dentist to British Antarctic Survey Medical Unit, UK

Dr Jonathan Leach
General Practitioner, Bromsgrove, UK

Dr Campbell MacKenzie
Specialist in Remote and Offshore Medicine, Bristol, UK

Dr Carey M. McLellan
Extended Scope Physiotherapist in Emergency Care, University Hospitals, Bristol, UK

Dr Iain McIntosh
Travel Health Consultant, St Ninians Travel Health Research Centre, Stirling, UK

Dr Alastair Miller
Consultant Physician (Infectious Diseases), Royal Liverpool University Hospital and University of Liverpool, UK

James Moore
Director and Nurse Specialist, Travel Health Consultancy, Exeter, UK

Clare Morgan
Sexual Health Adviser, University Hospitals, Bristol, UK

Dr Paddy Morgan
Consultant Anaesthetist, North Bristol NHS Trust, Westbury-on-Trym, Bristol, UK

Mr Daniel S. Morris
Consultant Ophthalmologist, Cardiff Eye Unit, University of Wales, UK

Dr Annabel H. Nickol
Clinical Lecturer in Respiratory and General Medicine, Oxford Centre for Respiratory Medicine, UK

Dr Howard Oakley
Associate Specialist in Environmental Medicine, Institute of Naval Medicine, Alverstoke, UK

Prof Andrew J. Pollard
Professor of Paediatric Infection and Immunity, Department of Paediatrics, University of Oxford, UK

Lt Col Harvey Pynn
Consultant in Emergency Medicine and Pre-Hospital Care, University Hospitals, Bristol; Medical Director, Wilderness Medical Training, UK

Dr Paul Richards
General Practitioner and Travel Medicine Specialist; Honorary Lecturer, Centre for Altitude, Space & Extreme Medicine (CASE), UCL, London, UK

Barry Roberts
Director, Wilderness Medical Training, UK

George W. Rodway
Assistant Professor, Division of Health Sciences, University of Nevada, Reno, NV, USA

Prof Marc Shaw
Travel and Geographical Medicine Consultant; Professor, School of Public Health, James Cook University, Townsville, Australia; Medical Director, Worldwise Travellers Health Centres, New Zealand

Dr Julian Thompson
Specialist Registrar in Anaesthesia and Intensive Care, Oxford University Hospitals, UK

Dr Lesley F. Thomson
Consultant Anaesthetist, Derriford Hospital, Plymouth, UK

Andrew Thurgood
Consultant Nurse—Prehospital Emergency Medicine, Mercia Accident Rescue Service and West Midlands CARE Team, UK

Prof David A. Warrell
International Director, Royal College of Physicians; Emeritus Professor of Tropical Medicine, University of Oxford, UK

Dr Andy Watt
Consultant Physician, Ayrshire and Arran NHS, UK

Dr Jane Wilson-Howarth
General Practitioner and Medical Director, Travel Clinic Ltd., Cambridge and Ipswich, UK

Dr Jeremy Windsor
Consultant in Anaesthesia and Intensive Care, Chesterfield Royal Hospital, Derbyshire, UK

Shane Winser

Geography Outdoors: the centre supporting field research, exploration and outdoor learning, Royal Geographical Society (with IBG), London, UK

Contributors to the first edition

Mr James Calder

Trauma and Orthopaedic Consultant, North Hampshire Hospital, and Clinical Senior Lecturer, Imperial College, London, UK

Dr Charles Clarke

Honorary Consultant Neurologist, National Hospital for Neurology and Neurosurgery, Queen Square, London, UK and President of the British Mountaineering Council, UK

David Geddes

Dental Surgeon

Dr Mike Grocott

Senior Lecturer in Intensive Care Medicine, Centre for Altitude Space and Extreme Environment Medicine, UCL Institute of Human Health and Performance, London, UK

Dr Stephen Hearns

Consultant in Emergency Medicine, Lead Consultant Emergency Medical Retrieval Service, Royal Alexandra Hospital Paisley, UK

Dr Michael E. Jones

Consultant Physician, Regional Infectious Diseases Unit, Western General Hospital, Edinburgh, UK; HealthLink360 Edinburgh International Health Centre Carberry, Musselburgh, UK

Dr Akbar Lalani

Royal Army Medical Corps

Christina Lalani

Trainee in Anaesthesia, Frimley Park NHS Foundation Trust, UK

Nick Lewis

Environmental Consultant, Poles Apart, Cambridge, UK

Prof David Lockey

Professor of Trauma and Pre-Hospital Emergency Medicine, North Bristol NHS Trust, UK

Prof Hugh Montgomery

Director, Institute for Human Health and Performance, University College London, UK

Dr Christopher Moxon

Research Associate, Malawi-Liverpool-Wellcome Clinical Research Programme, Honorary Paediatric Registrar, College of Medicine, Malawi

Prof Ian Palmer

Professor of Military Psychiatry, Head of Medical Assessment Programme, MoDUK, St Thomas' Hospital, London, UK

Dr Andy Pitkin

Department of Anesthesiology, University of Florida, Gainesville, FL, USA

Dr Tariq Qureshi

Department of Emergency Medicine, John Radcliffe Hospital, Oxford Radcliffe Hospitals, NHS Trust, UK

Dr Charlie Siderfin

General Practitioner, Heilendi Family Medical Practice, Kirkwall, Orkney, UK

Dr Joe Silsby

Consultant in Anaesthesia and ICM Taunton and Somerset NHS Foundation Trust, UK

James Watson

Physiotherapy Officer, Medical Support Unit, Headquarters, Hereford Garrison, UK

Symbols and abbreviations

➜	cross-reference
~	approximately
>	greater than
<	less than
⏾	website
±	with or without
ABC	airway, breathing, circulation
ACE	angiotensin-converting enzyme
ACL	anterior cruciate ligament (knee)
ACVPU	Scale to evaluate conscious level (awake/verbal/pain/unresponsive)
ADHD	attention deficit hyperactivity disorder
ADL	activity of daily living (disability)
AED	automated external defibrillator
AGE	arterial gas embolism
AIDS	acquired immunodeficiency syndrome
ALS	advanced life support
AMS	acute mountain sickness
AMTS	Abbreviated Mental Test Score
ARDS	acute respiratory distress syndrome
ASAP	as soon as possible!
ATLS	Advanced Trauma Life Support
BCG	bacillus Calmette–Guérin
BLS	basic life support
BMI	body mass index
BNF	British National Formulary
BP	blood pressure
BS	British Standard
BTS	British Thoracic Society
CABC	catastrophic haemorrhage, airway, breathing, circulation
CABCD	catastrophic haemorrhage, airway, breathing, circulation, disability
CABCDE	catastrophic haemorrhage, airway, breathing, circulation, disability, environment/exposure
CAGE	cerebral arterial gas embolism
CES	cauda equina syndrome
CMV	cytomegalovirus
CNS	central nervous system
CO	carbon monoxide
CO_2	carbon dioxide
COPD	chronic obstructive pulmonary disease
COVID-19	coronavirus disease 2019
CPAP	continuous positive airway pressure
CPP	cerebral perfusion pressure
CPR	cardiopulmonary resuscitation
CRT	capillary refill time
CSF	cerebrospinal fluid
DCI	decompression illness
DCS	decompression sickness
DEET	diethyltoluamide
DIC	disseminated intravascular coagulation
DIPJ	distal interphalangeal joint
DKA	diabetic ketoacidosis
DSH	deliberate self-harm
DTI	Department of Trade & Industry
DVT	deep venous thrombosis
EAV	expired air ventilation
EBV	Epstein–Barr virus
ECC	extracorporeal circulation
ECG	electrocardiogram
EHS	exertional heat stroke
ELISA	enzyme-linked immunosorbent assay
ELT	emergency locator transmitter (aircraft)
ENT	ear, nose, and throat
EPA	Environmental Protection Agency (US)
EPIRB	emergency position-indicating radio beacon
ERP	emergency response plan
ETEC	enterotoxigenic *Escherichia coli*
EU	European Union
FCDO	Foreign, Commonwealth & Development Office (UK)

FG	French gauge
g	gram
G	gauge
G6PD	glucose-6-phosphate dehydrogenase
GCS	Glasgow Coma Scale
GI	gastrointestinal
GMC	General Medical Council (UK)
GORD	gastro-oesophageal reflux disease
GP	general practitioner
GPS	global positioning system
GSM	global system for mobile communications
GTN	glyceryl trinitrate
HAART	highly active anti-retroviral therapy
HACE	high-altitude cerebral oedema
HAPE	high-altitude pulmonary oedema
HAR	high-altitude retinopathy
HAV	hepatitis A virus
HELP	heat escape lessening posture
HBV	hepatitis B virus
HCV	hepatitis C virus
HDV	hepatitis D virus
HEV	hepatitis A virus
HiB	*Haemophilus influenzae* b
HIV	human immunodeficiency virus
HPV	human papillomavirus
HR	heart rate
HRI	heat-related illness
HSV	herpes simplex virus
IBG	Institute of British
ICP	intracranial pressure
ID	intradermal
Ig	immunoglobulin
IM	intramuscular (drug administration)
IPJ	interphalangeal joint (digits)
IPO	immersion pulmonary oedema
IRM	intermediate restorative material (dental)
IUCD	intrauterine contraceptive device
IV	intravenous
LA	local anaesthesia/anaesthetic (e.g. lidocaine)
LIF	left iliac fossa of abdomen
LMA	laryngeal mask airway

LMIC	low- and middle-income countries
LRTI	lower respiratory tract infection
LZ	landing zone (aircraft)
MAP	mean arterial pressure
MCA	Marine and Coastguard Agency
MCPJ	metacarpophalangeal joint (digits)
MERS	Middle East respiratory syndrome
mg	milligram
MI	myocardial infarction
mL	millilitre
MMR	mumps, measles, rubella
MO	medical officer
MOB	man overboard
MRI	magnetic resonance imaging
NAAT	nucleic acid amplification test
NaTHNaC	National Travel Health Network and Centre
NEWS	National Early Warning Score
NEXUS	National Emergency X-Radiography Utilization Study
NGO	non-governmental organization
NHS	National Health Service (UK)
NICE	National Institute for Health and Care Excellence (UK)
NPA	nasopharyngeal airway
NSAID	non-steroidal anti-inflammatory drug (e.g. ibuprofen)
O_2	oxygen
OPA	oropharyngeal airway
OSA	obstructive sleep apnoea
P	pulse
PBI	pressure bandage immobilization
PCL	posterior cruciate ligament (knee)
PCR	polymerase chain reaction
PE	pulmonary embolism
PEFR	peak expiratory flow rate
PEPSE	post-exposure prophylaxis following sexual exposure
PF	peak flow (asthma)
PFD	Personal flotation device
pH	acid/base scale
PID	pelvic inflammatory disease

PIPJ	proximal interphalangeal joint	SCUBA	self-contained underwater breathing apparatus
PLB	personal locator beacon (ground personnel)	SPC	summary of product characteristics
PO	oral (drug administration)	SPF	sun protection factor (sunscreen)
PPE	personal protective equipment	STI	sexually transmitted infection
PPI	proton pump inhibitor *or* pressure pad immobilization	SUP	stand-up paddleboard
PR	rectal (drug administration)	T	temperature
PTSD	post-traumatic stress disorder	TB	tuberculosis
RGS	Royal Geographical Society	TBE	tick-borne encephalitis
RICE	rest, ice, compression, elevation	TMJ	temporomandibular joint
RIF	right iliac fossa of abdomen	UC	ulcerative colitis
RIG	rabies immune globulin	UK	United Kingdom
RR	respiratory rate	URTI	upper respiratory tract infection
RTC	road traffic collision	US	United States
rt-PA	recombinant tissue plasminogen activator	UTI	urinary tract infection
RUQ	right upper quadrant	UV	ultraviolet
SaO_2	arterial oxygen saturation	UVR (UVA, UVB)	ultraviolet radiation (types A and B)
SAR	search and rescue	VEGF	vascular endothelial growth factor
SARA	sexually acquired reactive arthritis	VHF	very high frequency (radio waveband)
SARS	severe acute respiratory syndrome	WBGT	wet bulb globe temperature
SBET	standby emergency treatment	WHO	World Health Organization
SC	subcutaneous (drug administration)	WMS	Wilderness Medical Society
		YF	yellow fever

Chapter 1

Expedition medicine

Chapter editor
Chris Johnson

Contributors
Sarah R. Anderson
Chris Johnson
Shane Winser
David A. Warrell (1st and 2nd editions)
Linda Dykes (2nd edition)

Reviewer
Richard Griffiths

A global change

The third edition of this handbook is being written amid huge global uncertainty and disruption. Coronavirus disease 2019 (COVID-19), the first pandemic for a century, has disrupted life for most of the world's 8 billion people. The pandemic struck a world that was becoming increasingly aware of the consequences of an exponential rise in human population, with its effects on global warming, resource depletion, and ecosystem destruction. Travel to exotic places, until half a century ago undertaken by a privileged few, has become a mass-market industry creating wealth and employment, but in popular locations has become unsustainable as excessive numbers of visitors cram into the most popular destinations.

Doomsday has been predicted many times, whether it be through plague, nuclear holocaust, global warming, or mass migration. Ecologists now predict the possibility of a mass extinction event and it is far from certain whether there is the will to make the necessary social, economic, and environmental changes to avoid such a catastrophe. The internet means that debates on almost anything can rapidly become vitriolic and divorced from science. Writing in the midst of the pandemic we cannot be sure of the future for travel and expeditions but do so in the hope of again being able to visit the world's remote and extreme environments.

Wilderness travel

This handbook is about the healthcare of travellers to remote areas. Remote areas are defined as places where access to sophisticated medical services is difficult or impossible, and the responsibility for dealing with medical problems falls on expedition members. In Europe this branch of medicine is usually called 'expedition medicine', while in North America it is called 'wilderness medicine'.

An expedition is an organized journey with a purpose. Early expeditions sought new lands to claim, develop, and exploit. In the twentieth century, as blanks on maps shrank, geologists, naturalists, and ecologists added detail to the knowledge, while physiologists explored human responses to extreme environments. Today, new scientific knowledge generally requires a highly technological approach and considerable funding, and personal development, cultural exchange, and charity fundraising have become an increasingly important justification for travel.

Adventure travel organizations send tens of thousands of people overseas each year to areas that 30 years ago could only be reached by a well-equipped expedition. Given sufficient funding, journeys to both Poles, the summit of Everest, and even into space can be purchased. Age is no longer a bar to travel, with both healthy and less-fit elderly clients expecting to reach remote and often physically demanding destinations—an octogenarian has reached the top of Everest, while expedition ships will take travellers with significant health problems to remote polar destinations. Attitudes to physical and mental disabilities have also changed enormously. A blind climber has summited Everest and limbless military veterans walked to the South Pole. The distinction between an expedition and a recreational journey is no longer obvious, but the challenges of caring for people far from a base hospital remain.

Technology has shrunk the world: superjeeps and helicopters enable ready access to previously isolated parts of the globe, while satellite navigation systems enable anyone with a smartphone or watch to locate their position precisely. Relatively inexpensive equipment enables global access to the internet and the progress of an expedition team can be monitored remotely and help summoned in the event of an accident. Increasingly, the wilderness is used as a playground for sporting endeavours that push the limits of human physiology.

> **Groups travelling to remote areas now include**
> - Well-organized and -funded expeditions.
> - Film crews documenting ecosystems or adventurous pursuits.
> - Small groups of independent travellers.
> - Commercial trips to remote destinations.
> - Charity fundraising treks to exotic destinations.
> - Participants in 'adventure' holidays.
> - Competitors in extreme sporting events.
> - Gap-year travellers.

Despite the improvements in communications and technology, the physical, environmental, and health risks of remote areas remain. This handbook is about helping travellers understand and prepare for those hazards. It is designed to assist doctors, nurses, and paramedics who support groups far from formal medical facilities.

Increasingly over the past two decades, military and disaster-relief organizations have developed the capability to provide portable but remarkably sophisticated healthcare in remote locations. This has been a response both to war in difficult environments such as the Middle East, and to better assist countries following major natural disasters such as tsunamis, earthquakes, or epidemic disease. These capabilities rely on skilled personnel and costly logistic support, and this handbook does not deal with this type of healthcare.[1]

---

1 See instead, for example: Partridge RA, Proano L, Marcozzi D (eds). *Oxford American Handbook of Disaster Medicine*. New York: Oxford University Press; 2012.

The scope of expedition medicine

Expedition medicine is about:
- Preparing for an expedition—to minimize ill health and maximize expedition achievements.
- Working during the expedition—in a professional capacity to diagnose, treat, and manage health problems.
- Managing expedition emergencies and potential evacuations.
- Finally, advising on health issues once the expedition has returned home.

Organizing the medical care of an expedition takes time and includes tasks such as:
- The assessment and reduction of risk and therefore injury.
- Team selection.
- First-aid training.
- Preventive medicine, including dentistry, both before departure and in the field.
- Organization and transport of a suitable medical kit.
- Knowledge of particular health problems in the area of the visit.
- Provision of medical skills in the field.
- Arrangements for medical back-up and evacuation.
- Organization of health insurance.
- Crisis management.

Each of these aspects will be covered later in this handbook.

Expedition medicine is not just about the treatment of disease or coping with injuries—it should permeate all facets of the expedition. Health criteria must be considered when the location of the base camp is selected and the activities of the trip planned. Food, sanitation, and psychology are part of the expedition medic's work. The medic will fulfil many roles and will certainly be expected to be nurse as well as doctor. Sometimes the work will involve listening to and encouraging those who are finding the expedition emotionally challenging, either due to the remote environment or interpersonal conflicts. The obligation of the medic to care for the sick or accompany a casualty during evacuation may mean that certain personal goals are not attained.

Not all expeditions will include a trained doctor, nurse, or paramedic, but all expeditions must consider how they can prevent disease, and cope with illness or trauma. Correctly practised, expedition medicine should not constrain the enthusiasms and ambitions of an expedition but, by anticipating preventable medical problems, facilitate the achievements and enjoyment of all participants.

Surveys of medicine in remote areas

Several research studies have provided information about the nature and frequency of medical problems in remote environments. Their size, methodologies, and environments vary but some common themes emerge (Table 1.1).

Expedition destinations

Expedition medicine requires an understanding of how humans can physiologically acclimatize and technologically adapt to extreme environments.

Contemporary travel can within a few hours take someone from a relatively benign to a potentially life-threatening environment. Newcomers may have no idea of the hazards they face and inadvertently place themselves in danger. Within an organized group, it is the role of the leader, local guides, and the medic to ensure that participants know how to behave to maintain safety, and that expedition plans match the physical and emotional capabilities of all the team members.

The Royal Geographical Society and Institute of British Geographers (RGS-IBG) surveyed a large number of expeditions in the late 1990s[2] and at that time mountainous terrain and tropical jungles were the most popular geographical areas for expeditions to visit (Fig. 1.1).

Other destinations have increased in popularity and accessibility. During the 1970s, only a handful of tourists visited Antarctica. In the 1980s, numbers increased to around 2000 a year, and this expansion has continued to the current level (2019/2020) of 74,000 visitors. Iceland is a very popular adventure destination and saw a dramatic climb in visitor numbers from 250,000 per year in 2000 to 2.3 million a year in 2018. Nepal has seen a similar although less dramatic rise from 460,000 tourists in 2000 to 1.2 million a year in 2019. However, even before the COVID-19 epidemic halted mass tourism, there were signs that visits to some areas were levelling off or dropping due both to environmental concerns and overcrowding at popular destinations.

Numerous holidays are marketed as 'adventure trips' with >400,000 'adventure holiday' packages sold in the UK in 2019. These may range from expedition level trips to the great mountain ranges through to less extreme trekking or cycling tours in low- or middle-income countries.

In 2018, 242,000 passengers visited remote destinations on 'Expedition cruises' in small vessels capable of carrying 50–200 passengers. Such trips are relatively expensive and attract a high proportion of mature travellers, who may have associated health problems. While large cruise liners now have comprehensively equipped medical facilities, the smaller vessels usually carry a medic and basic equipment but very limited diagnostic and treatment facilities.

Adventurous outdoor education trips have been available for >60 years and share characteristics with more remote overseas travel. They offer youngsters the opportunity to participate in camping, trekking, cycling, canoeing, and other pastimes, often culminating in a supervised but independent expedition.

Given the number of opportunities now on offer for people of all ages to head into the wilderness, it is probable that a family practitioner will be consulted about the preparations required for travel to remote areas. While expedition participants 30 years ago were generally reasonably fit, experienced, and skilled, it is now very easy for a naïve traveller to visit an extreme environment. ➲ Chapters 20–27 of this handbook provide information about human health and physiology in such extreme environments.

2 Anderson SR, Johnson CJH. Expedition health and safety: a risk assessment. *J R Soc Med.* 2000:93:557–562. https://doi.org/10.1177/014107680009301102

Table 1.1 Surveys of expedition medicine incidents

Lead author	Year	Expedition type	Person days	Deaths	Evacuations	Hospitalization	Reported incidents	Rate
Anderson[1]	2000	Small groups expeditions	130,000	0	25	13	835	6.4/1000 days
Price[2]	2002	Ocean yacht racing	2380	0	3	3	685	288/1000 days
Sadnicka[3]	2004	Youth expeditions	70,583	1	6	24	3099	44/1000 days
Lyon[4]	2010	Charity treks	42,482	0	21	c.10	1564	37/1000 days
Schutz[5]	2014	Antarctic expedition cruises	34,501	1	4	4	680	16/1000 days
Wells[6]	2018	Outdoor education (USA)	59,058	0	75	Not stated	143	2.4/1000 days

1. Anderson SR, Johnson CJH. Expedition health and safety: a risk assessment. *J R Soc Med.* 2000;93:557–562. https://doi.org/10.1177/014107680009301102

2. Price CJS, Spalding TJW, McKenzie C. Patterns of illness and injury encountered in amateur ocean yacht racing. *Br J Sports Med.* 2002;36:457–462. https://doi.org/10.1136/bjsm.36.6.457

3. Sadnicka A, Walker R, Dallimore J. Morbidity and determinants of health on youth expeditions. *Wilderness Environ Med.* 2004;15:181–187. https://doi.org/10.1580/1080-6032(2004)15[181:MADOHO]2.0.CO;2

4. Lyon RM, Wiggins CM. Expedition Medicine—the risk of illness and injury. *Wilderness Environ Med.* 2010;21:318–324. https://doi.org/10.1016/j.wem.2010.09.002

5. Schutz L, Zak D, Homes J. Pattern of passenger injury and illness on expedition cruise ships to Antarctica. *J Travel Med.* 2014;21:228–234. https://doi.org/10.1111/jtm.12126

6. Wells FC, Warder CR. Medical incidents and evacuations and wilderness expeditions for the NW Outward Bound school. *Wilderness Environ Med.* 2018;29:479–487. https://doi.org/10.1016/j.wem.2018.07.004

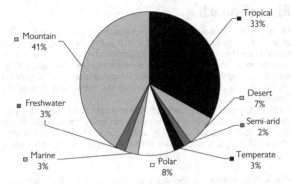

Fig. 1.1 Expedition destinations. Source: Royal Geographical Society Medical Database.

Risk of death

The explorer's worst nightmare may be to catch a dreadful tropical disease or to be attacked by a ferocious wild animal, but for most expeditions the reality is more mundane. Stomach upsets, sprains, bruises, and insomnia are the common problems. The risks of catching insect-borne diseases such as malaria or dengue or being involved in a vehicle collision on the way to the expedition area are usually far greater than the more exotic risks of the wilderness.

Death during an expedition is rare and tragic but should be kept in perspective. The media love dramatic stories but ignore the hazards of daily life. Fatal road collisions, drowning, or falls can occur anywhere; effective advance planning can reduce their incidence. Proper briefing of travellers, together with good risk management, can reduce harm.

> **Expeditions are getting safer …**
>   *But* society is less tolerant of risk.
> Deaths occur on expeditions …
>   *But* deaths also occur at home and receive less publicity.
> All deaths are a tragedy …
>   *But*—by not travelling do you reduce the number of deaths?
> *Only join a trip if you know, understand, and accept the risks.*

Expeditions are becoming safer. In the 18th and 19th centuries, complete expeditions such as Sir John Franklin's ill-fated Arctic Voyage, would disappear into the wilderness and never be heard from again. Between 1943 and 1983, 26 staff of the British Antarctic Survey died (1% of those who overwintered); in the 40 years since 1983 there has been only one death.

In the twentieth century, the ratio of successful summit attempts to deaths on Mount Everest was 1:7 (170 deaths/1169 summits); in the period 2000–2018, the ratio improved to 1:65 (123 deaths/7990 summits). However, this reduction in relative risk has been associated with far greater numbers of people tackling the challenge, not a reduction in the absolute numbers of deaths—with 12 climbers dying on the mountain in 2018 out of 891 climbers.

Fatalities among young people are always tragic and the dramatic circumstances in which they occur mean that deaths on an expedition are often highly publicized, giving the impression that such travel is more hazardous than it really is. Well-publicized deaths of UK nationals during youth expeditions in the past decade include cases of hyperthermia, drowning, wild animal attack, electrocution, anaphylaxis, and exercise-associated hyponatraemia.

In the studies listed in ➲ Table 1.1 (p.8) there were two deaths recorded, one a heart attack on an Antarctic cruise and the other a youngster who fell from height during a mountain trek.

Better weather forecasting, equipment, communications, training, and rescue services have all contributed to reducing the risk of remote areas travel, but safety should not be taken for granted, and travellers to remote areas must strive to minimize risk and be self-sufficient.

In a world where many aspects of life have become much safer, people are less willing to accept risk and keener to attribute blame to an organization if something goes wrong. However, risky behaviour by individuals remains widespread, with 259 people worldwide dying between 2011 and 2017 while taking a 'selfie' picture, about eight times the number of fatalities from shark attacks.

Journeys to remote places can never be completely safe but travelling in a group of motivated people who have carefully considered their plans is likely to be much safer than independently roaming the world.

Illness on expeditions

Gathering and collating information about health on expeditions is now-adays very difficult owing to concerns about confidentiality and data protection, but ➔ Table 1.1 (➔ p. 8) lists studies of this type. Fig. 1.2 shows a summary of diagnoses from the largest study.[3]

The incidence of medical issues reported varies widely depending upon the methodology of the study. For example, whether the administration of prophylactic drugs for sea-sickness or malaria was included, and/or whether relatively trivial problems such as headache or mild gastrointestinal (GI) upset were recorded. However, 70% of all expeditions encounter at least one significant medical problem and appropriate preparation is essential.

Gastrointestinal upsets

(See ➔ p. 420.) All surveys indicate that the commonest problems encountered are GI. On land, diarrhoea and vomiting are an inevitable hazard of travel and are usually self-limiting but serious cases lead to dehydration and hospitalization. Dysentery, cholera, giardiasis, and leptospirosis can infect the unwary. Offshore, sea sickness is a major problem while small boats and expedition ships are at risk of norovirus outbreaks. Meticulous hygiene measures, especially around dining areas, can reduce the incidence of problems, but all travellers need to carry basic remedies for days when travel is unavoidable, and larger expeditions ought to have the facilities to rehydrate a seriously affected member.

Medical problems

Simple medical problems such as mild respiratory infections and headache are very common and usually easily treated. Insect-borne diseases such as malaria and dengue fever can be incapacitating and sometimes fatal, while water-borne infections such as bilharzia and onchocerciasis need to be considered during travel to the tropics. Zika and Middle East respiratory syndrome (MERS) caused concern for travellers in particular areas before the COVID-19 pandemic.

Orthopaedic and trauma

(See ➔ p. 437.) Patterns of injury will depend upon the environment visited and the activities undertaken. Lower limb sprains and strains are common on walking and mountaineering treks. Upper body trauma is commoner on cycling and mountain biking trips. Offshore voyages on both yachts and expedition ships are associated with upper limb and head injuries, while falls in older passengers may result in hip, pelvic, or rib fractures.

Environmental problems

Environmental extremes may cause problems for the unprepared. Altitude sickness affects many travellers ascending rapidly. Heat exhaustion and heatstroke can be serious problems, while at the other extreme, frostbite and non-freezing cold injury may result in long-term disability. When

---

3 Anderson SR, Johnson CJH. Expedition health and safety: a risk assessment. *J R Soc Med.* 2000:93:557–562. https://doi.org/10.1177/014107680009301102

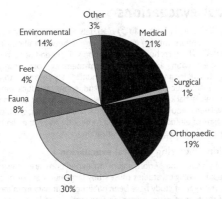

Fig. 1.2 Categories of 1263 medical problems recorded by the Royal Geographic Society Survey 1995–2000.

environmental problems occur, they can be serious, and require urgent treatment and evacuation, often in difficult circumstances.

Fauna

Unfamiliarity with local animal life can lead to injury. Scorpions and sea urchins commonly cause problems. Wherever rabies is endemic, dogs should be regarded with caution. Anaphylaxis to insect stings may occur at home or abroad. Although attacks are rare, large animals throughout the world present a hazard both directly and as a cause of road collisions.

Feet

Good foot care is always essential. Blisters cause misery and can become infected. Regular cleansing and use of foot powder reduce fungal infections and sores. Especial care is required in tropical forests where skin damage may lead to ulceration.

Surgical problems

(See p. 405.) Acute abdominal crises, severe gynaecological pain, and renal stones are very alarming and often require evacuation of the patient, but fortunately are rare.

Dental

(See p. 359.) Dental issues including lost fillings, displaced crowns, and abscesses become commoner with increasing trip duration. Medics should take a dental first-aid kit and know how to deal with basic problems.

Medical evacuations

All the studies listed in Table 1.1 (➔ p. 8) demonstrated a need to evacuate expedition members with an incidence varying between about 1:800 and 1:11,800 days. The threshold for evacuation will depend upon the ease of its logistics: evacuating an expedition team member from a campsite in a 4×4 is much simpler and safer than the multiagency response to an emergency on an Antarctic cruise vessel. On land, some casualties were able to walk themselves back to base camp, while others had to be transported. Not all evacuees require hospitalization; particularly during climbing expeditions, victims of altitude sickness could frequently rejoin the climbing team following a period of rest and acclimatization.

Conditions requiring hospital evacuation

Fortunately, death and serious injury on expeditions are nowadays very rare, so epidemiological studies must study large numbers of people. Few results of this type of study have been published, but data from the UK give an idea of the type of issues arising in a frequently visited mountainous area. The Ysbyty Gwynedd hospital in Bangor, North Wales, receives almost all the casualties from the mountains of the nearby Snowdonia National Park. The Park is a very popular destination for walkers, climbers, and tourists with around 4 million visitors spending 10 million days in the area annually. Military and civilian mountain rescue teams and helicopters provide search and rescue (SAR) cover to evacuate casualties beyond the reach of conventional ambulances.

The hospital receives >100 casualties a year who require rescue and urgent hospital treatment resulting from incidents in the mountains and its mountain medicine database[4] has logged >1700 admissions since 2004. 62% of the casualties were male, 10% were children, 19% were in the 18–28 years age group, 37% were aged 29–49 years, and 33% were >50 years. In recent years, the proportion of casualties aged >30 years has risen from 68% to 72%. 70% of injuries or illnesses were sustained while hill-walking, 6% while scrambling, 9% rock climbing, 3% mountain biking, and 2% trail running, with the remaining 9% unclassified.

Only 18% of the patients presented with medical conditions although the incidence of medical problems increases with age—in those aged >60 years, medical problems were the cause of more than a third of the admissions. 62% of those rescued presented with lower limb injuries, which was a single isolated injury in 44% of casualties.

Between 2004 and 2011 (the latest available figures), there were 70 fatalities in the mountains of the Snowdonia National Park, 93% of whom were male. This sex ratio reflects the predominance of male casualties in most other trauma registries. Owing to the remote locations of many accidents, skilled assistance takes time to arrive—typically between 45 minutes and an hour—and this delay has a triage effect: the most seriously injured do not survive. The majority of trauma victims who die within this initial period have non-survivable head or spinal cord injuries. Of those with serious spinal fractures, 73% had spinal cord disruption at postmortem.

---

4 The Bangor Mountain Medicine database (unpublished) is maintained by Linda Dykes, Ben Hall, Rhiannon Talbot, and Rich Griffiths, and is quoted with their permission.

The pattern of survivors is quite different. Half of Snowdonia mountain trauma casualties complain of back pain, or have a mechanism of injury that would mandate 'spinal packaging' in conventional pre-hospital practice. However, in the mountains, providing such care may delay evacuation and create additional hazards to both rescuers and casualty. Analysis suggests that while 14% of this group of casualties prove to have some form of spinal fracture, most are stable transverse process fractures that are painful, but clinically insignificant. <2% of mountain casualties found alive after a serious accident have an unstable spinal fracture—a comparable rate to most major trauma series in urban populations.

Pelvic fractures also cause concern to rescuers, because pelvic splints are difficult to apply in precarious locations. However, only 2% of the mountain trauma casualties had a pelvic fracture and severe pelvic disruption was only seen in those who died before help arrived.

Meeting the challenge

People enjoy the excitement and challenges of the great outdoors. Travels in remote areas will always carry risk, and if things go wrong, help may be far away. Expedition medicine involves many aspects of care unfamiliar to clinicians used to working in conventional hospital or family practice. Good planning and logistics, effective risk management, communication skills, and knowledge of hygiene and sanitation, together with an understanding of human health, physiology, and psychology in extreme environmental conditions, form the core of the specialist knowledge necessary to work effectively. The Royal College of Surgeons of Edinburgh has published a very helpful guide to the types of knowledge required to provide effective medical cover in remote areas.[5]

Many people attracted to remote areas are risk-takers. Effective planning and risk management is about ensuring that the risks encountered are managed and mitigated to the greatest possible degree. This is especially important when young or naïve clients join a group travelling to a remote area. Those with greater skills and knowledge have a 'duty of care' to the novices.

Many doctors and medics seek to participate in expeditions, and the authors hope that this handbook will provide a useful guide to the knowledge and skills that these medics will require as they head to distant parts.

5 The Royal College of Surgeons of Edinburgh. *Updated Guidance for Medical Provision for Wilderness Medicine.* 2020. ⅋ https://fphc.rcsed.ac.uk/media/2780/updated-guidance-for-medical-provision-for-wilderness-medicine.pdf

Chapter 2

Preparations

Chapter editors
Sarah R. Anderson
and James Moore

Contributors
Sarah R. Anderson
Jon Dallimore
Matthew Davies
Richard Dawood
Matthew Ellis
Peter Harvey
Iain McIntosh
James Moore
Barry Roberts
Jane Wilson-Howarth
Shane Winser
Tariq Qureshi (1st edition)
Claire Davies (2nd edition)
David A. Warrell (2nd edition)

Joining an expedition

The RGS (with IBG) estimates that many thousands of overseas expeditions leave the UK annually. These will range from solo travellers or teams of two up to expeditions involving 100 or more participants. Expeditions typically last for as short as 1–2 weeks to many months, if not years in the case of ongoing research programmes. The sheer volume of expedition traffic represents great scope for joining an expedition.

Potentially, there is a huge choice of where to go and what to do. To help narrow down your options:

First, think about your *motivation*:
• Science.
• Adventure.
• Personal challenge.
• Community involvement.

Second, think about your *personal circumstances*:
• Relevant skills and experience.
• The level of responsibility you desire.
• Time available.
• Financial commitments/resources.
• Personal interests.

Unless you fully appreciate the demands of expedition travel, as opposed to travelling independently, it is worth initially considering joining a short expedition before committing yourself to a prolonged and arduous journey in a very remote area, with little chance of repatriation if you find you cannot cope or hate the experience.

Expeditions are costly enterprises and normally each participant has to pay their way. At best you might get your costs covered by the expedition but it is unrealistic to expect a wage, unless you have a special skill and/or are vastly experienced.

Assessing an expedition opportunity

While you may be grateful to any expedition that accepts you, you are about to invest a considerable amount of time, effort, and possibly money, so research the organization offering the opportunity to satisfy yourself that it is likely to achieve its goals, and that the plans match your expectations.
• How long has the company/organization been trading and what is its financial structure and bonding system?
• Are they aligned to a standard, e.g. British Standard (BS) 8848 (Box 2.1), or screened via an external organization such as the RGS-IBG, or internally, e.g. by the Oxford University Expeditions Council?
• What are the credentials of the expedition leader(s)?
• How much do you have to pay and what does it include/exclude?
• How are participants selected and medically screened?
• What pre-expedition meeting/training plan is in place?
• What medical kit is provided?
• What insurance, risk assessment, and emergency back-up arrangements are in place?
• Will your medical defence organization cover you if there are Americans/Canadians or other internationals on the team?

- Will you be expected to treat locally employed staff or collaborators and therefore be required to register with the local government as a medical practitioner?
- Don't ignore your instinct or 'gut feeling'; sloppy administration might be a tell-tale sign of poor field organization.

Box 2.1 British Standard 8848 (2014)

BS 8848 is the British Standard for organizing and managing visits, field-work, expeditions, and adventurous activities outside the UK.

BS 8848 aims to reduce the risk of injury or illness on overseas ventures by specifying the safety requirements that have to be met by providers of these activities.

BS 8848 documents established good practice and specifies the processes needed to manage overseas ventures. These include adventurous and educational activities abroad such as university and academic field-work, gap year experiences, adventure holidays, charity challenges, and research expeditions. Providers, leaders, and participants need to know the risks involved, that they've been planned for, and that action has been taken to minimize them.

BS 8848 provides those that comply with the requirements of the standard with a way of being able to demonstrate to participants, leaders, and other interested parties that their venture provider is following good practice to manage safety on the venture. BS 8848 can also be used to identify areas for improvement in existing safety management procedures.

Following BS 8848 requirements will help ensure expedition providers:

- Assign clear roles and responsibilities to those involved.
- Plan a venture to help ensure that key elements are not missed.
- Provide clear and accurate information to participants on the safety issues and on the nature of the activities.
- Appoint competent staff with the right skills, training, and know-how.
- Prepare risk management plans and make staff aware of the risks associated with specific activities and locations.
- See ♫www.bsigroup.com/BS8848 for further details.

Role of the expedition medical officer

The expedition medical officer (MO) is key to the success of an expedition. Success is achieved by preventing expedition members becoming ill and treating them quickly and appropriately if they do. This does not mean that, as MO, you must treat everything that is presented to you, but rather you must use your knowledge to advise on the best course of action. As MO you are unlikely to be busy with medical problems but, if someone is ill or injured, you may be the only person who can deal with the situation. These can be stressful times, with limited or no advice available from seniors and no one to relieve you for a break. Good communication between you, your patient, and other expedition members is essential, as is strong decision-making, based on the knowledge and facilities available to you.

To prepare for the role of expedition medical officer

- Carefully research your expedition destination.
- Improve your knowledge of local medical problems.
- Attend relevant courses in expedition medicine, first aid, advanced life support, and basic dental skills.
- Consider a more formal qualification, e.g. a Diploma in Expedition Medicine or possibly a Diploma in Tropical Medicine and Hygiene.
- Prepare physically.

Pre-expedition roles

- Advise and brief the team on medical issues (general and specific to the expedition environment).
- Undertake medical screening of all expedition members (➔ p. 48).
- Ensure all participants have a pre-expedition dental check-up.
- Consider subscribing to the Blood Care Foundation to ensure access to safe blood and rabies treatment abroad (🕭 http://www.bloodcare.org.uk).
- Provide advice on immunizations and malaria prophylaxis (if medically qualified to do so); otherwise have an awareness of appropriate immunizations and antimalarials (➔ p. 28, p. 517).
- Organize appropriate first-aid training for all expedition members (➔ p. 44).
- Educate the team on health and hygiene issues.
- Obtain, pack, and transport medical supplies and kits (➔ p. 42).
- Undertake a risk assessment and prepare associated documents (➔ p. 70).
- Review local health services and medical facilities.
- Anticipate and plan evacuation of a severely ill or injured person.
- Prepare a communication network to support your medical diagnosis and decision-making in case of evacuation (➔ p. 160).
- Prepare an emergency response plan (ERP) (➔ p. 148).
- Organize medical insurance with full emergency evacuation cover (➔ p. 76).
- Confirm professional indemnity insurance will cover the role of an expedition MO.
- Liaise with and develop a good working relationship with expedition leaders.

Medical screening of expedition members is essential to ensure tailored pre-travel advice and to expand the expedition first-aid kit. Ask each member to complete a personal medical questionnaire and emphasize the need for full disclosure to enable proper preparation and appropriate insurance cover. Make three copies of the questionnaire: leave one in the UK with a nominated contact and take two on the expedition, in case an emergency evacuation is needed. In addition, consider having a cloud-based copy.

Pre-expedition medical questionnaire
Name:

Date of birth:

Address:

Next of kin:
  Name:
  Address:
  Tel./email contact details:
  Relationship:

General practitioner (GP) details:

Current medical problems:

Past medical history (including mental health problems):

Current medication:

Allergies:

Date of last dental check-up:

Blood group:

Immunizations:
Childhood vaccinations—did you receive all of your childhood vaccinations including MMR (Mumps, Measles, Rubella)?   Yes/No

Expedition-related vaccinations (against a list of recommended vaccinations for the expedition members should indicate date received):

Type: Date received:

Roles during the expedition

- Reiterate rules of camp and personal hygiene (➜ p. 22).
- Revisit and refresh these at regular intervals during the expedition.
- Ensure a safe, copious water supply.
- Undertake brief medical review of expedition members on arrival.
- Revise basic first aid and management of minor injuries with all expedition members.
- Place expedition medical kits in a designated place and inform all expedition members.
- Organize a routine for patient consultations (➜ p. 86).
- Oversee the safety of expedition members.
- Reassess the risks posed by the natural environment, instruct the team on prevention and early suspicion (e.g. heat illness, altitude sickness), and alter emergency plans as appropriate.
- Review evacuation plans.

- Consider visiting the local hospital early to introduce yourself.
- Practise a mock evacuation.
- Write up accident reports as necessary.
- Enjoy being part of the expedition.

Camp health and hygiene

As MO you are responsible for base camp health and hygiene—see ➲ Chapter 3 for full details. Contribute to the design of the camp layout to ensure water supplies and waste disposal are correct. Undertake regular checks of latrine and kitchen hygiene, food storage, and rubbish disposal. If anything is substandard, bring it to the attention of all expedition members and rectify. Strict adherence to the rules of camp and personal hygiene is essential to minimize gastroenteritis, the most common complaint on all expeditions.

Consultations

A consultation service for non-urgent problems is one of the main roles of an MO. For more details on how to run routine and emergency clinics, see ➲ p. 86.

Treatment

Size, weight, and cost considerations mean that most expedition medical kits are fairly basic, and the number of diagnostic aids limited. MOs should ensure that they have medical supplies sufficient for treating minor illnesses and are able to provide emergency care for more serious conditions until a patient can be evacuated.

Most problems are straightforward and can be dealt with on the spot. The role of the MO is therefore uncomplicated: to make a diagnosis and treat. In urban settings, help is available to confirm intuitive feelings or doubts; however, in the field it is not, and as expedition MO you therefore must assume the worst-case scenario. This may mean causing a lot of inconvenience, such as by sending someone with stomach ache to hospital with possible appendicitis, or making someone with a headache at altitude descend 1000 m, but you really have no choice other than to take the safest course of action.

MOs are also there to offer reassurance. People come with genuine symptoms, whether major or minor, and the significance may not always be apparent to the sufferer. You will not know what the situation is until you have made a serious attempt at a diagnosis, so *never fail to take this step*. If you think nothing is wrong, friendly reassurance is very important. Remember that psychological or psychiatric problems, fears, and tensions may manifest themselves as physical symptoms. Expeditioners tend to be self-sufficient people, and the circumstances of an expedition often reinforce this. MOs can overdo the self-sufficiency; this can lead them to try and solve all problems single-handedly. Always ask yourself whether extra advice is available and if it would be useful. More junior MOs should try and arrange for some 'senior cover' to discuss more worrying cases via whatever communications are available.

Confidentiality

All patients rightly expect that medical information will be confidential. People also have a right to refuse treatment, even if, in the MO's view, this will not be in their best interest. However, the General Medical Council (GMC) has made it clear that doctors also have a duty to the public at large. On expeditions, circumstances can arise where confidentiality may need to be broken so that the health and safety of other expedition members is not jeopardized. The expedition leader may need to be informed that an individual is concealing an illness or refusing treatment. General Data Protection Regulations (GDPR) came into law with the Data Protection Act 2018. It is likely that these will be applicable even on expedition.

Consent

Without consent, treatment is assault. Consent to emergency life-saving treatment is usually presumed by the law if the patient is unconscious or too ill to consent. The law presumes that a reasonable person would wish his/her life to be saved. In the case of a healthcare professional acting within his/her sphere of clinical competence, consent is usually implied, i.e. the patient does not resist the treatment and therefore is presumed to consent. In other situations where treatment carries considerable risk, or is controversial, informed expressed consent should be obtained. For consent to be informed, the individual must understand the proposed treatment and the risks involved in accepting or refusing that treatment. This means that the patient should be made aware of material risks and common or serious side effects, as well as the likely consequences should treatment be withheld. Verbal consent, especially in an expedition setting, is usually adequate.

For an individual >16 years of age, only that individual is able to give consent. Remember, patients have the right to refuse treatment. Children <16 years can consent to medical treatment themselves if, in the opinion of the doctor, they are capable of understanding the nature and consequences of that treatment (Gillick competence). The child should, however, be given information that is relevant to his/her age and understanding. When taking under-16s on an expedition it is wise to gain written permission from the parent or guardian that medical care can be given if it is thought to be in the child's best interest.

Duty of candour

This is an important concept to be aware of and is summarized here from the GMC and Nursing and Midwifery Council websites:

Every healthcare professional must be open and honest with patients when something that goes wrong with their treatment or care causes, or has the potential to cause, harm, or distress. This means that healthcare professionals must:

- Tell the patient (or, where appropriate, the patient's advocate, carer, or family) when something has gone wrong.
- Apologize to the patient (or, where appropriate, the patient's advocate, carer, or family).
- Offer an appropriate remedy or support to put matters right (if possible).
- Explain fully to the patient (or, where appropriate, the patient's advocate, carer, or family) the short- and long-term effects of what has happened.

Healthcare professionals must also be open and honest with their colleagues, employers, and relevant organizations, and take part in reviews and investigations when requested. They must also be open and honest with their regulators, raising concerns where appropriate. They must support and encourage each other to be open and honest, and not stop someone from raising concerns.

(See ℛ https://www.gmc-uk.org/ethical-guidance/ethical-guidance-for-doctors/candour---openness-and-honesty-when-things-go-wrong/the-professional-duty-of-candour and ℛ https://www.nmc.org.uk/standards/guidance/the-professional-duty-of-candour/read-the-professional-duty-of-candour/)

Incident reports

Incidents may happen. One of the roles of the expedition MO will be to write up an incident report if necessary and at an appropriate time. It is important that information collected is purely factual, and should include:

- The site and time of the incident/accident.
- The people involved.
- Who else was present (witnesses).
- What happened.
- What action was taken.
- The outcome.

Assessing health risk

Medical health risk management should form part of overall risk assessment (➜ p. 70). People who commonly encounter specific hazards, such as experienced climbers, cavers, or divers, should also contribute. In these activities, field leaders are usually well informed and often trained to advise less experienced individuals. Risks can be minimized by the use of sensible and simple precautions such as avoiding travelling at night, selecting appropriate equipment, wearing seat belts in vehicles, and wearing helmets while climbing. A crisis management plan should be prepared (➜ p. 146).

Once in the field, it is important to *reassess* the situation, particularly the hazards of local flora and fauna, the climate (e.g. both heat and humidity), activities, and the physical environment. Situations may arise in the field where the MO will either have to give an opinion about a proposed activity or give unsolicited warnings once activities have begun.

Evacuation

An essential role of the MO is the ability to make a decision on evacuation. Consider the following:

- The need to choose the safest option when diagnosis cannot be confirmed by colleagues or tests.
- The often-conflicting needs of the expedition leaders and other team members.
- Lack of privacy and confidentiality, all part of expedition life.

Plans should be prepared on communication and transportation methods in case an emergency or evacuation occurs. (See ➜ p. 160. for further details on evacuation.) If the evacuation is to be funded by an insurance company, it will be critical to liaise with the insurance company's medical assistance agent. This individual will hold the approval for financing evacuations. Failure to do this may result in the insurance company not paying for evacuation costs.

Local community interaction

Expeditions may employ local workers and will encounter local communities. MOs may be asked to assist with the medical care of someone who is sick or injured. ⬄ Chapter 4 discusses the ethical dilemmas associated with such situations.

At the end of the expedition

* When appropriate, repeat advice that expedition members should continue malaria prophylaxis for the full prescribed period.
* Warn members about non-healing skin lesions (e.g. tropical ulcers, eschars from typhus and leishmaniasis) and the vital importance of seeking medical help early if a fever develops within the first few weeks after return. Malaria can develop and kill rapidly (⬄ p. 512.).
* Provide continuing medical advice and support as necessary.

If participants are fit and healthy at the end of an expedition, they probably don't require any follow-up. For participants with symptoms, the MO should recommend urgent review by a doctor, to examine, investigate, and treat as appropriate. The most helpful post-expedition tests are:

* Full blood count with white cell differential to detect an increase in eosinophils (an eosinophilia is seen with parasitic disease).
* Urine dipstick for blood, protein, or sugar.
* Stool specimen for microscopy, culture, and antibiotic sensitivities plus ova, cysts, and parasites.
* Urine specimen and serology for schistosomiasis (>6 weeks after expedition) if they were exposed to fresh water in an endemic area (⬄ p. 530.).

Do not forget that tropical diseases such as malaria and schistosomiasis may present weeks, months, or even years after the expedition has ended. A single case in your expedition team should alert you to recommend the screening of other members, since they are likely to have shared the same risk of exposure. Usually, the role of the expedition MO post expedition will be to direct individuals to their local health provider to investigate and treat the problem. A useful diagnostic guide can be found at: ℘ www.fevertravel.ch

Creating expedition teams

Expeditions create their own unique social atmosphere. There can be enormous strain on individuals and the team, brought about by the intensity of living in a group, which is amplified by physical hardship, deprivation of normal western comforts, climatic and cultural demands, and the stress of striving to achieve the expedition's objectives. This is one of the great attractions of expedition life; to put oneself to the test and willingly forego the relative safety and security of home in exchange for the deep satisfaction, elevated self-esteem, and close human bonds that can be one of the greatest benefits of the expedition experience.

To optimize the expedition experience for all participants, particular attention must be paid to appropriate team selection, team building, effective leadership, and an understanding of the dynamics of groups in the field.

Team building

Time is well invested prior to the expedition in building the expedition members into an effective team so that the team is ready to handle the demands of the expedition. The time devoted to this should be proportional to the size of the team and the complexity and longevity of the expedition. For large multinational expeditions, it is impracticable to get the team together before the expedition; in these circumstances, a period of time should be devoted in-country to team building, skill development, and briefings, before the party is deployed to the field.

Group dynamics

A cohesive team is more likely to achieve the expedition aims than a fragmented group so it is desirable to promote this through pre-expedition team building and effective leadership. A cohesive team will be happier and more confident than a less cohesive group.

Morale and cohesion can be adversely affected under the following conditions
- Communication breakdowns.
- Illness or inability to cope with the demands of an expedition.
- Bad weather.
- Boredom—lack of structure and purpose.
- Splinter groups—cliques.
- Exclusive relationships in the group—who's in or out?
- Poor food.
- Unfairness and inequalities in food, assignments, accommodation, etc.
- Failure to achieve expedition objectives.
- Exhaustion, lack of recovery time, and recreation opportunities.
- Inappropriate leadership style, e.g. too dictatorial or too weak.

The performance of individual team members can also be adversely affected by
- Culture shock.
- Homesickness or bad news from home.
- Breakdown of close relationships within the team.
- Lack of fitness, poor health, and hygiene.
- Mental/psychological illness.

It is unrealistic to expect all team members to become great friends with each other. Team cohesion relies on trust, fairness, tolerance, and acceptance of different personalities, opinions, and habits within the framework of a workable team structure, an appropriate resource base, effective leadership, and a mutually agreed purpose that the team is motivated to achieve.

Immunization

Introduction

Vaccines offer safe, reliable protection against an increasing range of important disease hazards abroad. It is important to note that vaccine-preventable diseases account for only a tiny proportion of problems encountered on expeditions. Careful attention to the other health precautions covered in this handbook are of paramount importance, before, during, and after every successful expedition. An important benefit of going to be vaccinated is the opportunity to discuss a wider range of health concerns and precautions that may be even more beneficial than the vaccines themselves. It is important for those with an incomplete or absent vaccination history to understand that vaccinations are not only there to protect the individual, but also the indigenous population from imported disease.

Timing

Ideally, immunization should commence at least 8 weeks before departure, to allow time for vaccines requiring more than one dose and sufficient time for the vaccines to become effective. Vaccine supply problems do occur from time to time, and this can be a further reason for seeking protection well in advance.

Background

Everyone attending for immunization should bring with them any available records of previous vaccines received, to avoid unnecessary repeated doses.

Immunization schedules are becoming more complicated and especially where groups of young people are concerned, 'catch-up' protection may be necessary for any missed doses, notably MMR and diphtheria, tetanus, and polio.

Travel provides an important opportunity to ensure that the routine vaccination schedule is up to date. The UK childhood immunization schedule can be found at: ℘ http://www.nhs.uk/Conditions/vaccinations/Pages/vaccination-schedule-age-checklist.aspx

Where expedition participants are drawn from more than one country, it may be important to be aware of differences between national schedules.

Individuals with specific medical problems such as immunosuppression or those on certain medications will require more complex consultations.

Certificates and regulations

For many years, yellow fever (YF) has been the only disease for which international, World Health Organization (WHO)-approved vaccination certificates apply as a condition of entry to some countries. Occasionally, individual countries will enforce temporary certificate requirements, such as polio vaccination to Indonesia in 2020 or travellers to Saudi Arabia during the Haj or Umrah pilgrimage may be required to show proof of vaccination against meningitis ACWY. The 2005 International Health Regulations allow for other diseases to be added as needed, such as coronavirus disease 2019 (COVID-19) caused by severe acute respiratory syndrome coronavirus 2 (SARS-CoV-2). Most countries require evidence of COVID-19 vaccination prior to entry. A range of COVID-19 vaccinations is available. For the latest

guidance see: ॐ https://www.nhs.uk/conditions/coronavirus-covid-19/
coronavirus-vaccination/coronavirus-vaccine/

Choosing which vaccines to have

Most travel vaccines are not required formally as a condition of entry but
are 'optional'—the choice is based on an assessment of the likely health
risks such as locally prevalent diseases, the precise details of a trip or expedition, including its duration, conditions of accommodation, the likely level of
contact with local people, and the environment.

In England, Wales, and Northern Ireland, general guidelines are published by the National Travel Health Network and Centre (NaTHNaC) (ॐ
http://www.travelhealthpro.org.uk) and in Scotland, by Health Protection
Scotland; the WHO also issues information, and it may be helpful to consult resources from other countries, such as the US. Many medical practices, travel clinics, companies, and other organizations also formulate their
own policies. In the UK, the most up-to-date clinical information about vaccinations is available via the Public Health England publication 'The Green
Book'.[1] Information here supersedes the individual vaccine summary of
product characteristics (SPC) licence.

On an expedition, participants inevitably compare the vaccines and medication they have received; inconsistencies tend to be the rule rather than
the exception, which can lead to unnecessary anxiety and can undermine
confidence in the advice that has been given.

The best option is therefore for an expedition's MO to draw up some
general guidelines or a formal policy, seeking specialist advice if this is
needed. The best care comes when one clinic or practice takes responsibility for the entire group. If this is not possible, the MO should circulate
guidelines to all expedition members to give to the individual clinics or practices that will carry out immunization.

In the UK, only a small number of travel vaccines can be provided free of
charge on the National Health Service (NHS), and escalating development
costs mean that newer travel vaccines are costly—a factor that needs to be
considered in the context of an expedition's overall budget.

Previous vaccinations or interrupted schedules

Individuals may have received either a full or partial vaccine course in the
past. It is important to note that vaccine courses rarely require restarting,
irrespective of the time between doses. For example, if someone has received two hepatitis B vaccinations 3 years ago, they will only require a
single hepatitis B vaccination to complete the primary course.

Individual vaccines for travel

Meningococcal meningitis
(See ➔ p. 505.) Most travel clinics are able to provide up-to-date information about areas of risk. Travellers who have had their spleen removed may
be more vulnerable to this condition.

---

1 ॐ https://www.gov.uk/government/collections/immunisation-against-infectious-disease-the-
green-book

Table 2.1 Travel vaccine guide

Vaccine	No. of doses	Initial course — Primary course schedule	Notes	Duration of protection	Minimum age
Killed vaccines					
Cholera (Dukoral)	2	Adults & children 6–18 years: Day 0, 1–6 weeks		2 years	2 years
	3	Children 2–6 years: Day 0, 1–6 weeks, 1–6 weeks		6 months	
Diphtheria/ tetanus/ polio		Initial course usually completed in childhood		10 years	n/a
		Unvaccinated adults: 3 doses on month apart			
Hepatitis A	2	Day 0, then 6–12 months		25+ years	1 year
Hepatitis B-rapid schedule	4	Days 0,7, 21, and 12 months	A single Hep B booster at 5 years for those at continuing risk	Life	18 years
Hepatitis B-standard schedule	3	Months 0, 1, and 2 or 6		Life	Birth
Hepatitis A & B–combined	3	Months 0, 1, and 2 or 6		25+ years	1 year
Influenza	1	Children need a 2nd dose 4 weeks later if first ever flu vaccine course		1 year	6 months
Japanese encephalitis (Ixiaro)	2	Day 0 and 28	Booster at 1 year	Unknown	2 months
Meningitis ACWY (conjugated)	1	Single dose		Unknown	1 year
Meningitis B	2	Age 6 months to adults: Months 0 and 2	Booster between 12 & 24 monts	Unknown	
	3	Age 2–5 months: Months 0, 1, and 2			
Pneumonia (Prevenar, Pneumovax)	1	Single dose		5+ years	

Rabies (im or intradermal)	3	Days 0, 7, and 21 or 28	Life in most cases	Birth
Tickborne encephalitis	2 or 3	Days 0, and 28–42	3+ years	1 years
Typhoid/ Hepatitis A (combined)	1	Hepatitis A booster at 6–12 months Typhoid booster at 3 years	Hep A 1year, then 25+ Typhoid 3 years	16 years
Typhoid injected (Typhim Vi)	1	Single dose	3 years	2 years
Live vaccines				
MMR (measles/mumps/rubella) adults	2	Day 0 and 28	Life	
TB; BCG (mantoux first if anged 6+ years)	1	Single dose		Birth
Typhoid oral (Vivotif)	3	Day 0, 2, and 4	3 years	6 years
Varicella (chickenpox)	2	Months 0, and 1–2	Unknown	1 year
Yellow fever	1	Single dose	Certificate lasts for 10 years	Life	9 Months

Single dose vaccines require 10–14 days to become effective. Do NOT give live vaccines to immunosuppressed patients, and consider implications carefully during pregnancy. Vaccine schedules, indications, and booster recommendations are prone to change in the light of new evidence. For the most up-to-date information, including scheduling of live vaccines visit: ℞ http://nathnac.org/pro/index.htm

Adapted from Table 13.2.1 in Travellers' Health: how to stay healthy abroad (OUP),

Adapted from Table 13.2.1 in Dawood R (Ed). Travellers' Health: How to Stay Healthy Abroad, 5th ed. Oxford: Oxford University Press; 2012.

A conjugated vaccine offers robust protection against the A, C, W, and Y strains of the disease, and has now been added to the UK childhood routine vaccine schedule for children aged 14 years. For those at continued risk from these strains due to travel, a booster dose should be offered at 5 years.[2] A three-dose vaccine against meningitis B is now part of childhood immunization schedule in the UK and many other countries.

Vaccination is important for travellers at high risk (e.g. those who have had a splenectomy), and for travellers to high-risk destinations (Fig. 2.1), especially if they will be in close contact with local populations (e.g. in schools, hospitals, or refugee camps).

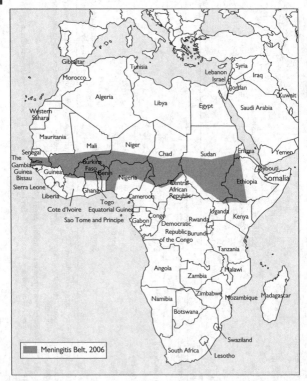

Meningitis Belt, 2006

Fig. 2.1 Distribution of annual epidemics of meningococcal meningitis in Africa: the 'meningitis belt'.

2 The Joint Committee on Vaccination and Immunisation: https://app.box.com/s/iddfb4ppw kmtjusir2tc

Cholera

Cholera is a disease of poor hygiene, transmitted via the faecal/oral route, usually by water. An oral vaccine is available that uses killed cholera bacteria and a modified form of the cholera toxin to generate localized antibody protection on the surface lining of the intestine. Other diarrhoea-causing organisms produce a very similar toxin, which is why this vaccine also provides a level of protection (for ~3 months) against some types of traveller's diarrhoea (notably enterotoxigenic *Escherichia coli*—ETEC—which accounts for as much as 40% of cases).

Cholera remains endemic in many parts of the world, but outbreaks tend now to be limited to settings with severe overcrowding, such as in refugee camps, or under conditions of extreme poverty. Improved ability to treat cholera with simple fluid replacement means that the consequences of infection are no longer as severe, though they can still sometimes be devastating. Cholera vaccine may be a sensible precaution for situations involving close contact with local communities in developing countries, though many people additionally use the vaccine for protection from ETEC.

- Symptoms range from minimal to catastrophic, watery diarrhoea. Cholera can be prevented by water purification, hygiene, and food and water precautions.
- The oral cholera vaccine available in the UK is Dukoral™.
- Dukoral™ is a suspension given in the form of a drink, in two doses, 1–6 weeks apart; protection is simple and safe.
- The course should be completed 1 week before departure.
- Protection lasts ~2 years.
- Other types of cholera vaccine are available in different countries.

Hepatitis A

(See ⟶ p. 486.) Hepatitis A is common in countries with poor hygiene and in certain populations, such as men who have sex with men (Fig. 2.2).

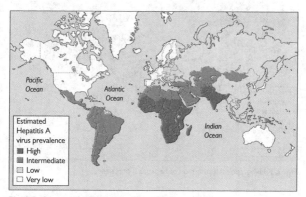

Fig. 2.2 Geographical distribution of hepatitis A prevalence.

A single hepatitis A vaccine lasts for ~1 year. A second vaccine provides reliable, long-lasting protection for up to 25 years or longer.

- The risk of a serious infection increases with age: during early childhood, complications are rare, but by the age of 40, there is a 2% risk of severe liver failure.
- Hepatitis A is one of the commonest vaccine-preventable diseases.
- Hepatitis A vaccine is safe, highly effective, and long lasting.

Hepatitis B

Hepatitis B is spread by sexual exposure, piercings, and tattoos. The most common method of transmission currently is through unsafe medical procedures, blood and blood product transfusions, and the use of non-sterile medical instruments; it is a hazard in all low- and middle-income countries (LMIC) (Fig. 2.3). It is a sensible precaution for anyone planning to spend a prolonged period abroad, particularly if they will be sexually active, in close contact with local communities, or at increased risk of needing medical treatment.

In addition to the standard regimen, a super-accelerated schedule can be used when less time is available prior to departure (given on days 0, 7, 21–28 with a final dose at 1 year), which conveniently also matches the schedule for rabies vaccination.

- Hepatitis B vaccination is now part of the standard childhood vaccination schedule in many countries, including the UK.
- Many consider it to be a sensible precaution for all sexually active young people.
- Hepatitis B vaccination should also be considered for long-term travellers, and anyone at increased risk of accident or injury abroad, who might need medical attention in circumstances where sterile medical instruments and screened blood transfusions might not be readily available.

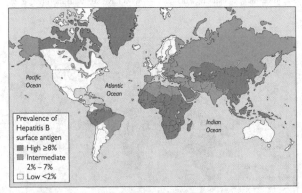

Fig. 2.3 Geographical distribution of hepatitis B prevalence.

Influenza

Seasonal influenza (flu) is one of the world's most highly prevalent vaccine-preventable diseases; it is certainly a disease of travel. Although it occurs seasonally during the winter months in the northern and southern hemispheres, it is a year-round problem in the tropics.

Expeditions, by their very nature, tend to involve groups of people spending much time together. It would seem sensible to protect members against this common, potentially serious problem. A further benefit of vaccination is that it reduces the risk of developing a fever that might be confused with other, more serious febrile illnesses associated with travel.

Japanese encephalitis

Japanese encephalitis is a viral disease transmitted by mosquito bites. It is rare in travellers (<1:1,000,000) but causes concern because it carries a high risk (~30%) of serious neurological side effects. It occurs throughout Asia (Fig. 2.4), with an estimated 30,000–50,000 cases occurring each year, accounting for at least 10,000 deaths and 15,000 cases of neurological complications. It occurs mostly in rural areas—farm animals are the source of the infection (baby pigs and wading birds). The vaccine should certainly be considered by anyone likely to spend much time in rural and some urban parts of Asia.

- An inactivated vaccine produced in cell culture (Ixiaro®), can be given to adults and children from the age of 2 months. Two doses are necessary, 28 days apart, with a further dose 1 year later for continued protection.
- A rapid schedule can be administered on days 0 and 7.
- Vaccination should be considered by anyone planning to spend time in rural parts of Asia; for further information, see: ℘ https://travelhealthpro.org.uk/factsheet/55/japanese-encephalitis

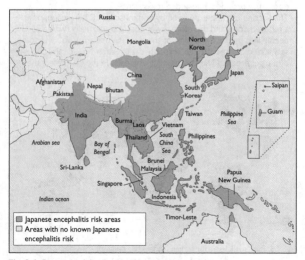

Fig. 2.4 Geographical distribution of Japanese encephalitis.

Rabies

(See ➲ p. 490.) Good-quality vaccine may not be available in a high proportion of the countries where rabies is a problem. Rabies immune globulin can be even more difficult to obtain and can be extremely expensive (~£1000–£2000 per person). Obtaining correct treatment may require a trip to be curtailed or abandoned.

Pre-exposure vaccination simplifies the treatment necessary after a bite: fewer vaccine doses, and no need for immune globulin injections. It is increasingly recommended for travellers likely to be exposed, particularly for travel to South-East Asia, Africa, and South America (Fig. 2.5). Modern rabies vaccines are safe and cause little or no reaction.

Three doses of vaccine on days 0, 7, and 21–28 will provide adequate pre-travel antibody titres, and there are other effective regimens in use, including a rapid schedule on days 0, 3, and 7, with an additional dose at 12 months. There is also evidence to show that four intradermal injections given at separate sites on the same day elicits significant antibody levels. This off-licence use of rabies vaccine could be used for high-risk travellers with no time to undertake the standard schedule.

- Pre-exposure vaccination is strongly recommended, particularly for long stays in countries with a high prevalence of animal rabies, or when taking part in activities that involve contact with animals.
- Vaccination is safe and highly effective.
- It is best to follow the standard vaccine three-dose course whenever possible, to avoid any doubts about protection.
- Most countries now accept that three doses of rabies vaccine confer life-long 'boostability'—with a rapid response to post-exposure vaccine and no immune globulin necessary: however, for individuals at continued risk, and where rabies vaccine is cheap and available, booster doses may provide some added reassurance.
- The vaccine can either be given by intramuscular (IM) injection, or at a reduced dose, and therefore lower cost, intradermally (with a 25 G needle into the topmost layer of the skin), an option available at some specialized centres. If given correctly the injection should raise a 'peau d'orange' papule. (The Department of Health in the UK prefers the

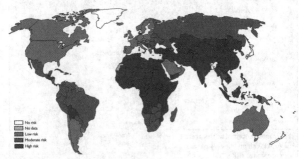

Fig. 2.5 Rabies risk levels for humans contracting rabies.

IM route but states that suitably qualified and experienced healthcare professionals may give the vaccine via the intradermal route. This method is known to be effective, is supported by the WHO, and is used routinely in many countries.)
- It is also acceptable to provide post-exposure prophylaxis by this method.

Tick-borne encephalitis

(See 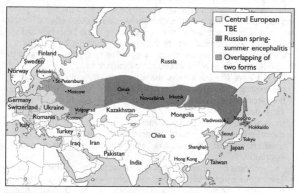 p. 488.) A safe vaccine is available, and medical experts in the affected regions strongly advise visitors to be vaccinated if they will be exposed to possible risk (Fig. 2.6). This immunization is part of the childhood schedule in many European countries. The vaccine requires two, or preferably three, doses for protection, starting at least 4 weeks prior to travel and given on months 0, 1–3, with the final vaccine given 5 months after the second. The first two doses can be given 2 weeks apart.
- Vaccination is strongly advised for people at risk, particularly those visiting forested areas in late spring, or those likely to drink unpasteurized milk from infected animals (e.g. Tibetan yaks). For short-term travellers, many advise tick avoidance measures only.

Tuberculosis (TB)

(See p. 508.) Immunization with bacillus Calmette–Guérin (BCG) is not routinely offered to children in the UK, though it is offered at birth to targeted risk groups. Expeditions involving travel to parts of the world that are highly endemic for TB (especially if there will also be close contact with local people) should consider the need for BCG or TB testing with a skin or blood test before and after return.

Typhoid

Typhoid remains common in all low-income countries, and in most hot countries with poor hygiene conditions. Vaccination is advisable for travel to Africa, Asia (especially the Indian subcontinent), and Latin America, and should also be considered for travel to Mexico and the Caribbean.

Fig. 2.6 Geographical distribution of tick-borne encephalitis (TBE).

An oral vaccine (Ty 21a) is available, consisting of three capsules to be swallowed on alternate days, that provides full protection for up to 5 years; and an (Vi antigen) injected vaccine. Both provide only 70–80% protection. A conjugated vaccine has been licensed in India and may be more effective and longer lasting but has not yet been licensed in the Europe or the US.

- The oral vaccine contains live, modified bacteria, so should not be taken at the same time as antibiotics (e.g. doxycycline used for bacterial infections and for malaria chemoprophylaxis).
- Current oral and injected vaccines are extremely safe with very low rates of side effects.

Yellow fever

(See ➔ p. 493.) Vaccination against YF is necessary for travel to many parts of Africa and South America (Fig. 2.7), as a certificate requirement and/or for personal protection. It is also a certificate requirement in many countries outside the YF endemic zones—notably in Asia, for travellers arriving from affected regions of Africa and South America. (Although YF does not occur in Asia, it has the potential to cause serious outbreaks if inadvertently introduced by an infected traveller.)

In July 2016, the rules regarding YF vaccination certificates were changed. New certificates will now state that they are valid 'for the life of the person vaccinated'.

Older YF certificates have a 'valid to' date 10 years after the most recent vaccination. This date can now be ignored, but do not cross it out or make any changes to your certificate as writing on the certificate can make it invalid. As a single dose of YF vaccine is considered to confer immunity in >95% of people vaccinated, if undertaking a project carrying a high risk of exposure, it may be appropriate to seek specialist advice on revaccination.

Increasing awareness of vaccine side effects has resulted in greater efforts to ensure safe and appropriate use of the vaccine. Two serious, life-threatening side effects are of special note—called YEL-AND and YEL-AVD (yellow fever-associated viscerotropic disease and yellow fever-associated neurological disease) They are particularly associated with older age (>60 years), immunosuppression, disease or surgery to the thymic gland, and having a close blood relative who has had one of these effects. For this reason, it is important to ensure that the vaccine is used carefully and appropriately. UK recommendations state that it should not be given for the first time to anyone over the age of 60 travelling to an area designated by the WHO to be of only low potential for exposure to YF.

- Do not leave YF vaccination to the last minute, especially if you have a pre-existing medical history that needs to be considered. Furthermore, the vaccination certificate does not become valid until 10 days after vaccination.
- Be aware that international regulations are aimed at protecting countries from importation of the virus rather than at protecting travellers, and that some countries apply these public health rules very vigorously.
- The vaccine is only given at designated YF vaccination centres.
- The vaccine contains live virus and therefore should not be given in pregnancy, to people with reduced immunity, or who are taking a range of medicine—including some steroids, cancer treatment, and 'biologics' such as new treatments for arthritis.

(a)

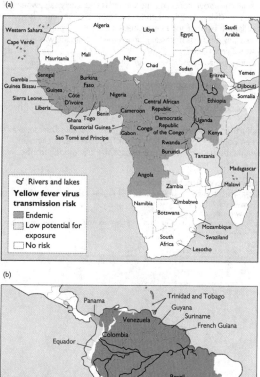

(b)

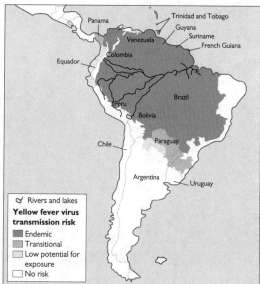

Fig. 2.7 Geographical distribution of yellow fever.

- Despite the above concerns, the vaccine is extremely safe, when used correctly: YF is a dangerous and preventable disease, and it is vital for travellers to be appropriately protected.
- Only a single dose is necessary, unless the first vaccine was given:
  - At <2 years old.
  - During pregnancy.
  - While infected with HIV.
  - When immune suppressed.
  - Before receiving a bone-marrow transplant.
- YF vaccine shortages do occur, so vaccinate well in advance of needing it.
- For further details see: *Immunisation Against Infectious Disease*, aka 'The Green Book' (ℛ https://www.gov.uk/government/publications/immunisation-against-infectious-disease-the-green-book-front-cover-and-contents-page).

Resources and further advice

Dawood R. (Ed.) Travellers' Health: How to Stay Healthy Abroad, 5th ed. Oxford: Oxford University Press; 2012.

ℛ http://www.nathnac.org
ℛ http://www.nhs.uk/Conditions/vaccinations/Pages/vaccination-schedule-age-checklist.aspx.
ℛ http://www.travax.nhs.uk
ℛ https://www.who.int/travel-advice/vaccines
ℛ https://wwwnc.cdc.gov/travel/

Medical kits and supplies

➲ Chapter 28 contains information about the type of supplies and drugs that need to be included in an expedition medical kit. The exact requirements will depend upon the:

- The size of the party, the duration of the trip, and its remoteness.
- The environments visited.
- Access to local medical assistance and its quality.
- The number of outlying camps.
- The likelihood of having to treat local staff and villagers.
- The medical knowledge of the team members/MO.
- Communications with other camps and remote medical help.
- Ease and speed of evacuation in event of a serious incident.
- Transportability.
- Cost.
- All equipment must be packed in suitably protective containers and clearly labelled. Security is important to minimize the risk of theft—especially of drugs that could be used for recreational purposes or resold in developing countries.

Obtaining supplies

Buying medical supplies from a retailer can be costly, and acquiring, packing, and labelling a medical kit can be time-consuming. UK drug companies may provide samples or donate medication, particularly if there is some formal recognition of the company's sponsorship. Technically, GPs should not give NHS prescriptions for illnesses which may be acquired outside the UK, but many do.

In some parts of the world, prescription drugs are available over the counter, but they may be counterfeit and the quality cannot be guaranteed.

Drug export

Expeditions carrying reasonable quantities of drugs are unlikely to encounter problems at customs when entering a country. However, it may be useful to have a doctor's letter stating that the drugs are for the personal use of the expedition team members and are not the subject of any commercial transaction.

Controlled drugs

Wherever possible, avoid taking 'controlled' drugs. A Home Office licence is required and must be returned within 28 days of return to the UK. (For more details see: ℛ www.gov.uk/controlled-drugs-licences-fees-and-returns) Any controlled drugs dispensed should be recorded in a controlled drug register. Local controls over drugs, especially painkillers, sedatives, and medicines for attention deficit hyperactivity disorder (ADHD) vary and it is important not to be found to be carrying inappropriate medications for that part of the world. The International Narcotics Control Board (ℛ www.incb.org) provides information on country regulations regarding the transfer of drugs across borders.

Useful resources

Home Office Drugs Branch: ℛ www.gov.uk/controlled-drugs-licences-fees-and-returns
Medicines Control Agency: ℛ www.mhra.gov.uk/#page=DynamicListMedicines
Nomad Medical Ltd: ℛ www.nomadmedicalsolutions.com/

Further reading

Auerbach PS, Constance BB, Freer L. *Field Guide to Wilderness Medicine*, 5th ed. *Philadelphia, PA: Elsevier; 2019.*

Du Pont HL, Steffen R. *Textbook of Travel Medicine and Health. Hamilton, Ontario, BC: Decker; 2000.*

Moore JK, Ladbrook M, Goodyer L, et al The provision of prescription-only medicines for use on UK-based overseas expeditions. *Wilderness Environ Med.* 2017;28(3):219–224.

Shaw MT, Dallimore J. The medical preparation of expeditions: the role of the medical officer. *Travel Med Infect Dis.* 2005;3:213–223.

Medical and first-aid training

Managing sudden illness or injury on an expedition is very different from giving conventional first aid in a developed country where there is rapid recourse to definitive care. It may be necessary to render first aid in difficult environmental conditions: desert heat, Siberian cold, at high altitude, in darkness, rain, or snow. Evacuating a patient to definitive medical care may take days because of a remote location, poor weather conditions, or lack of communications and suitable transport. This means that expedition team members need to be prepared to give first and second aid while on an expedition. Some medical conditions encountered on expeditions will be very unusual in the UK and are not covered in standard first-aid texts, e.g. malaria, altitude illness, and venomous bites and stings. Learning advanced first-aid techniques such as straightening broken limbs or using antibiotics to treat infections will be essential and the use of any special medical equipment or drugs will require careful training.

Ideally, all expedition team members should have a basic first-aid qualification. Basic first-aid training should cover:

- Scene assessment and safe approach to the injured casualty.
- Basic life support.
- Control of bleeding and the management of shock.
- Simple fracture treatment.
- Care of the unconscious patient.
- Safe movement of the injured patient.

If it is not possible to train all team members, then a trained first-aider should be available at each expedition project site.

Mental health

(See ➋ Chapter 16.) The recognition of the increasing frequency of mental health problems on expedition suggests that expedition medics should be able to provide basic mental health first aid. Mental health first-aid courses should include areas such as:

- Understanding of common mental health issues likely to present on expedition.
- Signs and symptoms of acute mental health problems.
- Basic assessment of patients with acute mental health problems.
- Development of mental health treatment or coping strategies.

First-aid courses

Basic first aid

This is best learnt by attending one of the many standard courses run by St John Ambulance or the British Red Cross. In addition, many other providers run courses aimed at those wanting to work in an outdoor environment.

See ℘ www.sja.org.uk and ℘ www.redcrossfirstaidtraining.co.uk

Aims of first aid
- To preserve life.
- To limit worsening of the condition.
- To promote recovery.

Specialist expedition medicine courses
📖 http://www.rgs.org/ExpeditionMedicine
📖 http://www.rgs.org/GOseminars
📖 https://mhfaengland.org

Expedition medical skills for the medical officer

The expedition MO (and as many of the expedition team as possible) should have basic first-aid skills, be able to measure vital signs, and be able to diagnose and treat important, common illnesses and injuries.

The Royal College of Surgeons of Edinburgh has produced updated medical guidance for the provision of medical care in wilderness situations. It is intended to give aspiring expedition medics and others a benchmark of skills they may need and facilitate expedition organizers in selecting the most appropriate medical provision for their planned activities.[3]

For an expedition MO, a summary of the minimum skills needed are listed in Box 2.2.

Box 2.2 Essential expedition medical skills

Knowledge and management of:
1. Common expedition complaints:
   • Blisters.
   • Bruises.
   • Sprains and strains.
   • Cuts/grazes.
   • Splinters.
   • Burns/scalds.
   • Bleeding.
2. Common medical conditions:
   • Infections, such as diarrhoea, upper respiratory tract infection (URTI), and urinary infections.
   • Asthma.
   • Fits.
   • Headaches.
3. Serious medical problems:
   • Anaphylaxis.
   • Chest and abdominal pain.
   • Shortness of breath and cough.
4. Important injuries:
   • Head and spinal injuries.
   • Fracture and dislocation reduction and splinting.
5. Environmental injuries:
   • Altitude-re lated illness— acute mountain sickness (AMS), high-altitude pulmonary oedema (HAPE), and high-altitude cerebral (o) edema (HACE) (➔ p. 692).
   • Heat illnesses—heat exhaustion and heatstroke.

(Continued)

---

3 📖 https://fphc.rcsed.ac.uk/media/2781/updated-guidance-on-medical-provision-for-wildern ess-medicine.pdf

Box 2.2 (Contd.)

- Cold injuries—frost bite, hypothermia.
- Diving injuries.
- Venomous bites and stings (➲ p. 571).

6. Patient handling:
   - Moving, lifting, and straightening of injured casualties.
   - Patient transportation, including improvised stretchers.
7. Mental health:
   - Basic assessment of acute mental health problems, such as deliberate self-harm (DSH), eating disorders, and psychosis.
8. Ability to provide remote advice and coach first-aiders through treatment.

Medical screening

Selection vs inclusiveness

Some potential expedition team members, including leaders, have pre-existing health problems or disabilities. Most of these people can still enjoy safe, successful trips with careful planning.

There are several issues:

- Team leaders and group members may be concerned that some disabilities or chronic illnesses may prevent individuals from participating fully in the physical and emotional challenges of an expedition.
- It is possible that the rigours of expedition life may worsen the underlying condition (and possibly compromise others).
- If the underlying condition does deteriorate, adequate facilities may not be available.

It is therefore essential to weigh up the possible risks against the potential benefits of travel for any individual who has significant pre-existing health problems. It would be nice to include all applicants, but for some the risk of serious illness, even death, may be unacceptable.

Non-declaration of medical information

Ensure all participants complete a health questionnaire—preferably at least 6 months before planned departure (Box 2.3). It can be worthwhile for the MO to interview expedition members face-to-face at the beginning of the expedition to check that their health questionnaire is accurate.

It is not unusual for individuals to deliberately omit information from a medical declaration form, potentially placing them and the team at greater risk, while possibly invalidating any insurance. Information omission occurs for a number of reasons, most commonly fear of exclusion, or stigma associated with a particular condition. Expedition participants should be encouraged to divulge all the information necessary for a safe expedition and this can be achieved through:

- Explaining the need for all medical information is primarily about safe preparation of team members and leaders *not* to exclude participants.
- Face-to-face reviews of medical forms (experienced communicators may ascertain that an individual has omitted information).
- Facilitating interview environments where individuals feel comfortable divulging sensitive information.

Minimizing the risks—things to consider

- Request the past medical history of participants sensitively. Encourage disclosure of key information that may be both important to the expedition medic and enable the traveller to enjoy their journey without medical problems. Follow up any significant issues with the patient and, if appropriate, request a report from a GP or specialist.
- How stable is the condition, and how severe can it become?
- What is the individual's knowledge of their condition and confidence to self-manage if needed?
- How well does the participant comply with their treatment?
- Exclude those with:
  - Unstable, severe mental illness, e.g. schizophrenia, bipolar disorder, hypomania, severe ongoing depression.
  - Any current untreated psychological disorder.

- Consider carefully whether to take or exclude those with:
  - Repeat episodes of anxiety or depression uncontrolled on medication.
  - Those in the early recovery stage of a mental illness.
  - Recent loss events.
  - Eating disorders.
  - DSH and previous suicide attempts.
  - Those with a recent-onset chronic health condition.
- Ask for any previous remote travel experience and how they coped.
- Ask about travel environment, expedition duration, medical back-up, communications in the field, and evacuation logistics.
- Make a decision—will this individual be travelling at unacceptable risk?
- Sometimes acceptance on a trip is provisional pending performance on training exercises or a full medical examination and review.
- Occasionally, significant pre-existing illness is not declared until the expedition is in the field. This can be a very risky situation where there is inadequate information about the condition, additional medication is not available, and the expedition is very remote from expert medical help. If the applicant is uninsured because the insurers will not cover this condition, it may be necessary to repatriate that person before an incident occurs.

Box 2.3 A health questionnaire for pre-existing conditions

1. Do you suffer from asthma, epilepsy, or diabetes?
2. Have you ever had any heart problems?
3. Do you suffer from recurring back or joint problems?
4. Do you have any condition that impairs your immune system?
5. Have you ever suffered from chronic fatigue syndrome or any other condition affecting your energy levels?
6. Do you have, or have you ever had any significant infectious disease e.g. hepatitis B, HIV, or TB?
7. Have you ever had any problems with your mental health, including an eating disorder, deliberate self-harm, overdoses, depression, anxiety or panic attacks, psychotic episodes, schizophrenia, or bipolar disorder?
8. Do you have any other current medical problems or are you on treatment for any condition?
9. Are you currently undergoing any medical investigations?
10. What medication are you taking, if any?
11. Are you allergic to anything?
12. Have you ever used recreational drugs or had a problem controlling your alcohol intake?
13. Do you have any objections to any form of treatment, including blood transfusions or immunizations?
14. How many days off sick have you had over the last year?
15. Please record your height and weight.

Generic pre-expedition advice

- Staff and other team members should have a working knowledge of any disability or illness and immediate treatment that may be necessary, such as management of hypoglycaemia, anaphylaxis, convulsions, or common mental health issues, such as anxiety.
- Review the group medical kit—will any extra items be required?
- Make contingency plans. Are there escape routes so that a journey can be curtailed if necessary?
- Ensure that the expedition's insurers are fully informed—some pre-existing medical conditions attract a higher insurance premium, and insurers are not required to meet a claim if they have not been informed of all material facts.

Pre-expedition advice for the participants

- The individual should be able to demonstrate a good level of fitness appropriate to expedition activities to be undertaken. Short, low-intensity trips to a similar environment with different activity levels will be particularly useful for people with conditions such as diabetes where the individual needs to learn to manage their illness in varied conditions.
- Optimize the illness and monitor with a diary of blood sugars, blood pressure, peak flow rates, etc.
- Each individual with a pre-existing medical condition should have a self-management plan after discussion with their GP, specialist nurse, or consultant. This can be summarized in a letter from the treating doctor together with any significant past illnesses and medications. Consider whether standby medications may be needed, e.g. prednisolone for acute asthma, antibiotics for those with immune suppression.
- Individuals need to carry their own medication with some in reserve.
- Discuss the risks openly, and ensure participants are prepared to accept them.

During the journey

- Flying west results in a long day, flying east a short day.
- People who take regular medication should discuss regimens with their specialist nurse or doctor.
- All travellers need to keep hydrated and mobile, particularly while flying.
- Pro-thrombotic conditions may benefit from compression stockings, even low-molecular-weight heparin injections on the advice of a haematologist.
- Where good communications exist, it may be possible to obtain advice from the home country and treating doctors.
- Encourage the 'buddy system', particularly for younger groups, so that all individuals are looking out for any problems.

After the expedition

- Encourage reassessment of any medical condition with the expeditioner's GP/specialist.
- Send a report of any significant problems to the GP.

Advising those with common pre-existing conditions

Asthma

(See ➲ p. 402.) One in 12 adults have asthma.
- Optimize control before departure to enable a good level of fitness.
- Consider carrying a peak flow meter and spacer (probably not a nebulizer as this is bulky and heavy but consider if on-board ship or on a larger expedition).
- Carry a supply of oral and injectable steroids.
- Consider standby antibiotics if an individual is prone to infections.
- Follow the British Thoracic Society (BTS) guidelines for management. See: ➱ http://www.brit-thoracic.org.uk/quality-improvement/guideli nes/asthma
- Each individual should discuss a treatment plan with their GP, asthma nurse, or respiratory specialist before departure.
- May need to exclude those with severe or brittle asthma. Those with numerous or recent exacerbations will also need to consider carefully the risks of travelling in areas remote from healthcare.
- High-altitude travel is not a provoking factor for asthma, but an asthma exacerbation at high altitude will be more serious because of the hypoxic environment and lack of access to medical care.
- Cold may trigger asthma attacks in some individuals.

The management of acute asthma is discussed elsewhere (➲ Asthma, p. 265.).

Diabetes

(See ➲ p. 274.) Diabetes need not be a contraindication to travel; however, a person with type 1 diabetes needs to be confident monitoring their blood sugars and adjusting their diabetes control. Those who have recently been diagnosed with diabetes should consider deferring a trip to a very remote area until they are completely confident that they can manage the disease safely without outside support.

The main concerns regarding travel with diabetes are:
- The risk of hypoglycaemia because of changes in time zones, food intake, and energy output. Some blood sugar monitors are less reliable in extreme conditions such as sub-zero temperatures.
- Infections are more likely and may be more serious, especially gastroenteritis.
- In those who have had diabetes for many years there is an increased risk of heart attack or stroke. Reduced kidney function, disturbances in skin sensation (particularly the feet), and ulceration should also be considered.

Diabetics: before the expedition

Antimalarials and immunizations should be advised as for other travellers. Consider how insulin will be stored on the expedition (Box 2.4).

It is useful to have the following information from the GP, diabetes nurse, or specialist:
- Date of diagnosis.

- How well controlled is the patient's diabetes (glycated haemoglobin (HbA1c) level)?
- Do they follow medical advice?
- Insulin type, dosage, frequency?
- Have there been episodes of hypoglycaemia/hyperglycaemia?
- Any complications—neuropathy, ulceration, eye problems, or insulin resistance?
- Has treatment varied over the last year?

This information can be written in a letter and given to the patient. If appropriate, it can also usefully mention the need for carrying needles and syringes. Even if not eating, people with diabetes continue to need regular insulin, and frequent blood sugar testing becomes even more important. Intravenous (IV) fluids and injectable antiemetics may be needed if vomiting occurs, and the use of these items may need special training or the presence of a suitably qualified healthcare professional.

Other group members should be trained in recognizing the symptoms of hypoglycaemia and the treatment needed—GlucoGel®, glucagon, or, rarely, IV glucose 10%.

Diabetics: during the expedition

It is important to consider:
- Will there be medical/nursing staff available to supervise/advise treatment?
- The expedition organizers need to consider the dietary needs of those with diabetes. Snacks should be readily available in case of delays or low blood sugar levels.
- 'Ideal' blood sugar levels may not be possible because of varying diet and activity levels. The main concern is preventing hypoglycaemia, so a little latitude is reasonable for a few weeks during the trip.
- People with diabetes are more susceptible to infections and should report any symptoms at an early stage before blood sugar levels become erratic. Foot infections may be particularly serious in those who do not have normal sensation. Particular importance should be paid to keeping feet clean, dry, and inspecting for problems. Wounds and fungal infections must be treated promptly to prevent ulceration and other complications.

Checklist for the individual diabetic

- Ensure adequate supplies of insulin, lancets, sugar testing sticks, syringes/pens, needles, sharps disposal, glucometer, GlucoGel®, and glucagon and plans for correct insulin storage as appropriate (Box 2.4).
- A talisman such as a MedicAlert® bracelet should be worn.
- Are the insurers aware, as diabetes is a significant pre-existing condition?
- If the individual suffers from travel sickness, consider an antiemetic to prevent vomiting/dehydration.
- Insulin storage (Box 2.4).
- Oral rehydration solutions should be available.

Box 2.4 Insulin storage

Ideally, insulin should be stored at 4–8°C. At these temperatures it will remain active for up to 2 years. Insulin that has been opened can be kept at room temperature, viability is usually 28 days, but individuals should check with the manufacturer of their insulin.

Frio® insulin storage pouches keep insulin vials cool in hot climates for up to 28 days (৫ http://www.friouk.com.

Insulin should be carried in hand luggage, although a medical letter of authorization should be obtained from the patients GP. X-rays do not affect insulin.

Vacuum flasks can be used to protect insulin from climatic extremes.

If insulin is 'clumped' or turbid it should not be used.

Other resources

৫ http://www.diabetes.org.uk
৫ http://www.diabetes-exercise.org
৫ https://www.diabetes.co.uk/travel.html

Hypertension

Isolated, well-controlled hypertension is not a problem for most people travelling to remote areas. However, if there is evidence of secondary organ damage due to hypertension (heart failure, renal failure) the risks of stroke or heart attack will be much higher. Consider:

• Blood pressure should be stable before travel.
• Whether there are other significant cardiovascular risk factors and whether they have been addressed.
• Check renal function before travel.
• Ensure that there is a good level of fitness and that individuals can cope with activity levels similar to those likely on the trip.
• Blood pressure may improve with weight loss and increased exercise during an expedition. Consider whether measuring blood pressure during the trip will be feasible or even sensible.
• Antihypertensive medication:
  • May affect exercise tolerance.
  • Beta-blockers can cause lethargy and limit maximum heart rate response. They also reduce the blood flow to the extremities, which may become important when travelling to cold areas. They can also predispose to heat illness.
  • Diuretics increase urine output, contribute to heat illness, and can lead to hypotension if an individual is already dehydrated.
  • Angiotensin-converting enzyme (ACE) inhibitors can also cause hypotension after exercising. They should be stopped during diarrhoeal illnesses.
  • Calcium channel blockers affect heart rate during exercise and side effects include ankle swelling and flushing which may be worse in hot climates.
  • Consider carrying aspirin 300 mg for angina or heart attacks, glyceryl trinitrate (GTN) spray for angina, and blood pressure monitoring equipment.
• After return, people with hypertension should be medically reassessed to check blood pressure and renal function.

Cardiovascular disease

A history of angina, previous myocardial infarction (MI), or claudication will be worrying. Similarly, those with multiple risk factors for cardiovascular disease (hypertension, hypercholesterolaemia, smokers and/or a strong family history of cardiovascular disease) need to consider carefully the risks of being remote from healthcare. Stresses of expedition life may provoke symptoms of chest pain (➔ p. 260) or breathlessness on exertion.

Six months after successful coronary artery bypass graft/angioplasty or stenting it is possible to undertake remote foreign travel provided there are no symptoms of chest pain or breathlessness while exercising to the level required on the expedition. The individual should be able to complete a full exercise electrocardiogram (ECG) without symptoms or undertake a stress echocardiogram to identify reversible ischaemia. There always remains the risk of recurrence and this must be accepted by the individual and team members. Ask the question: can the individual undertake vigorous activity at the same level as expected on the expedition (i.e. can they spend long days walking in the British hills)?

Epilepsy

(See ➔ p. 338.) The consequences of a seizure during an expedition activity could be very serious; for instance, falling from the back of an open vehicle, being tossed overboard during white water rafting, or collapsing on steep ground. Dehydration, alcohol, stress, and lack of sleep may all provoke convulsions. Gastroenteritis may affect antiepileptic levels and result in fitting.

Before the trip, more information will be required regarding the frequency, severity, preventive medication, and treatment of convulsions. Other team members need to be aware and know what to do in the event of a fit (➔ p. 272). Those whose epilepsy is poorly controlled may not be suitable for expeditions. Antiepileptic medication may interact with other drugs, particularly antimalarials and quinolones such as ciprofloxacin. Chloroquine and mefloquine may provoke seizures and should not be used in those with epilepsy.

Treatment of status epilepticus (a seizure lasting >5 min) is very difficult in a remote environment and the condition can be life-threatening. Those with epilepsy should follow guidance regarding swimming, driving, operating machinery, and dangerous activities such as diving and rock climbing as they would at home. Epilepsy is a significant pre-existing health problem and insurers must be aware of the diagnosis in the event of a claim. Consider taking rectal and IV diazepam or buccal midazolam together with an oropharyngeal airway and a hand-held suction device.

People with epilepsy are definitely travelling at increased risk but this can be minimized with preparation—some activities such as self-contained underwater breathing apparatus (SCUBA) diving may be unacceptably risky, and this should be understood before departure.

Allergy and anaphylaxis

Anaphylaxis is a severe form of allergic reaction (→ p. 256). It may be provoked by food, drugs, insect bites or stings. Knowledge of the allergy is essential for cooks, expedition staff, and other group members.

All expedition members need to be aware of the symptoms and signs of severe allergic reactions and should know how to give adrenaline (epinephrine), if required. A MedicAlert®/Medi-Tag® bracelet or similar should be worn at all times.

Adrenaline (epinephrine) autoinjectors in the form of an EpiPen® or Emerade®, if recommended by the GP or specialist, needs to be carried at all times and must be kept in hand luggage during air travel. It is important that the person at risk knows how to use it in an emergency. Consider taking extra drugs for anaphylaxis—adrenaline (epinephrine), prednisolone, chlorphenamine, hydrocortisone, and a salbutamol inhaler.

In those with severe allergies, consider oral antihistamine for the duration of the trip. This should be discussed with the GP or specialist. Remember that severe allergy can be induced by aspirin in some people, and that aspirin and non-steroidal anti-inflammatory agents, such as ibuprofen (Nurofen®) and diclofenac (Voltarol®), can cause or aggravate urticaria and angioedema.

Useful resources for allergies

⌖ http://allergyuk.org
⌖ http://resus.org.uk

> #### Suggested questions for those with allergies
>
> 1. What are you allergic to?
> 2. How do you react to this substance and how often?
> 3. When did you last have an allergic reaction?
> 4. What treatment is needed when you have an allergic reaction?
> 5. When, if ever, have you required hospital treatment for an allergic reaction?

Inflammatory bowel disease

Inflammatory bowel disease such as Crohn's disease or ulcerative colitis (UC) may predispose individuals to severe, possibly life-threatening diarrhoea and GI haemorrhage. Other complications such as anaemia, dehydration, and generalized infection may also occur. The drugs used to treat inflammatory bowel disease may have an effect on the immune system so that infections may be easier to acquire. Some drugs (e.g. azathioprine) require periodic monitoring of blood tests. Infectious diarrhoea may trigger a flare-up of the underlying condition. On expedition, it may be very difficult to differentiate between the two.

Individuals with inflammatory bowel disease should be fully aware of the potential risks. Severe, bloody diarrhoea, particularly if associated with a fever or abdominal pain, require prompt medical attention.

For those with inflammatory bowel disease:
• Be scrupulous with hand, food, and water hygiene.
• Inform the MO immediately if there is any flare-up of disease—particularly bloody stools, abdominal pain, and fever.

- The group should carry oral rehydration solutions, IV fluids, antibiotics, and steroids.
- A casualty evacuation plan should be in place.

Further information may be found at 🖰 http://www.crohns.org.uk and 🖰 http://www.crohnsandcolitis.org.uk/information-and-support

Mental health

(See ➲ Chapter 16.) Depression, anxiety, panic attacks, DSH, and eating disorders are all common. Non-disclosure happens occasionally and will affect insurance cover. There is a wide variety in severity and risk of each illness. Those with a single episode of depression and subsequent recovery in response to a significant life event pose a lower level of risk than those with recurrent or chronic problems.

A carefully worded pre-expedition questionnaire is needed to ensure that psychiatric and psychological illness is not overlooked. Anyone with a history of psychiatric illness should be followed up with a more detailed discussion of the problem.

Dehydration predisposes to lithium toxicity which may be fatal.

Low body mass index may mean that the individual has little physical reserve in the event of other illness.

Involve the GP and/or psychiatrist in making the decision regarding fitness to travel—an expedition is not the place to convalesce from a serious mental health problem.

If there is a history of psychotic illness, most psychiatrists recommend that the individual should have been stable for 2 years, is off medication, and can show evidence of coping with stressful situations, including foreign travel.

Disabilities

Remarkable achievements on expeditions have been made by those with significant disabilities. Appropriate challenges can be identified which help to maintain independence and dignity by the use of special adaptations. A multidisciplinary team (occupational therapists, physiotherapists, nurses, rehabilitation physicians, and prosthetists) can all contribute to identifying these challenges and advising on safe travel.

The needs of those with disabilities may be considered under the following headings:

- Mobility (prostheses, wheelchair, ability to transfer).
- Seating (are specialized cushions required?).
- Activities of daily living (ADLs)—what help is needed for ADLs, such as washing, feeding, shaving, and toileting?
- Communication—consider the safety aspects for those with hearing or visual impairment.
- Bladder/bowel control—self-catheterization, use of suppositories, and changing ileostomy bags are all possible issues which will need sensitive management.
- Skin—prolonged walking, immersion in sea water, and the effects of heat may affect the skin under a prosthetic limb or the prosthesis itself. Those with paraplegia may quickly develop pressure sores or blisters without realizing, so skin care in this group is very important.

- Cognitive and behavioural—are there any difficulties with thinking, understanding, behaviour, or psychological issues?

HIV and immunosuppression

Expedition members who are HIV positive or immunosuppressed for other reasons need specialist advice about immunizations well in advance.[4] Those who are immunosuppressed should be educated about the potential risks of infectious disease and there should be a low threshold for treatment as well as medical evacuation if needed. The individual risks of infectious disease in the location of the expedition need to be considered when deciding whether to accept a potential participant. Most immunosuppressed individuals are unable to receive 'live' vaccines including YF.

Those with HIV may need prophylaxis against opportunistic infections on the advice of their specialist. Those with a good CD4 count (>500 cells/mm³) are considered to be without significant immune compromise.[5] Consider whether any antiretroviral medication may need blood monitoring while away. Participants on immunosuppressive medications such as azathioprine may also require blood monitoring depending on the length of the expedition.

Splenectomized patients are at increased risk of bacterial infections caused by pneumococcus and meningococcus, as well as being more vulnerable to malaria. They should seek specialist pre-travel advice.

Those on prolonged courses of high-dose steroids (>20 mg prednisolone/day for >2 weeks) are at particularly high risk of infection.

Chronic fatigue syndrome

Participants with a history of chronic or post-viral fatigue should be able to demonstrate full recovery and ability to participate in normal daily activities for a significant period of time prior to the expedition. Infectious diseases or overexertion may contribute towards relapse.

Obesity

About 28% of adults in the UK are obese; some morbidly so (body mass index (BMI) >40 kg/m²). Obese travellers are at increased risk of heat acclimatization problems, dehydration, deep venous thrombosis (DVT), and musculoskeletal problems. In addition, there may be undiagnosed associated conditions such as hypertension and diabetes. Serious consideration should be given as to whether those with severe obesity are able to cope with the physical demands of an expedition. Encourage weight loss beforehand and consider assessment of physical capacity pre-expedition on training exercises.

4 ♬ https://travelhealthpro.org.uk/factsheet/66/immunosuppression
5 ♬ https://travelhealthpro.org.uk/factsheet/29/hiv-and-aids

The older traveller

Extended longevity and affluence encourage an increasing number of older people to visit remote and exotic places and participate in adventurous activities. Most travel without mishap. Advancing age, however, brings declining health and physical disability, which can increase health risk for the adventurous traveller. Pre-existing, chronic illness and medication increase overall health risk and older people are more likely to experience travel-related illness while abroad. Physical and clinical attributes and not age in years should determine fitness for challenging global travel.

Travellers aged >70 years may have specific health issues, with the potential to produce adverse effects on their global travel due to:
- Age-related physiological changes.
- Increased incidence of comorbidity.
- Atypical disease presentations.
- Increased incidence of iatrogenic illness.
- Functional and sensory disability.
- Decreased immunity to infection.

Effects of the ageing process
Adverse changes occur in:
- Renal function, water, and sodium regulation.
- Temperature regulation.
- Cardiopulmonary and GI function.
- Cell-mediated immune response.
- Neurological and sensory function.
- Metabolic response.

Health risks affected by ageing
- Reduced cardiac reserve decreases ability to cope with dehydration, high altitude, and physical exertion.
- Reduced lung capacity means less reserve to deal with reduced oxygen at altitude or from infections.
- Weakened immune system makes infection more likely.
- Deteriorating kidney function increases likelihood that dehydration will lead to kidney failure.
- Poor renal function diminishes ability for kidneys to cope with salt loss when diarrhoea occurs.
- Deteriorating brain function may result in confusion in stressful situations.
- Poor brain function causes difficulty in coping with new situations and can lead to serious anxiety.
- Poor vision and hearing can lead to accidents, or failure to see or hear public announcements.
- Poorer circulation and healing results in slower healing of injuries, wounds, and bites.
- Thinning bones from osteoporosis increase the risk of fractures with falls.
- Thinning skin increases the risk of nasty lacerations—especially over the shins.

- Reduced stomach acid increases risk from food poisoning and contaminated food and water.
- Impaired proprioception, vision, and muscle atrophy can disturb balance.

Pre-expedition considerations for older travellers

A personalized pre-travel health review can identify potential problems. Anticipation of hazards, prevention measures, and precautions can reduce overall risks to the older traveller's health. In terms of health risk, the potential older traveller can be grouped according to the following criteria:

1. *Group 1. Low risk*—the 'young' old includes:
   - Those travelling to low-risk destinations.
   - Those on short-haul journeys.
   - Those free from any pre-disposing illness.
2. *Group 2. Medium risk*—where travel involves:
   - Environmental extremes.
   - Travel to tropical countries.
   - The 'frail old'—those with pre-existing illness (e.g. diabetes).
3. Group 3. *High risk*:
   - The terminally ill.
   - Those with pre-existing illness *and* travelling to high-risk countries.
   - Pre-existing illness and visiting tropical countries or environmental extremes.

In addition to the regular pre-travel management plan, consider the following in relation to age, ability, and comorbidities:

- Identify and analyse health hazards of expedition (actual and potential).
- Minimize impact of potential health hazards (e.g. prophylaxis).
- Identify appropriate chemoprophylaxis/vaccination (include tetanus, influenza, and pneumococcal vaccination).
- Consider potential changes in routine drug medication.
- Review medication for potential interactions with antimalarials and prophylactics.
- Assess effects of pre-existing disease in foreign environment.
- Clinical evaluation at specialist travel health clinic/GP for groups 2 and 3.
- Consider: proximity to health facilities, quality of local medical resources, and availability of emergency evacuation.
- Ensure adequate travel health insurance including repatriation cover and protection for existing disease.
- Ask 'What if …?' and envisage worst-case scenarios en route and at the ultimate destination.

Expedition considerations for older travellers

While on expedition it is vitally important that both the individual traveller and expedition medic have a heightened awareness as to the age-related problems that might occur. Ensure:

- Expedition activities can be adjusted to match the physical capabilities of all the participants.
- Medications for those with comorbidities are stored appropriately.

- Changes to plans fall within acceptable and manageable risks for the whole team.
- Older individuals feel comfortable in voicing health concerns without feeling burdensome.
- A lower threshold for seeking medical advice when faced with illness in the older traveller.
- Availability of medical resources en route and at destination.
- Emergency evacuation facilities will be accessible.
- Acute awareness of the adverse effects of climatic and altitude effects on older travellers.

Post-expedition considerations for older travellers

As with any expeditioner, health problems can arise in the months following an expedition. Age-related physiological changes put the older traveller at greater potential risk for developing travel-related illness on return, the complications of which can be severe. Expedition members should be encouraged to seek medical advice on return if there are:

- Changes in bowel habits.
- An onset of fevers or flu-like symptoms.
- Changes in comorbidities (e.g. unstable blood glucose levels).
- Unusual rashes or dermatological changes.

Awareness of risk, sensible pre-travel preparation and a rapid response to problems while away will help ensure elderly travellers journey in good health. Very senior people now participate in adventures and expeditions across the globe, in all latitudes and at high altitude. They do so successfully to their personal benefit and that of fellow travellers and expedition leaders.

Resources for the older traveller

For further information see: ℰ https://travelhealthpro.org.uk/factsheet/70/older-travellers

McIntosh IB. Travel & Health: Management and Care of the Older Traveller. Exeter: Short Run Press; 2013.

McIntosh IB. Traveller's Health Problems: A Management Guide. British Global & Travel Health Association; 2019.

Child health in remote areas

Exploring with children and adolescents broadens everyone's horizons and facilitates introductions to people who might otherwise have been passed by. It does, however, often mean adapting the style and pace of travel. Goal-driven trips where the targets have been set by adults without consulting younger members can be disastrous. Involve everyone in the planning and allow time for everyone to indulge their interests. The trip will be most successful if the adults are performing well within their levels of competence. Children are often more adaptable and resourceful than the adults with whom they travel.

Diagnosing illness in children, especially in those <3 years, is difficult—even for paediatricians—and so any adult travelling to remote places with small children must be well prepared, well read, and have a good back-out plan. The commonest causes of problems in travelling children are accidents, scrapes and bumps, swallowing things they shouldn't have, traveller's diarrhoea, skin sepsis, and common infections as at home: tonsillitis, ear, and chest infections. The responsible adult should either be carrying the wherewithal to treat these problems or should know someone who can.

Immunization

Parents will need to ensure their child is up to date with the routine childhood vaccines (➲ p. 28) because, in less well-resourced regions, levels of local immunization will be low and thus 'herd' immunity is poor. Travellers are therefore at increased risk of measles, pertussis, diphtheria, etc. For other immunizations the family should consult a travel health expert. Intrepid children are more likely to get bitten by dogs and monkeys; rabies immunization is therefore especially relevant for any mobile child.

YF immunization is not given to infants under the age of 9 months so this might preclude family travel to regions where YF is common.

Parenteral typhoid immunization has poor efficacy in children under the age of 18 months and gives no cover at all against paratyphoid. Oral typhoid immunization offers some cover against paratyphoid but is only licensed for children >6 years. Parents must therefore be especially aware of the means of reducing the risk of these and other faecal/oral infections.

Antimalarials

Both mefloquine (Lariam®) and atovaquone/proguanil (Malarone®) can be given to small children. Mefloquine does not seem to cause the problems with mood that adults sometimes experience; the tablets crack easily into quarters for children's doses. It should be noted, however, that travel into highly malarious regions with small children or when pregnant is unwise, and expert advice should be sought before travel.

Unfamiliar environments

Odd and unexpected things can faze children and adolescents, including weird food, unfamiliar lavatorial arrangements (toddlers can't squat over long drops), and issues surrounding personal space. Small children prefer to be down at a level where they too can explore; they get bored if carried all day, and it is sobering to realize that every year in the Alps children die from hypothermia while being carried in backpacks by skiing or mountaineering parents. A thermometer is not necessary to assess if a baby or toddler is chilling dangerously. Compare their skin temperature on the limbs with trunk temperature; if the limbs feel colder then the child needs to be warmed in a place of shelter.

Sunshine

Sunburn in childhood increases the risk of skin cancer in adulthood. It also makes the whole family miserable. Severe sunburn can lead to hypothermia, disastrous loss of fluids, and secondary infection. It is crucial, therefore, that children are protected with long clothes, hats, sun-protective swimsuits, umbrellas (if carried in a backpack), sunscreens, and avoidance of exposure at the very hottest times of the day. So-called sun-blocks reduce exposure to the wavelengths that cause sunburn without necessarily giving adequate protection to cancer-causing wavelengths. Sun protection factors (SPFs) of 15–30 are therefore recommended; sunscreens need to be reapplied frequently (see also ➔ Solar skin damage, p. 284). Sunscreens need replacing each year.

A fine pimply, very itchy rash is probably *prickly heat*. Unlike many of the other causes of itching in children, this is not a histamine-mediated response and so it doesn't respond to antihistamines. The treatment is getting the child cool—either by immersing or splashing with cold water, dabbing (not rubbing) with a damp cloth, and/or retreating to a room with a fan or air conditioning. Calamine lotion is soothing. Dressing the child in loose fitting, 100% cotton clothes will help avoid the problem, and so will a rest during the hottest part of the day.

Bite prevention for children

(See ➔ p. 305). It is wise to embrace precautions that avoid insect and tick bites, not least because an itching bitten child is miserable but, in hot climates, scratched bites often lead to skin infections. Hydrocortisone 1% or Betnovate® RD ointments are the best treatment for bites and stings, although could promote sepsis if the skin is broken. Skin infections cause spreading redness, oozing, sometimes red tracking on the affected limb, and, later, fever.

Choosing the right clothes and footwear helps keep biters away, as does spraying these clothes with permethrin. At dusk, any remaining exposed skin can be covered in a repellent based on up to 30% DEET, or IR3535. Repellents that are based on citronella or lemon eucalyptus are less effective alternatives. If the child is small, then they can be protected under a cot net (preferably also proofed with permethrin). Further information on bite avoidance, bed nets, etc., is on ➔ p. 305.

The fretful small child—ill or bored?

When children become unwell, they can become precipitously ill within hours, and diagnosis can very difficult, especially if the patient isn't yet capable of explaining where it hurts. A toddler with tonsillitis, for example, will often point to their tummy when asked where the pain is. Many cautious paediatricians advise against intrepid travel with children who cannot yet talk because:

- It is difficult to distinguish boredom from disease.
- Small children are fearless and fall off things or drown.
- Children explore and swallow things they shouldn't.
- Bacillary dysentery can make them dangerously ill rapidly.
- Dehydration becomes an issue sooner and can be difficult to manage.
- Malaria is a huge risk and bite precautions are difficult to enforce.
- Small children taken to altitude are at risk of hypothermia and mountain sickness (→ p. 673).

Once a child has reached the age of 4 years they become fun to travel with, they'll enjoy sharing parental adventures, and are better able to communicate about any symptoms. Illness with fever can initially be treated with both paracetamol and ibuprofen. In a non-malarial region, it is probably safe to delay consulting a doctor if the child perks up, although meningitis or typhoid are always possible. In areas where malaria is a risk, a child with a fever >38°C should be evacuated to a clinic or hospital.

Diagnostic aids for an ill child

Diagnosis in an ill child is challenging whoever you are, and travel adds to the difficulties. The designated adult responsible for children would be well advised to travel with *urine dipsticks*, a *thermometer*, and a *child health book*. The *Baby Check* scoring system is invaluable for grading the severity of illness in babies <6 months (see 'Further reading'). The responsible adult should also know the location of the nearest competent medical facility.

Common causes of high fever in children

- Tonsillitis (toddlers usually refuse food).
- Middle ear infection (with earache on one side only).
- Pneumonia/lung infection (>40 breaths/min).
- Bacillary dysentery (fever can start before the diarrhoea; blood is sometimes visible in the stools).
- Sepsis arising from wound infections.
- Malaria (has the child been in a malarious region for >1 week?).
- Meningitis and meningococcal septicaemia.
- Dengue fever (children raised in temperate zones often avoid the severe 'breakbone' illness of adults).

Common causes of drowsiness in children

- Fatigue.
- Dehydration, especially secondary to diarrhoea.
- Malaria.
- Significant infection, including typhoid, meningitis, urinary tract infection (UTI), etc.
- The child has swallowed something noxious (e.g. someone's sleeping pills or spirit alcohol in a cola bottle).

Diarrhoea in children

In diarrhoea, fluids are lost through increased bowel actions and from sweating (especially if there is also fever), yet the appetite will be wanting and often it is difficult to get the child to drink. Standard oral rehydration salts and even fruit-flavoured oral rehydration solutions taste unpleasant because of the potassium content, and many children—even if somewhat dehydrated—will refuse them. In most situations all that the child needs is water with some kind of solute in it. Sugars and/or salts enhance fluid transport into the body, so that water is absorbed more efficiently than if pure water is drunk.

Examples of rehydration solutions include:
- Young coconut.
- Crackers and water.
- Thin soups.
- Colas (but not Diet Coke®); add a pinch of salt.
- Banana and water.
- Toast, jam, and fluids.
- Water or dilute squashes with honey or sugar added.
- Weak herb teas with sugar added.
- Blackcurrant juice.
- Sweet drinks that you can see through.
- Drinks made with Bovril®, Marmite®, or Oxo®.
- Plain carbohydrate foods such as boiled rice and noodles also enhance fluid absorption.

Dehydration in children

Paediatricians make meticulous calculations of what is required to rehydrate an ill child, but a child who is controlling fluid intake through drinking is most unlikely to overhydrate. An early sign of dehydration is to look at the lips and inside the mouth; if these areas look dry then the child needs more fluids. A child who is continuing to pass urine is not significantly dehydrated. Comparing the child's current weight with a recent reliable weight is a useful method of assessing whether there is dehydration. If the child becomes too drowsy to drink then IV or nasogastric fluids will be required.

Some causes of abdominal pain in children

- Diarrhoea/gastroenteritis (pain often relieved by passing wind or stool).
- Constipation (give more to drink, and lots of fruit; increasing pain often heralds stool passage).
- Tonsillitis (in the under-3s, antibiotics are recommended).
- Urinary tract ('bladder') infection (serious in the under-5s—treat with antibiotics and arrange further investigation on return).
- Fatigue (equivalent to a grown-up's migraine).
- Appendicitis (usually in children >5 years; pain starts around navel and moves to right lower abdomen; a child with an appetite does not have appendicitis, nor does one who can jump around, or sit up from lying without pain). Suspected appendicitis needs evacuation to a hospital.
- Meningitis, see ➲ p. 280 (an emergency—evacuate).
- Malaria, see ➲ p. 512 (an emergency—evacuate).

- Pneumonia (respiratory rate is usually increased to >40 breaths/min); antibiotics by mouth may cure. Hospital assessment is recommended.
- Typhoid or paratyphoid (note that paratyphoid is not covered by current injectable vaccines); this is a serious condition that needs expert treatment.
- Hepatitis A or E (often mild in small children) and some other viral infections.
- Intussusception (in child 3 months to 2 years; needs surgery).
- Threadworm (there will also be anal itching); treat with oral mebendazole and repeat dose after 1 week.
- Twisted testicle (some boys are too shy to mention where it hurts); needs urgent surgery.

Generally, the further away the pain is from the navel, the more likely it is to have a significant or serious cause. Pain that wakes a child at night suggests real illness and is seldom benign.

Breathing problems in children

Respiratory problems are common in travelling children. Perhaps a fifth will have asthmatic tendencies yet they may not have an inhaler with them. Chest infections are common too. Noisy breathing (grunting or wheezing) is a sign of illness, and the breathing rate will give some indication of the severity. Flaring of the nostrils on inspiration suggests that the child is struggling to get enough air into the lungs. Whistling or high-pitched musical noises, mostly on breathing out, suggest asthma, while deeper sounds, mostly on breathing in, are most likely to be due to croup or obstruction above the level of the lungs. Remember that asthma and croup can kill so, if in doubt, or if the child is small, evacuate to a hospital.

Normal breathing rates in children	
<1 year:	30–40 breaths/min.
2–5 years:	25–30 breaths/min.
5–12 years:	20–25 breaths/min.
>12 years:	15–20 breaths/min.

First-aid supplies for children

Those new to family travel tend to take too much. Probably the most important item is a knowledge base or book. Colourful dressings seem to have remarkable analgesic properties and so does chocolate: these are important items to have immediately to hand. Wound infections begin readily in hot climates and so an appropriate means of cleaning and dressing wounds is essential. Povidone iodine spray or 10% ointment is convenient, as are antiseptic wipes. For long periods in remote regions, potassium permanganate crystals are light, cheap, and portable; they are often available at the destination (make up to a rosé wine-coloured solution in water and use this to bathe wounds). Try to avoid using antiseptic creams since these promote infection. Other medication will depend upon the level of knowledge of the carers or medic.

Suggested medical kit for children

- Insect repellent (up to 30% DEET can be used, with care, on children).
- Sunscreen 15–30 SPF, broad-brimmed hat, and sun-protective clothes.
- Paracetamol and/or ibuprofen syrup (NB: if bought locally may not be so palatable).
- Digital thermometer.
- Steri-Strips™.
- Colourful sticking plasters.
- Betadine® ointment or povidone iodine spray or other drying antiseptic.
- Hydrocortisone or Betnovate® ointment (for itchy bites and eczema).
- Amoxicillin syrup (if confident in use of antibiotics and patient isn't penicillin allergic).
- Motion sickness preparation if child troubled by this (hyoscine is best for rapid onset one-dose situations or an antihistamine like cinnarizine if multi-dosing is likely).

Resources: children's health abroad

Baby Check. ℘ http://nicutools.org/
KidsTravelDoc. ℘ https://www.facebook.com/KidsTravelHealth/
Wilson-Howarth J. *Staying Healthy When You Travel: Avoiding Bugs, Bites, Bellyaches and More.* Chichester: Fox Chapel Publishing; 2020.
Wilson-Howarth J, Ellis M. *Your Child Abroad: A Travel Health Guide (3rd ed). Bradt Travel Guides; 2014.* ℘ https://www.bradtguides.com/product/your-child-abroad-3-pdf/

Risk management

The concept of managing risk is to identify potential hazards and use control measures to reduce significant risks. This process is only effective if all members of the expedition understand the necessity for these control measures to be in place and are willing to behave accordingly.

Risk can never be completely eliminated, and different people have different thresholds of 'acceptable risk'. Therefore, it is essential to include all expedition members in risk management planning. This ensures that members are fully aware of the risks the expedition is likely to encounter and are able to make an informed decision as to whether to take part in the expedition.

Risk assessments

At the heart of planning a safe and responsible expedition is the process of compiling the risk assessment. The concept is simple: hazards need to be identified and assessed for the severity of risk they represent to the people associated with the expedition (Tables 2.2–2.4).

Risks that are identified are ranked on the basis of the relationship between severity of impact and likelihood of occurrence; the significant risks are then accepted or reduced using appropriate precautions (control measures) such as those identified in Table 2.5.

Definitions from the UK Health and Safety Executive

- A *hazard* is anything that may cause harm, these can be hazards to physical or mental health.
- The *risk* is the chance, high or low, that somebody could be harmed by these and other hazards, together with an indication of how serious the harm could be.

Areas to cover in a risk assessment

- Competence of the leaders and participants, behaviour, and supervision.
- Geopolitical threats and local security.
- Health.
- Environmental hazards.
- The activities (e.g. glacier survey, white-water rafting).
- Transport and accommodation.
- Equipment

The UK Health and Safety Executive refers to the process as '*Five steps to risk assessment*'.[6] These are as follows:

1. Identify the hazards.
2. Decide who might be harmed and how.
3. Evaluate the risks and decide on precautions.
4. Record your significant findings.
5. Review your risk assessment and update if necessary.

6 ᗡ https://www.hse.gov.uk/risk/controlling-risks.htm

Table 2.2 Relationship between likelihood and severity of risk

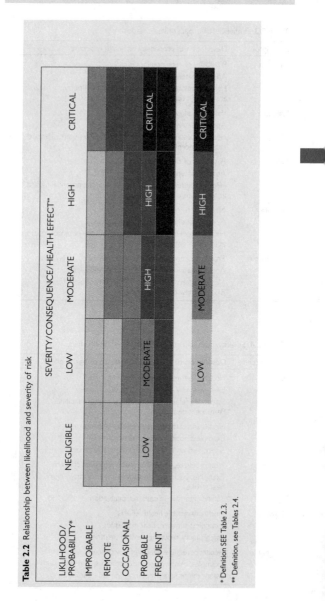

SEVERITY/CONSEQUENCE/HEALTH EFFECT**

LIKELIHOOD/ PROBABILITY**	NEGLIGIBLE	LOW	MODERATE	HIGH	CRITICAL
IMPROBABLE					
REMOTE					
OCCASIONAL					
PROBABLE	LOW	MODERATE	HIGH	HIGH	CRITICAL
FREQUENT					

* Definition SEE Table 2.3.
** Definition, see Tables 2.4.

Table 2.3 Probability of impact of health exposure

Descriptor	Description of probability or health exposure
Frequent	Possibility of repeated incidents
	Approximately once or more per week
	Health exposure: frequent contact with the potential hazard at very high concentrations
Probable	Possibility of isolated incidents
	Approximately once per month
	Health exposure: frequent contact with the potential hazard at high concentrations
Occasional	Possibility of occurring some time
	Approximately once per year
	Health exposure: frequent contact with the potential hazard at moderate concentrations
Remote	Not likely to occur
	Approximately once in 10 years or less
	Health exposure: frequent contact with the potential hazard at low concentrations
Improbable	Practically impossible
	Approximately once in 100 years or more
	Health exposure: infrequent contact with the potential hazard at low concentrations

Table 2.4 Severity/consequence of the impact or health effect

Descriptor	Description of severity/consequence or health effect
Critical	*Health:* life-threatening or disabling illness
	Examples: HIV/AIDS, hepatitis B
	Safety: any fatality or potential for multiple fatalities. Permanent disability
High	*Health:* irreversible health effects of concern
	Examples: noise-induced hearing loss
	Safety: serious injuries with potential for a fatality
Moderate	*Health:* severe, reversible health effects of concern
	Examples: back/muscle strain, repetitive strain injury, heat stroke
	Safety: extensive injuries, hospitalization
Low	*Health:* reversible health effects
	Examples: sunburn, heat exhaustion
	Safety: injury requiring medical treatment
Negligible	*Health:* reversible effects of low concern
	Examples: minor muscular discomfort, skin rash
	Safety: minor injury requiring first-aid treatment

Focus on the serious risks

To ensure risk assessments are effective, it is important to focus on hazards that present a serious risk to the group. Many models exist but simply by considering the severity of probable illness or injuries, it is then possible to judge the likelihood of a risk occurring (Table 2.2). TravelHealthPro highlight some of the main risks for travellers overseas (🕭 https://travelhealth pro.org.uk/factsheet/25/personal-safety).

Research

The best tool for compiling risk assessments is the experience of similar groups/expeditions to the same specific destination involving similar and proposed activities. Reports from past expeditions and networking with individuals who have relevant experience will be useful.

Sources of expedition reports include	
Royal Geographical Society with IBG:	🕭 www.rgs.org/expeditionreports
British Mountaineering Council:	🕭 https://www.thebmc.co.uk/expedition-reports/
Conservation Leadership Programme:	🕭 http://www.conservationleadershipprogramme.org/our-projects.asp
Royal Scottish Geographical Society:	🕭 http://www.rsgs.org/expeditions/

Expedition participants

Participants themselves create risk, e.g. through pre-existing medical conditions and inappropriate behaviour. People travel to remote places for various reasons, often involved with the wish to escape the confines and constraints of life at home and to take more risks. The data on increased levels of unprotected sexual contact by individuals on overseas visits reinforces this; however, extra risk-taking extends to all activities while on an expedition. It is the experience of many large expedition organizations that accidents tend to occur more often on days when expeditioners are relaxing (R-and-R 'off-duty' days), after hard work, and after drinking alcohol.

Assess the wider threats

Assessment of threat (including insurrection, political turmoil, anarchy, and lawlessness) can be completed via consultation with specialists or those who know the destination well. There are a number of commercial travel risk consultancies that can be used, such as Control Risks Group, Risk Advisory, and WorldAware.

Travel-related risks can also be researched using information sources provided by government representatives:

UK—Foreign, Commonwealth and Development Office:	http://www.gov.uk/foreign-travel-advice
Australia—Dept of Foreign Affairs and Trade:	http://www.dfat.gov.au
US—State Department:	http://www.travel.state.gov
Canada—Dept of Foreign Affairs and Trade:	http://www.voyage.gc.ca
World Health Organization:	http://www.who.int
Centres for Disease Control:	http://www.cdc.gov/travel
NaTHNaC:	www.travelhealthpro.org.uk

In-country contacts and agents.
Special interest clubs.
Local tourist board websites.
Guidebooks.

Control measures

Once the serious risks have been identified, each one must be reduced to an acceptable level using control measures (Table 2.5).

As Table 2.5 outlines, personal protective equipment (PPE; e.g. helmets) is one of the least effective methods of preventing risk and should not be used in isolation. A behavioural solution, such as avoiding areas of loose rock, should be used in combination with PPE.

Many control measures can be put in place by an expedition. For example:
- Providing first-aid training for all members.
- Getting immunized before exposure to disease.
- Preventing bites by disease-transmitting insects.

During the expedition, more control measures may need to be implemented that were not identified in the planning process. Reactive plans should aim to reduce the consequence of the incident via effective incident management and good crisis management.

Table 2.5 Proactive and reactive risk-reduction measures

	Method	Description
Most effective	Elimination	Do not do the activity
	Substitution	Do it in a different way; consider a 'Plan B'
	Engineering	Implement mechanical solution to reduce risk
	Behaviour	Change behaviour to minimize risk
	PPE	Reduce the severity and likelihood of injury using PPE
Least effective	Reactive plans	First aid and ERPs to reduce severity of incident

Educate the group

It is important to share the outcomes of the risk assessment with the participants. This also provides the background for participants to understand why control measures are in place.

Therefore, pre-expedition information should include the risk assessment or, as a minimum, a summary of the key risks and control measures in place to reduce them. Continual enforcement of control measures and frequent briefing of risks is considered good practice.

Group risk education should continue throughout the expedition, as many factors will be dynamic and prone to change.

Employ sensible flexible control measures

The key to effective control measures is to be flexible. Unnecessary overuse of control measures will produce a negative response from expedition members.

The level of controls used must reflect the seriousness of the risk. For example, drowning is more serious than new boots causing blisters. However, both these hazards can be highlighted in different ways. For example, a note about new boots in the pre-trip information coupled with group observation would be an effective way of reducing the likelihood of blisters.

The severity of drowning would require a different approach. This would include gathering data on whether participants can swim, providing appropriate life jackets, ensuring competent supervision, and, finally, having an ERP in case of capsize.

See also ➲ Emergency response plan, p. 148 and ➲ Crisis Management, p. 146 for further information.

Medical insurance

Making sure that there is adequate and appropriate insurance cover in place for all participants is an essential part of pre-expedition planning and integral to the ERP (➲ p. 148).

Most overseas visits will require insurance for the following elements:
- Medical treatment and additional expenses.
- Dental treatment.
- Repatriation.
- Personal accident.
- Search and rescue (SAR).
- Replacement/rearrangement.
- Public/personal liability.

You might also want to consider insurance for:
- Cancellation and curtailment.
- Loss of baggage and equipment (especially expensive medical equipment).

When buying insurance
- Read the policy/policies. This is essential, but not often done. Check the small print and make sure cover is in place for all aspects of the visit and what exclusions apply.
- Do not under-insure; the costs of in-country medical expenses and repatriation can be high.
- If you are travelling to North America or with North Americans, explicitly notify insurers of this and check whether your insurance covers you for this element, including for claims brought in North America, rather than just your own jurisdiction.
- Disclose all activities and risks to the insurer—including pre-existing medical conditions. Failure to do so may see you without cover.
- Ensure that specific risks are mentioned which concern your trip, e.g. death from hypothermia or altitude.
- If local staff are hired, make enquiries as to your responsibilities to them. Many countries have requirements for workers' compensation in the event of an accident or injury.
- Ensure that your policy will not expire if your expedition over-runs.
- For a group policy, be certain that the insurer has not limited the number of individuals covered in a single incident.
- The insurer should provide a 24 h phone number which can be called when an incident occurs.
- Report all claims in line with the requirements of the policy. Failure to notify insurers within time limits stated in the policy will likely lead to the insurer refusing to indemnify/pay out.
- Remember, if you travel to areas where the Foreign, Commonwealth & Development Office (FCDO) advises against all travel, your insurance may not cover you. Specialist insurance, via niche brokers, may be available for travel to certain high-risk countries.

Types of insurance

Medical and additional expenses

Medical insurance should pay for treatment and travel expenses incurred for individuals following accidental injury or illness. The insurance should have a 24 h contact number available for the insurer to guarantee payment to treatment centres or emergency services should their help be required. The level of medical cover for each member should reflect the cost of treatment. Medical expenses in the US can be particularly high, especially if surgery or intensive care is involved.[7] Any pre-existing medical conditions must be disclosed to the insurer. Non-disclosure invalidates cover.

Personal accident

This covers death and disablement due to an accident while on an expedition. An amount is paid to the injured party in the event of loss of use of limbs, eyes, disablement, or death.

Search and rescue considerations

Insurance may be found to fund a search and rescue, but SAR is very expensive, particularly if it involves aircraft, and the price of insurance will reflect this. The majority of SARs around the world are carried out via a mixture of police, army, and volunteers. Emergency funds or even a bond, paid in advance, may be required to initiate this process. Ensure the whole group is covered. The SAR insurance offerings associated with some emergency beacons may only cover the individual owning the beacon/named on the policy associated with the beacon.

Replacement and rearrangement

Insurance is available to cover the cost of replacing a key team member in the event of an expedition member being disabled or killed. It should also be possible to cover the costs of returning the injured person to the expedition when they have recovered.

Public/personal liability

Insurance against any legal liability incurred on the group or an individual or to a group or individual in the event of an incident is advisable. Leaders and medical professionals and expedition organizers have greater responsibilities than other members of the expedition.

Professional indemnity insurance

Doctors and other medical professionals should have a detailed discussion with their insurers or medical defence entity regarding their intended expedition, including nationality of participants and should confirm that their professional indemnity insurance company will cover them to work with all members of the expedition, in the country/countries in question and/or with host country nationals (➲ Legal liabilities, p. 78).

- If you are travelling to North America or with North Americans, explicitly notify insurers of this and check whether your insurance covers you for the expedition and for claims brought in North America, rather than just claims brought in your own jurisdiction.

7 🔗 https://www.gov.uk/guidance/foreign-travel-insurance

Legal liabilities and professional insurance

An introduction to legal liability in England and Wales

This section is based on the professional discharge of duties under the law of England and Wales. Scotland and Northern Ireland are separate jurisdictions and legal aspects and procedure may be different. Please be aware that the laws of the country in which the expedition takes place may apply to acts/omissions in that jurisdiction.

Whether you are an employee of the expedition company or are providing medical services as a third-party contractor may create additional/different legal obligations.

When reading this section please note the broad legal principles but seek specialist advice from your professional indemnity insurer regarding your specific circumstances and expedition. This is almost always beneficial and instructive. This is a complex area.

To date, there have been no reported cases where an expedition doctor has been successfully sued in a UK court. There have, however, been claims intimated against medical professionals operating in an expedition/remote area medical context. Naturally, it is difficult to have a full picture as some claims may be brought against the employer only, some cases do not advance to the issue of proceedings, and some claims may be settled. However, in what is perceived to be an increasingly litigious climate, no practitioner can afford to be complacent. The risk is real. That said, most cases turn on disputed facts—differing versions of events, rather than complex legal disputes. The law is generally well understood. *Keep thorough notes!*

Negligence

Negligence is a widely recognized concept in common law jurisdictions.

Medical professionals need to be aware that they may have responsibilities in both their non-medical roles as members of the leadership team (if operating in that capacity) and in their medical practitioner capacity as expedition medic.

The law of England and Wales places the burden of proof on the claimant and requires a claimant to prove their claim, on the balance of probabilities (i.e. more likely than not), by demonstrating the following:

- That the defendant owed the claimant a duty of care.
- That care fell below the standard of care reasonably expected, i.e. the duty of care was breached.
- That the claimant suffered harm and that this was caused or contributed to by the breach.

Duty of care

In the UK, an individual has no legal duty to assist random members of the public they encounter. The situation may differ in other countries/jurisdictions. In France, for example, there is a legal obligation on every person to give emergency assistance at the scene of an accident, and failure to do so has resulted in prosecution. You will need to comply with any local laws in the jurisdiction that your expedition will be undertaken in.

There may, however, be a professional obligation to render medical assistance. Even when off-duty, the GMC expects doctors to provide emergency assistance:

In an emergency, wherever it arises, you must offer assistance, taking account of your own safety, your competence, and the availability of other options for care.

GMC *Good Medical Practice* guide.

The Nursing and Midwifery Council has indicated in its professional Code of Conduct that it requires similar actions of its registrants.

These professional obligations do not carry the full force of law, but penalties for failing to comply may be serious (e.g. recently the GMC issued a formal reprimand to a doctor who failed to render assistance to an injured person at the scene of a road accident) and, in the absence of legal precedent, this may be taken as instructive by courts.

Any person treating a patient, advising a patient, or advising an expedition company has, in law, a clear duty of care. There has been a report in the literature of a claim intimated in relation to an expedition doctor regarding medical assistance provided to a member of a different expedition team. The company running the expedition to which the doctor was attached is reported to have declined to assist. The claim was ultimately discontinued.

Standard of care

Where a duty of care is owed, the obligation is to exercise reasonable care and skill in the circumstances. The case of *Bolam* v *Friern Hospital Management Committee* (1957) produced the following definition of what is reasonable:

The test is the standard of the ordinary skilled man exercising and professing to have that special skill. A man need not possess the highest expert skill at the risk of being found negligent . . . it is sufficient if he exercises the skill of an ordinary man exercising that particular art.

In *Bolam*, the Court made clear that a professional does not breach their duty of care if a responsible body of equivalent professionals would have treated the patient in the same way—this is so even if there are different 'schools of thought' and a majority of their fellow professionals would have treated the patient differently.

This legal test has been further refined by the Court in the case of *Bolitho* v *City and Hackney Health Authority* (1993)—a professional may still be liable even if a responsible body of equivalent professionals would have treated the patient in the same way if the Court finds that the 'school of thought' is irrational and cannot withstand logical scrutiny.

Courts have indicated that they will not allow inexperience as a defence in actions of professional negligence: if a doctor is unable to exercise reasonable care in carrying out a particular task, then they should not undertake this. Should a practitioner hold themselves out to be an expedition doctor (and as such having a 'specialist' skill), therefore, their actions would be judged against what might reasonably be expected of a reasonably competent expedition doctor even if this were the first time the individual had ever taken on such a role.

A resource-limited, remote environment is different to a fully equipped hospital. Those wanting to operate as expedition medics should evidence appropriate specialist expedition/remote area medical training from a reputable provider. As ever, continuing professional development is essential. These elements would be scrutinized in any court case.

At present, there are no definitive standards of care specifically for expeditions. Expert evidence from recognized experts in the expedition medicine field would be necessary, to assist the judge, in any court case. Both sides will likely advance their own expert evidence. The Faculty of Pre Hospital Care, Royal College of Surgeons Edinburgh guidance for the provision of medical care in wilderness situations offers a framework of recommended competencies.[8] BS 8848 has been used by Coroners (in the UK and overseas) inquiring into deaths on expeditions (➲ p. 184). The Faculty of Pre Hospital Care has also issued a document on the relevance of BS:8848 (2014) to new or inexperienced expedition 'medics'. These publications (and possibly this handbook) as well as Wilderness Medical Society Practice Guidelines (and updates) are likely to be referred to and relied upon by expert witnesses. They are an essential read.

Causation

A claimant must prove that the breach of duty caused the harm suffered. What has to be proved is illustrated by the case of *Barnett* v *Chelsea and Kensington Hospital Management Committee* (1969). A man was sent home from a hospital accident and emergency department after complaining of acute stomach pains and sickness. He died later that same day, of what later proved to be arsenic poisoning. The hospital admitted a breach of duty, but the widow failed to recover damages because the patient would have died whatever the doctor had done, i.e. causation could not be demonstrated.

In the context of an expedition, the requirement to demonstrate causation may prove to be the main obstacle to a claimant trying to sue a doctor for negligence. For example, in the case of a patient who suffered an intracranial bleed secondary to a head injury, it would be a challenge to show that it was a doctor's failure to site burr holes that led to long-term disability rather than the injury caused by a falling rock.

Bailey v *Ministry of Defence*, is the leading case on the law of material contribution as it relates to causation. *Bailey* provides, in essence, that where you have multiple causes of an injury and only one of the causes is negligent, the claimant is entitled to recover damages for the injury if the negligent cause probably made a material contribution to the injury. Each case turns on its own facts. If the doctor in the burr hole example described above had the means and equipment to do burr holes and negligently failed to do so, they could be liable if the delay was long enough to cause sustained raised intracranial pressure, even with the underlying head injury not being his/her fault.

Emergency situations

In an emergency, courts will take into account the specific circumstances, such as the need to act with speed in a hazardous situation and determine whether a practitioner had acted with reasonable care. The factual matrix will be highly relevant. A court will recognize the fact that medicine was being practised in a remote area and that medical resources would be limited. As one judge ruled:

I accept that full allowance must be made for the fact that certain aspects of treatment may have to be carried out in what one witness [. . .] called

8 ℘ https://fphc.rcsed.ac.uk/media/2781/updated-guidance-on-medical-provision-for-wilderness-medicine.pdf

'battle conditions'. An emergency may overburden the available resources, and, if an individual is forced by circumstances to do too many things at once, the fact that he does one of them incorrectly should not lightly be taken as negligence.

Wilsher v Essex Area Health Authority.

However, expedition members, as potential patients, must be informed of the skills and limitations of the expedition medic (such as equipment carried, distance to definitive care, evacuation times, etc.). Similarly, the risks that expedition members will be taking need to be clearly communicated.

Liability on commercial expeditions

Most of the medical indemnity organizations will provide 'Good Samaritan' cover for doctors acting in any part of the world. However, this would apply only where a team member just happens to be a doctor. It would certainly not cover a doctor receiving any form of inducement (e.g. a 10% discount on the trip fee) that may imply the doctor has an official medical role on the expedition.

Particular caution is required where citizens of the US or Canada are participating in the expedition. Indeed, it may be impossible for a UK-registered doctor to obtain professional indemnity insurance other than on a 'Good Samaritan' basis for treating or advising people who are ordinarily residents of North America. English courts have jurisdiction over the deaths of Britons wherever they occur and there is no formal time limit for criminal prosecutions for unlawful killing. There is little doubt that an American court would claim an analogous jurisdiction over the death of an American citizen. Even in civil claims, some US states will act contrary to jurisdiction clauses in expedition terms and conditions and agree to hear a case in that state, which arose from an incident during an expedition in another country. It is essential you make your insurer/indemnity body aware of involvement of North Americans on your expedition or if you will be acting as an expedition medic in North America. Their advice or limitations on coverage may be instructive. In these circumstances, check that your insurance covers you against a claim being brought in North America, not just your own jurisdiction.

Expedition companies have a responsibility in common law to ensure that any medic that they choose to employ is competent. In the event of a claim for negligence, any claim would likely follow the money and would usually be made against the expedition company in the first instance. It is likely that the claimant's solicitors would also include the medic as a party to the claim. The expedition company's insurers would then likely seek an indemnity from the medic and seek to pass the claim to the medic's insurers. Insurance coverage is absolutely essential to anyone operating as an expedition medic.

Expedition medics should check the insurance policy of any company engaging their services and should have a contract in place setting out each party's obligations.

Expeditions departing without a doctor

Many smaller expeditions may not have the resources to be able to take a doctor into the field. However, the team will still require medical advice and the supply of a suitable medical kit. In these cases, doctors may be approached to perform various services:

- Medical pre-screening of expeditioners and expedition staff.
- Assist with medical-related risk assessments (e.g. altitude).
- Provide advice on vaccinations or antimalarial chemoprophylaxis.
- Advise on contents of a suitable medical kit.
- Supply private prescriptions for an expedition[9] (NB: drugs may be used for the treatment of trip members previously unknown to the doctor).
- Medical advice and consultations by satellite phone to expedition medics.
- Delegate the responsibility for initiating treatment to a trip leader.

In these situations, the administration of medication should be via a written protocol or verbal consultation with a doctor (e.g. by phone, satellite phone, or email). All prescription medication should be accompanied by a letter from the prescribing doctor. It would also be prudent for the doctor to seek a written understanding from the person to whom prescriptions are supplied that the medication prescribed will only be used for the immediate treatment of expedition members while some distance from a hospital or clinic and not as a substitute for seeking professional medical advice where this is readily available.

Professional indemnity insurance

Most of the principal medical insurance bodies in the UK will extend the scope of their cover to include the practice of expedition medicine. However, this needs to be specifically requested (even if, depending on the grade and specialty of the practitioner, it were then provided at no extra cost) and, as mentioned earlier, may not extend to the care of North Americans or to claims brought in North America. Check this point carefully.

Other factors to discuss with insurers would include:

- The scope of the treatment you propose to provide (especially if this were to fall well outside your normal full-time specialty).
- Whether you intend to extend this beyond your expedition members (such as to local workers employed by your team, other members of the local population, and perhaps other travellers not involved with your own trip).

Be aware of the differing organizational structures of the principal medical insurance bodies—the scope of their services may differ.

Several organizations including the British Mountain Medicine Society have niche insurance schemes for expedition medics meeting certain criteria (see: https://thebmms.co.uk/).

Summary

- Expedition medicine is an interesting, highly rewarding vocation which can be challenging at times and one which needs to be practised with care.

9 Moore J, Ladbrook M, Goodyer L, et al. The provision of prescription-only medicines for use on UK-based overseas expeditions. *Wilderness Environ Med*. 2017;28(3):219–224.

- Before you accept the position, find out exactly what is expected of you. A clear, written agreement setting out your responsibilities as an MO is very important, particularly so where charity or commercial expeditions are concerned. Check that the jurisdiction clause in the contract relates to your own jurisdiction (i.e. will be interpreted in relation to the laws of the jurisdiction you habitually practise medicine in—you don't want to be held to a different standard).
- Check what the clients have been promised by the company in terms of medical coverage (look at the brochure/website).
- Check that the company has insurance that will cover you (including claims brought under the laws of and in North American jurisdictions). Get a copy of it, read it, keep it.
- Check what licences and approvals you need to operate locally.
- Keep thorough records. Contemporaneous evidence is worth its weight in gold.
- Drugs supplied to an expedition for administration or dispensing by non-medical personnel need to be prescribed via a written protocol or (preferably) by a doctor via a tele-medicine consultation.
- Irrespective of whether the expedition company provides you with insurance cover, you still need your own professional indemnity insurance. If you do not have insurance that covers the activities you are going to be doing, with the group you are engaged to be supporting, don't do it.
- Finally, many medics have undertaken the role of MO before you. Seek out advice—and, importantly, enjoy what may be the experience of a lifetime!

Chapter 3

Caring for people in the field

Chapter editor
Shane Winser

Contributors
Peter Bradley
Derek Evans
Larry Goodyer
James Moore
Shane Winser
Akbar Lalani (1st edition)
Christina Lalani (1st edition)
Paul Goodyer (2nd edition)

Expedition health clinics

Most health problems experienced on expedition are not emergencies and can be dealt with at set times during the day. Outside clinic times, emergency healthcare can be provided using a basic emergency first-aid kit.

Individuals should have a personal first-aid kit to enable self-care (➔ p. 854), although it is important for the medic to be aware of any self-administered medication.

Expedition health clinics described in this chapter are primarily concerned with providing healthcare for expedition team members and associates. The provision of healthcare dedicated to the indigenous population is complex and outside the remit of most expeditions (➔ p. 122).

Clinic times

Expedition health clinics can be structured to suit both mobile and static expeditions. All team members, including local employees, should be aware of how the clinic is to be accessed and the scope/limitations of available care.

Established expedition clinic times:
- Provide a structured daily timetable for medics and team members.
- Avoid the need to repeatedly open medical kits.
- Enable accurate stock control.
- Encourage self-care outside clinic hours.

Structure clinic times around the expedition working day. If involved in non-medical expedition activities, the medic can run a brief clinic in the morning before or after breakfast, during which there can be a review of ongoing problems and assessments of any new issues. Unless there are issues requiring simple answers or advice, or an emergency, individuals should be encouraged to attend clinics at the allotted times. A situation may arise where individuals wish to discuss a problem without the rest of the team becoming aware. The medic should ensure this is possible and that team members are aware of this option.

Clinic location

Medical clinics should be comfortable and well lit. Ideally, they should be away from communal areas and in a location that maximizes confidentiality and privacy. Clinics should not be on major camp thoroughfares where team members continually pass by.

If a dedicated clinic area is not possible, some expeditions may facilitate the medic having a slightly larger or independent sleeping area, e.g. a larger tent, where medical consultations can take place.

Depending on the expedition and camp layout, it may be preferable for the medic to visit individuals. Be aware that tents provide little sound insulation and sensitive information may be overheard.

Clinic layout

The ideal clinic should allow for patient examination to be conducted in a manner that closely resembles that of a healthcare facility at home.

Consider the following:
- Sufficient space for patient examination.
- Light—especially when assessing wounds/injuries.
- Protection from insects—e.g. a mosquito net.

- Ease of access—injured patients may struggle to access enclosed spaces.
- Safe and secure storage of medical equipment.
- A method of collecting waste.

Most patients can be examined in a seated position. If possible, a small chair or bench is a valuable piece of clinic furniture. However, if items like this are not present, improvise.

Within the clinic, clinicians should have access to:
- Medical kit.
- Handwashing/cleansing facilities.
- A method for sterilizing equipment.
- Medical notes.
- Basic reference textbooks such as this and, ideally, internet access or other method of communication.

Clinical areas should be kept as clean and free from dirt/waste as possible—especially food waste that attracts animal life. Surfaces should be wiped down with antibacterial/antiseptic solutions (e.g. Dettol®) after use. Clinical waste should be burned or disposed of appropriately. Sharps must be carefully stored and disposed on return from expedition.

Medical kits are expensive commodities and should be kept in a secure location. Access to medical kits should be limited to the clinician and specifically named individuals.

Sanatorium/sick bay

Most individuals suffering from illness or injury on expedition can continue to use their normal sleeping accommodation. Exceptions to this might include:
- Communicable disease requiring isolation.
- Where frequent or rapid access to toilet facilities is required.
- Where continual/regular patient monitoring is needed.

In these circumstances it will be beneficial to create a clinical area sufficient for the medic to provide care as dictated by the illness. This may necessitate the medic moving nearer the patient. In environmental extremes (such as polar blizzards), repeated visits between medic and patient will be impractical, even dangerous.

Sick or injured patients using their own accommodation should have a means of contacting the medic should their condition deteriorate. Where appropriate, this may include having an accommodation buddy. The medic's accommodation should be clearly marked and easily accessible.

Increased attention should be given to tidiness and hygiene in areas where patients are being looked after. Expedition patients often resort to the easier 'go behind the nearest tree' option, rather than utilize appropriate latrines. This behaviour should be discouraged.

Latrine hygiene is especially important during times of sickness. Creating a rota of cleaning responsibilities may be useful to ensure consistently high standards of hygiene. It is not uncommon for individuals suffering from traveller's diarrhoea to experience bouts of incontinence. In such situations, clothes will require careful laundering.

Field nursing care

Successful management of any illness or injury depends on the harmony between the clinical skills of medicine and the dedicated care and compassion of nursing. Good nursing skills should be employed in every aspect of patient care, for those in the acute phase of patient assessment and treatment as well as those awaiting either evacuation or being nursed back to health in the field.

Nursing care includes providing psychological reassurance, maintaining patient comfort, ensuring observations and interventions are carried out, and documenting the process.

Nursing a sick or injured patient is not something that comes naturally to everyone. Perhaps the best way of approaching patient care is to remember and emulate the care and compassion you received as a poorly child. Generally, the one individual any ill person wants to see when feeling unwell is their mother. Be their mother.

Psychological support

Being unwell while far from the safety and security of a domestic health service can be disconcerting at best, terrifying at worst, particularly for younger or less experienced team members. The knowledge that in-country healthcare systems may be inaccessible or inadequate will add to this stress. From initial assessment the clinician should seek to provide reassurance and encouragement. Keeping patients informed throughout procedures, treatments, and care planning will keep stress levels to a minimum and help patients feel involved.

The reaction of others will affect an individual's perception of the severity of their illness or injury. Looks of terror or disgust are likely to increase feelings of anxiety. This should be considered especially in those with little or no previous exposure to traumatic situations.

The power of touch is frequently overlooked in a modern, busy health service. The calm reassurance of someone holding a hand is often enough to help a patient relax. However, some patients will prefer not to be fussed over.

For the medic as well as the casualty this will be a very stressful time, especially if circumstances delay evacuation. The medic will require rest and other members of the group will have to help with basic nursing tasks up to the limits of their capability. If communications can be established, receiving knowledgeable advice and support from an expert will improve care and provide reassurance.

Prolonged field care

However ill a casualty is, it may be impossible to arrange immediate evacuation for reasons that could include breakdowns in communications, weather conditions, or lack of local logistic support. Isolated groups, often with little prior training, will then have to care for their sick or injured companion, possibly for a long time. The expedition medic will have to fulfil all the roles of an interdisciplinary healthcare team.

Prolonged field care kit

(See also ➔ Chapter 28.) Among risk management considerations prior to departure should be consideration of how an expedition would cope with caring for a casualty who cannot be immediately evacuated. Many factors will influence this, including the mobility of the group, the modes of transport, the budget, the expertise of the medic(s), and the size and weight available for the medical kit. Consider:

- *Monitoring and examination:* respiratory rate (RR), heart rate (HR), capillary refill, and peripheral pulses can all be assessed with no additional kit. Arterial oxygen saturation (SaO_2) and temperature monitors are light and portable. More sophisticated monitors such as portable ECG and ultrasound devices are becoming widely available at reasonable cost.
- *Fluid resuscitation:* consider whether to take IV fluids and in what quantities. Static expeditions should consider from where replacement supplies could be obtained.
- *Ventilation, oxygenation, and airway:* advanced airway kit for prolonged field care may be required on some expeditions. O_2 consumption vs time to definitive care will dictate whether this is a useful addition. Formula for amount of O_2 needed (L) = time to definitive care (min) × flow rate (L/min).
- *Medications:* medical kits should be stocked with enough basic drugs to last through any expected care timescales, and a day or so beyond. Key drugs such as antibiotics and painkillers should be available in various preparations (oral (PO)/rectal (PR)/IM/IV) such that they can be administered to vomiting or unconscious patients.

Rescue phase

See also ➔ Chapter 5.

Rescue

Following an accident, the site must be made safe, and the casualty extracted from hazardous surroundings as swiftly as practical. It is essential not to add to the number of casualties during this time.

Primary survey and secondary survey

(See ➔ p. 203 and ➔ p. 224.) Identify acute and ongoing care issues.

Request for support

(See ➔ p. 146.) If communications permit, identify if immediate evacuation to definitive medical care is practical, using local SAR facilities. If immediate support cannot be arranged, then:

Consider shelter

Carefully select the location where the patient will be cared for in the mean-time. Ideally this will be a well-constructed building but a bothy, tent, snow hole, tent, or bivvy bag might have to be considered. Getting there could involve use of a vehicle, boat, pack animal, or makeshift carry.

External communications

Once the rescue is complete and the casualty protected from the elements, external help must be sought. This could be from local agents or pre-arranged links in the country of origin. The expedition leader and medic need to communicate information on:
- The incident and subsequent diagnoses.
- The current state of the patient and anticipated progress.
- The plan for evacuation and requirement for external help.
- The likely timescale that care will be needed.
- Ensure the details of contacts are clearly detailed.
- Use standardized formats: SBAR, ATMIST, (M)ETHANE (➲ p. 159).

Continuing care

Depending on where you are caring for the patient, different challenges will be apparent. A tent or vehicle may be cramped and prevent easy access to parts of the patient for reassessment, access to monitoring devices, and interventions if the patient's condition suddenly deteriorates. Ongoing care must be provided to prevent secondary issues.

The acronym '*SHEEP VOMIT*' covers the nursing needs.

S: skin protection and hygiene

Skin breakdown or damage will lead to increased risk of infection, dehydration, pain, and discomfort. Remove jewellery and clothing that might cause problems.

Skin should be kept clean and dry. Start at the face and 'clean' areas and work your way outwards to 'dirtier' areas. Regularly wash your cloth before continuing to the next area to prevent the spread of contamination. Avoid uneven/rough ground and protect the skin with barrier creams and physical barriers; blister plasters, dressings, and incontinence pads. If necessary, protect eyes with moist covers to prevent drying out and corneal abrasion.
- Do not neglect body areas prone to infection such as groins and armpits.
- Ensure any soap used is rinsed off.
- Dry the patient thoroughly.
- Provide mouth and dental care.
- Maintain the highest level of dignity possible.
- Offer a chaperone.

H: hypo/hyperthermia

Aim for normothermia by appropriate heating or cooling (➲ p. 808).

E: elevation and positioning

Regularly reposition and check the patient, ensuring they are as comfortable as possible. Consider the recovery position if there is a need to protect the airway from vomit or other secretions, persistently low blood pressure (BP) may be helped by elevating the legs, while isolated head-injured patients may benefit from a sitting position.

E: exercise (active/passive)

Encourage patients to move themselves. If changing from a horizontal position, move slowly to reduce risk of syncope. Regular passive movements reduce the risk of stiffness and clot formation.

P: pressure points

A person lying in one position for too long may develop serious skin sores and muscle injuries that take months to heal. Regular turning and massage can reduce this risk. These patients may also require toileting assistance. The warning signs that a pressure injury is occurring will be changes in sensation or temperature in a blanching area of skin. A non-blanching erythematous area of skin indicates the first stage of injury has occurred. Any pressure injury accompanied by skin loss is significant. Pressure injuries can be eliminated by regular turning of patients, massage, well-cushioned pressure areas, and cleanliness. Remember, air mattresses can be too rigid due to over-inflation.

For details of safe movement of a spinal injury patient see: ♫ https://www.youtube.com/watch?v=9M1GOIzeF3s

V: vital signs

Depending on the nature of the illness or injury, regular clinical observations may be indicated (➔ p. 254). These must be documented in a manner that allows rapid interpretation and pattern recognition.

Minimum observations should include:
- RR.
- HR.
- Temperature (T).

In addition, the following may also be required:
- Fluid intake and output.
- Urinalysis.
- BP.
- O_2 saturations.
- Blood sugar.
- Pain scores. Use a scale of 0–10 where: 0 = no pain to 10 = the worst pain *the patient* has ever experienced.
- Neurological observations—using either the awake/verbal/pain/unresponsive (ACVPU) scale or Glasgow Coma Scale (GCS) (➔ p 223, 263).

These are conveniently recorded on an observation chart. See ➔ Fig. 8.7. Injury or illness severity will dictate the frequency of observations. As a basic rule, the further a patient's observations are from normal, or the more acute the injury or illness, the more frequent observations should be.

For example, a patient suffering from shock following a serious injury will require regular observations (RR, HR, BP, conscious level, pain score, fluid intake, and urine output) approximately every 10–15 min, until the shock has been corrected and the patient remains stable. A less unwell patient suffering from gastroenteritis will require basic observations (RR, HR, T, urine output) once or twice daily.

O: oral hygiene

Patients require regular oral care to prevent drying of mucous membranes, aspiration risk, and bacterial growth. Water on a sponge can be incredibly refreshing for those unable to tolerate food or fluids.

M: massage/DVT prophylaxis

If available, use thromboembolism deterrent stockings such as flight socks. Massage the limbs to give comfort and improve blood flow. Work distally to proximal, starting at the feet.

I: ins and outs (diet and fluids)

Conscious patients with no risk factors for aspiration should eat and drink as is appropriate. Do not risk aspiration of solids or liquids in semi-conscious patients, or those lying supine. Record fluid intake.

Urination

If there are any concerns about moving, encourage the careful use of a bottle or bed pan equivalent. Consider the use of urinary sheaths rather than urinary catheters. Measure urine volumes carefully. Aim for 0.5 mL/kg/h of urine.

Defaecation

Try to collect urine first to allow measurement. It is vitally important that patients are kept clean and dry, so use this time to examine and wash patients accordingly.

T: turn/cough/deep breath

When a patient is supine, has lower consciousness levels, or pain preventing deep inspiration, the lower airways can become poorly ventilated and risk of atelectasis and infection increase. Encouraging patients to breath in as far as possible, hold, then 'sniff' will help ventilate the peripheral alveoli. Encourage patients to cough up any secretions/sputum. If pain is preventing these manoeuvres make sure analgesia or support is given (hugging a pillow when coughing is helpful). Consider learning 'assisted coughing' techniques for those with limited or no muscle tone.

Documentation

Good documentation is important for the following reasons:
- Allows observation of illness progression/regression.
- Aids diagnosis.
- Increases handover accuracy and safety.
- Provides a record of what has/has not been done.
- Can be a source of reassurance for less experienced medics.
- Is vital during patient handover.
- Reduces clinical error.

Documentation should include medical assessments, diagnosis, and treatment along with ongoing care, which will include medicines administered, observations and interventions. It is preferable to write medical notes as soon as something has been done but do not delay interventions for the sake of documentation. Good medical records will allow a receiving clinician to have a clear understanding of the patient's illness, treatment, and progression, irrespective of their level of involvement.

Ensure all documentation is kept in the best possible condition. This may prove difficult in some environments, such as the tropics, where humidity or dirt invades every aspect of expedition life. Observation charts can be printed on waterproof paper (Toughprint®). Increasingly, dictation software such as Pages® can be used on smartphones to keep accurate, contemporaneous electronic notes.

Notes are confidential and should be kept securely and accessible only by those involved directly in patient care. Patient confidentiality extends beyond the expedition and any medical records should be stored securely on return home. Clinicians should retain a copy of the notes for reference purposes.

See Table 3.1 for a useful checklist in field care nursing.

Preparation for the evacuation

(See also ⊕ Chapter 5.) Identify and prepare for likely challenges to be faced once underway:
- O_2 requirements.
- Battery life of equipment/power sources available for equipment.
- Urinary catheter/waste collection options.
- Nasogastric tube/antiemetics/suction/safe positioning if patient does vomit.
- IV access visible and with backup.
- Fuel for vehicle—are stops required? Full vehicle check carried out? Contingency for flat tyre/engine failure?
- Uneven terrain/river crossing—effects on unstable patient?
- What actions will you realistically be able to carry out once packaged and in a vehicle?

Table 3.1 Field care nursing checklist

Clinical observations	
Essential	☐
Specific	☐
Clinical care	
Analgesia	☐
Antiemetics	☐
Other medicines	☐
Hydration and fluids	☐
Nutrition	☐
Wound care	☐
Dressing or splint care	☐
Patient care and comfort	
Warmth	☐
Pressure area care	☐
Patient hygiene	☐
Dental care	☐
Communication and mental health	☐
Documentation	☐

- How will observation equipment to be attached to the patient and remain visible?
- Does the medic or patient suffer with travel sickness?
- How often do you need to stop to reassess patient?
- Can equipment be used at altitude/in aircraft?

Once the patient has been evacuated, the rest of the team will still require time and space to reflect on the event. Some may want to continue with the initial goal, while others may wish to leave. Medical resources will have been depleted and need to be replaced. There may be requests for statements from the local authorities and the media, and team members may need psychological support (➔ p. 545). Considering the possibility of such contingencies during the planning of an expedition can reduce problems in the field and minimize the problems of post-event stress.

The ill or injured medic

The medic on expedition is at the same risk as everyone else from travel, illness, or accident. Consider how to cope if it is the medic who is incapacitated.

Medicines management

Before you give a drug to anyone, you should know about it. Information can be sourced from:
- The patient information leaflet (PIL) supplied with the drug.
- The SPC, available at: 🖉 http://www.medicines.org.uk/emc
- Freestanding apps such as the *British National Formulary* (BNF) or *Epocrates*.
- Online formularies or the internet.

Errors in drug prescribing and administration are frighteningly common even among trained hospital staff. Fig. 3.1 provides a flowchart of the things that require checking each time a drug is given to a patient.

Any other treatments such as dressing changes should be documented in the patient notes and relevant observations made (e.g. wound granulation, signs of infection). Documentation should be clear and unambiguous to avoid confusion and potential drug errors.

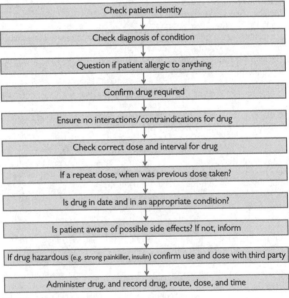

Check patient identity

Check diagnosis of condition

Question if patient allergic to anything

Confirm drug required

Ensure no interactions/contraindications for drug

Check correct dose and interval for drug

If a repeat dose, when was previous dose taken?

Is drug in date and in an appropriate condition?

Is patient aware of possible side effects? If not, inform

If drug hazardous (e.g. strong painkiller, insulin) confirm use and dose with third party

Administer drug, and record drug, route, dose, and time

Fig. 3.1 Drug administration.

Medicines storage

Expedition environments are unforgiving on equipment, and extremes of temperature and humidity will degrade less robust containers. A balance must be struck between container strength, durability, and weight. Medical kit containers should be strong enough to withstand all the rigours of transport, with delicate items such as glass vials packed in foam within rigid containers. Sterile packaging of items such as IV giving sets are particularly prone to damage through abrasion or moisture. Labels should be written in permanent ink or laminated, as text can become illegible in damp or humid conditions.

Medicine containers should be sealed sufficiently to keep out moisture, extremes of temperature, and animal or insect invasion. Try to keep the kits off the ground.

Most oral medications (tablet or syrup) are stable across a broad range of temperatures. Pre-mixed and injectable medicines can be less stable with some requiring refrigeration. Lyophilized (powdered, non-mixed) injectable medications (such as rabies vaccines) are generally very stable outside stated storage temperatures.

Medicine stability information can be found in the SPC, which can be obtained at: ✒ http://www.medicines.org.uk/emc The SPC will also contain a manufacturer's helpline. Pharmaceutical manufacturers will often have extra information not normally found on the SPC.

Certain medications such as snake antivenom will degrade if stored outside specified temperatures. If refrigeration of these substances is impossible, use a medicine pack designed specifically to insulate medications against extremes of temperatures such as a vacuum flask. In environments where a considerable temperature gradient exists between night and day, the flask can be cooled at night and sealed during daylight hours. Minimize access to these medications during daylight hours to preserve low temperatures.

Medical kits are one of the most important parts of expedition equipment. However, without care and discipline they will soon deteriorate. There have been instances where vital medical kit has been found unusable in emergencies due to poor care and maintenance—an unacceptable scenario. Aim to keep the medical kit in the condition you would like to receive it.

Administration of medicines

See Box 3.1. For registered medical professionals, administration of medicines on expedition carries with it the same legal and professional accountability as it would in your country of registration. Non-medics can also be held accountable for the mis-use or mis-administration of medicines, and not having a professional qualification is no defence. The Royal College of Nursing and Royal Pharmaceutical Society *Professional Guidance on the Administration of Medicines in Healthcare Settings*[1] should be a benchmark for practice and adhered to as closely as possible.

1 ✒ https://www.rpharms.com/Portals/0/RPS%20document%20library/Open%20access/Professional%20standards/SSHM%20and%20Admin/Admin%20of%20Meds%20prof%20guidance.pdf?ver=2019-01-23-145026-567

Box 3.1 Before administering any medication, remember these three key points

Give the right drug
- Check the drug is correct drug (names are similar).
- Check it is for the right condition.
- Check it is in date.
- Check it is in good condition.

To the right person
- Check you have the right patient.
- Check they have no allergies.
- Check they are happy and have consented to receiving the drug.

At the right time
- Do they need this drug?
- Check the drug dosing interval.
- Check when it was last given.
- Check if they are taking other medication and if there are interaction risks.

Treating pain (analgesia)

Ensuring patients are free from pain or discomfort will help them rest. Patients in pain should have their pain score monitored regularly (➔ p. 194). Before administering analgesic drugs (Table 3.2), consider other ways of relieving discomfort:
- Temperature—ensure the patient is not too hot or cold.
- Control of nausea and vomiting.
- Fatigue.
- Psychological stress.
- Other symptoms.
- Current techniques of pain relief depend upon the use of increasingly potent treatments, used in combination until the patient is comfortable. A low dose of several different drugs is preferable to a high dose of just one.
- *Simple physical measures* such as padding, rubbing, supporting, or splinting may reduce discomfort. Heat or cold, depending upon the nature of the injury, can relieve swelling and discomfort.
- A *simple analgesic* such as paracetamol (acetaminophen) will be safe for most people.
- A *non-steroidal anti-inflammatory drug* (NSAID) such as ibuprofen or diclofenac can be given PO or PR and may be available as a skin rub. About 15% of the population cannot take NSAIDs.
- *Codeine* is a drug that works very well in some people, but leaves others feeling spaced out and dreadful.

For further details, see ♫ Chapter 19.

Anxiety and stress make pain worse both psychologically and because muscles tense around the affected part of the body. Small doses of muscle relaxants (diazepam) can help but must be used with extreme caution if the patient has received potent painkillers as respiratory depression or deep sedation may result.

Table 3.2 Analgesic ladder

		Route	Usual adult dose	Contra-indications	Cautions/side-effects
Physical measures	Pad, support, strap, splint, elevate				Ensure circulation not affected by swelling. Monitor capillary return & colour
	Cold (ice packs)	Skin	Useful for: bruises, sprains, burns		Avoid freezing skin or deep tissues
	Heat	Skin	Useful for aching pains		Avoid burns
Mild pain	Paracetamol Acetaminophen (US)	Oral/ Rectal/IV	1g 4 times daily	Allergy (rare) Liver disease, Alcoholics	
Moderate pain	Ibuprofen	Oral	400mg 3 times daily For short periods: 600mg 4 times daily (MAX)	Allergy Peptic symptoms	Stomach pain (take with food or milk if possible) Increased bruising
	Diclofenac	Rectal Skin rub IV(diluted)	50mgPO 3 times a day	Some asthmatics Bleeding tendency Anticoagulants Renal disease Heart disease	
Severe pain	Codeine	Oral, IV, IM	30–60mgs 6 times day Max 240mg/day	Allergy	Drowsiness Confusion Nausea Dizziness
	Tramadol	Oral, IV, IM	Titrate to pain relief, then: 50–100mg 4 hourly. Max 400mg/day.	Allergy	Drowsiness Confusion Nausea Dizziness
	Morphine	Oral, IV, IM	Titrate to pain relief then: 10mg 2 to 4 hrly	Allergy	Respiratory depression (monitor). Drowsiness, giddiness, nausea, vomiting, confusion.

Healthy expedition living

Organization of a healthy base camp

Clean water, good food, and a comfortable place to sleep are essential for a happy and healthy expedition. Tired and hungry people are significantly more prone to accidents and illness and caring for people in a well-organized, safe environment is much easier as 'any fool can be uncomfortable'. Expeditions can base themselves anywhere from luxury hotels to bivouacs under the stars. Whichever type of accommodation is used it should offer:

- Refuge from the elements.
- Security from personal attack or theft.
- Protection from the local fauna and flora.
- An acceptable level of comfort and privacy.

Camp location

When choosing the site for an expedition camp, consider:
- Weather and prevailing wind.
- Providing shelter from stormy weather.
- Avoiding areas prone to snow accumulation.
- Use of available shade and breeze in hot climates.
- Avoiding areas at risk of lightning strike.
- Floods:
  - Avoiding tidal regions and flood plains.
  - Dry riverbeds that may be liable to flash flooding.
  - Narrow valleys in areas of high rainfall.
- Dangers from falling rocks and mud slides, avalanche (snow/ice), dead trees and branches, or animal attacks.
- Animal hazards:
  - Not placing camp between animals and their watering holes.
  - Avoiding large animal mating and breeding areas.
  - Avoiding areas of insect infestation.
  - Avoiding routes of migration/travel.

Animal risks (particularly from snakes and insects) are more likely when clearing vegetation and setting up camp. Arachnids also make temporary homes under groundsheets and tents should be moved and shaken before being packed away.

Local permissions and environmental impact

Permissions may need to be obtained from the landowner.
- Avoid placing a campsite in an area that has religious or spiritual significance for the local people.
- Many cultures will readily offer supplies and hospitality even when this leaves them with shortages. Ensure that your presence does not deplete local resources such as water, firewood, food, or fuel when these are in short supply.
- Ensure that your campsites create no long-term ecological damage. (➔ p. 126).

Re-supply and casualty evacuation

Investigate the logistics of:

- Evacuating an injured casualty (➜ p. 160).
- Access to re-supplies of food, water, and fuel.
- Reliable communications with local agencies and emergency services, or others upon whom you may rely.

Campsite identification

In unfamiliar surroundings or poor weather conditions, it is easy to become disorientated, even within the vicinity of base camp. To reduce the risk of members getting lost, clearly mark out key areas such as:

- Camp entrances, exits, and boundaries.
- Latrines.
- Washing areas.
- Refuse areas.
- Communication facilities.
- Medical and first-aid facilities.
- Fire extinguishing equipment, fire exits and fire assembly points.

When constructing a camp, consider the layout in relation to those with an illness or injury. Once sign-posted, ask the following question: 'Could I find who or what I need, in an emergency, in the dark or in poor visibility?'

Food hygiene and safe practice

One of the greatest contributing factors to the success or failure of an expedition is the standard of the food. Success depends not only on the provision of a nourishing and varied diet, but also on the prevention of diet-related illness and disease, probably the biggest cause of diarrhoea in travellers abroad.

The kitchen

The position and construction of a kitchen will vary according to the type, size, budget, and location of the expedition. The gold standard for a big base camp, one could argue, should be to reproduce a commercial kitchen, with all the regulations required to pass a health and hygiene examination. Ideally the kitchen should be located at least 30 m away from areas of possible contamination such as latrines, wash areas, and equipment stores.

Catering personnel

Some teams will employ local people for this role, while others will use expedition members and may opt for a rota system of cooking, cleaning, and washing up. It is important that everyone on the team is clear about their roles and responsibilities.

Beware of illnesses in all members of the expedition team. This might include chronic illnesses carried by locally hired staff such as:
- Diarrhoea or other GI upsets.
- Helminth or protozoal infections.
- Carriers of chronic diseases (e.g. *Salmonella typhi* and TB).

Ensure that both catering and expedition teams clearly understand what is required regarding:
- Standards of hygiene and cleanliness within the kitchen.
- Regular handwashing with soap.
- Use of equipment.
- Disposal of kitchen refuse.

Basic kitchen rules
- If you are ill, do not go in the kitchen. Do not prepare food until at least 48 h have passed since last vomit or loose stool.
- Wash hands regularly.
- All cooking utensils should be washed, dried, and stored appropriately.

The kitchen should always be kept scrupulously clean
- Clean work surfaces after use.
- Clean storage areas daily and when required.
- Clean and dry equipment immediately after use (including the cleaning equipment itself).
- Restrict the kitchen area to those involved in food preparation.
- Look after the chef, and the chef will look after you.

Food preparation

GI upsets are the commonest illnesses to affect travellers. Minimize problems by ensuring that water is clean (➜ p. 108), and that food preparation is as hygienic as possible.

Do not share cutlery, bowls, and other eating or drinking utensils. Sharing is one of the fastest ways of spreading germs around camp.

After eating:
- All cooking and eating utensils should be washed, dried, and stored cleanly and away from possible interference by insects and animals.
- Try to use a two-bowl system for washing up: one for washing, the other to rinse.
- Try to avoid the use of tea towels, air drying is preferable.
- Surfaces should be wiped clean, if possible, with a disinfectant, to reduce the chances of bacteria/viral contamination.
- Floors should be cleaned of even the smallest crumbs of food.
- Hands should be washed, again.

Washing hands

- Done properly, handwashing is one of the most effective ways to prevent the spread of disease. Assume all expedition team members are insufficiently skilled and arrange a training session at the start of any expedition. Use the equipment and facilities likely to be encountered while away.
- Ensure you have sufficient clean water (ideally clean enough to drink but does not have to be sterile).
- Provide soap—solid (on a cord) or liquid—and a nail brush.

If using a bowl for handwashing:
- Wet hands by scooping water out of the bowl to one side.
- Apply soap and wash hands thoroughly for 20 seconds, paying attention to fingertips, web spaces, and nails.
- Rinse by scooping water out of the bowl, preventing any dirty soap and water from re-entering the bowl.
- Air dry hands or use paper towels that can be burned.
- Dispose of any unused water.

Avoid a line of expedition members taking turns to wash their hands *in* the bowl. This will render the water dirty after the first person, while creating a huge infection risk should one team member be unwell.

Key handwashing times
- Before preparing food.
- Before mealtimes.
- After work.
- Following the touching of animals.
- After using the latrines.
- When noticeably dirty or at any point where appropriate.

Alcohol gels
The use of alcohol gels on expedition should be discouraged unless there is no alternative. Evidence has shown that individuals rarely use enough, while its use may provide false reassurance as alcohol gels alone are ineffective at killing norovirus, for example.

Maintaining a healthy diet

Most expeditions involve considerable physical exercise. A balanced and varied expedition diet is essential to enable expedition members to maintain health, fitness, and morale.

Growing teenagers have a high metabolic rate and will have a considerably higher calorific requirement in even the most mundane expedition environment.

Calorific requirements

The basic daily calorific requirement for a 75 kg person doing little physical work is 1500–1700 kcal; additional energy requirements are dependent upon the work undertaken. Fast walking burns 600–700 kcal/h, and running uses around 850 kcal/h. The duration of a task must be considered; working at low intensity for several hours requires more energy than short bursts of high-intensity exercise. The more food that is carried, the more energy is burnt in carrying food. Climbing carrying loads and hauling sledges are among the most energetic activities known, with around 10,000 kcal/day expended. On short expeditions, deficits in energy balance can be tolerated healthily; this is not the case on longer expeditions. Highly trained individuals can endure persistent energy deficits but at a cost of up to one-third of their lean body weight, and gradual decline in physical capabilities.[2]

Dietary components

Dietary balance

Individuals tolerate novel food to different degrees but providing the same menu each day will also discourage healthy eating. Simple sauces or condiments can make basic food more interesting. Fresh fruit and vegetables are always welcome but are difficult to preserve without refrigeration. Additional calorie intake is less important in the short term than the quality of nutrition and the distribution of nutrients (Table 3.3).

2 Stroud M. *Survival of the Fittest: The Anatomy of Peak Physical Performance*. London: Vintage; 2010.

Table 3.3 Food types: pros and cons

Food type	Advantages	Disadvantages
Prepared food, e.g. sandwiches	Pleasing to the palate	Requires prior preparation Not practical on longer expeditions Short shelf life
Tinned produce	Very long shelf life High liquid content Can be eaten cold	Bulky and heavy Non-biodegradable waste product
Local produce	May be readily available Part of cultural experience of travel	Risk of infections and gastroenteritis Longer preparation time
Dried produce, e.g. pasta and sauce	Pleasing to the palate	Time-consuming Requires large amount of fuel to prepare Bulky compared to finished product
'Boil in the bag' or MRE (meal ready to eat)	Easy to prepare Can taste good Long shelf life Can be cooked in dirty water or even eaten cold Requires no pan washing	Expensive Limited choice of meals Lower energy density than dried products
Dehydrated meals	Some can be made with hot water added to bag and not prepared on a stove Energy dense	Others require cooking over stove for 6–8 min Uses significant amounts of water
Powdered synthetic foods, e.g. sports drinks	Easy to prepare, no cooking utensils required Energy-dense (several thousand kcal can be carried in <1 kg)	Taste Unbalanced diet, lack of fibre

Water purification

A safe water supply is essential. Adults in temperate conditions need to drink about 3 L a day, but in very hot climates an individual can lose up to 15 L of fluid a day. If walking all day in the desert, up to 10 L of water may need to be carried per individual. A further 4 L of clean water per person per day will be needed for cooking and washing up. Sufficient safe water must be provided both at base camp and for use by field parties. Often water from taps and wells, as well as that from rivers, lakes, and ponds, can be contaminated. Spring water, i.e. clear 'pristine water collected away from human habitation', may be safer, but it is still sensible to treat it.

Water must be treated:

- To remove silt.
- To remove harmful organic matter and other pollutants.
- To kill all forms of organism.

Sediment must be removed initially if sterilization procedures are to be effective. Removing silt can pose considerable problems if you are trying to obtain supplies for a large expedition, and sedimentation tanks may be required. If the expedition is close to mines or factories, chemical pollution must be foreseen, and appropriate filtration methods used.

Some methods of water purification are more suitable for base camp and others for field workers (➔ p. 108). Before choosing a system, consider the likely infective organisms and the risk posed by them.

Transmission of disease by water

Organisms such as bacteria, viruses, protozoa, and other parasites (including schistosomes, guinea worm larvae, and leeches) can transmit infections. Two types of organisms contracted through drinking surface waters which are of particular concern are *Giardia* and *Cryptosporidium*; their characteristics are summarized in Table 3.4. It is important to consider methods of disinfecting water to the full range of potential organism.

Table 3.4 Treating water infected by *Giardia lamblia* or *Cryptosporidium* spp.

	Transmission	Symptoms	Treatment	Water treatment
Giardia lamblia	Consumption of contaminated food/water Cysts deposited in water/food and reinfection. Only low numbers of cysts required to cause infection Human and animals (domestic and wild) can be hosts	1–4 weeks' incubation Malabsorption of food Frothy foul-melling diarrhoea Abdominal discomfort, flatulence, and bloating Symptoms last 1–2 weeks Sometimes chronic disease with malabsorption	Antiparasitic: metro-nidazole, tinidazole, albendazole	Filtration methods High doses of chemical agents with long contact times
Cryptosporidium spp.	Usually waterborne through humans or livestock Spores can remain dormant in soil for many years. Low numbers of cysts don't always result in infection	2–14 days' incubation Profuse watery diarrhoea Abdominal pain, low-grade fever, cramps Symptoms last for 7 days May relapse after 14 days Dangerous for those with impaired immune systems and elderly	No specific treatment Aggressive rehydration	Filtration methods Chlorine not effective Chlorine dioxide claimed to be effective

Camp water purification arrangements

Providing enough treated water from a natural source for a camp of 20 people is time-consuming, but exceedingly important. The best approach is to incorporate a strict regimen from the start by appointing one person as 'water chief' to supervise the sterilization, safe storage, and use of the water. The appointed person should also make sure that every member of the expedition can sterilize his or her own drinking water effectively.

Rigid plastic containers with a tap and handle are the best for water. These come in 10 or 25 L sizes, but the larger size container is heavy when full of water so keep in mind distances to water source and terrain. If you do not have a method of removing the taste of chemicals, water will taste better when cold. Storing water in special canvas bags will keep it cool through evaporation from the small pores of the canvas. If they can be obtained, army surplus bags are excellent and come in sizes suitable for storage of large volumes in camp or for tying to the back of a vehicle.

Water treatment could be split into sessions if it is necessary to reduce the number of containers in use. To avoid confusion, have a good system of marking containers for the three different types of water treatment:
- Untreated for storage, sedimentation, or settling process.
- Strained ready for treatment.
- Fit for drinking.

Each field party member should also carry personal equipment for sterilizing water; metal cups are preferable to plastic as the latter often break.

If travelling by vehicle, do not use one large container for storing water; a single puncture may have disastrous consequences. Jerry cans or the canvas bags as described above are the best option but try to adopt the same system of markings as employed in base camp.

Removal of sediment and organic matter

If water is cloudy or contains suspended matter, it must be cleared before further treatment.

Settling tanks

Cloudy water can be left to stand for some hours for solids to settle, either in a jerry can or in sedimentation tanks depending on the volume to be treated. Very fine particles, such as 'rock flour' in glacial outflow and mica flakes, are GI irritants and must be removed by a ceramic filter. Simply clearing water does not sterilize it and further treatment will be needed before it may be drunk.

Fabric pre-filters

A convenient method for removing sediment in relatively small volumes is to pass the water through a tightly woven cloth material. Useful for this is the Millbank bag, which is a sock-shaped bag woven so that solids are retained but water flows by gravity through the weave.

Coagulation–flocculation

Small amounts of certain chemicals can be added to cause an aggregation of particles which will sink to the bottom of the container. The flocculate is then strained off through a tightly woven cloth or Millbank bag. A potential advantage is that larger organisms such as *Giardia* or *Cryptosporidium* are removed by this technique, although it is not as reliable as an appropriate mechanical filter. The most easily obtained chemical is alum, of which about an eighth of a teaspoonful is added to 4 L of water, more if it remains cloudy. The water is then stirred for 5 min and allowed to settle for 30 min. A newer system, developed by Procter & Gamble, consists of sachets containing chemical disinfectant and substances that cause flocculation of particles. This has been very effective in field trials and may also be useful against *Cryptosporidium*. The product goes under the name of Purifier of Water™ and each sachet treats 10 L of water.

Methods of water disinfection

These are presented in Fig. 3.2 with notes on use and indicating situations where they are most useful.

Boiling

This is undoubtedly the best method but is often inconvenient and wasteful of fuel supplies or natural resources. Water should be kept boiling continuously for 5 min, which is sufficient at any altitude, although some experts state that 1 min is adequate. The water should be covered when cooling to prevent recontamination.

Chemicals

Chlorine is the most commonly used chemical and commercial tablets for treating a range of volumes of water are widely available. The effectiveness of chlorine is reduced by several factors that may not be easy to control, such as alkaline water, very cold water, or the presence of organic matter—hence the need for prior filtering. Treated water should be left for at least half an hour before drinking and longer if it is very cold. As it is less effective in removing parasitic cysts (*Giardia*, amoebic cysts, and *Cryptosporidium*) these could be removed by pre-filtering through a simple coffee filter paper, or an efficient sedimentation/flocculation method. Adding ascorbic acid or sodium thiosulphate can improve the taste but will inactivate the chlorine, so it should be added by individuals only at the time the water is drunk and never be added to a storage receptacle such as a canteen or jerry can. Chlorine in water will tend to lose efficacy after 24 h so is not so useful for long-term storage, unless retreated regularly.

Chlorine dioxide is one of the most popular chemical methods for sterilizing water among wilderness travellers but is more expensive than chlorine tablets. Several commercial products are available but tablets can only treat relatively small volumes for personal use.

Chloramination (chloramine T) is sometimes used to treat large volumes of water and prevents recontamination. However, it must be left for many hours to be effective, and some safety concerns have been raised in recent years.

Katadyn silver, available as tablets and granules, is only effective against bacteria. It does not impart a bad taste and it is claimed to be able to prevent recontamination of water by bacteria for many months. It should not be added to water previously treated with chlorine or iodine.

Iodine has been a popular choice of chemical for water purification for wilderness travellers for many years, being more tolerant to the presence of organic matter than is chlorine, but due to European Union (EU) biocide regulations unavailable in the EU/UK.

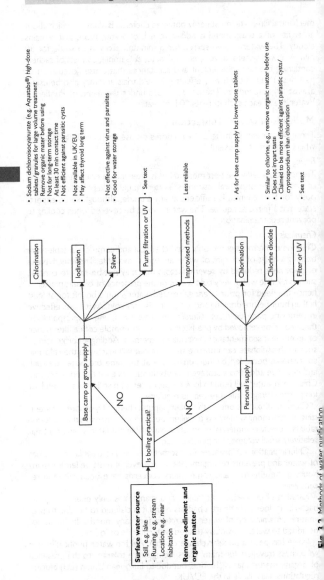

Surface water source
- Still, e.g. lake
- Running, e.g. stream
- Location, e.g. near habitation

Remove sediment and organic matter

Is boiling practical?

NO

Base camp or group supply

NO

Personal supply

Chlorination
- Sodium dichloroisocyanurate (e.g. Aquatabs®) high-dose tablets/granules for large volume treatment
- Remove organic matter before using
- Not for long-term storage
- At least 30 min contact time
- Not efficient against parasitic cysts

Iodination
- Not available in UK/EU
- May affect thyroid long term

Silver
- Not effective against virus and parasites
- Good for water storage

Pump filtration or UV
- See text

Improvised methods
- Less reliable

Chlorination
- As for base camp supply but lower-dose tablets

Chlorine dioxide
- Similar to chlorine, e.g., remove organic matter before use
- Does not impart taste
- Claimed to be more efficient against parasitic cysts/cryptosporidium than chlorination

Filter or UV
- See text

Fig. 3.2 Methods of water purification

Less reliable methods

There are several methods that can be employed when the previously mentioned disinfection methods are not available. These include improvising a sand and/or charcoal filter or filtering through very tightly woven material. For a full description see Küpper et al. (2012).[3]

Water filter and ultraviolet (UV) treatment

Water filters are one of the easiest systems to purify water with the highest water clearance rate. For personal use (<1 L), the principles are very similar between the various types in that contaminated water can be passed through the filter which removes some of the pathogenic material and chemicals.

The main variance between the filters is their composition which affects the ability of what can be removed and establishes the effectiveness of the filter. Filters containing carbon, silica, and alumina such as AquaPure® and Water to Go® remove viruses, bacteria, and protozoa from water sources. Filters containing hollow fibres/micro tubes (Life Straw®, Sawyer®) are only able to remove bacteria and protozoa. The efficiency of the removal is measured by reference to the international standards of the US Environmental Protection Agency (EPA). These standards express the minimum removal of viruses to be 99.99 % (log coefficient 4), bacteria 99.9999% (log coefficient 6), and protozoa 99.9% (log coefficient 3). Therefore, in the selection and choice of personal water filter systems, the advertising should be checked that these standards are met or exceeded. Note also that many do not remove viruses and hepatitis A might be of the most concern, emphasizing the importance of hepatitis A immunization for wilderness travel.

Potential filtration systems for larger groups at base camps are pump-based filters, gravity-fed filters, and UV systems. The simplest to use is a gravity-fed system (Katadyn Base Camp Pro®, Platypus® GravityWorks™) which can be suspended from a tree and gravity allowed to push the water through the in-built filter. Filters can last for up to 1500 L.

Pump action filters (e.g. MSR SweetWater®) can be purchased with filters which are small enough to remove viruses. These are efficient, but require a lot of pumping to produce even a small amount of water. UV systems are reliant on the water being clear before purification and therefore often require an additional method of filtration. Therefore, to produce large volumes of clean water, the gravity-fed systems are the primary choice.

See Tables 3.5 and 3.6 for comparisons.

See also ℘ Fluids and electrolytes p. 804, and ℘ Diarrhoea and vomiting, p. 420.

3 ℘ https://www.theuiaa.org/documents/mountainmedicine/English_UIAA_MedCom_Rec_No_6_Water_Disinfection_2012_V3-1.pdf

Table 3.5 Comparison of personal use water filters

Type of filter	Mechanically advanced disinfection	Carbon, silica	Hollow fibre
Example	AquaPure®	Water To Go®	Life Straw®
Provides reduction of:			
Viruses	Yes	No*	No
Bacteria	Yes	Yes	Yes
Protozoa	Yes	Yes	Yes
Tested to EPA standards at LSHTM	Yes	Yes	No

* This standard is only met after the filter has been primed. LSHTM, London School of Hygiene & Tropical Medicine.

Table 3.6 Comparison of high-volume water filters

Type of system	Gravity fed	Pump based	Ultraviolet
Example	Katadyn Base Camp Pro®	MSR SweetWater®	Steripen Aqua®
Provides reduction of:			
Viruses	No	No	Yes
Bacteria	Yes	Yes	Yes
Protozoa	Yes	Yes	Yes
Change of filter/ equipment	1500 L	750 L	3000 L per lamp 50 L per battery set
Flow rate of clean water	2 L/min	1 L/min	0.5 L/min

Sanitation and latrines

The health and hygiene surrounding the waste that we generate is as important to the prevention of illness as are the standards of cleanliness we apply to the preparation and consumption of food.

The management of waste on an expedition is a balancing act between factors such as location, available facilities, and personal adherence to standards or procedures, with an overall aim to minimize ecological and environmental impact.[4]

Latrines

The disposal of human waste on expedition can be separated into its two forms:

Urine disposal

Unless infection is present, urine is sterile and therefore provides less of a problem in its disposal. However, large quantities of urine can smell offensive in a short space of time and affect fragile ecosystems.

When siting a urinal:
- Choose an area 50–100 m from the camp.
- Make sure it is downstream of any water collection point.
- Avoid caves or other areas where urine will remain stagnant.
- Avoid rocks or gravel, where urine lingers.
- Clearly mark the path to the urinal and the urinal itself.
- Re-site the urinal on a regular basis to avoid large collections of urine.

Latrine placement

The latrines must be far enough from camp to pose no infection or contamination risk, yet close enough to be used with convenience. Thus:
- Place it 100 m from the camp.
- Place it 100 m from any lakes, rivers, or streams:
  - Look for high water marks.
  - Consider local water tables.
- Consider water run-off channels in the event of:
  - Heavy rain.
  - Flash floods.
- Consider hazards posed by fauna and flora—especially at night.
- Use a flag or other system to notify others when it is in use.
- Identify latrine boundaries clearly.
- Ensure that everyone is familiar with latrine etiquette.

Other human waste disposal options

Burying

This is only an option in environments where there is enough bacterial activity within the soil. Bacterial activity normally occurs only within the first 20 cm of topsoil, therefore only a shallow scrape is required.

When re-filling the scrape, use a stick to 'stir' in faeces, ensuring greater contact with soil enzymes, and then cover over with topsoil.

Group latrines should consist of a long trench, approximately 15 cm wide and 20 cm deep.

When the first trench is filled in, site another one. Mark the previously used trench.

4 Meyer K. How to Shit in the Woods, 4th ed. Berkeley, CA: Ten Speed Press; 2020.

Treating/sterilizing
Chemically treating faecal waste on expedition is a complicated process. It can be costly and requires equipment and proper faecal storage facilities.

In strictly limited circumstances where expeditions find themselves in remote locations away from human or animal populations, it is possible to use the sun's UV rays to break down faecal matter with a method known as 'frosting a rock' or 'icing a cake'.

Carrying out
• The last method requires a suitable container which should be either disposable or reusable (and therefore cleanable), durable, portable, an appropriate size for expedition length, and size of the expedition population.
• There should be a definitive plan regarding final disposal of effluent. 'Carrying out' is sometimes used for forward camps in ecologically sensitive environments. On return to a base camp in a more hospitable environment, the waste can be disposed of appropriately.

Sanitary towels/tampons and toilet paper
These should never be buried as they do not biodegrade effectively in the wild. Store them with used toilet paper, then burn at the end of the day or carry out to dispose of after the expedition.

For alternatives to sanitary towels/tampons, see ➲ p. 433.

Ethics and professional responsibilities

Chapter editor
Shane Winser

Contributors
Jim Bond
Rebecca Harris
Amy Hughes
Nick Lewis
James Moore

Ethics of expeditions

The importance of ethical considerations and behaviour on an expedition cannot be overstated. Despite its achievements—be they adventurous goals or scientific discoveries—it is often how an expedition is approached or conducted which leaves the most lasting impression.

Each of us should be individually guided by a conscience and a sense of social, cultural, and environmental responsibility.

There are, however, at least four other sets of ethical standards operating on an expedition:

- The personal ethics of other individuals.
- Group ethics that the team adopts, deliberately or subconsciously.
- The religious beliefs, values, and cultural customs of the people in whose territory you are journeying.
- Universal human rights.

Principles

The 'four principles plus scope' model of biomedical ethics[1] is a recognized framework that helps make some of these standards explicit—and defendable. It should be familiar to most recent medical graduates and can, if thought through, be applied to almost any situation.

The 'four principles' of ethical debate and behaviour

1. *Autonomy*: the right to individual self-determination.
2. *Beneficence*: the doing of good.
3. *Non-maleficence*: the avoidance of doing harm.
4. *Respect for Justice*: equity, fairness, etc.

Note: there is no hierarchy to the 'four principles'. They simply form a 'checklist' for assessing the ethical dimensions of a decision or dilemma.

The task of the responsible person is to consider a question from each perspective, and then to make a judgement on balance.

What do the four principles mean in practice (and in plain English)?

Autonomy (A)

Autonomy involves respecting an individual's right to choose or refuse to do something. Respect for the autonomy of others carries with it the moral obligation to maintain (appropriate) confidentiality, to keep one's promises, not to deceive, and, by extension, to communicate with clarity.

Beneficence (B) and non-maleficence (N)

Beneficence ('doing good') and non-maleficence ('not doing harm') are complementary obligations. Examples include ensuring that all team members, including the expedition medic, have adequate training and experience for what they would reasonably be expected to do in the field.

1 Gillon R. Medical ethics: four principles plus attention to scope'. *BMJ*. 1994;309:184.

Justice (J)

Respect for *justice* is the moral obligation to act on the basis of fair adjudication between competing claims. This can be to do with:

- The fair distribution of scarce resources (distributive justice).
- Respect for different peoples' rights (rights-based justice).
- Respect for morally acceptable laws (legal justice).

Empowerment, whether of individuals or local communities, can be seen as an overlap of all four principles (A, B, N, and J). Arguably, it is a core function of any expedition.

Scope

When applying the 'four principles', you also need to determine the boundaries within which your ethical question lies. One rule of thumb for expeditions is to consider all people directly affected by the expedition's presence. For environmental impacts, the scope may need to be much wider.

There are often no easy or right answers for what constitutes ethical practice. Part of the fun of an expedition is the new and unexpected challenges that make you think about, or rethink, your position. Acknowledge your mistakes, apologize if you have got it wrong and learn from them.

> The remainder of this chapter includes several examples relevant on expeditions, with the appropriate A, B, N, or J annotation used as previously described.

Cultural sensitivity

Respecting and being observant to the cultures of the expedition team and the community the team will be engaging with, and the individuals within the team, is fundamentally important.

Any situation where a mixed group of people is working together under arduous conditions has some potential for a cultural clash. Cultural miscommunication, leading to loss of mutual respect and trust, may be exacerbated by:

- A history of colonialism in either the host or guest peoples.
- Apartness (or *apartheid*), in eating, sleeping, travelling, or other living arrangements. (N)
- Inappropriate behaviour including arrogance, inappropriate dress, or failure to respect local customs or religious codes. (N)
- Imparting your own, or your team's, opinions and beliefs on a community (or each other) in a disrespectful or forceful manner. (N)

The hazards of such situations can be minimized by effective communication including:

- Awareness that you are operating in a different cultural norm. (A)
- Good translation skills that, for instance, make implicit meanings explicit. (A)
- Good listening skills, including non-verbal communication. (A)
- Serious efforts to understand socially and culturally determined references and attitudes. (A, B)
- Openness, honesty, good humour, and inclusiveness at all times. (B)

- Appropriate behaviour: especially the avoidance of drugs, alcohol, and sexual licentiousness. (N)
- Personal values: such as humility, respect for differing beliefs, taboos, and strong work ethic. (B)

Personal and professional clashes

Even with the best of intentions and a shared common purpose, people do not always get on well with each other during expeditions. Hardships and physical challenges, close working conditions, and interdependency may turn minor irritations into resentments, and lead to arguments. If everyone on the team has a clear role to play, it may be easier to respect each other's contribution, while accepting joint responsibility for helping out in any way possible when things are not going well.

Causes of interpersonal disharmony

- Poor communication: both expressive and receptive.
- Unrealistic or mismatched expectations: which may in themselves be a result of poor communication.
- Conflict based on pre-conceived ideas/notions surrounding professional hierarchies and relationships.
- Personal clashes sometimes masquerade as professional clashes and vice versa.

Leadership styles vary, and people respond in different ways to the same style. Usually, inclusive leadership styles in which problems are talked through in groups are more likely to lead to effective understanding and solution of problems.

Regular group meetings to discuss progress and effective debriefing after activities can help bridge gaps. Such meetings should ensure that everyone continues to support the goals of the expedition and feels that risks are being minimized in the most effective manner.

Regardless of any personal views, the medic should try to remain removed from interpersonal conflicts so that everyone on the expedition remains able to communicate their concerns and worries, confident that they will be listened to sympathetically. (B)

Preventing interpersonal disharmony

- *Before setting off:* choose your team carefully. Consider team-building exercises, e.g. imaginary worst-case scenarios. (B) Ensure there are clear and unambiguous leadership roles—especially within the medical and leadership team.
- *Ensure there is clarity and harmony over aims, objectives, and expectations of the expedition.* (S)
- *At the start:* establish ground rules, e.g. no criticism of people behind their backs (N); respect for personal space. (B) Acknowledge the potential for falling(s) out and identify beforehand clear ways to air grievances and resolve disputes. (B, J)
- *During:* aim to build on shared group values and develop a sense of group responsibility. (B) Communicate with each other; no one should be expected to carry all the weight of their individual role alone. Mix up the group socially to avoid cliques.

- *In a crisis:* depending on the anticipated hazards of the expedition, you may ultimately need to have a formal chain of command. This should be pre-agreed, and understood from the outset.
- *After:* be self-critical and prepared to learn from your mistakes for next time.

Management of disputes

Although the management of disharmony should ideally be a group responsibility, it often falls on the leader or the expedition medic (respecting each individual's right to confidentiality) to sort such conflicts out. Allowing everyone to have their say is important; however, 'time-out' may need to be called first before a resolution is attempted.

In some instances, it may be useful to use an arbitrator external to the expedition, perhaps via satellite phone, who can make the final decision, redirecting conflict away from the clinician or leadership team.

Interacting with local communities

Understanding the life of those who live in the areas visited by an expedition can be very rewarding, and some researchers (e.g. ethnobotanists) rely almost exclusively for their data on what they can learn from working with local guides and their communities.

General approach

The wisdom of being open, honest, warm-hearted, and respectful in all your dealings cannot be overstressed. All people hate it if they think you are trying to deceive them. Local customs and hierarchy should be observed. For example:

- Avoid arriving at a village at daybreak. (N)
- Wait to be properly introduced and accepted by the headman and elders. (B, N)
- Seek permission before taking any photos. (N)
- Listen and learn. Local people can be a fount of knowledge to keep you safe and well. Local practices/customs are often there for a reason.

Put yourselves in their position:

- How would you wish to be treated by a group of wealthy foreign visitors who decide to come and spend some time in your community? Would you wish to be ignored, kept at a polite distance, or invited into their camp?
- How would you respond to their curiosity about your way of life?
- Would you prefer them to have at least mastered a few basic civilities in your language, such as greetings, 'thank you', 'delicious', etc.?
- How would you feel if they were overpaying staff and upsetting the economy of the village?

Hospitality is very important to most societies and is never to be rebuffed or abused. It should always be met with grace and gratitude.

Treating local people not part of the expedition

In many parts of the world, expeditions are perceived by local people to be rich and endowed with clinical skills and drugs. The apparently universal human desire to take medication may be stimulated by the arrival of the expedition, and the slightest hint that you will treat people in the local community may lead to a queue of 'ill' people outside the medic's tent. It is tempting to try to 'help' and to establish goodwill by offering medicines to all but, before you do, consider the potential harm:

- You may not understand local people's health problems and therefore misdiagnose. (N)
- You may endanger your own expedition members by using drugs intended for them. (N)
- You may be blamed unreasonably for adverse outcomes. (N)
- You may offend local healers (and other health services). (N)
- Treatment may be incomplete and thus ineffective or harmful. (N)
- You might be exploited for your novelty value.
- You may not be able to follow up treatment.
- You may encourage expectations among local people that the local medical services cannot meet. (N)

Nevertheless, sometimes you cannot, *and should not*, avoid doing what you can to help other people. If you have appropriate time and facilities, it could appear churlish not to see and examine anyone who presents, if only to re-assure yourself and others whether it is a genuine emergency. (B)

Ethically, as a trained medic or doctor, you have an obligation to act as a 'Good Samaritan' in situations where there is an acute emergency. When setting off to work in very remote communities, it is therefore worth budgeting a little extra for such scenarios when preparing the medical kit. (B)

Local people, particularly children, who are severely ill or injured, should be treated—but not necessarily by you; try to evacuate these patients if possible. Your authority may help to achieve this.

As the expedition medic, you should not treat chronic disease. You will not have the resources or the time, and it will be better for everyone if pa-tients are treated by the local health service. (N)

You also have an ethical duty to empower people, i.e. to manage their own illness, wherever possible, and to strengthen, rather than undermine, existing healthcare systems, including traditional healers (Box 4.1). (A, B, N, J)

Examples of emergency situations encountered on expeditions in Madagascar
- A villager with cerebral malaria.
- An infant of a nomadic, forest people, with a severe chest infection.
- A fisherman, stung by a stonefish, who had a necrotic dorsum of foot, requiring surgical debridement and antibiotics, to help it heal.

What if things go wrong?

As medical practitioners, we should be used to taking appropriate risks for our patients, *with their full and informed consent* (see: ℘ https://www.gmc-uk.org/). Good communication is thus paramount, particularly when warning of possible adverse effects. (A) Know and admit your limita-tions; don't attempt heroic procedures when you're out of your depth. (N) A useful maxim is 'always treat each patient as you would if they were a member of your own family'.

Public, national, and international health

Occasionally, it may be clear that the whole population of a village or sur-rounding area could potentially benefit from an intervention to address a common threat to health, e.g. dirty water, malaria, trachoma. (B)

Public health interventions, working with a local population, can appear seductively simple, but should not be undertaken lightly. They require a good deal of sensitive groundwork to work well. An ongoing project in the same area has many advantages over a 'one-off' expedition, by being able to build up trust and demonstrating commitment. It may be more empowering and effective in the long term to sow the seed of an idea, ra-ther than to raise false expectations. You should also feedback any relevant findings to key, local public health providers.

In the light of the recent COVID-19 pandemic, expeditions also have an obligation to consider the potential risks of contributing to the import of illness ranging from vaccine preventable disease through to public health emergencies of international concern.

Working with local healthcare providers

The nature of some expeditions may bring them into contact with local healthcare providers, including indigenous healers who provide roughly 80% of the medical services used worldwide.[2] Beyond their wealth of local knowledge, trained and untrained healthcare providers usually have a strong sense of clinical duty towards their constituency and a great deal of influence. This is an often-overlooked potential resource, particularly in public health (see case study in Box 4.1).

As an expedition medic, working in the territory of local healthcare providers, one might anticipate that you could be viewed as competition, or worse, a threat. This should not put you off going the extra mile to seek out and pay one's respects to a fellow healthcare professional. (B) You might be surprised at the reception and level of cooperation you subsequently receive for showing this simple courtesy.

The Tropical Health and Education Trust (THET) has eight 'Principles of Partnership'[3] which are widely acknowledged as forming the bedrock of any healthcare collaboration.

1. Strategic.
2. Harmonized and aligned.
3. Effective and sustainable.
4. Respectful and reciprocal.
5. Organized and accountable.
6. Responsible.
7. Flexible, resourceful, and innovative.
8. Committed to joint learning.

Box 4.1 Community-led TB treatment in SW Madagascar

Case study: Project Renala

On an ethnobotanical research project, working with the Mikea, an elusive, forest people, the expedition doctor/botanist was approached by local healers to advise on how to deal with an outbreak of TB, which was affecting their (apparently TB-naïve) population. Because of cultural differences, a nearby mission's TB programme was finding it hard to reach the Mikea people effectively in their forest home.

Over the next few years, the project helped to bridge the gap between the two healthcare systems, by providing backup and training. A special, fully ambulatory TB treatment regimen/arrangement for the Mikea was worked out with traditional healers and other notables taking full responsibility for initial case detection, and treatment supervision in the forest, and the mission's healthcare workers confirming diagnoses and managing any complications.

In this way, a responsible directly observed therapy, short-course (DOTS)-TB treatment programme was extended to include the Mikea on their terms, but without compromising their semi-nomadic, hunter-gatherer lifestyle, and without undermining the authority or undervaluing the clinical acumen of either set of healers. (A, B, N, J)

2 WHO. *Traditional Medicine. Fact Sheet No. 134.* Geneva: World Health Organization; 2008.

3 THET. *Principles of Partnership.* ℞ https://www.thet.org/principles-of-partnership/

Environmental impact

Environmental management requires you to analyse and then minimize, whenever possible, the consequences of an expedition's activities. Larger expeditions inevitably have a greater environmental impact as a result of increases in:

- Transportation requirements.
- Quantities of supplies to be transported.
- Need for local staff.
- Requirement for local supplies, including food, water, fuel, etc.
- Amount of waste and sewage produced.

Economic effects can be complex and are largely dependent upon how much money an expedition spends locally.

Assessing an expedition's environmental footprint

Ideally, each group should appoint an environmental manager, whose responsibilities should include:

- Researching the environmental requirements of the host country.
- Ensuring that these are considered during permit and grant applications.
- Looking into the specific environmental impacts of the expedition, such as path erosion, environmentally sensitive areas, problems from existing waste accumulation, social and economic impacts on local communities, etc. (N)

The environmental manager should work closely with the other members of the expedition to consider:

- Transport options to and from the destination: can public transport be used? (N)
- Accommodation options: do the hotels or guesthouses subscribe to a reputable environmental initiative?
- Local employment cooperatives: will the expedition's employees get a fair deal? (B, N, J)
- Expedition support agencies (guides, trekking companies, boat charters): what is their environmental policy?
- Local vendors: where will local supplies come from? What is the impact on the local community?
- Waste management procedures during the expedition, including the packaging on food and equipment, the type of waste handling structures available in the expedition area, and any documentation required for waste disposal in the country. (N)

Everything should be considered from the point of view of reducing the amount of unnecessary resources that the expedition will use. Good use of locally provided, sustainable resources can also benefit the local economy. (B)

Making an environmental mitigation plan

An environmental plan needs to be drawn up to explain how the impacts already highlighted will be mitigated. The environmental plan should include the following:

- The expedition's environmental statement. Say what it is you are trying to achieve from an environmental point of view.

- A summary of the environmental problems that may already be present in the area.
- The impacts that will be generated by you.
- How you will mitigate them, listing the different responsibilities.
- The waste management options available to you.
- What environmental permits or applications are required to visit your chosen area.
- Your arrangements for local employment: you need to work with any local expedition employees (e.g. cooks and porters) sympathetically and diplomatically about the importance of avoiding environmental damage. For example, use wood fires as little as possible, as deforestation is a serious problem in many expedition areas. Supply fuel-efficient stoves and encourage their use. (B, N, J)
- Any reporting requirements upon completion of the expedition.

The plan should be succinct and easy-to-understand.

Working with other expeditions

The same basic rules about ethical conduct apply when interacting with other expeditions; for instance, avoid negative criticism of another expedition's methods or style. (N)

In the field, your expedition will inevitably be scrutinized and compared with others by local people. Overt displays of friendliness towards another group, e.g. of the same mother tongue/nationality as your own, that is *different from your interactions with local people*, will not go unnoticed.

Expeditions are not competitions. If you hear, in advance, that another expedition is planning something similar, or might coincide with yours, the 'right' thing to do is to take the initiative and start talking things over with them. You might find that the ground you are each planning to cover is actually somewhat different, or even complementary, from a research perspective. Aside from the possibility of sharing data, there may be the opportunity to pool certain resources, such as medical expertise or use of a satellite phone for medevac. For obvious reasons, this kind of arrangement is preferably discussed in advance.

If another expedition has already set up camp at the site you had intended to use, normal etiquette would be for your, second, group to find another suitable location at a comfortable distance, if possible. Establishing good relations should be a priority, once *local* formalities have been completed.

Your interaction with other expeditions visiting the area may continue long after the expedition is over. Keep in contact, learn from each other's successes and mistakes, never misrepresent others' efforts, and share your expedition findings. (B, N)

Care of local staff

Duty of care

An expedition's 'duty of care' extends to all participants. (J) A participant should be defined as *'anyone who would not be in a given situation if it were not for the expedition'*, for instance: local drivers, porters, guides, and cooks. (N, S) Factors that should be considered include:

- The basic essentials of life: are your local staff appropriately fed, watered, clothed, shod, and sheltered at night? (N, J)
- The right to be consulted, and to say no. (A)
- Fair recompense for any work carried out, or extra risks taken. (B) Payments should be commensurate with local wages and costs, so as not to distort the local economy. (N, J)
- Health and safety:
  - Is there enough basic protective gear such as life jackets and helmets to go round, and does everyone know how to use them? (B)
  - Are some participants expected to take greater risks than others; e.g. local people riding in the back of a pick-up truck, while expats sit inside (with seat belts)? (N)
  - Are your local team members as well protected against significant medical risks (e.g. rabies) as you are? (B, N, J)
- Access to appropriate medical attention: standards of medical care for everyone on the expedition should be similar. This does not necessarily mean expatriation for treatment of serious injury or illness but could well entail having to arrange casualty evacuation for local personnel to appropriate in-country medical facilities. (J)
- Respect for home and family life. Setting off at a certain time may mean someone can't milk their goats and instead has to arrange for someone else to do it. (A, N)
- Respect for feast or fasting days, providing time to pray. (A)
- Long-term consequences for local participants:
  - Are you empowering them? (A, B, N, J)
  - Is anything you're asking them to do (e.g. to translate) likely to compromise their social standing in the community? (N)

Good practice

Duty of care, whether moral or legal, is only a minimal requirement. Good practice, enabling you and your team to get the most out of the expedition, demands a lot more.

When an expedition is embedded within an isolated community for an extended period, the boundaries between expedition participants, their dependents, and the rest of the local population may become rather blurred at times. (S) The limits to this need to be defined as the expedition may find that large numbers of people become dependent upon it and potentially a huge drain on resources.

Clinical competence

As in other areas of professional practice, there is pressure to improve the defined clinical competencies of those providing medical support to expeditions. Individual clinicians have a responsibility—both professional and ethical—to ensure they are capable of providing appropriate medical expertise in an autonomous, decision-making situation far removed from the support systems present at home.[4]

Patients must be able to trust doctors with their lives and health. To justify that trust you must show respect for human life and make sure your practice meets the standards expected of you in each of four domains (Box 4.2):

As a sole or lead clinician you may find yourself dealing with a serious clinical or logistical problem, without recourse to senior support, with few or no diagnostic adjuncts to aid decision-making, which is further complicated by hostile environmental conditions. This is a level of responsibility and stress often not anticipated in the initial excitement of joining an expedition.

Medics should ensure they are appropriately qualified for the anticipated role, and have completed appropriate training. (B, N) Hosting organizations and distant advisers should be aware of the level of medical expertise able to be provided by the clinician, and expedition members need to know what sort of medical support they can expect while abroad, both from staff on the expedition and from the local medical services.

Hosting organizations and expedition doctors may not agree entirely with each other on the priorities of what should and should not be included in the group kit, or whether additional training might be required e.g. how to manage particular bites from venomous snakes. Clarity on who is the lead medic should be established, and any differences of professional opinion resolved well in advance. While responsibilities may be shared, it may still be the expedition medic who is summoned to face cross-questioning in court about their preparations, should something go wrong in the field that should arguably have been anticipated.

By itself, the label 'expedition medic' does not explain one's level of competency and it would be misleading to use this title—giving the impression of great competence—if one only has minimal medical knowledge, skills, or experience in the field.

> **Box 4.2 Duties of a doctor (GMC)**
>
> *Knowledge skills and performance*
> - Make the care of your patient your first concern.
> - Provide a good standard of practice and care.
> - Keep your professional knowledge and skills up to date.
> - Recognize and work within the limits of your competence.
>
> *Safety and quality*
> - Take prompt action if you think that patient safety, dignity, or comfort is being compromised. Protect and promote the health of patients and the public.

4 ℘ https://www.gmc-uk.org/ethical-guidance/ethical-guidance-for-doctors/good-medical-practice/duties-of-a-doctor

Communication, partnership, and teamwork
- Treat patients as individuals and respect their dignity.
- Treat patients politely and considerately.
- Respect patients' right to confidentiality.
- Work in partnership with patients.
- Listen to, and respond to, their concerns and preferences.
- Give patients the information they want or need in a way they can understand.
- Respect patients' right to reach decisions with you about their treatment and care.
- Support patients in caring for themselves to improve and maintain their health.
- Work with colleagues in the ways that best serve patients' interests.

Maintaining trust
- Be honest and open and act with integrity.
- Never discriminate unfairly against patients or colleagues.
- Never abuse your patients' trust in you or the public's trust in the profession.

You are personally accountable for your professional practice and must always be prepared to justify your decisions and actions.

Decision-making

The combination of unfamiliar medical pathologies, difficult logistics, and lack of diagnostic aids on an expedition can make medical decision-making incredibly difficult. Inexperienced clinicians will not have the breadth of knowledge to make informed choices, and may struggle with decisions such as:
- How and when do you decide to medevac a patient? (A, B, N)
- When do you stop a group ascent or jungle trek if you think that environmental conditions are inappropriate, or the journey will exceed individuals' capabilities? (N)
- How and when do you remove an individual from an expedition if they have health issues, are physically unable to cope, or do not gel with the rest of the group? (B, N)
- How do you manage communication both with the group, with local people, and with those back home?

Medics may be pressurized by an individual or the whole team to take decisions based on factors beyond the purely medical situation. For instance, clinical judgements about whether to evacuate a patient following an injury might be being influenced by issues such as:
- The proximity of the expedition to its goals—e.g. a summit within reach.
- Financial implications—loss of sponsorship, inadequate insurance cover.
- Logistic difficulties in evacuating the individual.
- The continuing viability of the team having lost a key member.

In addition to such external pressures, the medic may be taking decisions based purely on clinical judgement, lacking the usual diagnostic equipment available at home. Given the numerous unknowns, medics should usually err on the side of caution, assume the worst, and arrange evacuation. They ought not be criticized for this, even if the eventual diagnosis is of a benign rather than a serious medical condition.

Throughout, the responsibility lies with the clinician and the aftermath of a wrong decision can be catastrophic both for the patient and for the medic, who may suffer professionally, personally, and medico-legally. Clinical experience, appropriate training, familiarity with the 'pre-hospital' environment, and time spent in remote environments travelling or in global health settings eases the path to decision-making and most likely improves outcomes for all those involved.

Obtaining experience

Expedition medicine can be, without doubt, one of the most exciting clinical areas in which to practise. As such, it often attracts young, enthusiastic healthcare professionals who, unhindered by the responsibilities of marriage, mortgage, and multiple offspring, find it easier to take time out of regular career pathways. While in an ideal world one would prefer expedition medics to have many years of training in an acute specialty, preferably with pre-hospital experience, this is not always possible. Enshrined within their prospective codes of conduct,[5,6,7] clinicians from all disciplines are expected to work within their known scope of competency. Therefore, expedition medics should constantly check the levels of autonomy and judgement required of them, against the standards of their education, training, and experience. For first expeditions, junior medics will benefit from:

- Completing a good-quality course on expedition medicine, relevant to the environment that they will visit (➋ p. 44).
- Shadowing experienced medics.
- Working on less remote expeditions.
- Ensuring they have access to good communications and telemedicine (➋ p. 176).

It is worth remembering that good clinical skills make up about only one-third of the skills required to be a good expedition medic; personal and expedition skills are just as important. As one gains experience and knowledge, the boundaries can be pushed—the moral responsibility of the medic is to know when and how hard to push.

5 ℘ http://www.gmc-uk.org/guidance/good_medical_practice/knowledge_skills_performance.asp

6 ℘ http://www.nmc-uk.org/standards/code/

7 ℘ http://www.hpc-uk.org/standards/standards-of-proficiency/

Medical registration

Medical registration overseas—a checklist from the GMC for UK doctors

You must recognize and work within the limits of your competence:
* Are you physically fit enough to undertake the role?
* Have you considered the impact of any break in practice—revalidation requirements and restoring your licence to practise and registration?
* What do you need to do to register with the in-country regulator?
  On returning to the UK:
* Can the GMC verify your registration with the in-country regulator?
* If not, is there any other acceptable evidence?
* Is this break in practice relevant to your application to restore your registration/licence?
* Will there be any impact on your revalidation?

Revalidation

If you have a responsible officer or suitable person, speak to them about your plans as early as possible. They may be able to help identify any action to take before your break, as well as any support you'll need to help you return to medical work in the future.

During your break, it will be important to keep up to date with changes and new developments. Think about how you can do this.

If you plan to take a longer break from UK practice, consider whether you can give up your licence to practise but maintain your registration. If you do this, you'll pay a reduced fee and you won't need to revalidate.

If you need your licence back at a later date, it is a straightforward process that takes around 3 weeks. The GMC has guidance on giving up and restoring your licence.

If you need to keep your licence, you must continue to participate in revalidation. Your connection details may change and you may no longer have access to the appraisal systems you have been using. Check your contract or employment details and explore your options. In some circumstances, you may need to find your own appraiser. In others, it may be acceptable to miss an appraisal.

The GMC does not need you to catch up on appraisals you miss because of a break in practice but you should agree this and the best way to fulfil any local requirements with your responsible officer or suitable person before the break begins. If you don't have a connection, you should speak to the GMC.

Maintaining registration

The GMC recognizes that doctors may wish to temporarily relinquish their UK licence to practise while abroad. They have produced guidance for overseas regulators and overseas organizations about revalidation and the licence to practise for doctors working wholly outside the UK.

However, many international medical organizations such as Doctors Without Borders continue to require that their medical volunteers maintain a licence in their home country.

If doctors return to the UK within 5 years of being registered overseas and can produce a 'certificate of good standing' from the appropriate overseas regulator, it can be relatively straightforward to regain a licence to practise upon return. If the volunteer was not locally registered, the doctor would need to supply a form (UD8) from the organization they volunteered for, instead of a certificate of good standing.

Working with the media

Providing medical support alongside a film or television production company can offer exciting opportunities for an expedition medic. These include paid employment while doing a 'glamorous' job, the chance of working on location in remote and exciting settings, possibly with celebrities, and even the opportunity to appear on-screen.

However, the appealing nature of these opportunities often belies the very real and unique risks associated with working in this field. Before signing up as a medic for a television or media company, it is important to consider these risks and obtain a comprehensive understanding of the situations likely to be encountered and the probable ability of the production company to deal with them.

Medics are only likely to be recruited if filming will involve a remote or dangerous assignment, where if something were to go wrong the harm would be considerable. Although some production companies undertaking this type of work are well informed and produce detailed risk assessments, such attention to detail isn't guaranteed. Remote filming trips often experience 'expedition' conditions, yet many media companies, often more through inexperience than malpractice, do not do the detailed planning needed or one would expect. This occurs despite the strict health and safety regulations governing their business.[8]

Regardless of personal performance, the high-profile nature of these trips means that should something go seriously wrong, the medic is at risk not merely of questions from the regulatory authorities, but could end up experiencing 'trial by media', which can be immensely stressful and equally damaging.

There are various types of media production styles. These include:
- Wildlife/factual documentaries.
- News/current affairs.
- Reality TV/light entertainment.
- Feature films.
- Commercial (advertising/promos/charity).

Understanding the aims, goals, and experience of the production and the previous work of the production company will give an indication as to potential health risks. For example, highly experienced news and current affairs programmes might film in areas of conflict or famine where there is the ever-present risk of physical and psychological trauma, whereas 'reality TV' programmes, with little hostile environment experience, may potentially place contributors in increasingly hazardous or challenging situations in an attempt to obtain 'exciting TV'.

Risks can be considered in terms of those affecting the medic the film crew (behind the camera), presenters/celebrities (in front of the camera), and the production team (director/producer on location).

Medic-specific risks
- Limited involvement in pre-travel team screening, leading to:
  - Unknown pre-existing medical problems and fitness levels.
  - Poor team medical preparation.

---

8 Health and Safety Executive. *Audio-Visual Production: Legal Duties.* ℅ https://www.hse.gov.uk/pubns/indg360.pdf

- Limited involvement in pre-travel risk assessment, including:
  - Little/no knowledge about in-country medical facilities.
  - Little/no knowledge about emergency procedures.
  - Limited knowledge of insurance cover details—such as your own cover, as well as medevac for remote locations (e.g. is it only available from major cities?).
  - Little/no knowledge of filming details, including schedule, logistics, and locations.
- Unclear definitions of roles and responsibilities, including:
  - When medical intervention is deemed appropriate.
  - Levels of control and input into decision-making, particularly in relation to schedules, filming locations, and leadership.
- Lack of personal knowledge about the illnesses/injuries likely to be encountered (including psychological stress).

Production crew risks

Although all crew are issued with a production risk assessment prior to filming, to protect them on location, sometimes it can be issued so late, they have little time to read it or they can overlook their own personal safety.

- Media crews are focused on filming and less on personal day-to-day health issues such as hydration, hygiene, sun exposure, and protection against vector-borne diseases such as malaria.
- While filming, camera operators have a narrow field of vision. If the majority of filming is 'handheld' (without a tripod) with camera operators often walking backwards, they may not see physical hazards such as uneven ground, dangerous flora (e.g. rattan), or dangerous fauna (e.g. snakes/spiders).
- Sound recordists, wearing headphones, may be insulated from their physical surroundings. With their sound levels amplified, injury can occur through unexpected loud noises.
- The nature and pressure to achieve the 'once-in-a-career' shot can place crew in harm's way with limited chance of regress (e.g. in exposed, hazardous positions), even while being swarmed by insects or charged by larger animals.
- Camera crew carry heavy kit, for long periods of time, in all weathers and terrains and so are occupationally vulnerable to certain types of injury (e.g. to neck, back, shoulders, and knees).
- Filming has the potential to draw large crowds, putting the crew in a vulnerable position physically, especially with expensive kit.
- Crew can often be asked to 'split' location, with little thought given to provision of a medical kit for every filming location.
- A director/producer may make last-minute filming changes, without fully taking into account the health or safety of crew.

Contributors/presenter/celebrity healthcare risks

- Tight production schedules increase pressure on contributors, presenters, and celebrities to 'deliver', despite the presence of illness or injury. (N)
- Contributors take part without the skills/expertise or fitness required of the film location. (A, N)

- Contributors are placed in situations hazardous to their physical/mental well-being in order to obtain 'exciting TV'. (B vs N)
- Production crews are often used to working in difficult conditions, while contributors can have little/no experience—leaving them physically and emotionally vulnerable in demanding situations. (N)

Production and general team risks

- Tight filming schedules caused by budgetary constraints, permits/visas, and availability of crew/presenters lead to reduced environmental acclimatization. This in turn results in an increased risk of environmental health issues such as heat exhaustion and acute mountain sickness.
- Poor preparation for living and working in hostile environments.
- The production team (director/producers) are often the 'silent' workers—continuing to work when the crews, presenters, and contributors have finished filming. Tiredness can make them vulnerable to health risks.
- Regular health risks associated with working in foreign/hostile environments.

Issues with working in television

Certain types of programmes, such as reality TV, can raise ethical concerns for a medic as the programme's objective is often to stress participants to breaking point, through physical and mental challenges, or in some cases to use the rigours of expedition life to deal with traumatic personal issues not being faced at home. As a medic, you are responsible for both the physical and psychological well-being of the team.

Before embarking on such a project, ensure you are clear in your own mind as to where your boundaries lie, and how far you are willing to let individuals be pushed. Your ethical standards (including environmental and treatment of wildlife) may well differ from those of the production team. While filming, there is a risk that film crews focus more on production, schedules, and personal needs, rather than the welfare of porters, staff, and local communities. Some local communities have had bad experiences with film crews, but medics have the advantage of being separate from the filming process and can help to prevent this from happening, by setting a good example.

Teamwork

An alert and attentive expedition medic will predict and prevent problems before they materialize. For the majority of the time, the medic will not be involved in providing medical care. However, on a daily basis, a medic can have a valuable role as a 'second pair of eyes' for the health and safety of the team. It is important that the medic is seen as an active member of the team, contributing to the smooth running of the production. Smaller film crews may ask medics to take on an additional role (e.g. photographer/driver).

The nature of filming can result in excessive periods of waiting—for subjects to appear or during repeated takes of the same shot. Keeping alert during these periods will help ensure the medic is not caught out.

Celebrities

The role of a medic on a film shoot may include working alongside famous faces. This can present challenges. An on-screen character may be a very different person in real life—the charismatic comedian may be an introvert and nervous traveller. This may make it harder to detect either health or psychological issues as they arise. As a medic it is important to take everyone as you find them, without preconception, and to treat them equally. It's advisable to build a rapport with everyone before departure and to be aware of confidentiality clauses in your contract. Celebrities/presenters may also travel under a different name for security/privacy.

Disaster medicine

Disasters can occur anywhere in the world, often having the greatest impact on a community and country infrastructure in low-income countries, where needs significantly outweigh resources.

To many, they appear exciting and often appeal to a medic's natural instinct of wanting to help others and utilize skills less frequently used in the UK. Raw and emotive media coverage helps fuel this desire to travel to catastrophes across the globe, from providing relief work after natural disasters with organized agencies, through to leaving a postgraduate training programme and travelling independently to a war zone.

Although opportunities to provide assistance in a disaster are frequent, there are many ethical issues that surround this type of medical provision. Medics travelling independently to disaster zones, even with the best intentions, are at great risk of becoming a hindrance to local and international healthcare efforts, in addition they can be a drain on local resources and an infrastructure already under great pressure. Issues that often draw criticism include:

- *Language:* Western healthcare workers have been found providing medical care without interpreters or the ability to communicate effectively with the local population.
- *Continuity:* teams provide treatment (e.g. basic surgical procedures, splinting of fractures) but with no arrangements for ongoing care.
- *Documentation:* care is often provided without medical records.
- *Coordination:* there is often little or no coordination between various healthcare providers; a situation made worse with multiple, international teams.
- *Credentials/suitability:* independent workers may provide care unsupervised, and without any formal checking of credentials may lack any authority to practise in country.

Historically, there has been a trend for medics embarking on disaster relief projects to be more junior and less experienced. As such, not only are they likely to lack the relevant clinical competencies and accountability required for such work, they are likely to be unaccustomed to the scale and magnitude of suffering visited on populations during periods of disaster. This inexperience can place personal health and well-being at risk, as well as that of the local population. (N)

Being part of a team providing medical care following natural or man-made disasters is exciting, challenging, and incredibly rewarding. However, it is also a complicated, multifaceted process, in which even global governmental and non-governmental organizations sometimes struggle. It is now widely accepted that professionally, clinically, and perhaps even ethically, the most appropriate way is through well-established and regulated bodies that can provide suitable training and direction. (B, N, J)

UK International Emergency Trauma Register (UKIETR)
The UKIETR has been established as a register aiming to draw together clinicians interested in deploying as part of a team in response to sudden-onset disasters and humanitarian emergencies. Its aim is to provide structured and standardized training to individuals and teams, promoting a governed, coordinated, accountable, clinically competent, and guided approach to medical and logistical team response in disasters. For more information see: ℜ www.uk-med.org

Crisis management

Chapter editor
Shane Winser

Contributors
Rose Buckley
Peter Harvey
Stephen Jones
Marc Shaw
Kristina Birch (1st and 2nd editions)
Chris Johnson (1st and 2nd editions)
Clare Morgan (2nd edition)

Medical crisis management

A medical crisis on an expedition can result from illness, injury, or accident to team members. The expedition planning team has a duty to foresee and try to prevent a crisis by developing a *risk analysis and management system* (RAMS). If an emergency develops, an *emergency response plan* (ERP) will provide the team with the information and resources necessary to manage the situation effectively.

Medical aspects of the safety management system include:
- Organizing medical training for all participants (➔ p. 44).
- Providing appropriate medical kits (➔ p. 851).
- Organizing medical insurance with full emergency evacuation cover (➔ p. 76).
- Contracting a service providing medical consultations via the insurance medical assistance company or an alternative.
- Planning for evacuation and repatriation of a severely ill or injured person (➔ p. 160 and ➔ p. 174).
- Preparing a communication network in case of evacuation (➔ p. 149).
- Investigating medical facilities and support available both locally and remotely (e.g. using telemedicine, ➔ p. 176).
- Maintaining medical records and compiling accident reports.

During an emergency the team are likely to be involved in:
- Preventing additional illness or injury.
- Locating and accessing the ill or injured parties.
- Providing medical care.
- Expediting evacuations using effective logistics and communications.
- Managing and supporting the rescue team.
- Communicating accurately and effectively with key individuals.
- Considering how to minimize long-term psychological effects on casualties and other team members (➔ p. 556).

Emergency response plan

An ERP, associated with each phase of the expedition, should be developed. This reference document includes information to enable any member of the team to respond appropriately to an emergency. Elements of an ERP are summarized in Fig. 5.1.

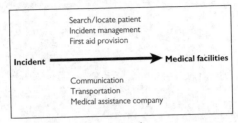

Search/locate patient
Incident management
First aid provision

Incident ➡ **Medical facilities**

Communication
Transportation
Medical assistance company

Fig. 5.1 Elements of an emergency response plan.

All these elements are important in expediting an evacuation. A rapid and timely response to a crisis may save a life; prior research, training, and resourcing are vital. Global communication is now relatively easy and satellite phones enable medical consultations from the field, so long as the medic has ready access to a medical specialist.

The most reliable source of help in an emergency is your expedition team. As far as possible aim to be self-contained. Reliance on third parties in home countries is not robust and the best solutions are often local and simple. Therefore, do your research and know the transport, medical, and SAR options for the region in which you are working. Once collated, everyone involved in the expedition should know the plan, and their responsibilities in implementing it.

Components of an emergency response plan

An ERP should include as a minimum:

Section 1. Roles and responsibilities in an emergency situation

This should clarify roles and responsibilities, focusing on the initial priorities as outlined in Table 5.1. Simplicity is critical. Consider who is trained and competent for each nominated role.

Section 2. Initial response steps

Ensure that the initial response of the team is quick and effective. The generic steps outlined below can be applied to diverse situations:

- STOP—Stop, Think, Observe, and Plan.
- Manage the scene.
- Remain calm.
- Assess hazards.
- Preserve life and prevent further injury.
- Delegate roles.
- Inform the expedition leader.

Table 5.1 Roles/responsibilities in an emergency

Role	Tasks
Leader	Overall coordination
Incident manager	Scene safety
Logistics	Evacuation/transportation
Communication	Radio/telephone links and information transfer
First aid	Provision of temporary immediate care

- Ask expedition members not to contact home or use any social media.
- Contact appropriate medical assistance company.
- Contact on-call team with details, location, and contact number.
- Minimize damage to property/environment.

An example of an initial response plan is given in Fig. 5.2.

Section 3. Emergency services—contact numbers

This should contain important telephone, email contacts, and addresses, and include:

- All team members' mobile/satellite phone numbers.
- 24 h on-call contact details.
- In-country contact details.
- Service providing medical consultations.
- Emergency medical support company details.
- Insurance companies.
- Response organizations you may need to call, such as air charter companies, the host country air force, police, air ambulance, local mountain rescue teams, coastguard, etc.
- There are likely to be different transport options for day and for night evacuations to medical facilities. The risks of transporting patients at night should be assessed before proceeding.

Section 4. Medical facility information

This section should list in-country medical facilities to enable effective evacuation of ill or injured participants. Each facility should be listed with its name, address, directions (including maps), telephone numbers, capabilities, and hours of operation. Hospitals and clinics vary around the world and it is important to assess what capabilities exist in the vicinity of your expedition. People are not always safer in a local clinic or hospital. By knowing the capabilities of local medical facilities beforehand you can plan transport to the most appropriate for the circumstances you are dealing with.

Screened blood

In countries where blood is unavailable or there are concerns over its quality, arrangements can be made to obtain supplies of blood in an emergency. The Blood Care Foundation provides screened blood and emergency deliveries of human rabies immunoglobulin and/or rabies vaccine to its members around the world (ℐ www.bloodcare.org.uk).

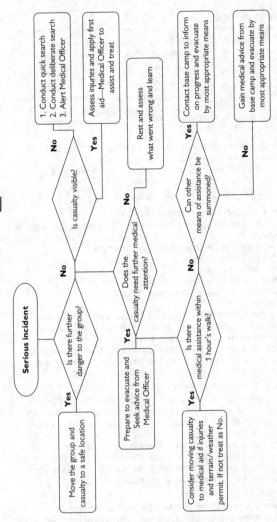

Fig. 5.2 Initial response plan.

Section 5. Trip itinerary and evacuation options

This section enables the on-call contact to locate the group if there is an emergency at home or a breakdown in communications. This should include a protocol for the expedition to either call in to the on-call contact at the same time every day, or to use their communications equipment at a pre-agreed time every day to collect messages.

The itinerary should include enough detail and contact numbers to enable the on-call contact to locate the group. As a minimum this must include a list of dates of where the group will be staying, including addresses, phone numbers, and geo-references. The itinerary can be supplemented with the use of satellite trackers which are becoming common and more affordable.

In addition, this section should briefly outline the emergency evacuation route for an injured participant from each phase of the expedition. Note that night-time evacuation options may be more difficult and more hazardous than day-time options.

Section 6. Participant emergency contact list

In emergency situations it may be necessary to contact a participant's next of kin. To enable this, each participant will need to supply the name and contact details for minimum of two individuals to be stored in the ERP. It is good practice for the home on-call team to deal with next of kin to leave the expedition team to handle the incident.

Section 7. Plans to deal with death or critical injury

These are discussed in Fig. 5.2 (➔ p. 150) and Death on an expedition (➔ p. 184).

Section 8. Media plan

The media plan should establish the procedures and resources needed to respond to the press in the event of a serious incident and/or death. It might include a draft press release outlining the intentions and purpose of the expedition, the framework for reporting the incident, and who to contact for further information.

Have a contingency to separate the on-call team from the personnel responding to the media, otherwise all phones and communications can be swamped by media, leaving no channels of communications between the expedition and the on-call team.

Search and rescue

Searching involves looking for a person whose location is unknown; rescuing is the evacuation of someone from a known location, generally a more straightforward task.

SAR services typically consist of groups of volunteers supported by logistics from police, ambulance, or coastguard, and may be integrated into the national civil defence system. The volunteers usually have extensive local knowledge and may have specialist skills in marine, cliff, mountain, or cave rescue. Effective SAR systems will bring manpower, communications, appropriate transport, and tools such as thermal imaging, sniffer dogs, and rescue stretchers. Equipment and personnel have to be transported to site in a manner appropriate to the terrain, this could involve the use of boats, four-wheel drive, superjeeps, tracked vehicles, skidoos, hovercraft, or animals. Casualty evacuation may eventually involve a helicopter or a fixed-wing or float plane, but one cannot rely on aerial support as it may be restricted by range, height, or weather conditions. Casualties may have to be transported to a suitable landing zone (LZ).

SAR services are expensive, sometimes hazardous for the personnel involved, and take time to assemble. The quality and availability of service varies worldwide; in LMIC, expeditions may have to be fully self-sufficient. Risk management plans should include determining the capability of SAR services available, methods of contact, and insurance requirements—as aerial support is frequently charged to the user. In some countries (e.g. Nepal and Pakistan), payment of a bond in advance is required if there is a possibility that air evacuation will be requested.

Missing persons

Finding that an individual or small group are not where they should be, is worrying. The cause may be innocent—poor timekeeping or an unexpectedly arduous trip—but the concern may be that someone has become injured, lost, or detained. Anxieties will be heightened if those missing are young, elderly, or unfamiliar with the terrain and conditions. People are more likely to become separated in dense vegetation, fog, or driving rain, or if leaders set a very fast pace. Navigation is harder at night, in snow which masks the contours, and shifting desert sand.

Don't get lost

- Avoidance is always best.
- Teach survival skills. Maps and compasses are invaluable, but only if you know how to use them.
- GPS is nowadays readily and cheaply available on phones and cameras, equipping everyone is worthwhile, but once again only if people can use the resulting information. Small power packs are invaluable to recharge mobile phones and other devices.
- Ensure everyone in the group knows the plan for the day.
- Designate a leader and back marker, keep everyone else between the two. Do not permit weaker members of the party to drop behind. Ensure the back marker can communicate with the leader.
- If groups separate, designate obvious rendezvous places and specify time. If in doubt, stop and wait to be found.
- Some countries with comprehensive mobile networks provide Apps (e.g. *112 Iceland, what3words.com*) that can link travellers direct to SAR services.

Initial actions

- Ensure the main party remains safe: seek shelter, fluids, and warmth wherever possible.
- Attempt to contact missing persons by phone, radio, or visual or auditory signals.
- Ensure searchers are properly equipped, have means of communication, and a rendezvous place and time.
- Retrace route, most people will be found close to last known position.

Lost persons

If an initial search fails, a more comprehensive search will be needed. Time is important, external SAR agencies using appropriate technologies will be able to cover the ground more quickly and effectively. Analyses of rescues have indicated common patterns of behaviour, which while not individually predictive, give an indication of how individuals may behave.[1] Skilled SAR leaders use knowledge of the situation and locality to plan their search strategy. The International Search & Rescue Database collects data on missing persons, the terrain, and methods of search.

Search scenarios can be categorized (Box 5.1).

---

1 Koestler RJ. *Lost Person Behavior*. Charlottesville, VA: Dbs Productions; 2008.

Box 5.1 Causes of missing persons

- Avalanche.
- Immersion and drowning.
- Despondency.
- Overdue, but unharmed.
- Criminal activity including abduction.
- Medical problems.
- Evasion.
- Stranded.
- Trauma.
- Lost.

Becoming lost and disoriented is not unusual; even highly experienced orienteers and backwoods travellers will admit to becoming lost on occasions. A lost person may adopt one of a number of strategies to re-locate:

- *Random travelling.* Confused and frightened, the lost person moves around randomly taking the apparently easiest route. An ineffective strategy, most people other than youngsters try to adopt a more purposeful method.
- *Route travelling.* The lost person follows a linear feature such as a path, trail, or drainage, even though the route and destination are unknown. This is not usually an effective method.
- *Direction travelling.* Travellers aim in a direction and persist on this route. Direction travelling may be worthwhile if a major target such as a road or river is well used but following a compass bearing may lead to a cliff top or impassable terrain.
- *Backtracking.* The traveller attempts to follow their exact route back to its origin. This can be very effective, especially for those with good terrain memory, but requires skill, patience, and an acceptance of delay. Surprisingly, few people follow this strategy.
- *Route sampling.* The lost person starts at a path junction and samples each track in the hope of finding a more familiar or obvious feature, returning to the junction, and trying again if a path fades away or proves unfamiliar. Technique may be used in conjunction with backtracking.
- *Direction sampling.* Like route sampling, but in featureless terrain. Beginning at a unique feature such as a hill or obvious tree the traveller heads out on compass bearings until all main directions have been tested. If original base point proves valueless, the person moves to a second base and repeats the process.
- *View enhancing.* Heading uphill permits a better view of the surrounding terrain and may enable acquisition of a mobile phone signal. It is a popular way to attempt to re-locate, especially among those able to read a map, but is an unpredictable strategy. Weather conditions may be worse and it can take you away from water.
- *Heading downhill.* Following a valley or watercourse downhill works well in some terrain, especially in areas of high population density as habitation clusters around water. In remote areas this is a hazardous strategy as streams may go over falls or enter gorges before possibly terminating in a trackless bog, muskeg, or dry wadi.
- *Staying put.* Survival teaching emphasizes the benefits of staying put especially in thick terrain or if a vehicle has broken down in a remote area; it is often an effective strategy provided that the climate is benign. But few active people have the patience to simply stay put and wait

to be rescued, and most move around for at least the first 24 h after
becoming lost. Many SAR callouts in urban areas of Scandinavia and
North America involve people suffering from depression or dementia
who move less than more active individuals.

Understanding how people may respond to being lost helps limit the area
that needs to be searched. Offering a sensible strategy in advance aids
decision-making. Generally this will involve 'staying put', but might, for instance state 'head due south until you reach the road, then walk east'.

Making contact
Mobile phones are a great help if within range of masts. Police or SAR
services may be able to obtain an approximate fix on a casualty by triangu-
lating their signal or interrogating their position. Some helicopters have
the ability to locate and fly down to a mobile phone signal. Elsewhere—
especially in thick terrain such as the New Zealand bush—lost individuals
have phoned for help and then directed a helicopter to directly above their
location—saving rescue groups from much effort struggling through thick
vegetation. When possible maximize battery life by turning off unused apps,
Wi-Fi, and Bluetooth. Extra batteries/chargers may be very helpful.

Satellite tracking beacons, such as the Garmin inReach®, are superb items
of equipment that enable two-way messaging, global positioning system
(GPS) functions, location tracking, and an SOS function. They are one of
the most useful developments for expedition communications.

Satellite rescue beacons (➔ p. 179) carried by aircraft as emergency locator transmitters (ELTs), by ships as emergency position-indicating radio
beacon (EPIRBS), and by ground personnel as personal locator beacons
(PLBs) are a transmit-only means of transmitting an SOS signal. For ground
personnel, they have been largely superseded by satellite tracking beacons.

Avalanche transceivers (➔ p. 680) should be worn during winter travel in
backcountry mountain areas.

The rescue
Even if uninjured, a person lost for some time is likely to be frightened,
cold, hungry, and thirsty; they need appropriate support. Occasionally, individuals on adventure treks appear totally naïve to hazards and must be
watched to ensure they do not get into further difficulties.

Scene management

Management of a serious wilderness incident may be complex. Excellent leadership, teamwork, communications, and forward thinking are necessary. If resources allow, the expedition leader should stand back from the actual rescue and coordinate the overall situation, dynamically assessing and managing potential hazards.

Patients who have been injured are often in hazardous environments. The safety of the rescuers should have paramount importance. Stop and assess the risks of the situation. A minute spent on this task is vital for the safety and efficiency of the rescue operation, and the delay rarely leads to an adverse outcome for the patient.

In *steep ground*, place a belay (anchor) above the incident to secure both patient and rescuers. Consider the potential for rock fall or avalanche.

At *road traffic collision* (RTC) sites, deploy two members of the team to stop the traffic in both directions. To protect rescuers from further collisions, park vehicles back from the site at an angled 'fend-off' position. Once the crash vehicle can be approached (avoiding danger of fire, explosion, rollover, etc.), the vehicle ignition should be turned off and the handbrake applied. Vehicle stabilization procedures should be improvised as soon as possible.

If there is a continuing significant risk to rescuers or patients, it may be necessary to extricate the patient rapidly from the hazardous zone before a primary survey has been completed and, in some cases, before spinal care has been optimized (➲ p. 218).

Equipment should be organized in a kit dump a few metres from the accident scene. This ensures the equipment is readily located when needed but does not get trampled or damaged by those managing the casualty.

Whenever possible, external help should be sought. While the casualty is being assessed and treated, ideally by medics, the leader should plan the different stages of the evacuation; effective logistics facilitate rapid and effective evacuation.

Meanwhile the rest of the group will also need to be supported and cared for (particularly true with commercial and youth expeditions). While ensuring their safety, try to involve those nearby as much as possible in the rescue. Keep everyone informed about what is happening, even if they were not directly involved.

Structured communications

Effective, succinct communications reduce misunderstandings. The nature and position of an incident must be accurately reported.

Major incident priorities and tasks—CSCATTT
- **C**ommand.
- **S**afety.
- **C**ommunication.
- **A**ssessment.
- **T**riage.
- **T**reatment.
- **T**ransport.

Initial incident reporting—ETHANE
- **E**xact location.
- **T**ype of incident.
- **H**azards.
- **A**ccess.
- **N**umber of casualties.
- **E**mergency services on scene and required.

Patient handover report—ATMIST
- **A**ge and sex.
- **T**ime of incident.
- **M**echanism of injury.
- **I**njuries sustained.
- **S**igns and symptoms.
- **T**reatment to date.

Team communication report—SBAR
- **S**ituation.
- **B**ackground.
- **A**ssessment.
- **R**ecommendation.

Evacuation

Medical evacuation (medevac) is defined as the movement of a sick or injured expedition member to appropriate local medical facilities. Transfer may be by land, water, or air. Repatriation is the return of an expedition member home following initial treatment.

Advance planning reduces the stress of a difficult situation and should allow an evacuation to proceed as smoothly and safely as possible, with minimum risk to the sick or injured person and their companions. The aim is to get the casualty to the right care at an appropriate speed; too much haste may increase hazard without benefit to the victim.

Many expeditions visit areas with sophisticated SAR facilities. If visiting such areas, determine the capabilities of the local rescue services, their requirements, and the costs. Night-time evacuations can be particularly difficult, so alternative evacuation plans for day and night are recommended.

Considerations in planning a specific evacuation

Medical
- Is the patient's condition time-critical?
- Can the patient receive further treatment in their current location?
- Can care be provided in a local clinic or hospital, or should they be transferred to a major hospital?
- Might they be able to rejoin the expedition after treatment?
- Could the patient safely undertake a road/water journey or is air transport a better option? Is the patient safe to travel by air at the altitudes involved?
- Is medical supervision available for the journey?

Logistics
- What is the capacity, availability, and suitability of procurable local transport to travel to the various medical facility options?
- What risks are associated with the evacuation? Do the benefits outweigh the risks?
- Can the evacuation be completed in daylight, and if not, what are the relative risks of delaying evacuation until next morning, or travelling at night?

Financial
- Does the team have adequate access to finances to trigger the evacuation?
- Will costs incurred be covered by insurance? If not does the team have funds to cover costs? It is essential to involve the insurers as soon as possible.

The answers to these questions vary depending on the location of the incident, the nature of the injuries, and the treatment required. A serious head injury, for example, will require a different response from a fractured wrist.

Moving an injured person

Incidents often occur at locations remote from good transport links; initially the patient must be transferred to a location from which evacuation is possible. Anyone in danger should be moved at once by whatever means possible. Patients not in immediate danger should first be stabilized and positioned to prevent aggravating their injuries during transport. Once a safe location is reached, fully assess their condition to determine the urgency of evacuation.

Urgent movement

If an injured person must be moved immediately from a life-threatening situation (damaged building, fire, avalanche, or rock fall), the greatest danger is the possibility of aggravating a spinal injury (Fig. 5.3) or compromising the airway. Try to pull the patient in the direction of the long axis of the body to provide as much protection to the spine as possible.

If on the ground, pull the patient's clothing in the neck or shoulder area. If several people are available, straddle the patient and lift on to an improvised stretcher (sleeping bag, blanket, or air mattress) and drag the material head first with the patient's head and shoulders off the ground to prevent further injury. See: ℘ https://vimeopro.com/healthandcarevideos/mount ain-rescue-england-and-wales/video/226716256 for a short video to demonstrate the straddle lift technique.

If nothing is available to support the patient, place your hands under the armpits (from the back) and grasp the forearms to drag the patient (Fig. 5.4).

If not on the ground, move the patient by any means possible, but do not pull a patient's head away from the neck or the rest of the body.

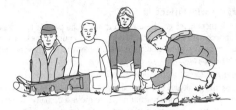

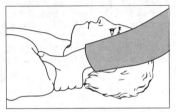

Always support the neck (never release)

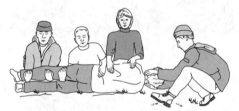

Everyone works together, with the person
at the head directing movement

Fig. 5.3 The log-roll method of turning a casualty with a suspected spinal injury.

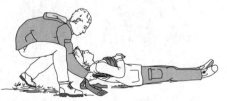

Fig. 5.4 Reverse drag.

Non-urgent movement

A variety of techniques can be used to transfer the patient to the nearest piece of appropriate equipment. Carrying a heavy human is exhausting, especially over rough ground, and the more people who are involved the safer it will be for everyone.

Single rescuer

A single rescuer is always at risk of injuring themselves, but there may be circumstances where a lone rescuer needs to move a casualty. Traditionally, the way to carry an unconscious person is the fireman's carry, but there is a high risk of back injury to the rescuer and it should be avoided if the injuries involve the arms, legs, ribs, neck, or back. If the patient is able to assist, a sling carry may be attempted (Fig. 5.5). Walking poles may assist with balance.

The tied hands crawl (Fig. 5.6) may be used to drag someone who is unconscious under low structures. The injured person's head is not supported.

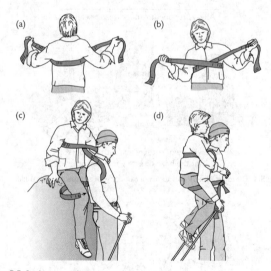

Fig. 5.5 Single-person sling carry.

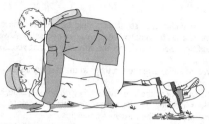

Fig. 5.6 Tied hands crawl.

The chair carry is good for going up or down stairs or through narrow passages. This should not be attempted in a patient with neck, back, or pelvic problems. Variations of this lift can be used without a chair with two rescuers.

Rope sling (Fig. 5.7) using two rescuers relieves some strain over longer distances but increases the risk of falling in rough ground.

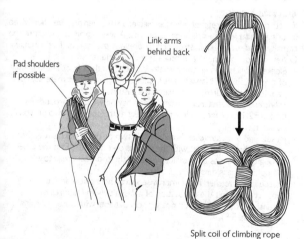

Pad shoulders if possible

Link arms behind back

Split coil of climbing rope

Fig. 5.7 Two-person sling carry.

Stretchers

If available, a manufactured stretcher should be used to transport a casualty. If none is available, improvisation may be necessary. Always ensure there are sufficient people to carry the stretcher so that you do not drop the casualty.

- Whenever possible, take the stretcher to the casualty instead of the casualty to the stretcher.
- Fasten the casualty to the stretcher so they do not slip, slide, or fall off.
- Use blankets, clothing, a group shelter, or other materials to pad the stretcher and protect the casualty from exposure.
- Try to splint broken limbs before movement and provide appropriate pain relief to minimize distress and reduce shock.
- Lay the casualty on their back for transport unless this may cause further injury.
- Ensure that the airway will remain open and unblocked.
- Move the casualty feet first so that the rear bearer may watch the patient for signs of difficulty or distress.
- Always brief the personnel carrying the stretcher and the casualty themselves, if applicable, about the procedure to be employed. Ensure one person is designated as team leader.

Improvising a stretcher

If a custom-made stretcher is not available, a stretcher may be improvised by using available materials such as boards. Always attempt to secure the casualty to the makeshift stretcher to prevent the risk of further injury. Other methods for manufacturing a stretcher include:

- *Blanket/fabric stretcher*: the casualty is placed on their back in the middle of a group shelter, blanket, tent flysheet, or similar fabric material. Four people roll the side edges towards the casualty and lift.
- *Fabric and poles stretcher*: a fabric sheet may be wrapped around two poles (~2.1 m (7 feet) in length) to make a stretcher that two persons can carry.
- *Jackets and poles stretcher*: button or zip two or three jackets together and turn them inside out with the sleeves on the inside. Pass the poles through the sleeves after making holes in the shoulder areas to allow the poles to pass through (Fig. 5.8).
- *Roscoe rope stretcher*: most improvised stretchers give inadequate support to permit the evacuation of a casualty with fractures or extensive wounds. They do not support patients with potential spinal injuries (Fig. 5.9).

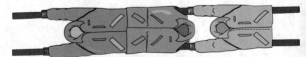

Fig. 5.8 Improvised jacket and poles stretcher.

Roscoe Rope Stretcher

1 Find centre of the rope.
2 Leave enough rope for a carrying loop (to go over head and shoulder of carrier).
3 Make a loop with one of the ends using an overhand knot.
4 Make a slip knot in the rope on the opposite side.
5 Thread the loop through the slip knot, then pull the slip knot inside out, to form a sheet bend. (The end of the loop should be long enough to tie a half-hitch, once the stretcher is finished, and be used as a small handle.)

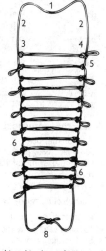

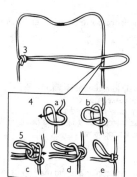

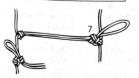

6 Repeat this, taking loops from alternate sides, until the stretcher is the required length. The knots should be about 4" apart at weight-bearing parts of the stretcher (where shoulders, head and hips will be); if short of rope they can be further apart on legs.
7 Adjust width of stretcher to fit patient. Tie off ends of loops with half-hitches. (These can then be used as small handles.)
8 Tie ends of rope to form a carrying loop at foot of stretcher. Pad stretcher before loading patient.

Fig. 5.9 Rope stretcher.

Priority for evacuation of a casualty

A system commonly used to communicate the priority required for evacuation of the patient is outlined in Table 5.2.

Table 5.2 Priority classification

Priority 1A	Immediate evacuation of the casualty required, if possible from the accident site
Priority 1B	Immediate evacuation required but the casualty can be moved from the accident site
Priority 2	Evacuation required within 12 h
Priority 3	Evacuation required within 12–24 h
Priority 4	Evacuation required but is not time sensitive

Evacuation transport and considerations

Evacuation may be by:
- Air—fixed-wing plane or helicopter.
- Land—usually motor vehicle, but mules or porters can be better over rough ground.
- Water—boat or raft.

Evacuation of a casualty by air

Advantages of air evacuation
- Casualty can be transported relatively long distances quickly.
- Sophisticated medical care can be accessed quickly.
- Air transport allows difficult terrain to be traversed safely.
- Rotary wing aircraft can reach areas inaccessible to ground or water transport, especially if they have winch facilities.

Disadvantages of air evacuation
- Aircraft are very expensive to run.
- They cannot fly in very adverse weather conditions and maybe not in the dark. Not all operators have night vision capability.
- Fixed-wing aircraft require a landing strip, while helicopters usually require a suitable LZ, unless they are equipped with winching facilities.
- Noise and vibration may make monitoring of and communication with the casualty impossible. Ear defenders for the patient and any person accompanying them are preferable. Diagnosis is difficult.
- Air sickness can be a significant problem.
- Helicopters work inefficiently at high altitude and trade payload for altitude. Do not rely on helicopter rescue from high altitudes; it will only be possible in ideal weather using the best available aircraft. See also Helicopter evacuation, p. 170.
- Altitude: as altitude increases and pressure decreases, air will expand. If air is trapped in a confined space, severe problems may result. At 5500 m the atmospheric pressure is half that of sea level, but the drop is not linear, with the decrease in pressure greater closer to sea level.

Creating a temporary helicopter landing zone
- A LZ may have to be improvised if casualty evacuation by rotary wing (helicopter) aircraft is planned.
- Try to keep the LZ at least 150 m downwind of base areas or the casualty to prevent blowing dust and debris affecting the patient or operations. The LZ should be level and free of obstacles such as cables, wires, rocks, or ruts. Obstacles that cannot be moved should be clearly marked with items that cannot be affected by prop wash or gusting winds. Mark the wind direction to assist the pilot in landing into wind.
- Light signals should be planned. For example, the headlights of two downwind vehicles converging on the LZ, or four people with flashlights marking each corner of the LZ. The lights must be bright enough to be visible during the day, but not so bright they blind the pilot.
- A designated person should guide the aircraft in with land-to-air communication and direct the pilot by standing with their back to the wind and arms outstretched to indicate the LZ.
- Never approach a helicopter unless signalled to do so by the crewman. If a crewman is not on board, only approach in the pilot's field of frontal vision so they may indicate when and how to approach the aircraft. See Fig. 5.10.

Potential problems include:
- Development of tension pneumothorax.
- Distension of gas in stomach or bowel.
- Intracranial air expansion if pneumoencephaly.
- Over-pressure of air in endotracheal tube cuffs.
- Ambient temperature falls by about 5°C per 1000 m increase in altitude (depending on the humidity).
- Hypobaric hypoxia: the reduction in partial pressure of oxygen in inspired air produced by ascent to altitude is a serious potential risk during flight at high altitude, particularly if the patient's oxygenation is critical (→ Humans at altitude, p. 686).

Helicopter evacuation from offshore craft
See → Helicopter evacuation, p. 756.

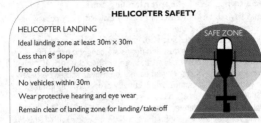

HELICOPTER SAFETY

HELICOPTER LANDING

Ideal landing zone at least 30m × 30m

Less than 8° slope

Free of obstacles/loose objects

No vehicles within 30m

Wear protective hearing and eye wear

Remain clear of landing zone for landing/take-off

SAFE ZONE

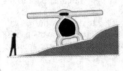

BOARDING THE AIRCRAFT

Approach only with flight team or when signalled

Usual approach from front/side of helicopter

Do not walk behind aircraft near tail rota

Approach from downhill side on uneven terrain

Fig. 5.10 Helicopter safety.

Evacuation of the casualty by land

Advantages of evacuation over land

Vehicles, either propelled mechanically or by animals, are usually more available than aircraft, and in locations with road access permit immediate evacuation to medical facilities. Vehicles can travel in conditions that impede boats and aircraft.

Disadvantages of evacuation over land

Speed and range may be limited. Rough terrain and winding roads may prevent immediate access to the casualty and make evacuation a slow, painful, or nauseating journey for the casualty.

Evacuation of the casualty by water

Advantages of evacuation by water

In tropical forests and marine archipelagos, water is the main communication route. Evacuation by boat or seaplane becomes possible. Boat transport can be quite quick and smooth, with good access to the patient during transfer. Care must be taken to ensure that a restless or confused patient does not upset the boat or plunge overboard.

Disadvantages of evacuation by water

Boats should be big enough and stable enough to be capable of transporting a patient. Weather, geographical, and biological hazards must be considered before the evacuation begins.

Documentation for a medevac

It is desirable that a companion travels with a casualty to ensure that they are properly supervised and to enable their condition to be communicated back to the expedition and to relatives at home. However, there are circumstances such as helicopter transfers where this will not be possible and it is essential that appropriate paperwork travels with the casualty. This should include:

- Passport and travel documents.
- Expedition and next of kin contact details.
- Insurance documents.
- Copy of any medical documents (e.g. pre-expedition medical questionnaire, and any assessment notes) (→ p. 21, p. 194).
- Incident report.
- Medical assessment and records of external advice received.
- Record of procedures.
- Medication chart and history of allergy.
- Investigations (e.g. malaria rapid diagnostic test).
- Observations and fluid balance chart and pain charts.
- Written instructions to accompanying personnel (if relevant) (→ ATMIST report, p. 159).

Other evacuation considerations

- Ensure you know the whole evacuation plan, from the patient leaving your location to arriving at a facility that can offer adequate care. Ensure any escort is aware of the planned destination. If possible, try to confirm the arrival of the casualty at a medical facility.
- If accompanying the patient, try not to do so alone. It can be a long and very tiring process. Try not to leave the casualty alone if medical facilities are basic. Carry enough money or credit cards with you to cover accommodation and travel; you can always be reimbursed later and, if possible, take communications such as a radio, mobile phone, or satellite tracking unit such as a Garmin inReach®.
- Take a translator with you if available and required.
- Take a medical kit.
- Take a grab bag with food, water, spare clothes, and wash kit. This will make the journey more comfortable.

Nursing and emotional care awaiting evacuation

Patients requiring evacuation need nursing care which might include:
- Clinical observations and patient monitoring.
- Assistance with personal hygiene.
- Assistance with nutrition/fluids.
- Pressure area care for unconscious/spinal injured patients.
- Dressing changes.
- Administration of medicines or IV fluids.
- Psychological and emotional support.

When nursing patients, try to provide care in a structured routine as this is both reassuring for the patient and helpful clinically.

- Clinical observations should be taken and documented as dictated by the severity of the illness/injury.
- Adhering to regular daily patterns, such as washing and mealtimes, normalizes the daily routine.
- Time the administration of medicines to maximize their clinical effectiveness (e.g. providing analgesia and antiemetics prior to sleep).
- Administration of fluids is generally easier when patients are normally awake.

Medical evacuation from an expedition has the potential to be a psychologically stressful event, for both patient and clinician. Stress can be caused by:

- Medevac method.
- Delays.
- Duration.
- Sick or unstable patients.
- Discomfort during medevac (e.g. overland transfers for patients with fractures).

Patients being evacuated from an expedition may feel dismayed over the prospect of permanently leaving the project site. Contributing to an expedition may have considerable financial implications and this financial loss may compound feelings of distress or frustration. In some instances, patients will dispute the need to be evacuated, or even refuse to leave (e.g. patients with psychosis or more determined personalities). Do not let these issues cloud clinical judgement or distract from the need for evacuation. Inexperienced medics or those providing care in 'high-pressure' situations should be especially aware of the potential for this issue.

It is advisable for the medic to work with the broader leadership team to make this decision, balancing medical needs with logistical realities and financial considerations. The use of independent advice to support these, often difficult, decisions is recommended.

Patients should be made as comfortable as possible during the evacuation. Keeping patients well informed will generally reduce stress levels, as will honesty over events, conditions, and treatment. Where appropriate, facilitating communication with home may help lessen fear and anxiety while at the same time provide reassurance through contact with loved ones. However, this should be balanced with minimizing the psychological stress likely to be caused to friends and relatives at home who are unlikely to know the full clinical picture.

During a medical evacuation, the overall aim is to maximize a patient's clinical condition and comfort, minimize or eliminate clinical deterioration, and ensure a thorough handover to definitive care.

See also ➔ Chapter 3.

Repatriation

Repatriation may use a dedicated air ambulance or a commercial airline. The patient will usually need to be escorted by an experienced aeromedical doctor or nurse. Such transfers are very expensive and it is essential that insurance covers this possibility.

Medical assistance companies

Because assistance companies will not start an evacuation or repatriation without guarantee of payment, most expeditions will initially contact a medical assistance company through their insurers. Most of the work of medevac organizations involves tourists and businessmen in destinations with good travel links rather than expeditions in remote regions, so their databases may not contain information on the capabilities of remote clinics/ hospitals, or on the logistical solutions to remote evacuations. Medevac organizations should be relied upon as a third level of support after help has been sought from the group's own medical expertise and the medical resources in-country.

Expeditions should do their own research on local medical facilities and the logistics and transport necessary to ensure a patient can get to an internationally recognized airstrip capable of receiving a medical team.

> *Medical Assistance companies include*
> - International SOS: ✍ http://www.internationalsos.com
> - Royal Flying Doctor Service of Australia: ✍ https://www.rfds.org.au/
> - AMREF: ✍ http://www.flydoc.org/
> - CEGA: ✍ http://www.cegagroup.com/
> - Healix: ✍ https://healix.com/
> - International Assistance Group: ✍ http://www.international-assistance-group.com/

Establishing a direct relationship with a medical assistance company is recommended, although this can be difficult as one normally is forced to negotiate through the insurance company. Once in direct contact, it is important to confirm the organization's capabilities and limitations. Check all contact numbers before departing on the trip and consider running a test to ensure the system works.

Telemedicine and communications

Telemedicine refers to the use of information and communication technology (ICT) to facilitate in the delivery of healthcare between two people at a distance from each other. It can be as simple as a phone call between medical practitioners about a case. Other examples include live videoconferencing between a patient and specialists, or a radiologist reporting an MRI scan sent by email from the other side of the world.

Telemedicine is a rapidly evolving area of medicine as access to the internet increases globally, the cost of ICT reduces, and more types of media can be digitalized. It has well-established uses in remote and developing areas of the world where healthcare is hard to access. Telemedicine can avoid the cost of patient transfers and specialist travel expenses, while in technologically advanced areas of the world patients can now have their blood sugar levels or cardiac rhythms monitored from home by specialists. In recent times, we have seen its use in attempts to slow down the spread of viral epidemics by reducing face-to-face contact and also in reducing the environmental impact of multiple car journeys to and from hospitals for appointments.

As telemedicine is expanding and changing quickly, caution is required by its users. It is an area of medicine with limited legislation and lacks international consensus on areas such as liability and cross-border jurisdiction where advice comes from a country with different health laws and standards to the country where the patient is based. There are also issues with information management and patient confidentiality. On a more practical level, telemedicine relies on having a reliable means of communication, which can be a problem if there are poor radio links or a very slow internet connection. There may also be problems maintaining equipment and finding adequately trained staff.

Telemedicine has exciting possibilities and it is conceivable that it will result in many more aspects of healthcare delivery moving away from clinical settings and into patients' homes.

Uses of telemedicine in expedition medicine

Telemedicine has obvious advantages for expeditions. Its use may avoid the cost of an evacuation and the disruption that arises from potentially losing key members of the expedition. It can reassuringly support relatively inexperienced expedition medics by giving them access to senior and specialist advice. The reality for most expeditions is that the budget and location will mean that the options for telemedicine will involve a relatively low-tech approach. Examples of its use in the field include:
- A non-medic on the expedition radioing from a satellite camp back to base camp to get advice from the expedition doctor.
- The expedition doctor emailing a specialist back home with a photo or video attachment for help with diagnosis.

Telemedicine—preparations before departure

A contact point for obtaining senior or specialist advice should be organized before departure. It may be a personal contact, ready made in the form of a senior medic that works for the expedition company, or from a commercial company that provides a telemedicine service.

It is important that the person giving advice understands the nature of the expedition and what facilities are available to you on the expedition. It is unhelpful being advised to get a CT scan as the investigation of choice by a specialist when you are a week away from the nearest hospital.

Before departure, ensure that the communication equipment that you are taking is working, and that you know how to use it. Consider battery life and whether it is robust enough for the environment and expedition. Ensure that you understand and can use any medical equipment supplied to you for the expedition in case you are advised to use it. It is worth training up at least one other member of the expedition to use the kit in case of your absence, or if you become the patient. Leave a definitive list of your equipment and medicines with your home base or telemedicine contacts so they can advise you knowing your actual resources (e.g. a list of the antibiotics you have in the group medical kit).

Telemedicine—in the field

Once you have arrived in country, test the systems that you have put in place—checking both that the communication equipment works and that your telemedicine contact is contactable.

Ensure that non-medics who might have to contact you for advice have a guide to assist in their questioning and examination of patients (→ p. 194) and that, to avoid unnecessary delay during the call, they know what sort of information you will seek from them.

Arranging a set report format makes communications as efficient as possible (see → ETHANE and ATMIST, p. 159). This may be useful for getting information to telemedicine contacts as well as receiving information from non-medics on expedition. Keep good records of telemedicine consultations, consider recording the call if able to do so. The use of dictation software on smartphones such as Pages® can be invaluable for keeping contemporaneous records. Remember the issue of confidentiality and think about what methods of communication are secure and which are not. Note what advice was given and by whom. These are as important as any other clinical record.

Contact with seniors back home may be on an as-required basis only, or it may be that a regular time is set to report back. Ensure both parties know what frequency of communication to expect and what to do in the event of a scheduled communication being missed.

Technologies for telemedicine

Radio

Likely to only be of use within the expedition itself but a useful way for the expedition medic to communicate with other parties in the expedition. Readability is not always reliable so it is important to have a pre-formatted report procedure to avoid loss of information. Radio use requires training and is not a secure method of communication, with other members of the expedition and outside parties potentially able to listen in.

Telephone

Could be landline, mobile, or satellite. Has the advantage of familiarity of use and with increasing global coverage likely to be the first port of call for many telemedicine consultations especially for when emergency advice is needed. As with talking to specialists on the phone at work back home, remember to orientate the caller to who you are, why you are calling, and keep information brief and to the point.

Satellite messaging

Garmin InReach® devices, which are satellite communication devices, can send and receive text messages with cell phones or email addresses anywhere in the world. They are a small, light, low-cost option for two-way communications without the voice calls that a phone or satellite phone provides.

Email and internet

May be an option out in the field and likely to be available from fixed base camps. Good option for when routine advice is required that can wait a day or two before a reply. Not all email accounts are secure so consider anonymizing information about individuals.

Attaching photos to emails is an excellent way to get information across for another opinion:

- Consider compressing photo files to reduce the time it takes for the recipient on the other end to download the attachment. However, ensure enough detail is left for them to study the photo properly.
- If photographing an injury or rash, for example, consider using a hand, ruler, or familiar object to portray scale to the reviewer.
- Plain X-rays can be photographed easily with a camera to create a digital form that can be emailed on for further opinion.
- In dental cases, the use of mirrors is invaluable in allowing the most hidden of tooth surfaces to be photographed.

If the internet bandwidth is wide enough, video files can be shared. This can be a useful way for someone to demonstrate how to perform a procedure to an expedition medic. Remember that there are many clinical demonstrations on video sharing websites.

Satellite phones

Satellite phones work in remote locations beyond the coverage of normal telephony and cellular networks. Satellite phones complement the use of international roaming on GSM cellular phones or the use of locally bought SIM cards to access in-country cellular networks.

Satellite phones work with one of three basic systems. A stationary phone can be aligned with a specific satellite (Inmarsat, BGAN); a mobile satellite phone can communicate with a specific satellite overhead (e.g. GlobalStar and Thuraya); or a satellite phone can transmit and receive to an array of orbiting satellites to give global coverage (e.g. Iridium). The Iridium network has been upgraded and bandwidths significantly improved in recent years.

Considerations before rental or purchase of satellite phones:

- Location: compare the coverage maps to see which system will work where you are going.
- Applications: decide what you need, from two-way voice communication to email and video conferencing, and then see which are supported.

- Accounts structure: decide on pre-pay or on account options and check how easy it is to top up a prepaid SIM card while you are away.
- Running cost: compare the airtime costs per minute.
- Power supply: plan a recharging system suitable for your planned area of usage, such as solar panels or lithium batteries in areas where mains electricity is not available.

Plan to protect your equipment from water, dust, and shock hazards with padded or waterproof cases. Pelican Products® cases and micro-cases are excellent.

If your project is dependent on satellite phone communications take more than one, and spare ancillaries.

Improve the functionality of email over slow satellite phone connections by using a specialist satellite email service such as UUPlus or other compression service. Check before departure whether the expedition is equipped to use a satellite phone as a modem to send emails or pictures so you know in advance the telemedicine capabilities.

Satellite phones are subject to restrictions or additional controls in some countries, including China, Cuba, India, Myanmar, and Russia. Check before leaving home. In some jurisdictions, possession of a satellite phone can result in a prison sentence.

Satellite tracking beacons

Satellite tracking beacons such as a Garmin inReach® allow remote tracking and two-way messaging. They can send and receive text messages with cell phones or email addresses anywhere in the world. They are a small, light, low-cost option for two-way communications without the voice calls that a phone or satellite phone provides. They are paired with a smartphone for ease of typing messages. They also have an SOS function and it is important to update the contact information for this as part of your trip planning.

Pocket Wi-Fi

Pocket Wi-Fi devices are another option to upgrade the utility of cellular phones while away on expedition. They enable Wi-Fi calling and provide increased security to your data compared to local public networks and work in 170 countries, but not everywhere.

Global cell phone

Cell phone systems work on different radio frequencies in different countries. Not all cell phones will work in every country even with a local SIM. Global cell phones allow you to use one phone number on your travels and mean you don't need to buy a local SIM.

Emergency beacons

The use of COSPAS-SARSAT emergency beacons as a method for expedition SOS alerting has been largely superseded by the development of satellite tracking beacons such as the Garmin inReach® which have many more functions.

COSPAS-SARSAT emergency beacons

The joint American–Russian SAR satellite system called COSPAS-SARSAT provides an international SAR network with global coverage for transmission-only emergency beacons. They use the 406 MHz frequency and the frequency is a useful way of identifying the type of beacon. The technology has a different name depending on where it is used:

- Aircraft carry ELTs.
- Ships carry EPIRBs.
- Personnel on the ground carry PLBs.

When a beacon is turned on to transmit its emergency distress signal, its signal is transmitted to a network of Mission Control Centres and then on to a Rescue Control Centre near the beacon's location. In some cases, no action will be taken so it is critical to ascertain what action will be taken and by whom in advance. These are for emergency use only, transmit-only alerting beacons and the response is organized by governmental agencies.

Along with location information, 406 MHz beacons transmit *information on* the type of beacon, the country code, and identification of the beacon. Using this information, SAR bodies can access contact details and information on the aircraft/ship from a beacon database.

All 406 MHz emergency beacons need to be registered before use. In the UK this is to the *EPIRB* Registry of the Maritime and Coastguard Agency. For countries that do not have a registration system, beacons can be registered at the International Beacon Registration Database (IBRD) at https://www.406registration.com

PLBs should only be used for life-threatening emergencies, as no qualifying information can be added. They are a useful item of last resort as a back-up to satellite phones.

Tracking beacons

Tracking beacons such as the Garmin inReach® can be used for GPS navigation, two-way messaging, non-emergency reporting, location monitoring and tracking, as well as having an SOS emergency distress signal. The key difference with the emergency distress signal is that with the non-governmental tracking beacons, the SOS goes to a private operations centre rather than government-run Rescue Control Centres. They will alert the pre-notified call list of your situation and the initial response can be arranged by the expedition's on-call contact in accordance with your expedition ERP.

Their low cost, small size, and utility of tracking beacons means that they have become a key item of equipment for wilderness and back-country use. Consider equipping each subgroup or team within an expedition with them, rather than just as an item of expedition leader equipment.

Before the expedition, check the emergency contacts are up to date, check the subscription and account settings, and check the privacy settings so the on-call contact and other home contacts can see where the unit is and message it.

VHF and HF radios

Two-way voice communications by radio are an important part of the communications system on many expeditions. VHF radios are for short-range local use; the range can be extended by using a more powerful base station at one site with handheld radios being used to call back to base, or to shore. VHF radios require little training, and some are licence-free in many countries. HF radios can be used over very large distances but require more training to operate and licensing.

If the expedition involves mobile subgroups working in the same area, then VHF radios will be very useful. In some situations, such as mountaineering on a peak with more than one team present at the same time, it is good practice to have a shared radio frequency so different teams can alert everyone on the mountain about a problem and a response can be coordinated.

Radio communications are not private, anyone in range on the same frequency can listen, so for medical communications or for passing confidential information it is useful to be able to switch to satellite phones or use the messaging of tracking beacons which, in normal use, are more secure.

Sexual assault

A sexual assault is defined as any type of sexual act committed without the informed consent of one of the parties. Incidents of this type are highly distressing to all involved. Both men and women can be subject of an assault, which may come from within the expedition group or occur during travel.

Expeditions—especially those involving groups of teenagers or young adults—should consider how they would respond if a member of the group claims to have been sexually assaulted. The response of local authorities in different jurisdictions can vary considerably and may not always be sympathetic to the complainant.

Management

Consider the four Ps as described in Table 5.3.

Table 5.3 The four Ps—management of sexual assault

Four Ps	Consider
Police	If patient wants police involvement this *must* be done first (any examination may compromise forensic examination). Consider asking your government representative for local help and advice
Pregnancy	Emergency contraception: • levonorgestrel as soon as possible (up to 72 h) • ulipristal acetate as soon as possible (up to 120 h) • Emergency intrauterine contraceptive device (IUCD) fitted up to 5 days (or day 19 of 28-day cycle)
Prophylaxis	Post-exposure prophylaxis following sexual exposure (PEPSE) for HIV (⊃ p. 543). Start within 72 h Consider prophylactic antibiotics to cover chlamydia, gonorrhoea, and trichomoniasis Doxycycline 100 mg twice daily for 1 week *or* azithromycin 1 g PO stat Ceftriaxone 500 mg IM stat (or other third-generation cephalosporin) *or* cefixime 400 mg stat *or* ciprofloxacin 500 mg stat *but* beware of high resistance worldwide Metronidazole 400 mg twice daily for 5 days *or* metronidazole 2 g stat If not vaccinated against hepatitis B, first dose can be given within 3 weeks to cover retrospectively. Rapid course of vaccine preferred (0, 7, 21 days, and 6 months)
Psychological	Strongly consider repatriation owing to likely physical and emotional trauma. Ongoing counselling may be required (⊃ p. 556)

Death on an expedition

Although death during an expedition is rare, expeditions need to have a follow through process for this eventuality included in their ERP (➲ p. 148). If an expedition member should die, then it is important that the death is dealt with sensitively, expeditiously, and in accordance with the legislative requirements of both the deceased's home country and the country where the death occurred. Local police and judiciary should be informed as quickly as possible—in some countries the location of an unexpected death will be considered to be a potential crime scene until the circumstances have been confirmed. Your local embassy or consulate should be able to offer support, advice, legal assistance, and communication links. The psychological sequelae following the death must be considered, with all the surviving team members involved in measures to minimize and prevent their immediate and long-term distress.

Following the death, a designated person within the group, in all likelihood the expedition MO, should coordinate the necessary actions:
- *Locate the body.* Take responsibility for locating the body and, if retrieval is possible, if advised by the local police, collect it and deliver it to the appropriate authorities to obtain a death certificate. This may involve packaging and transporting the body some considerable distance, a process that should be done quickly and with dignity. Other expedition members will be noting the response of the MO to the event.
- *Ensure there are no further injuries.* Make sure that the team is at no increased risk as a result of the death. If the death has occurred in a difficult physical location, then retrieval of the body may be necessary, but there should be minimal risk to the rest of the team in attempting recovery of the body.
- *Find out what happened.* Record the details as they are given and then check with all available sources to establish any other details that are known or gradually learned and compile these together into an accurate 'diary of events'.
- *Prevent possible infection.* If the person died of an infectious (or potentially infectious) disease, or if the cause of death is unknown, handle the body in a manner that minimizes the risk of infection spreading to other members of the expedition.

Reaction to the fatality

The MO needs to be aware of, and respond to, the impact of the fatality on the other expedition members.
- Symptoms develop after experiencing a stressful event of an exceptionally threatening or catastrophic nature.
- Sufferers involuntarily re-experience the event or aspects of this and this may be very real, frightening, and distressing.
- Victims have flashbacks/nightmares and may avoid triggers reminding them *or* return continuously to 'wonder why' it happened and how it could have been avoided (➲ Post-traumatic stress disorder, p. 558).

Practical considerations following the death

Once death has been confirmed

Communication needs to be sent to the expedition's headquarters informing them of the tragedy. Importantly for the families of other surviving members of the expedition, the information needs to note that other team members are safe and well.

Other expedition members need to be informed of the death (➔ Breaking bad news, p. 560) as soon as possible and collectively in a group so that the information is uniform and that there can be minimal misunderstanding.

The next of kin must be notified at the earliest opportunity. This should be done in person by two people representing the expedition; two people because the person advising of the death will need support and both together have a greater chance of giving support to the deceased's relatives. In many cases, police in the home country will inform the next of kin.

The family of the deceased should be offered immediate access to practical and social support, whether this be psychological to deal with the event, practical help with the funeral or, where possible, financial assistance via the insurers.

Legal responsibilities

- Urgently inform the embassy or consulate representative of the deceased person of the circumstances surrounding the death.
- Inform the embassy or consulate representative of other expedition members' situation and safety.
- Inform the police, particularly if there are legal issues about the death.
- Obtain a police report, for medical and legal purposes. This may be required by the deceased person's family at some later date.
- An autopsy may be required by the authorities.
- Contact insurance companies.
- Issue an appropriate report on the tragedy, for insurance purposes. This will need to be done in conjunction with the expedition leader.
- The MO will need to make comprehensive medical notes relating specifically to the death.
- Develop contacts between the insurance company and the local authorities who can organize repatriation.

Repatriation of the body

- Often the local embassy or consulate will assist with this process.
- It will include negotiations with local authorities, insurance, and transport companies.
- Keep an accurate diary of all events, the persons who were communicated with, and the times of these communications.

Dealing with the media

Prepare a statement or press release that can be used to respond to any media enquiries and prevent any incorrect reportage. This should be made available as quickly as possible to avoid mis-information about the tragedy.

Self-care for the medical officer and expedition leader

MOs and expedition leaders need to be proactive in caring for themselves should any untoward tragedy occur. This ideally could involve personal psychological first aid, and pre-travel counselling for untoward eventualities.

Caring for the group

(See also ➜ Psychological reactions to traumatic events, p. 558.)

- Consider needs of surviving team members and their families.
- Consider needs of concerned outsiders.
- Ensure regular opportunities for communication between team members and their families while on the expedition but try to discourage use of social media. It is better for families to receive information in a controlled and supportive manner than through poorly regulated social media.

After the expedition, ensure members are followed up at least twice over the following 2 months to ensure that there are no adverse psychological responses. Screen for symptoms of depression, excessive arousal, avoidance behaviours, intrusive phenomena, and dissociation. The emphasis here is on recognizing 'at-risk' individuals. If involved in the care of the deceased, the MO may have feelings of responsibility, guilt, or failure that need to be recognized.

Chapter 6

Emergencies: diagnosis

Chapter editor
Jon Dallimore

Contributors
Edi Albert
Jon Dallimore
Charlie Siderfin (1st edition)

This guide to the medical history taking, examination, and measurement of vital signs is designed to assist someone without medical training to obtain the necessary information to communicate effectively with a doctor over the radio, telephone, or internet.

For information on the initial management of an injured person, see ➲ Chapter 7.

For the initial management of serious medical conditions, see ➲ Chapter 8.

History and examination: an introduction for non-clinicians

There are three important aspects to the assessment of the ill patient:
- History—an account of how the illness developed.
- Examination—three modalities are used to examine:
  - Look.
  - Feel.
  - Listen.
- Monitoring—'vital signs' are measured to assess an individual's status and progress.

History

- Patient details—name, date of birth, and location/altitude.
- Document the time and date of examination.
- Write down the main problems.
- Use the patient's own words. Avoid technical medical terms—there is a danger of them being used incorrectly.
- Short history of the illness—a description of how the illness evolved over time. Give more details about any pain. Start from when the patient was last completely well and relate each symptom to time. For instance:
  - Last completely well yesterday.
  - Started to vomit 3 hours ago. Vomited five times—initially food.
  - Last vomit 15 min ago—yellow fluid.
  - Right-sided abdominal pain for 2 h.

Apparently unrelated symptoms can be important in reaching a diagnosis. A list of important questions can be found in Fig. 6.1 (⊃ p. 194).

Examination

Answer these questions from your own observations, not by asking the patient. Prior to the expedition, obtain training in the techniques of examination. Practise examining normal individuals so you can recognize abnormality. Try not to feel shy or embarrassed—you will do a sick person no favours if you fail to spot an important sign when examining. Examine the whole person carefully in the following order:
- General appearance.
- Hands.
- Face.
- Neck.
- Chest.
- Abdomen.
- Limbs.
- Nervous system.

- Look:
  - General well-being. Make an assessment as to whether the patient is generally well or unwell. Expose the patient and observe. Compare the left and right sides of the body for any asymmetry.

- Feel:
  - Warm your hands, be gentle but firm. While feeling, watch the patient's face for signs of pain.
- Listen:
  - Use a stethoscope or put your ear on the body to listen for breath and bowel sounds.
- Measure:
  - You should be able to make simple measurements to gauge the patient's condition. These include conscious level (ACVPU), breathing rate, oxygen saturations (using a pulse oximeter), temperature, pulse rate, and BP, if possible (⊃ p. 192).

General appearance

- Look:
  - At patient's expression—in pain, anxious, or confused.
  - At body posture—holding head, curled up in a ball, etc.
  - Condition of skin—pale, blue, sweating.
  - Assess breathing effort—struggling to breathe or weak.

Hands

- Look:
  - Sweating.
  - Temperature.
  - Shaking.
- Feel:
  - Skin—does it feel cold or sweaty?
- Measure:
  - Radial (wrist) pulse for rate, rhythm, and character (normal, bounding, or thready).

Face

- Look:
  - For abnormal colour or swelling of face and lips.
  - Inspect mouth and throat for ulcers, blisters, and redness.
  - Look at the tongue—is it dry, coated, or moist?

Neck

- Look:
  - For distended neck veins.
- Feel:
  - For lymph nodes and swellings in neck, cheeks, and back of head.
- Listen:
  - For abnormal sounds associated with breathing—snoring, stridor when breathing in, or wheeze.

Chest

Examine front and back of the chest:

- Look:
  - Breathing rate.
  - Compare chest movement on both sides.
  - Check for injuries to the chest wall.

- Feel:
  - Irregularities or crepitus (grating) of chest wall indicating broken ribs.
  - Chest wall tenderness (be gentle!).
- Listen:
  - Place stethoscope under the collar bone and then outside each nipple. Compare the sounds on each side.
  - Listen over the lungs at the back with the stethoscope and compare the sounds:
    o Normal.
    o Added sounds—wheeze or crackles?
    o Absent.

Abdomen

Make sure that your hands are warm. Ensure the patient is relaxed, lying on their back, head on one or two pillows, and the abdomen exposed:

- Look:
  - Swelling, discoloration, or bruising (especially over flank), scars from previous surgery, lumps (hernias) in the groins.
- Feel:
  - Place hand flat on abdomen and gently apply pressure with all four fingers by bending at the knuckles, keeping the fingers flat and straight.
  - Begin away from region of tenderness and move towards the area. Move methodically around the entire abdomen.
  - Feel for tenderness while watching the patient's face. Facial expression will often signal tenderness.
  - Tensing of the abdominal muscles (guarding) sometimes occurs with tenderness.
  - Ascertain if guarding is localized or generalized. In severe cases, the abdominal wall will be rigid, implying inflammation within the abdominal cavity (peritonitis) owing to bowel perforation or bleeding.
  - Be gentle but firm. If the patient is unable to relax their abdominal muscles, ensure your hands are warm and ask them to bend their knees up to relax the abdominal muscles.
- Listen:
  - Place the stethoscope 1 cm below the umbilicus (belly button) and listen for bowel sounds for 1 min.
  - Normal—gentle gurgling a few times per minute.
  - Increased—overactive bowel (e.g. diarrhoea or bowel obstruction).
  - Absent—may be observed in the later stages of peritonitis.

Limbs

- Look:
  - Areas of redness, swelling, or bruising.
  - Deformity—particularly shortening or abnormal position.
  - Joint swelling.
  - Pain on movement.
- Feel:
  - Tenderness.
  - Creaking or grating sensations.

Nervous system
- Look:
  - Assess ACVPU (➜ Disability, p. 222).
  - Note any speech difficulty. Ask the patient to say 'The early bird catches the worm'.
  - Check both eyes can move in all directions.
  - Look for asymmetry of the face—'Please show me your teeth'.
  - Assess pupils for size, asymmetry, and reaction to light.
  - Test power and sensation in all limbs. Place your hands in the patient's hands and ask them to squeeze your hands. Assess the strength of grip on each side. Ask the patient to lift their legs, then press up and down with their feet and again assess the strength of movements. Check that they can feel you touching their arms and legs.

Clinical measurements

Measuring body temperature
(See also ➡ p. 796.)
- Normal temperature: 36.5–37.5°C.
- Hypothermia: <35°C.
- Significant fever: >38.5°C.

Taking the pulse

Press gently with the pulp of the middle and index fingers. Count beats for a timed minute, or half a minute and multiply by two. Evaluate whether regular or irregular and note the pulse strength.
- Normal adult pulse at rest: 51–90 beats/min.

Radial (wrist) pulse
Feel with the fingers on the thumb side of the wrist.

Carotid (neck) pulse
Locate the larynx (Adam's apple) with your fingertips. Move your fingers across the neck until reaching the groove between the trachea (windpipe) and muscle edge. *Press gently.* Never feel the pulse on both sides of the neck at the same time as this will reduce the blood supply to the brain.

Femoral (groin) pulse
Press in the skin crease at the top of the leg halfway between the midline and the iliac crest (front of the pelvis).

Blood pressure

There is large variability in BP between different situations and individuals. It is an important measurement for monitoring a patient's progress over time.

Use of the sphygmomanometer
Automated BP measuring devices are reasonably inexpensive and widely available. However, basic versions of such machines will struggle to measure the BP if a patient has low BP or a slow pulse.

For those who have been taught how to use a manual sphygmomanometer, the following will act as a reminder:
- Wrap the sphygmomanometer cuff around the upper arm.
- Straighten the arm, palm up, and locate the brachial pulse on the inner aspect of the front of the elbow.
- Inflate cuff 20–30 mmHg above the point that the pulse disappears. Hold the stethoscope gently over the pulse. Listen for pulse and release cuff 3–5 mmHg per second.
  - Systolic pressure = level when pulse first heard.
  - Diastolic pressure = level when pulse muffles and disappears.

Estimating blood pressure using presence of pulses
- Radial pulse palpable: systolic BP >80 mmHg.
- Femoral pulse palpable: systolic BP >70 mmHg.
- Carotid pulse palpable: systolic BP >60 mmHg.

Capillary refill time (CRT)
Firmly press your thumb on a fingernail, toenail, or bony prominence such as the breastbone for 5 s. When the thumb is removed, the area will appear

white. If it takes >2 s for the colour to return, reduced circulation is im-plied. NB: this is not reliable when the patient is cold (compare with your own finger).

Measuring respiratory (breathing) rate

Count the RR over 1 min. Feel the pulse at the same time as the RR may alter if the patient is aware the RR is being measured.
• Normal adult RR at rest: 12–20 breaths/min.

Reduced level of consciousness

In the case of head injury, the ACVPU scale (→ Disability, p. 222) is a rough initial assessment. To monitor a patient's progress, chart the GCS (→ Table 7.2, p. 223). Minimum GCS score is 3, with maximum score of 15.

Three areas of basic brain function are tested and scored: eye opening, speech, and movement:
• Use increasing level of stimulus to obtain response.
• Speak.
• Tap the shoulders gently.
• Apply pain—squeeze the muscles at the base of the neck (trapezius).
• For scoring, see → p. 92.

A decrease in the GCS score indicates a deterioration in the patient's con-dition. Causes include:
• Bleeding.
• Brain swelling.
• Infection.
• Low oxygen levels.
• Shock.
• Abnormal blood sugar levels.
• Drugs that affect breathing.
• Stroke.
• Hypothermia.

Remember, if the patient deteriorates during your assessment, *immediately* re-check the ABC and rectify any life-threatening problems.

Monitoring
• Keep timed, written notes of the patient's condition.
• Chart vital signs hourly or more frequently. If very unwell, monitor every 15 min.
• Pulse.
• Temperature.
• BP.
• Saturations.
• RR.
• GCS—if previous head injury or concerns about level of consciousness.
• A model chart is given in Fig. 8.7 (→ p. 254).

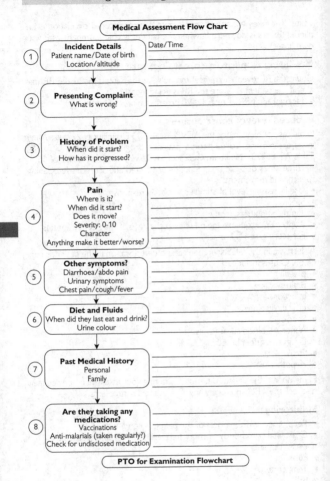

Medical Assessment Flow Chart

Date/Time

(1) Incident Details
Patient name/Date of birth
Location/altitude

(2) Presenting Complaint
What is wrong?

(3) History of Problem
When did it start?
How has it progressed?

(4) Pain
Where is it?
When did it start?
Does it move?
Severity: 0–10
Character
Anything make it better/worse?

(5) Other symptoms?
Diarrhoea/abdo pain
Urinary symptoms
Chest pain/cough/fever

(6) Diet and Fluids
When did they last eat and drink?
Urine colour

(7) Past Medical History
Personal
Family

(8) Are they taking any medications?
Vaccinations
Anti-malarials (taken regularly?)
Check for undisclosed medication

PTO for Examination Flowchart

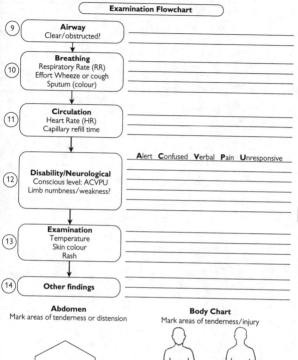

Examination Flowchart

⑨ **Airway**
Clear/obstructed?

⑩ **Breathing**
Respiratory Rate (RR)
Effort Wheeze or cough
Sputum (colour)

⑪ **Circulation**
Heart Rate (HR)
Capillary refill time

Alert **C**onfused **V**erbal **P**ain **U**nresponsive

⑫ **Disability/Neurological**
Conscious level: ACVPU
Limb numbness/weakness?

⑬ **Examination**
Temperature
Skin colour
Rash

⑭ **Other findings**

Abdomen
Mark areas of tenderness or distension

Body Chart
Mark areas of tenderness/injury

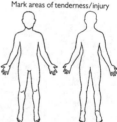

Fig. 6.1 Medical assessment flowchart.

Chapter 7

Emergencies: trauma

Chapter editor
Jon Dallimore

Contributors
Edi Albert
Spike Briggs
Jon Dallimore
Sundeep Dhillon (1st edition)
Stephen Hearns (1st edition)
David Lockey (1st edition)
Julian Thompson (1st edition)

Reviewer
Harvey Pynn

Initial response to an incident

(See also ➲ Chapter 5.) The ABC approach to patient assessment ensures that the most important life-threatening conditions are dealt with in the correct order.

- Ensure safety of scene, self, and casualty.
- Triage casualties if multiple victims.
- Control catastrophic bleeding.
- Airway (and cervical spine control where appropriate).
- Breathing and ventilation.
- Circulation.
- Disability.
- Environmental control and evacuation.

Triage

A major incident involving several casualties, such as an avalanche or RTC, stretches the resources of fully equipped emergency services. In the wilderness, it is easy to feel overwhelmed and helpless. However, developing and practising an effective triage and treatment system will enable as many people as possible to be treated and give later reassurance that everything possible was done.

The triage process aims to prioritize patients according to their medical needs given the resources available. This approach ensures that those requiring immediate treatment receive appropriate care, but also that limited resources are not diverted to treating an irreversible condition at the expense of other casualties. Triage principles should be applied whenever the number of casualties exceeds the resources of skilled rescuers available. It is a dynamic process where the state of the patients and environment may change, and available equipment will dictate the level of care available.

Priorities

Several systems are used internationally. The four priority groups are defined as follows (Table 7.1):

- P1. Immediate priority—casualties who require immediate life-saving interventions.
- P2. Urgent priority—casualties who require surgical or medical intervention within 2–4 h.
- P3. Delayed priority—less serious cases whose treatment can safely be delayed beyond 4 h.
- P1 Hold. Expectant priority—casualties whose condition is so severe that they cannot survive despite the best available care and whose treatment would divert medical resources from salvageable patients who may then be compromised.

When multiple casualties occur, remember that it is usually the still and silent person that needs the most urgent attention. Someone who is calling out may be distressed and in pain, but at least is conscious and has a clear airway.

Table 7.1 Triage classifications

Priority	Description	Label colour
P1	Immediate	Red
P2	Urgent	Yellow
P3	Delayed	Green
P1 Hold	Expectant	Blue
Dead	Dead	White or black

Casualties should, if possible, be regularly re-triaged. Triage categories can change at any time and are not fixed.

Triage sieve

This is a rapid, simple, safe, and reproducible method of prioritization based upon the Catastrophic haemorrhage, Airway, Breathing, Circulation (CABC) approach of resuscitation (Fig. 7.1).

Mobility
- Walking patients are initially categorized as P3, delayed priority.
- If the patient is not walking, then apply the ABC approach.

Airway
- Patients who cannot breathe despite simple airway manoeuvres (chin lift or jaw thrust) are dead.
- If breathing starts on opening the airway, the patient is P1, immediate.

Breathing
- Check RR. If RR >30 or <10 breaths/min then patient is P1, immediate.

Circulation
- Check capillary refill time (CRT) (➡ p 439).
- If >2 s then patient is P1, immediate.
- If CRT <2 s then patient is P2, urgent.
- Cold conditions may prolong CRT and comparison with the rescuer's CRT will allow adjustment.
- In extreme conditions or in the dark, CRT may be impossible to assess and a pulse rate of 120 beats/min can be used as the circulatory assessment or the presence/absence of a radial pulse.

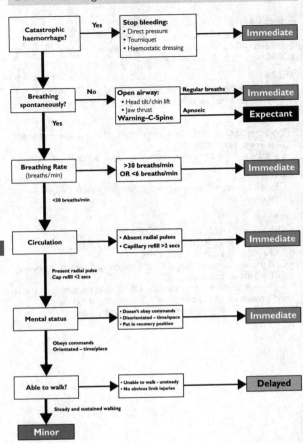

Fig. 7.1 Triage sieve.

Assessment of a casualty

Once the incident scene has been made safe, approach and evaluate the casualty. If you have the skills, follow Pre-hospital Trauma Life Support (PHTLS) guidelines. This text offers guidance to those without advanced resuscitation skills and suggests courses of action appropriate to the wilderness setting.

Assessment of the trauma victim

The assessment and management of the seriously injured patient in remote wilderness environments is extremely challenging. Problems include:

- Lack of equipment.
- Lack of skilled assistance.
- Prolonged transfer times to definitive care.

It should be made clear to everyone in the expedition group that the clinical interventions possible in remote environments are extremely limited compared to those that one would expect in urban environments in a developed country.

The key to managing any pre-hospital trauma is to perform basic assessments and interventions well and then transport the casualty safely and rapidly to a centre capable of providing definitive surgical and critical care. A properly prepared evacuation plan (medevac) will facilitate this process (→ p. 160).

Catastrophic bleeding

There may be major bleeding following some injuries, particularly ballistic trauma. In these rare cases, bleeding should be managed immediately using:
- Direct pressure.
- Topical haemostatic dressings.
- Tourniquets for limb haemorrhage.
- Pelvic binders for suspected pelvic fractures.

Airway

Provided there is no catastrophic haemorrhage, assessment and management of the airway is the first priority in the management of an injured casualty.

The main causes of airway obstruction are:
- Loss of muscle tone because of reduced conscious level, which can lead to the tongue falling back and blocking the throat.
- Blood and/or vomit in the airway.
- Anatomical distortion or swelling caused by direct facial trauma or burns.
- Think 'four Ts'—tongue, teeth, tissues, trauma.
- Trismus (tightly clenched jaw) during seizures or hypoxia.
- Initially ask the patient a question or get them to stick their tongue out. If they can speak or protrude their tongue, then the airway is patent and protected; and usually no further intervention is required. If you think there is a problem with breathing:
  - Look.
  - Listen.
  - Examine.

Inspection of the chest and neck may reveal that the patient is working hard to move air through a partially obstructed airway. If the airway is seriously blocked, the casualty, particularly their lips, may appear blue from cyanosis.

When listening to the airway one may hear gurgling or stridor (noise on breathing in). If the airway is obstructed and the patient is unconscious, the first thing to do is attempt to clear the obstruction with a jaw thrust. With both thumbs on the patient's cheek bones place the index fingers of both hands behind the angle of the jaw. Firmly lifting the jaw upwards will move the tongue away from the back of the throat, opening the airway. Try to minimize neck movements during this manoeuvre (Fig. 7.2).

Examine the airway. If there is fluid or vomit in the mouth or throat, this should be gently removed using a portable suction device. Alternatively, the patient should be log-rolled onto their side (➔ p. 163) while maintaining in-line cervical spine immobilization, to allow the fluid to drain with gravity. Inspect the mouth to see if there is foreign material in the throat.

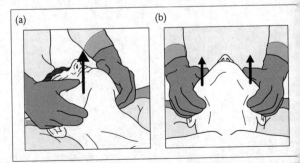

Fig. 7.2 Jaw thrust for airway management in trauma. Reproduced from Deakin CD et al. *Resuscitation.* 2010;81:1317, with permission from Elsevier.

Maintaining an open airway

Nasopharyngeal airways (NPAs)

Such airways are ideal during seizures when the teeth are clenched, preventing the use of oropharyngeal airways (OPAs). A 6–7 mm internal diameter airway is appropriate for most adults (use the size of the patient's nostril as a guide). Lubricate the tube well before insertion and apply gentle continuous pressure straight towards the back of the head, not upwards parallel to the ridge of the nose. Insertion can cause slight bleeding, but this should stop once the airway is in place. If one nostril seems very tight, try the other as nasal cavities are rarely symmetrical, or use a smaller size. Gentle rotation may help if the airway gets stuck at the back of the nose. The NPA is extremely useful in semi-conscious patients who will not tolerate an oral airway. Insertion of an OPA or NPA does not guarantee that the patient's airway will remain clear and the patient should be carefully observed. Jaw thrust may be needed in addition.

Oropharyngeal airways (OPAs)

Two types of basic airway adjuncts can be used to keep the airway open. The Guedel OPA is inserted into the mouth with the tip lying between the tongue and the back wall of the throat. An airway of this type is measured by placing it against the side of the patient's face before insertion. The length of the airway should be the same as the distance from the central incisor teeth (mouth in the midline at the front) to the corner of the jaw under the ear. Slide the curve of the airway over the tongue until the flange is against the lips. Do not trap lips or tongue between teeth and airway. If the victim's mouth is dry, it may be easier to insert the airway inverted, and then rotate gently as the tip reaches the back of the mouth. A size 2 (9 cm) is usually appropriate for adult females and a size 3 (10 cm) for males.

A semi-conscious patient may not tolerate an OPA; do not persist in trying to insert the device as it may cause the patient to vomit. Consider removing the OPA and placing the patient in the recovery position or use a nasopharyngeal airway instead.

Endotracheal tubes/supraglottic airways (LMAs, i-gel™)

Airway manoeuvres and basic adjuncts help to maintain the airway in the majority of seriously injured patients but do nothing to prevent aspiration of regurgitated stomach contents. Definitive airway maintenance and protection can only be achieved by the insertion of a cuffed endotracheal tube, or to a lesser extent, by the insertion of a supraglottic device. If an injured patient is so obtunded that an endotracheal tube or supraglottic device can be inserted without the use of anaesthetic drugs, the patient's chance of survival is very low. Endotracheal tubes and supraglottic airways can be misplaced, leading to airway obstruction, spasm of the vocal cords, vomiting, bradycardia, and raised intracranial pressure.

Only personnel who both understand and can correct these problems should use these airway adjuncts.

Surgical airways

Surgical cricothyroidotomies, or tracheostomies, are indicated in patients whose upper airway obstruction cannot be relieved by other means, such as victims of burns or serious facial injuries. Cricothyroidotomy should only be performed by appropriately trained personnel but its need can be anticipated in circumstances where the clinical situation typically deteriorates steadily, such as serious airway burns. An expedition medical kit is unlikely to include a cricothyrotomy kit; in dire circumstances consider using a narrow-bladed knife or scalpel together with the barrel of a ball-point pen or the sharp end of an IV fluid giving set.

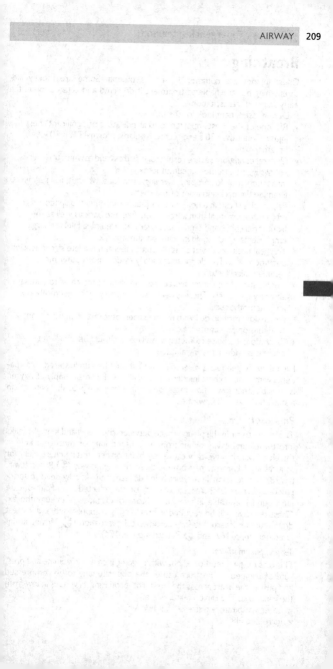

Breathing

Chest injuries are common in serious trauma. Some are rapidly life-threatening but amenable to treatment if detected and acted upon in the early stages of resuscitation.

During assessment look for the following:

- RR: one of the most important clinical indicators of significant chest injury. Count over 30 s and record regularly. Normal RR is 10–20 breaths/min.
- General condition: severe respiratory distress and asymmetrical air entry suggest a tension pneumothorax.
- Inspection: look for bruising, swelling, abrasions, wounds, flail segments. Examine the back and front of the chest.
- Palpate the chest: in a noisy pre-hospital environment, palpation is often more practical than auscultation. Feel the back as well as the front for crepitus and tenderness over fractured ribs. Feel for surgical emphysema which could indicate pneumothorax.
- Tracheal position: deviation is difficult to feel and is a late sign in tension pneumothorax. The diagnosis is usually evident from other more reliable clinical features.
- Auscultation: listen in the axillae, not the front of the chest to compare air entry effectively. There is decreased air entry with pneumothorax and haemothorax.
- Percussion: may be dull with massive haemothorax. Hyper-resonant with tension pneumothorax.
- Saturation: if a pulse oximeter is available—should be >95% but decreases with increasing altitude.

High-flow oxygen (via a reservoir mask) should be administered to all patients with serious chest injuries if it is available. If a small supply of oxygen is available, then lower flow rates for a longer time are probably better than a short burst at high flow rates.

Pneumothorax

This refers to air in the pleural space between chest wall and lung. Air leaks into the pleural cavity either from a damaged lung or through a hole in the chest wall. It is typically caused by blunt or penetrating chest injury, or as a result of barotrauma from rapid ascent when diving (→ Barotrauma, p. 778), but occasionally—typically in tall, lean men—it may develop spontaneously. There is decreased air entry on the affected side. Point-of-care ultrasound, if available, is a very useful tool for diagnosis of pneumothorax. Chest drainage will be required if breathing is compromised and a chest drain must be inserted before aeromedical evacuation (→ Moving an injured person, p. 162, and → Repatriation, p. 174).

Tension pneumothorax

This is as for pneumothorax, but with ongoing increase in volume and pressure of trapped air. Pressure causes the opposite lung to be compressed and pushes the heart across the chest, compromising its venous inflow from the vena cava. The clinical features are:

- Severe respiratory distress—'air hunger'.
- Increased HR.

- Reduction in BP.
- Hyper-resonance when percussing the affected side.
- Cyanosis may develop when the condition is severe.

Tension pneumothorax requires urgent needle decompression followed by formal chest drainage.

Needle decompression of tension pneumothorax

Use a large-bore cannula attached to a syringe partially filled with fluid. Insert the cannula at right angles to the skin, through the second intercostal space in the midclavicular line, just above the third rib, to avoid the vessels and nerve that run immediately below the second rib.

Aspiration of air indicates that the cannula tip has entered the pneumothorax.

If no air is aspirated:

- Either the diagnosis was wrong.
- Or the cannula has been occluded by a 'fat plug' (blow a few millilitres of air or sterile saline through the cannula).
- Or the chest wall is deeper than the needle is long. If the diagnosis is still suspected, then try again in the fourth or fifth intercostal space in the anterior–axillary line.

After aspiration of air, remove the syringe and tape the cannula in position. If available, insert a formal chest drain attached to an underwater seal or a Heimlich valve (Fig. 7.3).

ThoraQuik® is a purpose-built device for decompressing a tension pneumothorax in the pre-hospital environment. This may be available in certain situations and is straightforward to use after very little training (% http://www.youtube.com/watch?v=4aAXDbOUCeg).

Other devices are also available—Russell PneumoFix®-8 or PneumoFix®. A tension pneumothorax can often redevelop, especially when the patient is moved, and may require further decompression—leave the original cannula *in situ*.

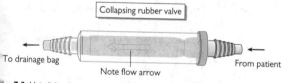

Fig. 7.3 Heimlich valve.

Chest drain insertion

This procedure should only be undertaken by those with prior training and experience and where essential, e.g. prior to air evacuation.

- Equipment required: local anaesthetic (lidocaine 1%), syringes, needles, scalpel, antiseptic solution, sterile gloves, artery forceps for blunt dissection, adhesive tape, chest drain (size 28–32), Heimlich valve or underwater seal set with water, suture material.
- Place the patient at 30–60° with patient's arm above head.
- Identify the site for incision—the fourth or fifth intercostal space in the anterior axillary line. Avoid breast tissue.
- Clean the skin and infiltrate local anaesthetic down to the pleura.
- Using the scalpel make a 3 cm incision directly above the rib.
- Bluntly dissect down to the pleura with artery forceps and insert a gloved finger through the pleura.
- While keeping the finger in the hole, slide the chest tube beside the finger (trocar removed). This is easier if the end of the chest tube is attached to one jaw of an artery forceps.
- Push the tube into the chest and direct the tip towards the apex of the lung. Ensure all the drain holes are in the pleural cavity.
- Attach the Heimlich valve or underwater seal (Fig. 7.4). Look for condensation in the tube or swinging of water in the underwater seal apparatus.
- Fix the tube firmly to the skin using sutures. Avoid a purse suture which may cause unsightly scarring.
- Apply gauze swabs to the skin at the base of the tube and tape in position.

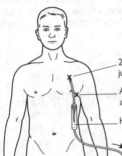

2nd intercostal space mid-clavicular line just above 3rd rib

Alternative position 5th intercostal space anterior axillary line

Heimlich valve

To drainage bag

Fig. 7.4 Chest drain with Heimlich valve.

Haemothorax

Following blunt or penetrating chest injury, blood leaks into the space between the chest wall and lung, usually from damaged intercostal vessels. The bleeding often stops following formal chest drainage and re-inflation of the lung. The bleeding may be associated with a pneumothorax—the chest may be dull to percussion over the blood-filled area; bleeding can be massive and lead to hypotension.

Flail chest

If multiple adjacent ribs are fractured in two or more places, there is a free-floating segment of chest wall that moves inwards with inspiration instead of outwards (paradoxical movement). This injury is typically caused by blunt chest trauma and is always associated with significant underlying pulmonary contusion.

Clinical features:
- Increased RR.
- Visible flail segment (may not be obvious clinically).
- Palpable crepitus.
- Painful breathing—use paracetamol and NSAIDs for pain relief.

Splinting the flail segment with tape may improve both discomfort and breathing. Lidocaine patches may help to relieve pain.

Urgent evacuation from the field will be required as bleeding and lung infection are common.

Sucking chest wound

This refers to an open wound through the chest wall as a result of penetrating chest injury. Air preferentially moves through the hole rather than the trachea with inspiration if the diameter of the hole is ≥2/3 of the diameter of the trachea (typically around 1 cm).

Clinical features:
- Sucking wound.
- Decreased air entry on the affected side.
- Severe respiratory distress.

Cover the wound with an occlusive dressing sealed on three sides to prevent tension pneumothorax developing. The Bolin Chest Seal®, Russell Chest Seal™, and Asherman Chest Seal® are designed for sucking chest wounds in the pre-hospital environment.

Insert a chest drain then seal the wound completely.

All patients with suspected or actual chest injury will require evacuation. *All patients with a real risk of pneumothorax must have a chest drain inserted before air evacuation.*

Circulation

Major haemorrhage in the seriously injured casualty can be from any of five places: 'blood on the floor and four more', i.e. external bleeding or bleeding into the chest, abdomen, pelvis, or thighs. Much can be done to arrest bleeding from wounds or closed long bone fractures but little can be done outside of the operating theatre to arrest haemorrhage in the other three sites. Rapid evacuation to a hospital with surgical facilities is therefore essential in these patient groups.

Assessment of circulatory status:
- HR: may be raised with blood loss (≥120 beats/min) but may be raised in the absence of blood loss due to pain or anxiety.
- BP: owing to compensatory mechanisms in young healthy adults, there may be significant blood loss before the BP falls. Beware of a false sense of security with a normal BP.
- Peripheral perfusion: very useful in a warm environment to indicate circulatory failure. It is not as useful in cold environments as this may be a response to the environment rather than any blood loss.
- Peripheral pulses: absence of a palpable radial pulse indicates significant blood loss.
- Mental status: hypovolaemia leading to reduced cerebral perfusion leads to confusion and reduced conscious level.
- Bleeding source: look for wounds and haematomas. Examine chest, abdomen, and pelvis. Examine long bones, especially femurs. Don't forget the back and scalp.

All patients should receive oxygen if available, at least initially. Minimize movement by planning the 'patient packaging' process in advance. Unnecessary movements may cause blood clots which have formed to dislodge, worsening haemorrhage. Most clotting factors are used in the formation of the initial clot. Give adequate pain relief and attempt to reassure the patient; this will reduce catecholamine release. Keep the patient warm. Hypothermia worsens clotting and increases haemorrhage.

Arrest external haemorrhage with direct pressure, dressings, and elevation (Box 7.1). Bleeding wounds, especially scalp wounds, may require urgent suturing. In cases of life-threatening bleeding from limb injuries, initially apply very firm pressure over the wound but, if this fails to stem the flow, apply a proximal tourniquet such as the Combat Application Tourniquet® (CAT®). A number of commercially available compounds are available which can be applied to wounds to promote clotting. They are currently in use with many military medical services and may be of use in certain remote expedition settings (e.g. Celox® and QuickClot®). These are used in combination with direct pressure.

Limb injuries should be splinted to promote clot formation and decrease pain. Femoral fractures can result in up to 1.5 L of blood loss. Traction splints act to reduce haemorrhage by reducing soft tissue damage and reducing the volume of the thigh compartment, hence increasing pressure and reducing bleeding.

Open fractures should be reduced if possible. They should be covered with clean, saline-soaked dressings and broad-spectrum antibiotics administered, e.g. co-amoxiclav or ceftriaxone (➜ Table 28.1, p. 856).

Pelvic fractures can cause fatal haemorrhage. Examination and movement should be minimized to promote clot formation. A splint should be applied to stabilize the fracture. These can be commercially designed splints (e.g. SAM Sling®) which should be placed at the level of the greater trochanters or improvised with a sheet wrapped firmly around the pelvis. The aim is to return the pelvis to its normal anatomical position, not to tighten the splint as much as possible. First, secure the ankles with feet pointing upwards using a figure of eight, then the knees should be slightly flexed and tied together (with padding between). If a pelvic fracture is suspected it should be treated as such, splinted, and not re-examined until the patient reaches hospital. For an improvised pelvic binder, see: ℘ https://www.crisis-medic ine.com/improvised-pant-leg-pelvic-binder/ and colour plates 21–23.

In recent years there has been a shift away from routinely administering large amounts of IV fluids to injured patients. A normal physiological response to bleeding is for the BP to fall, reducing flow through damaged vessels and tissues and so allowing clots to form. The remaining blood circulating has a high concentration of haemoglobin and may be sufficient in volume to allow perfusion of the vital organs if peripheral vasoconstriction has occurred. Administering IV fluids does not increase the oxygen-carrying capacity of the blood but does increase the BP. This may dislodge clots which have formed, causing further loss of haemoglobin. IV fluids, especially colloids, also adversely affect coagulation, again increasing bleeding.

Established pre-hospital trauma management practice is *not* to administer fluids if the patient has a palpable radial pulse. If the radial pulse is not palpable, normal saline is titrated in 250 mL boluses until the radial pulse returns (NICE guidelines, 2004). The evidence supporting this 'permissive hypotension' is mostly based in urban environments with short times from injury to definitive surgical care to arrest bleeding. Its use in remote environments is not proven but is likely to be appropriate when blood transfusion is not available and fluid supplies are limited.[1]

Tranexamic acid (TXA) has been shown to reduce mortality in major trauma provided that it is administered in the first 3 h after injury. Do not give to anyone with known sensitivity to the drug. Give a loading dose of 1 g (10 mL) 1 mL at a time over 10 min. Faster injection can cause nausea, vomiting, or convulsions. Subsequent doses may be given by infusion, but seek advice from a base hospital as the casualty will require urgent evacuation. TXA can be given to children of any age involved in trauma—the dose is 15 mg/kg.

Box 7.1 Control of haemorrhage

1. Direct pressure to the bleeding point

This should be tried first for all external bleeding and is effective in most cases. It may be ineffective if the bleeding vessel is not 'within reach' of pressure (e.g. deep in a wound). In this case, consider 'packing' the wound firmly from the base upwards using gauze/sterile bandage material.

2. Elevation of the affected limb/site of bleeding may also slow flow

Elevation is less effective when big vessels are damaged. Avoid raising legs if there are suspected pelvic, lumbar spine, or leg fractures/injuries.

3. Using a tourniquet

A tourniquet is indicated when direct pressure to a bleeding point may be ineffective for any reason. It can be used to 'free hands' from having to apply such sustained direct pressure. It is generally used when major arteries have been severed and have retracted beyond reach or where the area of tissue disruption in a limb is extensive (e.g. avulsions or ballistic injury).

Always apply above the knee (for lower limb injuries).

You can increase efficacy by helping apply directed pressure (i.e. a packed pad over the artery). Pad a little beneath the tourniquet to prevent skin damage.

Use a commercial tourniquet or improvise:

- A strip of cloth 5–10 cm wide. A waist belt could be used.
- Tie around limb loosely and tie a half-knot.
- Slip to 5–10 cm above the wound (and above the joint if the injury is distal).
- Put a stick over the half-knot and complete the tie.
- Rotate the stick as a 'windlass' until the bleeding stops.
- Leave on for at least 30 min. Use this time to try to identify the bleeding point and directly pack/compress. Do not 'dig and dab'; clot must be left to stabilize.
- Slowly release the tourniquet and observe. If bleeding continues, reapply the tourniquet.

Neck and other spinal injuries

Neck and other spinal injuries

Suspected spinal injuries cause great anxiety for mountain rescue teams and during expeditions to remote areas. Data from the Bangor Mountain Medicine Project indicate that half of mountain trauma casualties in Snowdonia have a mechanism of injury that would mandate spinal immobilization in urban pre-hospital practice. However, only about 2% of mountain casualties *found alive* after a significant mechanism of injury had an unstable spinal fracture.

Spinal cord injury is relatively rare, but remains a potentially devastating injury. However, irrational fear should not overrule clinical judgement and the use of common sense. There are a number of key messages that any practitioner in a remote or wilderness setting must understand.

- 'Neck injury', 'broken neck', and 'spinal cord injury' are not synonymous.
- Most victims sustaining a neck injury will simply have a soft tissue injury (⊃ p. 326).
- A small minority may have a stable compression or avulsion type fracture with no threat to the spinal cord.
- An even smaller proportion will have an unstable fracture that has caused damage to the spinal cord.

Spinal injuries most frequently occur at junctions of mobile and fixed sections of the spine (C6,7/T1, T12/L1). In patients with multiple injuries who have a spinal injury, over half will have a cervical spinal injury. Approximately 10–15% of patients with one spinal fracture will be found to have another.

Spinal cord injury must be considered in the following circumstances:

- High-speed injuries (RTCs, falls, or falling objects striking the victim's head).
- Patients with multiple injuries.
- Patients with head injuries.
- Unresponsive patients who have suffered trauma.

It is now known that damage to the spinal cord takes place either at the time of the injury or during a later phase as a result of bleeding and soft tissue swelling at the site of the fracture. While victims with suspected spinal injury must be handled carefully, unfounded fears of making the damage worse should not prevent the rescuer or medic from making sensible on-site decisions. In an expedition or wilderness setting, the decision to immobilize and evacuate a patient should not be made lightly as it can have significant resource and safety implications for the patient's companions and for organized rescuers. The patient may initially be treated for a spinal injury, but this can be reviewed once other injuries have been treated and the patient is warm and comfortable. However, clearing the spine clinically, especially in higher-risk patients, must not be undertaken lightly.

Assessment

Assessment of the cervical spine in a conscious patient takes place as an extension of the primary survey described previously. Remember that Advanced Trauma Life Support (ATLS) guidelines clearly state that airway management takes precedence over cervical spine control. Two prospectively validated decision-making tools are commonly used to assess the cervical spine: Canadian C-spine, and National Emergency X-Radiography Utilization Study (NEXUS) guidelines. While the former has been shown to have a slightly higher sensitivity in a conventional setting, the more restrictive criteria, and the differing context and population, make the latter the more logical choice for the expedition or wilderness context. See Fig. 7.5.

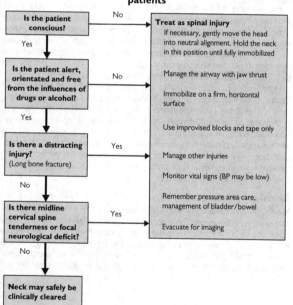

NEXUS low-risk criteria for trauma patients

Is the patient conscious? — No → **Treat as spinal injury**
If necessary, gently move the head into neutral alignment. Hold the neck in this position until fully immobilized

Yes ↓

Is the patient alert, orientated and free from the influences of drugs or alcohol? — No → Manage the airway with jaw thrust

Immobilize on a firm, horizontal surface

Yes ↓

Is there a distracting injury? (Long bone fracture) — Yes → Use improvised blocks and tape only

Manage other injuries

No ↓

Monitor vital signs (BP may be low)

Is there midline cervical spine tenderness or focal neurological deficit? — Yes → Remember pressure area care, management of bladder/bowel

Evacuate for imaging

No ↓

Neck may safely be clinically cleared

Fig. 7.5 Assessment of patients with trauma using NEXUS low-risk criteria.

Using the NEXUS low-risk criteria
- Exercise extreme caution using this approach in young children or the elderly.
- *Distracting injury* means an injury where the pain is sufficiently severe that it distracts the patient from the assessment process. If the patient can cooperate with your assessment without difficulty, then no distracting injury is present.
- Often it is the 'mid-line tenderness' criterion that clinicians find the most difficult to assess. Many patients with neck pain will have tenderness in the para-spinal muscles. Ensure that it is mid-line bony tenderness that you are testing. If in doubt act conservatively and reassess later.
- Neurological assessment for NEXUS purposes is limited to assessing upper and lower limb motor function.

Patients who are clinically cleared should be managed as for a neck sprain (→ p. 327).

Patients who fail the NEXUS criteria must be assumed to have a cervical spine injury. Avoid turning these patients unless penetrating trauma or significant haemorrhage is suspected as the outcome of the examination will not change management. If examination of the back is indicated, they should be lifted vertically with a 'straddle lift' with spinal alignment carefully maintained. Further neurological assessment can be delayed until the patient reaches definitive care as it does not change management.

In patients who can be cleared clinically, the question of a thoracic or lumbar spine fracture is still valid. Patients with a fracture will complain of severe pain in the back, and those with lumbar spine fractures may have complained of pain and difficulty performing a straight leg raise during assessment. A log roll should be performed unless pelvic or femoral fractures are suspected. Midline bony tenderness would be expected with a fracture, but may be absent in anterior wedge fractures of the vertebral body. Patients with neurological signs or suspected fracture must be immobilized, preferably with a vacuum mattress.

Spinal immobilization

Ideally, cervical spine immobilization should consist of blocks or sand bags and tape, with the patient lying supine on a firm but padded surface. Rigid spine boards are for short-term use to extricate patients only. They should not be used for long-term transport or ongoing patient care as they are uncomfortable and may cause pressure areas. Improvised spinal immobilization must be effective—inadequate splinting is falsely reassuring for rescuers.

Hazards of spinal immobilization

Spinal immobilization has been a component of immediate aid protocols for many years. However, an evidence-based review by the Wilderness Medical Society (2013) has highlighted the paucity of evidence for its benefits, and the potential risks of the procedure in remote areas when transfer to hospital care will take time. A spinal board or neck collar may force a casualty into inappropriate positions, and increase the risks of inhalation of vomit, pain, pressures sores, and breathing problems. Those interested in learning more should read the full guidelines.[2]

2 http://www.wemjournal.org/article/S1080-6032(13)00071-9/pdf

Disability

Assess the casualty's level of consciousness (disability) using the ACVPU scale:
- Awake and alert.
- Confused—new confusion
- Verbal—responds to voice ('Squeeze my hand').
- Pain—responds to pain.
- Unresponsive—no response to painful stimulus.

To monitor a patient's progress, chart the GCS (Table 7.2). Minimum GCS score = 3, with maximum score of 15. Three areas of brain function are tested and scored: eye opening, speech, and movement. Use an increasing level of stimulus to obtain a response:
- Speak: 'Are you okay? What's your name?'
- Tap the shoulders gently: 'Squeeze my hand'
- Apply pain: press firmly over the muscles at the side of the neck—trapezius squeeze.

Any decrease in the GCS score is significant and may indicate deterioration in the patient's condition. Motor responses <4 are very significant. Causes of reduced conscious level include:
- Bleeding.
- Swelling.
- Infection.

Remember, if the patient deteriorates during your assessment *immediately* re-check the ABC and rectify any life-threatening problems.

Table 7.2 Glasgow Coma Scale

	Score
Eye opening	
Open spontaneously	4
Open to verbal command	3
Open to pain	2
No response	1
Verbal response	
Talking and orientated	5
Confused, not orientated	4
Inappropriate words	3
Incomprehensible sounds	2
No response	1
Motor response	
Obeys commands	6
Localizes pain	5
Flexion/withdrawal	4
Abnormal flexion	3
Extension	2
No response	1

Reproduced from *The Lancet*, 304:7872, Teasdale G, Jennett B. Assessment of coma and impaired consciousness, pp.81–84, Copyright (1974), with permission from Elsevier.

Exposure and environmental control

It is important to examine the patient thoroughly and protect them from exposure to the elements.

A seriously injured patient, especially one with a reduced conscious level, may have life-changing injuries which are not obvious during the initial stages of resuscitation. This is because pain from them may be masked by more serious injuries, or the clinician involved is concentrating on immediately life-threatening problems. Such injuries might include peripheral joint dislocations or eye injuries which may lead to lifelong disability if not detected and corrected in the early stages. A systematic head-to-toe examination ('secondary survey') is necessary to seek and identify these injuries.

During and after the secondary survey the patient should be adequately insulated, particularly from the cold ground, and protected from the external environment using a group shelter.

Secondary survey

The aim of a primary survey is to simultaneously identify and treat life-threatening problems. A secondary survey is a methodical head-to-toe search for all the injuries that may be present. It may be possible to conduct a full secondary survey where the patient is found, but in a wilderness setting it is likely that the patient will need to be protected from the environment using a group shelter or tent. If the patient must be moved remember the possibility of spinal injury and try to conduct a limited secondary survey first.

In injury cases take a brief history. Remember:

AMPLE

- **A**—allergies.
- **M**—medicines.
- **P**—past medical history.
- **L**—last meal time.
- **E**—events leading to the injury.

Examination

When in a warm, dry, and safe environment, the casualty should be undressed to enable a complete head-to-toe examination. Examine the whole body: front, back, and sides in the following order:

1. Head.
2. Neck.
3. Chest.
4. Abdomen.
5. Pelvis.
6. Legs.
7. Arms.
8. Spine.

General appearance

- Skin colour—pale or blue (cyanosed).
- Dehydration.
- Sweating.
- Body temperature.

Examination of the head

- Scalp: bleeding, swelling, bruising.
- Conscious level: assess ACVPU or measure the GCS (➲ Table 7.2, p. 223).
- Eyes: pupil size/reaction to light. Normal vision?
- Nose: look for deformity, discharge (?cerebrospinal fluid (CSF) leak), bleeding (➲ p. 357).
- Ears: discharge (?CSF leak), bleeding.
- Face: feel face on both sides looking for deformities and tenderness. Is there a fractured jaw?
- Mouth: does the breath smell (alcohol)? Any broken teeth?

Examination of the neck

- The patient may complain of limited or painful neck movements or limb tingling/weakness.
- Look and feel for any 'step', swelling, or midline tenderness.

Examination of the chest

- Look for laboured breathing, tracheal deviation, asymmetrical chest movements (flail chest), open wounds, bruising, impaled objects, or signs of a tension pneumothorax (➲ p. 210).
- Is there tenderness on gentle rib springing? Only do this if there is no obvious external injury.
- Listen for reduced air entry, listen under the collarbone and outside the nipple on each side.

Examination of the abdomen/pelvis

- Look for bruising, open wounds.
- Feel in all four quadrants for localized tenderness.
- Listen for bowel sounds.
- Gently feel the pelvis *once only* to elicit pain/movement.

Examination of the limbs

- Look for bruising, swelling, deformity, wounds, shortening, crepitus.
- If injuries are found check Movement, Circulation (pulses), and Sensation: M, C, + S.

Examination of the spine

- If a spinal injury is suspected do not move the patient unnecessarily— log roll and use in-line spinal immobilization (➲ p. 163).
- Look for loss of movement or sensation. Feel for swelling, tenderness, 'step'.
- In high neck injuries, diaphragmatic breathing may be present and in males an involuntary erection of the penis (priapism) indicates a high-level spinal injury (above T6).

Continuing care

(See also ➋ Chapters 3 and 5.) Subsequent care will depend upon:
- Severity of the injuries.
- Condition of the patient.
- Urgency of evacuation.
- Ease of evacuation.

Isolation or adverse weather conditions will mean that the expedition team may have to care for a casualty for several days. During this time, you will have to provide effective nursing care:
- Regular observations to give warning if the patient's condition deteriorates and they develop shock (➋ p. 250).
- Pain relief (➋ p. 616).
- Nutrition and fluids as possible.
- Warmth.
- Personal needs and hygiene, including toileting.
- Good nursing to avoid pressure areas.
- Psychological support (➋ p. 556).

Blast and gunshot injuries

Blast and gunshot injuries are common in some parts of the world. Explosions can be caused by vehicle accidents, gas cylinders, in some industrial environments (e.g. mining), or, more commonly, in wars and acts of terrorism. There may be multiple casualties after an explosion.

Safety is paramount at the scene of a bombing or shooting incident. Ensure that there is no ongoing threat to the patient or rescuers.

Explosions cause injury in six ways:
1. Blast wave.
2. Blast winds.
3. Fragmentation.
4. Flash burns.
5. Crush.
6. Psychological.

Blast wave

This is a momentary front of overpressure formed by compression of air at the interface of the rapidly expanding sphere of hot gases. Injuries are caused by a combination of body compression followed by disruption of tissues at air/tissue interfaces—particularly in the lungs, gut, and ears. The lungs are commonly affected in two ways—intra-alveolar haemorrhage and pneumothoraces (→ p. 211). These can be rapidly fatal or lead to adult respiratory distress syndrome. Bowel haemorrhage and perforation may develop several days after the initial injury. The ear drums are often ruptured but will depend on the angle of the blast wave.

The overpressure can be multiplied several times over when the pressure wave is reflected by walls, ceilings, or water.

Air can enter the pulmonary circulation and result in fatal air emboli.

Blast winds

These are rapidly moving columns of air which follow the blast wave. They can be powerful enough to dismember or even disintegrate a person close to the explosion. Casualties further away can sustain traumatic amputations and can be thrown against solid objects which will cause deceleration injuries and fractures from the impact.

Blast injuries should be treated following the usual principles of Catastrophic haemorrhage, Airway, Breathing, Circulation, Disability, Exposure and environmental control (CABCDE) assessment and management.

Fragmentation missiles and bullets

Most injuries after an explosion are caused by fragmentation. The missiles are primary (from the bomb casing or nails, bolts, or nuts packed around the explosive) or secondary (stones, glass, or wood from the environment). These missiles, like bullets, can cause lacerations, fractures, contusions, and penetrating wounds.

Injuries from ballistic trauma—missiles and bullets—should be assessed and treated as for all major trauma.

Flash burns

The hot gases from the explosion can cause smoke inhalation injuries to the airway and exposed skin may be burned. Burns tend to be superficial. For management of burns, see ➲ p. 300.

Crush injuries

Falling debris and building collapse can cause crushing injuries (➲ p. 837).

Psychological injuries

These may be the main objective in terrorist attacks. Explosions result in panic, fear, and widespread destruction. In the long term, some will experience post-traumatic stress disorder (PTSD; ➲ p. 558).

Lightning

The voltage in a bolt of lightning is between 200 million and 2 billion volts of direct current. A bolt of lightning can reach temperatures approaching 28,000°C and lasts microseconds. Lightning strikes can injure humans in different ways:

- Direct strike—where the electrical charge hits the person.
- Splash hits—the lightning jumps from a nearby object and strikes the victim on its way to the ground.
- Ground strike—the lightning bolt lands near to the victim and is conducted through the ground. The energy transmitted depends on the resistance of the ground material—dry sand is a poor conductor and wet spongy earth is a better conductor.
- Electromagnetic pulse—a burst of electromagnetic energy which produces high currents and voltages.

On average, two people are killed and 30 injured by lightning in the UK each year. Between 1988 and 2012, 7% had cardiopulmonary resuscitation (CPR) and survived; 16% had serious injuries (fractures, burns and unconsciousness); while 56% had minor injuries (minor burns, temporary damage to eyes or ears, transient numbness). Most survivors have no significant long-term disabilities. Similar figures have been found in studies of lightning injuries in the US.

Lightning injuries

- Cardiopulmonary arrest. Cardiac arrest tends to be brief because of the heart's intrinsic automaticity; however, paralysis of the respiratory centre in the medulla may lead to prolonged respiratory arrest.
- Burns. There may be characteristic feathering burns (Lichtenberg figures) or linear or punctate burns (→ Colour plate 1).
- Neurological injuries. Victims may be confused, have convulsions, paralysis, or amnesia.
- Ear and eye trauma. Tympanic membrane rupture is very common (>50%) and blindness occurs. Cataracts can develop as a late complication.
- Other injuries. Fractures, muscle aches, chest pains, and contusions may be seen and clothing/footwear can be damaged.
- Long-term injuries. These are usually neurological, including memory problems, sleep disturbance, dizziness, and chronic pains.

Treatment

Some victims suffer immediate cardiac arrest and will not survive without immediate emergency care:

- Assess scene safety, ABC, and commence CPR if indicated. Prolonged resuscitation may be required because of temporary damage to the respiratory centre in the medulla.
- Consider the possibility of spinal injuries and other injuries as the victim may have been thrown a considerable distance by the strike.
- Reduce and splint any fractures.
- Evacuate for cardiac monitoring and observation. Cardiac failure can occur as a late complication.

Prevention of lightning injuries

- Avoid power lines, boat masts, ski lifts, and wire fences.
- If in a tent, stay away from the poles and wet canvas.
- Avoid tall trees in open areas or hilltops and ridges.
- Move away from open water and metal boats.
- Stay away from isolated small structures in open areas.
- In forests, seek low areas under small trees.
- Do not shelter in the entrances of caves.
- If in the open, seek low ground and stay away from single trees. Do not lie flat on the ground. If possible, insulate yourself from the ground with sleeping mats and bend forwards on your knees keeping hands off the ground.
- Hair standing on end, blue haloes around objects, and crackling noises all indicate an imminent strike. Leave the area if possible or crouch down on the balls of your feet with head tucked down.[3]

Emergencies: collapse and serious illness

Chapter editor
Jon Dallimore

Contributors
Edi Albert
Spike Briggs
Jon Dallimore
Sundeep Dhillon (1st edition)
Mike Grocott (1st edition)
Stephen Hearns (1st edition)
Hugh Montgomery (1st edition)
Julian Thompson (1st edition)
David A. Warrell (1st and 2nd editions)

The collapsed patient

Management of injured patients follows a well-established sequence (➔ Chapter 7). However, when an individual suddenly becomes unwell ('collapses'), their basic life functions must be supported, a likely diagnosis made, the appropriate treatment instituted, and the patient stabilized before evacuation can be considered.

Collapse in young adults is very rare but is generally very serious; infectious disease or environmentally induced conditions are the most likely causes. Psychological causes must be considered, but only after medical ones have been excluded. In older travellers the likelihood of cardiovascular disease increases.

Medical emergencies

Before attempting to examine any seriously ill person look for life-threatening hazards so as to avoid further injury to the patient and any danger to the rescuers. If absolutely necessary, rapidly and carefully move the casualty to a safer place.

Rapid primary assessment and resuscitation

This is the simultaneous assessment, identification, and management of immediate life-threatening problems. Rapid primary assessment should follow the ABC model.

- **A** Safe Approach and Assessment.
- **A** Airway (consider the neck if there is a history of injury).
- **B** Breathing.
- **C** Circulation (control bleeding and manage shock).
- **D** Disability of the nervous system.
- **E** Exposure and environmental control.

Primary assessment should be repeated following any change in the patient's condition. It is important to treat life-threatening conditions, such as hypoxia, before a firm diagnosis is made.

Approach and assessment

When it is safe to approach, check the casualty's level of responsiveness. Tap or gently shake the shoulders and say 'Are you okay?' If there is no response, call for help and proceed to check the airway.

Airway

- Assess without moving the neck more than necessary—particularly if the patient has fallen and might have injured the head or neck. Remember, airway takes precedence over neck control.
- Open the airway using chin lift or jaw thrust (→ p. 206).
- Look for and remove any obvious obstruction, consider the use of airway adjuncts such as NPAs or OPAs (→ p. 207). Remember that OPAs can provoke vomiting. Where possible, place the patient on their side.

Breathing

- Once the airway has been checked and opened, assess breathing. If conscious, ask if there is chest pain or shortness of breath.
- Look, listen, and feel for breathing (10 s). Abdominal movements may be easier to see than chest movements.
- Give oxygen if available, particularly to those who are shocked, bleeding, or who have breathing difficulties.
- If respiration is absent, impaired, or inadequate, commence CPR (→ p. 242).
- Is the breathing rate normal?
- Can the patient count to ten in one breath?
- If you suspect a chest problem, examine the chest for movement and breath sounds—normal, crackles, wheeze, or absent?

Circulation care with haemorrhage control

The aim is to detect and treat shock. Look for and control any external bleeding (consider direct pressure and elevation). Consider the possibility of internal bleeding such as GI haemorrhage.

- Look at the patient's skin colour and assess the skin temperature.
- Measure pulse rate and assess pulse character (normal, thready, or bounding).
- Estimate the BP by feeling the pulse:
  - Carotid (neck): systolic BP >60 mmHg.
  - Femoral (groin): systolic BP >70 mmHg.
  - Radial (wrist): systolic BP >80 mmHg.
- CRT should be <2 s in a warm casualty (➔ p. 192).
- Treat shock:
  - Lie the patient flat, elevate legs.
  - Keep warm and reassure.
  - Consider IV fluids, replacement amounts and rate will depend upon the cause of the shock (➔ p. 252).

Disability

- Assess the patient's neurological status using the ACVPU scale:
  - **A**—alert.
  - **C**—new confusion.
  - **V**—responds to verbal command.
  - **P**—responds to pain.
  - **U**—unresponsive.
- Pupils—assess size and reaction to light.
- Look for neck stiffness.
- Check blood glucose levels if possible.
- If the patient is fitting, place them in the recovery position.
- Is patient's speech normal or slurred?
- Look for facial or limb weakness.

Exposure and environmental control

Where possible, examine the patient in a warm, light environment such as a tent or group shelter. Insulate from the ground in the cold and protect from the sun if in hot environments. Be gentle—unnecessary roughness may aggravate the problem. Examine the patient carefully but always prevent the development of hypothermia which will worsen shock. Measure body temperature and look for a rash.

Rapid history

The patient or bystanders may be able to give brief details to aid diagnosis:
- Patient's symptoms.
- Events leading up to the illness, any history of injury.
- Past history, particularly known cardiac or respiratory illness, diabetes, epilepsy, alcohol/drug abuse, head injury.
- Medication taken on a regular or occasional basis.
- Allergies.

Secondary assessment

Secondary survey is a methodical search for all signs of disease which may be present (➔ p. 224). On an expedition this should be delayed until the casualty is in a warm, dry environment such as in a tent or building or under a group shelter, and lying on an inflatable mattress or sleeping bag.

History taking and examination are covered in ➔ Chapter 6.

Resuscitation in the wilderness

Survival from a cardiac arrest depends upon the cause of the arrest, the previous health of the patient, the rapidity of the initial response, and the availability of medical and transport facilities to ensure the *chain of survival* (Fig. 8.1).

Chain of Survival

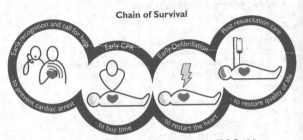

Fig. 8.1 Chain of survival. Reproduced from JP Nolan et al. ERC Guidelines 2010: *Resuscitation*. 2010;81:1223, with permission from Elsevier.

The basic life support (BLS) algorithm (➔ Fig. 8.2, p. 242) remains the default response for a collapsed, unresponsive patient. However, current BLS and advanced life support (ALS) guidelines have been developed for the patient who has had a cardiac arrest, most likely due to a MI, and who collapses in an environment where early defibrillation and timely transfer to a facility for post-resuscitation care are possible.

Resuscitation in the wilderness presents issues that do not normally need to be considered in a conventional healthcare setting and may require some difficult decision-making. Rescuers must consider their own safety both at the time of arrival on scene and for potential dangers arising during the re-suscitation and rescue process, and be prepared to either not commence resuscitation, or abandon it. The expedition medic and leader must con-sider not only the medical needs of the victim, but also recognize that there is a duty of care to other expedition members. A prolonged resuscitation and rescue may expose others to unacceptable environmental risks, es-pecially if the other members are children. The physical location of the victim and the available rescue equipment may mean that it is not possible to rescue the victim *and* continue CPR effectively.

Guidelines from UK search and rescue

Do not initiate CPR

- If unsafe for rescuer to approach the scene.
- Unable to perform CPR or maintain it.
- Obvious injuries incompatible with life.
- Cardiac arrest >15 min ago with no bystander CPR and no reversible causes.
- Avalanche burial >60 min and airway packed with snow.

Discontinue CPR

- If spontaneous pulse and breathing return.
- If no reversible causes—hypothermia, hypoxia, hypovolaemia, toxins, tension pneumothorax, thrombosis (e.g. MI).
- If no signs of life after 20 min of CPR.
- Rescuers become exhausted.
- Rescuers are placed in danger.

Recognition of life extinct

- No attempts at breathing.
- Absence of breath sounds.
- No palpable carotid pulse—check for 1 min.
- No spontaneous movement.
- Pupils fixed and dilated.
- No corneal reflex.
- No motor response.

Special circumstances

Rescuers must consider if the following circumstances apply and modify their approach accordingly:

- *Hypothermia* (➔ p. 654)—airway protection and CPR should be commenced as soon as possible. However, CPR *must* be continued until the patient is either 'warm and dead' or return of spontaneous circulation (ROSC) occurs. See: ℔ https://cprguidelines.eu
- *Avalanche burial* (➔ p. 679)—CPR should not be continued in buried victims with a blocked airway on extrication and a burial time >60 min.
- *Snake bite or marine envenomation*—prolonged CPR is sometimes successful.
- *Electrocution* (lightning strike) (➔ p. 230)—prolonged CPR is worthwhile, especially after lightning strike. Late defibrillation may be successful.
- *Drowning, including cold water immersion* (➔ p. 720)—commence CPR, but discontinue after 20 min unless timely evacuation to a medical facility is possible. Submersion for >60 min in non-icy water or submersion for >90 min in icy water are incompatible with life.
- *Cardiac arrest secondary to trauma/haemorrhage*—mean survival rate in conventional practice is 5%. Survival in a wilderness setting is extremely unlikely.

If none of these circumstances apply then conventional BLS and ALS guidelines should be followed where possible. Recovery from a ventricular fibrillation arrest requires timely defibrillation. If defibrillation occurs in a pre-hospital setting within 4 min of arrest with subsequent transfer to hospital, then long-term survival is 60%, at 20 min it is <1%.

Automated external defibrillators (AEDs)

AEDs are compact, light, and relatively inexpensive, they can be used by lay people with little additional training, and in theory could be carried on many types of expedition. However, there are two major potential breaks in the chain of survival that render this approach of little value in most expedition contexts. Firstly, it is unlikely that the victim will have their cardiac arrest close to the medical kit where the defibrillator is kept. Secondly, long-term survival is usually dependent on the ability to identify and correct secondary complications such as arrhythmias, acidosis, and electrolyte disturbance.

Dangers of resuscitation

There is understandable concern about the possibility of transmission of blood-borne and airborne diseases during resuscitation—particularly HIV, hepatitis, and COVID-19. To minimize the risk of acquiring infection, rescuers should wear PPE and use barriers whenever possible, and great care must be taken with sharps.

Basic life support (CPR)

For any seriously ill or collapsed patient it is important to assess for level of response and to start cardiopulmonary resuscitation (CPR) if the patient is unconscious and not breathing normally.

(UK Resuscitation Guidelines 2021).

Initial management of adult patients
See Fig. 8.2.

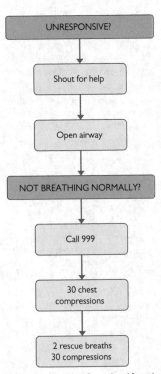

Fig. 8.2 Adult basic life support algorithm. Reproduced from the Resuscitation Council (UK) Guidelines 2010, with permission.

- Check for a response:
  - Gently shake the shoulders. Ask loudly 'Are you alright?'
- If patient responds:
  - If the individual is able to speak, the airway is open and maintained.
  - Leave them in the position you find them, provided there is no further danger.
  - Stabilize the head and neck if there is a possibility of injury (➲ p. 220).
  - Find out what is wrong and get help (ideally via radio, telephone or inReach® device), if available.
- If patient is unresponsive:
  - Shout/call for help.
  - Turn the casualty on their back, while minimizing neck movements.

Assess, open, and manage the airway as described on ➲ p. 206. Check the airway for 10 s.

If the casualty is not breathing *normally* start CPR (Fig. 8.3):
- Start with 30 chest compressions at a rate of 100–120/min:
  - Kneel beside victim.
  - Place heel of one hand in centre of victim's chest.
  - Place heel of other hand on top of the first hand.
  - Interlock fingers of the hands and ensure pressure is not applied over the victim's ribs, upper abdomen, or bottom end of the bony sternum See figure 8.3.
  - Position yourself vertically above the victim's chest and, with straight arms, press down on sternum 5–6 cm.
  - Release pressure without losing contact between your hands and the sternum. Compression and release should take equal time.
- After 30 compressions give two rescue breaths, if trained and able. This is particularly important in children and immersion victims when five rescue breaths should be given *before* chest compressions:
  - Open airway with chin lift and head tilt.
  - Pinch soft part of the victim's nose closed with the index finger and thumb of your hand on their forehead.
  - Allow patient's mouth to open while maintaining chin lift.
  - Take a normal breath and place lips around their mouth. Ensure a good seal.
  - Blow steadily into the mouth for about 1 s and watch the chest rise.
  - Maintaining head tilt and chin lift, take your mouth away and watch for the chest to fall as air comes out.
  - Take another normal breath and blow into the victim's mouth to give two effective rescue breaths. Immediately return your hands to the sternum and give a further 30 compressions.
- If rescue breaths do not make the chest rise and fall, before next attempt:
  - Check victim's mouth and remove any visible obstruction.
  - Recheck there is adequate head tilt and chin lift.
  - Do not attempt more than two rescue breaths before returning to 30 chest compressions.
- Chest compressions: rescue breath ratio 30:2.

Continue CPR until:
- Normal breathing resumes.
- You become exhausted.
- The team agrees that the resuscitation should be discontinued.
- See also notes above regarding prolonged resuscitation attempts (➔ p. 239).
- Performing CPR in a remote location can be daunting. Use a team-based approach to make decisions, this includes relatives, friends, and other team members. Consider the need for debriefing after a resuscitation attempt—➔ p. 557.

Core rules of CPR
- Call for assistance.
- Push hard (effective cardiac compressions).
- Push fast (maintain regular cardiac compressions).
- Breathe slowly (excessive ventilation is unnecessary).
- Don't stop (gaps in compression reduce survival).
- Follow automated defibrillator commands (if available).

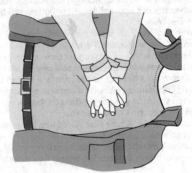

Fig. 8.3 Hand position for CPR.

Choking

Recognition

Foreign bodies may cause either mild or severe airway obstruction. Choking usually occurs during eating and the victim may clutch their neck.

Ask the conscious victim 'Are you choking?'

Mild airway obstruction

- Victim is able to speak, cough, and breathe.

Severe airway obstruction

- Victim unable to speak.
- Victim unable to breathe.
- Attempts at coughing are silent.
- Victim may become unconscious.

Management

See Fig. 8.4.

Mild airway obstruction

Encourage them to continue coughing but do nothing else.

Severe airway obstruction

- Give up to five back blows.
- Stand to the side and slightly behind the victim.
- Support the chest with one hand and lean the victim forwards.
- Give up to five sharp blows between the shoulder blades with the heel of your other hand.

If five back blows fail to relieve the airway obstruction, give up to five abdominal thrusts:

- Stand behind the victim and put both arms round the upper part of their abdomen.
- Lean the victim forwards and clench your fist and place it between the umbilicus (navel) and the bottom end of the breastbone.
- Grasp hand with your other hand and pull sharply inwards and upwards. Repeat up to five times.
- If the obstruction is still not relieved, continue alternating five back blows with five abdominal thrusts.

If the victim becomes unconscious:

- Support the victim carefully to the ground.
- Begin CPR which often relieves the obstruction (➲ p. 242).
- If this is unsuccessful, consider a surgical airway.

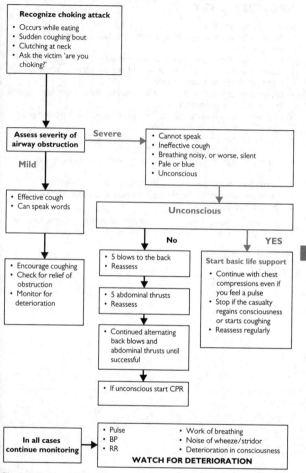

Fig. 8.4 Choking algorithm.

Recovery position

See Fig. 8.5 and Fig. 8.6.
- Remove the victim's spectacles, if worn, and take any object from the pockets.
- Kneel beside the victim and make sure that both their legs are straight.
- Place the arm nearest to you out at right angles to their body, elbow bent with the hand palm uppermost.
- Bring the far arm across the chest and hold the back of the hand against the victim's cheek nearest to you.
- With your other hand, grasp the far leg just above the knee and pull it up, keeping the foot on the ground.
- Keeping the hand pressed against the cheek, pull on the far leg to roll the victim towards you onto their side.
- Adjust the upper leg so that both the hip and knee are bent at right angles.
- Tilt the head back to make sure the airway remains open.
- Adjust the hand under the cheek, if necessary, to keep the head tilted.
- Check breathing regularly.

If the victim has to be kept in the recovery position for >30 min, turn them to the opposite side to relieve the pressure on the lower arm.

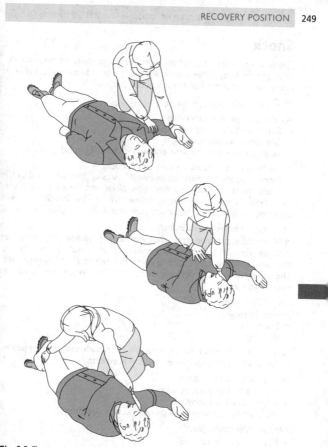

Fig. 8.5 Turning into the recovery position.

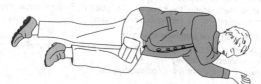

Fig. 8.6 The recovery position.

Shock

Shock occurs when the circulation is inadequate to meet the metabolic demands of the body. When key organs such as the kidneys, heart, and brain are relatively underperfused their function fails.

Clinical presentation and types of shock

All 'shocked' patients may exhibit:
- Cerebral effects—irritable, drowsy, yawning.
- GI effects—nausea, vomiting.
- Renal effects—reduced urine output, (>0.5 mL/kg/h being 'normal').

Other findings will depend on the type of shock.

Shock is usually accompanied by low BP. Arterial BP is governed by the combination of cardiac output driving the blood into the arteries and peripheral vascular resistance resisting its forward flow. Thus, low BP may result either from a *reduction in cardiac output* or from a *fall in peripheral resistance*.

Shock caused by low cardiac output

A fall in cardiac output leads to a reflex increase in sympathetic activity—an increase in HR, RR, peripheral vasoconstriction, and sweating. Cold, clammy skin, fast pulse, and rapid breathing will be common to all underlying causes. Underfilling of the main pumping chamber of the heart, the left ventricle, may result from:

Loss of fluids from the body:
- Haemorrhage.
- Diarrhoea.
- Vomiting.

Skin turgor (elasticity of the tissues) is low, the mouth is dry, and the patient is thirsty. With blood loss alone, sweating is expected.

Loss of fluids into tissue spaces:
- Burns (including severe sunburn).
- Allergic shock—anaphylaxis.
- Profound hypoproteinaemia (as may occur in dysentery).

Obstruction to cardiac filling:
- Pulmonary embolism (PE).
- Cardiac tamponade.

When fluids have been lost from the body or moved into tissue spaces, neck veins will be empty: when there is obstruction to blood flow from PE or cardiac tamponade, the neck veins will be full. Breathlessness may be most profound with PE (as hypoxia contributes).

Shock caused by low peripheral resistance

This occurs in any major systemic inflammatory response, including:
- Severe infection (sepsis).
- Toxins (stings, venom) and/or anaphylaxis.

Blood vessels dilate, peripheral resistance decreases, and therefore BP falls. The inflammatory response directly affects the peripheral blood vessels and so the compensatory sympathetic response cannot cause the blood vessels to constrict—BP remains low. The skin may be warm, hot, or 'patchy'. In sepsis, such 'patchiness' may alter with time (legs freezing one minute, and warm the next). Neck veins will be collapsed, and the skin may sweat due to fever but will not be 'cold and shut down' (i.e. clammy). Pulse rate and cardiac output will be high.

Catches in the wilderness

- The young and fit can maintain BP for a very long time through sympathetic activity. Sometimes BP may not fall until around 50% of the circulating volume has been lost.
- Underlying dehydration may be common.
- Urine output may already be low.
- Sweating responses may be reduced—sweating thresholds are altered by acclimatization to ambient temperature and to exercise loads (➲ p. 798).
- In the heat, most people are vasodilated. In 'heat stroke' (➲ p. 791), severe inflammation coupled with volume loss may lead to a 'shivering clammy' patient, despite a very high central temperature.
- In the cold, most people are vasoconstricted.

Management of the shocked patient

See Fig. 8.7 and Fig. 8.8.

- As for all major emergencies—make sure that the environment is safe, summon help, and attend to *CABC* (→ Chapter p. 198). Assess conscious level.
- Control any massive external haemorrhage first. Apply direct pressure to the bleeding area. Use a tourniquet for limb trauma and consider Celox® or QuikClot® (→ p. 214). Pack deep large wounds and bind firmly.
- Treat anaphylaxis immediately (→ p. 256). Look/listen for signs of airway obstruction such as wheeze, stridor, facial and neck swelling, or/ and urticarial (nettles-type) rash.
- Give oxygen if available.
- Consider a cardiac cause and give aspirin 300 mg crushed with a small amount of water and GTN if available. See → p. 262.
- If the patient is more than mildly unwell, establish venous access at once. You may find it a lot harder later!
- Give tranexamic acid IV in trauma, particularly head injuries (→ p. 215).
- Stop the losses and treat the causes:
  - If septic, seek the source (including the rare, but often missed, retained tampon—which must be removed) and treat at once with broad-spectrum antibiotics such as ceftriaxone IV.
  - Give fluids. Most wilderness victims will be depleted of intravascular volume, as will most with shock of any cause (→ p. 215). The rate and route will be determined by a number of factors: if you have an uncontrolled source of blood loss, internal or external, give fluids cautiously until the source of bleeding is controlled. Raising pressure by rapid resuscitation will make bleeding worse. If fluid supplies are limited, use 'permissive hypotension' (maintain a just palpable radial pulse or 'titrate to talking').
  - Consider intraosseous administration if oral or venous routes are unavailable, and you have the kit (and are trained to use it!).
  - During fluid resuscitation, give fluids by 'bolus' of 250 mL, and observe response, especially HR. For maintenance, calculate losses (blood loss, diarrhoea, vomiting, from skin in burns), including insensible losses (sweating and breathing, 10–20 mL/kg/day). Once resuscitated with boluses, spread this 'maintenance' over 24 h.
  - If the patient is conscious and able to swallow (without GI tract injury), let the patient drink as a means of conserving IV fluids.
  - Stop all sources of loss (e.g. use antidiarrhoeals, antiemetics, cooling with sponging and fanning, keeping in the shade, light-reflective clothing if sun unavoidable).
  - For collapse in the heat, consider exercise-associated hyponatraemia (→ p. 806).
- Indicators of successful treatment:
  - Improvements in observations—HR within normal range and RR falling, BP rising.
  - Control of fluid losses.
  - Patient is alert and orientated, urine output >0.5 mL/kg/h.

Neurogenic shock

Neurogenic shock is a very rare situation, in which severe damage to the spinal cord disrupts the transmission of nerve impulses to the small arteries. The blood vessels therefore dilate, and 'low resistance shock' results. This is usually caused by spinal cord injury (usually trauma, although inflammatory/ infective causes are possible).

The signs are those of 'low peripheral resistance shock': tachycardia, high-volume pulse, warm skin, low BP. Casualty may develop priapism—an involuntary erection of the penis in males (seen with high spinal cord injuries above T6). Other signs of spinal cord injury (sensory loss, weakness, or paralysis).

Neurogenic shock requires careful administration of IV fluids (as the intestines usually stop moving with high spinal cord injury) using 250 mL fluid challenges. Evacuate as soon as possible. The patient may need a nasogastric tube. Remember pressure area care and immobilization of the entire spine, ideally using a vacuum mattress.

Monitoring shock in the wilderness

BP may be well maintained at first. Look for trends over time and any postural drop (measured while lying then sitting or standing).
- What is happening to:
  - Breathing rate?
  - Pulse rate?
  - Oxygen saturations?
  - Skin colour and body temperature?
  - Conscious level—alert/orientated?
  - Urine output? Prolonged drops in BP can affect kidney function. Consider a urinary catheter (if you have one) and measure hourly urine output. You can measure with a cup or Nalgene™ bottle if no catheter.
- Fig. 8.7 reproduces the NHS observations chart including the National Early Warning Score (NEWS). Patients whose observations fall outside the normal range require increased monitoring, and deterioration in the score will highlight the need for increased frequency of observations and may guide urgency of a medevac. Expeditions are recommended to obtain equivalent charts to these at full size and in colour as part of their medical stores. Online instructions on the use of NEWS can be found at: ℅ https://news.ocbmedia.com

Prevention and preparation
- Decide on the volume of fluids you will carry, depending on logistic constraints (weight, bulk), duration of trip, evacuation times.
- Take antibiotics for infections and adrenaline (epinephrine), steroids, and antihistamines for anaphylaxis.
- Find out how to access safe local blood supplies.
- Avoid GI tract infection if possible, and all the other recognized environmental causes.
- Make sure your cannulation skills are current.

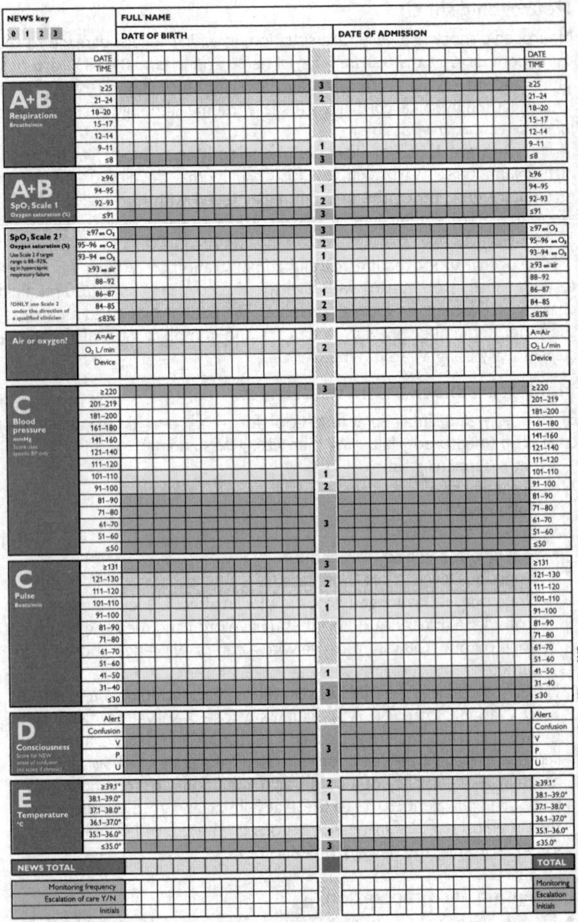

Fig. 8.7 Observations chart including National Early Warning Score (NEWS).

Physiological parameter	3	2	1	Score 0	1	2	3
Respiration rate (per minute)	≤8		9–11	12–20		21–24	≥25
SpO₂ Scale 1 (%)	≤91	92–93	94–95	≥96			
SpO₂ Scale 2 (%)	≤83	84–85	86–87	88–92 ≥93 on air	93–94 on oxygen	95–96 on oxygen	≥97 on oxygen
Air or oxygen?		Oxygen		Air			
Systolic blood pressure (mmHg)	≤90	91–100	101–100	111–219			≥220
Pulse (per minute)	≤40		41–50	51–90	91–110	111–130	≥131
Consciousness				Alert			CVPU
Temperature (°C)	≤35.0		35.1–36.0	36.1–38.0	38.1–39.0	≥39.1	

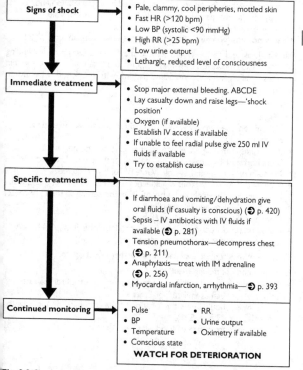

Signs of shock	• Pale, clammy, cool peripheries, mottled skin • Fast HR (>120 bpm) • Low BP (systolic <90 mmHg) • High RR (>25 bpm) • Low urine output • Lethargic, reduced level of consciousness
Immediate treatment	• Stop major external bleeding. ABCDE • Lay casualty down and raise legs—'shock position' • Oxygen (if available) • Establish IV access if available • If unable to feel radial pulse give 250 ml IV fluids if available • Try to establish cause
Specific treatments	• If diarrhoea and vomiting/dehydration give oral fluids (if casualty is conscious) (➲ p. 420) • Sepsis – IV antibiotics with IV fluids if available (➲ p. 281) • Tension pneumothorax—decompress chest (➲ p. 211) • Anaphylaxis—treat with IM adrenaline (➲ p. 256) • Myocardial infarction, arrhythmia— ➲ p. 393
Continued monitoring	• Pulse • RR • BP • Urine output • Temperature • Oximetry if available • Conscious state **WATCH FOR DETERIORATION**

Fig. 8.8 Shock algorithm.

Anaphylaxis and anaphylactic shock

Anaphylaxis is a rapidly evolving clinical syndrome, usually precipitated by recent exposure to a substance (allergen) to which the patient is allergic, e.g.:
* Drugs: any, especially penicillins.
* Foods: especially nuts, fruits, sea food.
* Environmental factors: animal venoms (e.g. wasp, hornet, bee, ant, or snake), plant substances (latex).

Examination

Anaphylaxis is characterized by one or more of the following features in any combination:
* Rash and/or mucous membrane involvement: urticaria ('hives'), flushing, itching, generalized erythema and swelling owing to massive extravasation of fluid and swelling of the lips, tongue, gums, and uvula.
* Life-threatening airway obstruction: lower airways—bronchoconstriction,/asthma or, less often, upper airway—angioedema of the larynx. The signs include wheeze, tachypnoea, stridor ('croup'), and cyanosis.
* Life-threatening circulatory collapse caused by vasodilatation and/or hypovolaemia: early features include dizziness, loss of vision, tachycardia, falling BP, and loss of consciousness.
* GI symptoms (vomiting, diarrhoea, retrosternal pain, abdominal colic).

Patients look and feel very unwell and may have a feeling of impending doom. In extreme cases, they may collapse and lose consciousness within minutes of allergen exposure. Some present with shock and hypotension alone.

Treatment

See Fig. 8.9.
* Maintain an open airway with head position and airway adjuncts as necessary.
* *If bronchospasm is severe or persistent* despite adrenaline, give a bronchodilator by inhalation (salbutamol, ipratropium). Use a spacer.
* Maintain BP >90 mmHg systolic. Give IV fluids as required.
* *If cardiac arrest occurs:* follow guidelines for CPR. Early ALS is essential. IM adrenaline is unlikely to be beneficial in this setting so try an IV route.
* Monitor vital signs and urine output.
* Continue chlorphenamine 4 mg/8 h PO.
* Consider a short course of steroids—prednisolone 40 mg/24 h for 5 days to prevent recurrent anaphylaxis.

The patient may require evacuation for further investigation.

Prevention and risk management

* Those with known allergy should carry an epinephrine (adrenaline) auto-injector such as EpiPen®, or Emerade®.
* Companions should know the location of the auto-injector and how to use it (➜ Fig. 17.7, p. 591).
* Ensure cooks are aware of food allergies.

Useful resources

- British Society for Allergy and Clinical Immunology: ℑ http://www.bsacii.org
- European Academy of Allergology and Clinical Immunology: ℑ http://www.eaaci.net
- European Resuscitation Council: ℑ http://www.cprguidelines.eu
- Resuscitation Council UK: ℑ http://www.resus.org.uk

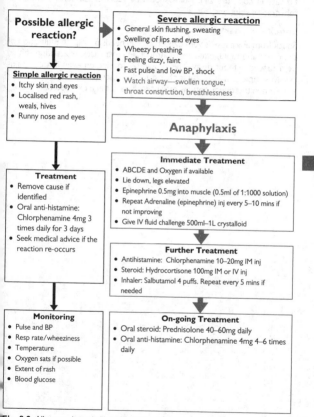

Possible allergic reaction?

Simple allergic reaction
- Itchy skin and eyes
- Localised red rash, weals, hives
- Runny nose and eyes

Severe allergic reaction
- General skin flushing, sweating
- Swelling of lips and eyes
- Wheezy breathing
- Feeling dizzy, faint
- Fast pulse and low BP, shock
- Watch airway—swollen tongue, throat constriction, breathlessness

Anaphylaxis

Treatment
- Remove cause if identified
- Oral anti-histamine: Chlorphenamine 4mg 3 times daily for 3 days
- Seek medical advice if the reaction re-occurs

Immediate Treatment
- ABCDE and Oxygen if available
- Lie down, legs elevated
- Epinephrine 0.5mg into muscle (0.5ml of 1:1000 solution)
- Repeat Adrenaline (epinephrine) inj every 5–10 mins if not improving
- Give IV fluid challenge 500ml–1L crystalloid

Further Treatment
- Antihistamine: Chlorphenamine 10–20mg IM inj
- Steroid: Hydrocortisone 100mg IM or IV inj
- Inhaler: Salbutamol 4 puffs. Repeat every 5 mins if needed

Monitoring
- Pulse and BP
- Resp rate/wheeziness
- Temperature
- Oxygen sats if possible
- Extent of rash
- Blood glucose

On-going Treatment
- Oral steroid: Prednisolone 40–60mg daily
- Oral anti-histamine: Chlorphenamine 4mg 4–6 times daily

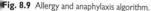

Fig. 8.9 Allergy and anaphylaxis algorithm.

Heat illnesses, dehydration, and shock

Exertional heat exhaustion, exercise-associated hyponatraemia, and exertional heat stroke may present with a shivering shocked patient. Patients need active cooling and fluids. Isotonic fluids should be given with caution if exercise-associated hyponatraemia is suspected (➔ p. 806).

Dehydration is common in all wilderness environments, owing to the effects of the heat, exercise and sweating, and high breathing rates (particularly in cold, dry air). Fluids should be replaced, preferably with oral rehydration solutions.

Shock summary

Shock from any cause is very dangerous and needs prompt identification of the cause and rapid, effective treatment. In most cases, evacuation should be arranged without delay. This should be considered even if anaphylaxis resolves rapidly. It is possible that a further allergic challenge may occur again when treatment options may have already been exhausted.

Chest pain

See Fig. 8.10.

History

- *Site* of pain and any radiation to arms, neck, jaw, or back.
- *Character* of pain—heavy, sharp, tight, tearing, pleuritic (worse on inspiration).
- *Severity*—out of ten.
- *Onset*—at rest or during exertion.
- *Nature*—whether constant and aggravated by exertion, position, eating, breathing, or relieved by analgesics, antacids, or GTN.
- *Associated symptoms*—sweating, breathlessness, nausea, palpitations, fever.
- *Trauma*—nature of any injury.
- *Past history*—cardiac or respiratory problems, acid indigestion.
- *Drugs*—cardiac or respiratory drugs, antacids.
- *Social and environmental factors*—alcohol/drugs, smoking status, recent stressors.

Cardiac disease risk factors

- Previous ischaemic heart disease, smoking, hypertension, obesity, diabetes, family history of ischaemic heart disease, hypercholesterolaemia.

Venous thrombosis or pulmonary embolism risk factors

- Previous thromboembolic disease (DVT or PE), smoking, immobility, dehydration, prothrombotic conditions, oestrogen-containing medication—hormone replacement therapy/oral contraceptive pill, recent surgery/long travel/leg injuries.

Gastrointestinal risk factors

- Gastro-oesophageal reflux disease (GORD).
- Previous peptic ulceration.
- Alcohol excess.

Examination

- Temperature, pulse, RR, BP in both arms, conscious level.
- General condition—cyanosis, pallor, sweating.
- Pulse rate, rhythm, character, BP, look for elevation and dilatation of the neck veins, listen to the heart sounds (any murmurs?), look for signs of cardiac failure (basal crackles in the lungs and swelling of the ankles), look for calf swelling or redness/tenderness.
- Feel for chest wall tenderness.
- Feel the abdomen for localized tenderness or a pulsatile mass (abdominal aortic aneurysm).
- Check blood glucose.

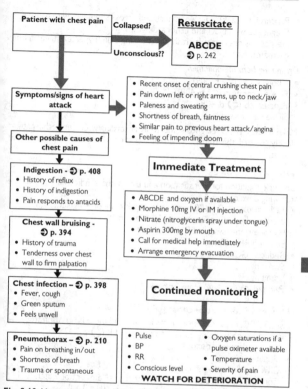

Fig. 8.10 Management of chest pain.

Differential diagnosis

Originating from the chest
- MI/angina (➔ p. 393).
- Tension pneumothorax (➔ p. 211).
- PE (➔ p. 260).
- Pneumonia (➔ p. 398).
- Pleurisy.
- Aortic dissection—tearing pain between the shoulder blades.
- Chest wall pain—reproduced by chest wall pressure but doesn't rule out other causes.
- GORD (➔ p. 408).

- Pericarditis—stabbing, pain in neck and across shoulders with nausea. Diagnosed with ECG and echocardiogram.
- Herpes zoster—vesicular rash with burning pain/hypersensitivity in one dermatome.

Originating from the abdomen
- Cholecystitis (➔ p. 409).
- Peptic ulceration (➔ p. 408).
- Pancreatitis (➔ p. 409).
- Sickle cell crisis.

Make a 'best guess' diagnosis and treat accordingly. Observe the patient closely, record the details on an observation chart, and monitor urine output.

Worrying features

Urgent evacuation for investigation and treatment is indicated if any of the following develop:
- Tachycardia—HR >100 beats/min persistently or irregular rhythm.
- Bradycardia—HR persistently <50 beats/min.
- Hypotension—systolic BP <90 mmHg.
- Elevated RR >25 breaths/min.
- Reduced GCS.
- Sweating.
- Vomiting.
- Pain radiating to jaw, arms, or back.

Urgent treatment of chest pain

Assess ABC. If the patient is unresponsive and there is no respiratory effort and/or no palpable pulse, commence CPR (➔ p. 242).

If the patient is conscious:
- Sit patient up.
- Give high-flow oxygen if available.
- Consider 300 mg aspirin crushed with a small amount of water, GTN, and IV analgesia if cardiac cause seems likely (Fig. 8.10).
- Monitor pulse, BP and RR.

Shortness of breath (dyspnoea)

See Fig. 8.11.

History

- *Dyspnoea*—speed of onset, at rest, cough, wheeze.
- *Sputum* (colour, quantity, any blood).
- *Chest pain*—characterize any pain (➔ Chest pain, p. 260).
- *Associated symptoms*—sweating, nausea, palpitations.
- *Trauma*—nature of any injury.
- *Past history*—cardiac or respiratory problems.
- *Drugs*—inhalers, respiratory or cardiac drugs.
- *Allergies*—medication and environmental, food, other allergens.
- *Social/environmental*—smoking status, travel history (➔ p. 280).
- *Risk factors for PE/DVT*—previous thromboembolic disease, smoking, obesity, immobility, dehydration, high altitude, prothrombotic conditions (e.g. factor V Leiden), hormone replacement therapy/oral contraceptive pill, recent surgery or long travel, leg injuries.

Examination

- Temperature, pulse, saturations, RR, BP, conscious level.
- General condition—confusion, cyanosis, pallor, cool peripheries, sweating, tremor, use of accessory muscles. Can the patient count to ten in one breath/talk in full sentences?
- Pulse rate, rhythm, BP, look for elevation and dilatation of the neck veins. Measure peak expiratory flow rate if possible, look for tracheal tug, percuss the chest, listen for air entry and breath sounds—normal, crackles, wheezes, or absent. Look for calf swelling/redness/tenderness or ankle swelling (DVT).
- Feel the abdomen for localized tenderness or a pulsatile mass (abdominal aortic aneurysm).

Differential diagnosis

Wheeze present:
- Asthma or chronic obstructive pulmonary disease (➔ p. 402).
- Anaphylaxis (➔ p. 256).

No clinical signs:
- PE.
- Hyperventilation (➔ p. 341).
- Diabetic ketoacidosis (➔ p. 274).

Crackles audible:
- Pneumonia (➔ p. 398.).
- High-altitude pulmonary oedema (➔ p. 695).
- Heart failure.

Stridor present:
- Anaphylaxis (➔ p. 256).
- Foreign body (➔ p. 246).

Absent breath sounds:
- Pneumothorax (➔ p. 396).

Make a 'best guess' diagnosis and treat accordingly. Observe the patient closely; record the details on an observation chart.

Worrying features

Urgent evacuation for investigation and treatment is indicated if any of the following develop:

- RR >25 breaths/min.
- Tachycardia or bradycardia (<50, >120 beats/min).
- Core temperature >39°C.
- Hypotension (<systolic 90 mmHg).
- Reduced conscious level.
- Exhaustion or agitated.
- Pale, clammy skin. Cyanosis.

Urgent treatment of shortness of breath

Assess ABC. If the patient is unresponsive and there is no respiratory effort and/or no palpable pulse, commence CPR (➔ p. 242).
If the patient is conscious:

- Sit patient up.
- Give high-flow oxygen if available.
- Consider specific treatment—adrenaline, salbutamol, antibiotics, and steroids. Treat pain.
- Monitor saturations, pulse, BP, RR, and conscious level.

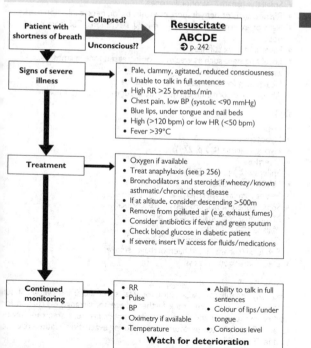

Fig. 8.11 Shortness of breath algorithm.

Coma

Unrousable unresponsiveness. See Fig. 8.12.

History (from bystanders)

- How/where found.
- Sudden or gradual onset.
- Seizure activity, incontinence.
- Any trauma, particularly to the head.
- Recent illness—headache, chest pain, breathlessness, palpitations, fever, confusion, depression, sinusitis, seizures, vomiting.
- Past history—cardiac, respiratory, diabetes, hypertension, epilepsy, psychiatric illness.
- Drugs—overdose? Sedative or hypnotic medication.
- Social/environmental—alcohol, illicit drugs, travel to malarial area.

Examination

- Check for danger and assess ABCDE.
- Assess conscious level—ACVPU or GCS. See ➔ p. 223.
- Record pulse, saturations, BP, RR.
- Check pupil responses frequently.
- Smell the breath—alcohol, ketones.
- Rashes, signs of dehydration, cyanosis, pallor, needle injection marks.
- Signs of external head injury—bruising, lacerations, CSF from ears/nose.
- Fever and neck stiffness.
- Localizing signs such as weakness or increased tone in limbs, asymmetrical reflexes.
- Heart/lung for murmurs, wheeze, crackles.
- Abdomen for organomegaly, aortic aneurysm, bruising, melaena.

Differential diagnosis

- Hypoxia.
- Hypotension.
- Hypoglycaemia (➔ p. 274).
- Overdose.
- Epilepsy (➔ p. 341, 566).
- HACE (➔ p. 698).
- Hypothermia/hyperthermia.
- Sepsis (pneumonia, uro-sepsis, toxic shock).
- Meningitis/encephalitis (➔ p. 505).
- Malaria (➔ p. 512).
- Carbon monoxide poisoning (➔ p. 647).
- Subdural/subarachnoid haemorrhage, stroke.
- Decompression sickness.

Treatment

Treat any identifiable cause. Monitor vital signs and urine output. If full recovery does not occur, seek further advice and arrange evacuation for further investigation and treatment. Remember pressure area care, maintenance fluids, and temperature control during evacuation. Catheterize the bladder if possible.

Urgent treatment
- ABC.
- Place in recovery position.
- Consider OPA or NPA.
- Give high-flow oxygen, if available guided by saturations.
- Stabilize the cervical spine if there is a history of trauma.
- Measure blood glucose and body temperature.
- Obtain venous access and consider IV fluids.
- Control seizures, treat hypoglycaemia (blood sugar <4 mmol/L).
- Treat life-threatening infection if suspected.
- Keep the casualty warm and dry.
- Monitor vital signs: pulse, saturations, BP, RR, GCS. See NEWS chart (➲ Fig. 8.7, p. 254).

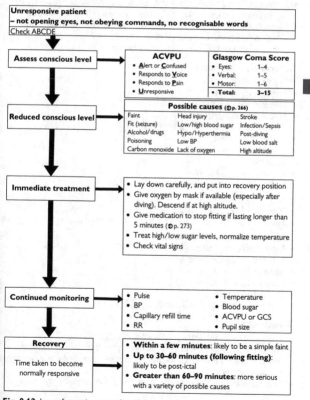

Unresponsive patient
– not opening eyes, not obeying commands, no recognisable words
Check ABCDE

Assess conscious level	**ACVPU**	**Glasgow Coma Score**
	• **A**lert or **C**onfused	• Eyes: 1–4
	• Responds to **V**oice	• Verbal: 1–5
	• Responds to **P**ain	• Motor: 1–6
	• **U**nresponsive	• **Total: 3–15**

Reduced conscious level — **Possible causes** (➲p. 266)

Faint	Head injury	Stroke
Fit (seizure)	Low/high blood sugar	Infection/Sepsis
Alcohol/drugs	Hypo/Hyperthermia	Post-diving
Poisoning	Low BP	Low blood salt
Carbon monoxide	Lack of oxygen	High altitude

Immediate treatment
- Lay down carefully, and put into recovery position
- Give oxygen by mask if available (especially after diving). Descend if at high altitude.
- Give medication to stop fitting if lasting longer than 5 minutes (➲ p. 273)
- Treat high/low sugar levels, normalize temperature
- Check vital signs

Continued monitoring
- Pulse
- BP
- Capillary refill time
- RR
- Temperature
- Blood sugar
- ACVPU or GCS
- Pupil size

Recovery

Time taken to become normally responsive

- **Within a few minutes**: likely to be a simple faint
- **Up to 30–60 minutes (following fitting)**: likely to be post-ictal
- **Greater than 60–90 minutes**: more serious with a variety of possible causes

Fig. 8.12 Loss of consciousness algorithm.

Headache

See Fig. 8.13.

History

- Headache—severity, location, character, speed of onset, nausea/vomiting, head injury?
- Direct questions—dizziness, blackouts/fits, visual changes.
- Past history—previous headaches, migraine.
- Drugs—recent change in medication.
- Social/environmental — alcohol/drugs, recent stressors, post-diving or change in elevation.

Examination

- Temperature, pulse, BP, blood sugar, GCS score.
- Evidence of head injury? Neck stiffness, photophobia, Kernig's (fully flex hip and passively extend knee. Positive if painful in head or neck). Look for any focal neurology—weakness/paralysis or changes in sensation.
- Check whole body for purpuric rash.
- Look for signs of URTI, including ear infection or sinus tenderness.

Differential diagnosis

- Tension headache.
- Migraine (➜ p. 342).
- Dehydration.
- Heat exhaustion/stroke.
- Acute mountain sickness (➜ p. 692).
- HACE (➜ p. 698).
- Carbon monoxide poisoning (➜ p. 773).
- Sinusitis.
- Dengue fever (➜ p. 494).
- Malaria and other febrile illnesses (➜ p. 512).

If signs of meningism:
- Meningitis/encephalitis (➜ p. 505).
- Subarachnoid haemorrhage with 'thunderclap' headache.

Decreased conscious level/localizing signs:
- Meningitis/encephalitis (➜ p. 505).
- Subarachnoid haemorrhage.
- Stroke.
- Malaria (➜ p. 512).
- HACE (➜ p. 698).
- Post-traumatic (extradural, subdural) (➜ p. 334).

Treatment

- If reduced GCS, see management of coma (➜ p. 267).
- Focal neurology or possibility of meningitis/encephalitis: give oxygen, broad-spectrum antibiotics such as IV ceftriaxone or oral ciprofloxacin, evacuate urgently.
- Give fluids and regular analgesia. Advise rest. Observe closely.

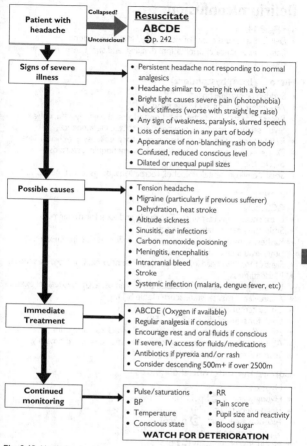

Fig. 8.13 Headache algorithm.

Delirium/confusion

See Fig. 8.14.

- *Delirium*: an acute onset of confusion with hallucinations.
- *Confusion*: a deficit in orientation, thinking, and short-term memory with reduced awareness.

History (from bystanders)

- Sudden or gradual onset.
- Any injury, particularly to the head.
- Recent illness—headache, chest or abdominal pain, dysuria, cough, fever, seizures, vomiting, dizziness, diarrhoea, incontinence.
- Past history—diabetes, cardiac, respiratory, epilepsy, psychiatric illness.
- Drugs—overdose, sedatives/hypnotics, mefloquine, steroids, psychiatric medication.
- Social/environmental—alcohol, recreational drugs, usual mental state.

Examination

- GCS score.
- Eyes: check pupil responses frequently and look for nystagmus.
- Smell the breath—alcohol, ketones.
- Rashes, signs of dehydration, cyanosis, pallor, needle injection marks or other evidence of illicit drug use.
- Signs of external head injury—bruising, haematoma, CSF from ears/nose.
- Neck stiffness.
- Localizing signs such as increased tone in limbs, asymmetrical reflexes.
- Abbreviated mental state score (Table 8.1).
- Check temperature.
- Look for signs of shock (➔ p. 250).
- Heart/lung for murmurs, rubs, wheeze, crackles, or injuries.
- Abdomen for tenderness, signs of injury, melaena, organomegaly.
- Test the urine and check blood glucose.

Confusion—differential diagnosis

- Hypoxia.
- Hypoglycaemia (➔ p. 274).
- Head injury (➔ p. 334).
- Alcohol/illicit drugs (➔ p. 566).
- Sepsis (commonly chest or urine infection).
- Meningitis/encephalitis (➔ p. 505).
- Intracranial bleed.
- Stroke.
- Drug toxicity.
- Malaria (➔ p. 512).
- HACE (➔ p. 698).
- Post-ictal (➔ p. 340).

Treatment

Treat any identifiable cause. Do not leave patient alone. Sedate only with great caution: lorazepam 1–2 mg PO/IM/IV. This may allow more detailed examination if the patient is very agitated/confused. Observe closely and evacuate for further investigation/treatment if complete recovery is delayed.

Table 8.1 Abbreviated Mental Test Score (AMTS)

Age	1
Date of birth	1
Repeat '42 West Street'	0
Year	1
Time (nearest hour)	1
Current location	1
Recognize two people	1
Year World War II ended	1
Name of the monarch	1
Count backward from 20 to 1	1
Recall '42 West Street'	1
Total	10

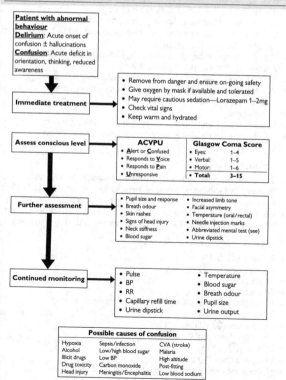

Patient with abnormal behaviour
Delirium: Acute onset of confusion ± hallucinations
Confusion: Acute deficit in orientation, thinking, reduced awareness

Immediate treatment
- Remove from danger and ensure on-going safety
- Give oxygen by mask if available and tolerated
- May require cautious sedation—Lorazepam 1–2mg
- Check vital signs
- Keep warm and hydrated

Assess conscious level

ACVPU	Glasgow Coma Score
• **A**lert or **C**onfused	• Eyes: 1–4
• Responds to **V**oice	• Verbal: 1–5
• Responds to **P**ain	• Motor: 1–6
• **U**nresponsive	• **Total: 3–15**

Further assessment
- Pupil size and response
- Breath odour
- Skin rashes
- Signs of head injury
- Neck stiffness
- Blood sugar
- Increased limb tone
- Facial asymmetry
- Temperature (oral/rectal)
- Needle injection marks
- Abbreviated mental test (see)
- Urine dipstick

Continued monitoring
- Pulse
- BP
- RR
- Capillary refill time
- Urine dipstick
- Temperature
- Blood sugar
- Breath odour
- Pupil size
- Urine output

Possible causes of confusion		
Hypoxia	Sepsis/infection	CVA (stroke)
Alcohol	Low/high blood sugar	Malaria
Illicit drugs	Low BP	High altitude
Drug toxicity	Carbon monoxide	Post-fitting
Head injury	Meningitis/Encephalitis	Low blood sodium

Fig. 8.14 Delirium/confusion algorithm.

Convulsions

See Fig. 8.15.

Urgent treatment

- Airway: roll patient into the recovery position, protect from further harm but do not restrain. Consider oxygen and a NPA.
- Breathing: if no respiratory effort, commence CPR.
- Circulation and drugs: attempt venous access. Measure blood glucose; if <3.5 mmol/L give 100 mL glucose 10% by infusion. Recheck levels subsequently. Give lorazepam 4 mg IV over 2 min or midazolam 10 mg via buccal route.
- If fits continue for >20 min, consider diazepam by infusion 100 mg in 500 mL of 5% glucose; infuse 40 mL/h. Phenytoin or IV levetiracetam are unlikely to be available.
- If seizures continue, make arrangements for urgent evacuation.

History

Get a detailed description of the seizure or fit:

- Onset—activity, position, warning, tonic, starting in one limb?
- During fit—sounds, cyanosis, breathing, eye, facial and limb movements, incontinence, time the duration.
- Post-fit—tongue injury, post-ictal state, limb weakness, muscle pain/ injuries, headache. Dislocated shoulder.
- Preceding illness—headache, chest pain, palpitations, dyspnoea.
- Past history—previous seizures, diabetes, alcoholism, pregnancy, cardiac, respiratory, or renal disease.
- Head injury.
- Drugs—antiepileptics, oral hypoglycaemics, medication compliance.
- Social/environmental—alcohol/drugs, recent feverish illness, post-diving.

Examination

- Temperature, pulse, saturations, BP, blood sugar, conscious level.
- Evidence of head injury? Sweating, neck stiffness, photophobia. Look for any focal neurology—weakness/paralysis or changes in sensation.
- Check whole body for injury—posterior dislocation of the shoulder is often missed (check for full, pain-free movements of both shoulders).

Convulsions—possible causes

- Epilepsy (➔ p. 340).
- Hypoglycaemia (➔ p. 274).
- Hypoxia.
- Alcohol withdrawal.
- Metabolic (low calcium, hyponatraemia/hypernatraemia, hypomagnesaemia).
- Head injury (➔ p. 334).
- Meningitis/encephalitis (➔ p. 305).
- Malaria (➔ p. 512).
- Drug overdose (➔ p. 566).
- Hypertension/eclampsia of pregnancy after 28 weeks.

Treatment after convulsion

- If reduced GCS, see management of coma (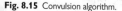 p. 267).
- Focal neurology or possibility of meningitis/encephalitis evacuate urgently.
- Otherwise give fluids and regular analgesia. Advise rest. Observe closely. If a first fit, evacuate for hospital investigations including a blood screen and CT head scan.

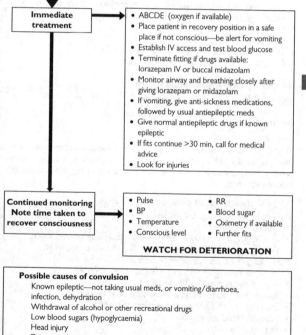

Types of convulsion
- Generalized ('grand-mal')—all body shaking
- Partial—shaking only in part of body or face
- Absence—unresponsive, unaware
- Other types—myoclonic, tonic, atonic

Immediate treatment
- ABCDE (oxygen if available)
- Place patient in recovery position in a safe place if not conscious—be alert for vomiting
- Establish IV access and test blood glucose
- Terminate fitting if drugs available: lorazepam IV or buccal midazolam
- Monitor airway and breathing closely after giving lorazepam or midazolam
- If vomiting, give anti-sickness medications, followed by usual antiepileptic meds
- Give normal antiepileptic drugs if known epileptic
- If fits continue >30 min, call for medical advice
- Look for injuries

Continued monitoring
Note time taken to recover consciousness
- Pulse
- BP
- Temperature
- Conscious level
- RR
- Blood sugar
- Oximetry if available
- Further fits

WATCH FOR DETERIORATION

Possible causes of convulsion
Known epileptic—not taking usual meds, or vomiting/diarrhoea, infection, dehydration
Withdrawal of alcohol or other recreational drugs
Low blood sugars (hypoglycaemia)
Head injury
Drug overdose
Infections—meningitis/encephalitis/malaria
Hyperthermia—febrile convulsions in children
Low or high blood sodium
Post—diving (decompression sickness)

Fig. 8.15 Convulsion algorithm.

Diabetic emergencies

Hypoglycaemia

- Coma or reduced conscious level with blood sugar <4 mmol/L.
- Can occur in non-diabetics—sepsis, alcohol excess, liver failure, exhaustion, malaria, quinine therapy.

History

- Sweating, hunger, anxiety, inappropriate behaviour, exercise, seizure, last meal, previous hypos, usual blood sugar levels.
- Past history—diabetes, liver disease.
- Recent infection.
- Drugs—insulin dose, other hypoglycaemics.
- Social/environmental—alcohol excess.

Examination

- Pallor, sweating, tremor, slurred speech, confusion/aggression, focal neurology, poor coordination, convulsions.
- Check observations: pulse, BP, RR.
- GCS score.
- Examine for cause of sepsis: see **⊃** Fever, p. 280.
- Consider a rapid diagnostic test for malaria.

> **Urgent treatment of hypoglycaemia**
> See Fig. 8.16.

Treatment

Diabetes

Most likely cause is excess insulin, particularly if the patient has been undertaking unusually high levels of activity on the expedition. If hypos are recurrent, reduce insulin doses. Monitor blood sugars regularly, preferably before each meal.

> **Urgent treatment of diabetic ketoacidosis**
> - Give high-flow oxygen, if available.
> - Obtain venous access.
> - Insulin: give 20 units soluble insulin IM followed by 10 units IM/h. When patient has improved and is eating change to insulin SC.
> - Fluids: give 1 L normal saline IV, then 250 mL/h for 4–6 h.
> - When blood sugars <15 mmol/L change to glucose 5% 250 mL/h for 4–6 h (continue insulin 10 units IM/h).
> - Start a fluid balance chart and measure urine output.
> - Start antibiotics if any cause for infection identified.
> - Monitor blood sugars hourly.
> - See Fig. 8.16.
> - See also ♒ https://www.diabetes.co.uk/

Alcohol

Hypoglycaemia may recur if further excess alcohol is taken. Monitor blood sugars until patient is sober and eating/drinking normally.

Other causes

Evacuate from the field for further investigations/treatment.

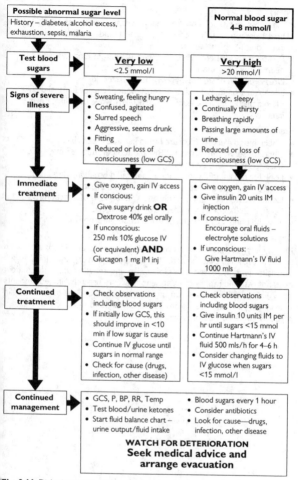

Possible abnormal sugar level History – diabetes, alcohol excess, exhaustion, sepsis, malaria		Normal blood sugar 4–8 mmol/l
Test blood sugars	**Very low** <2.5 mmol/l	**Very high** >20 mmol/l
Signs of severe illness	• Sweating, feeling hungry • Confused, agitated • Slurred speech • Aggressive, seems drunk • Fitting • Reduced or loss of consciousness (low GCS)	• Lethargic, sleepy • Continually thirsty • Breathing rapidly • Passing large amounts of urine • Reduced or loss of consciousness (low GCS)

Immediate treatment	• Give oxygen, gain IV access
	• If conscious:
	  Give sugary drink **OR** Dextrose 40% gel orally
	• If unconscious:
	  250 mls 10% glucose IV (or equivalent) **AND** Glucagon 1 mg IM inj
		• Give oxygen, gain IV access
		• Give insulin 20 units IM injection
		• If conscious:
		  Encourage oral fluids – electrolyte solutions
		• If unconscious:
		  Give Hartmann's IV fluid 1000 mls

Continued treatment	• Check observations including blood sugars • If initially low GCS, this should improve in <10 min if low sugar is cause • Continue IV glucose until sugars in normal range • Check for cause (drugs, infection, other disease)	• Check observations including blood sugars • Give insulin 10 units IM per hr until sugars <15 mmol • Continue Hartmann's IV fluid 500 mls/h for 4–6 h • Consider changing fluids to IV glucose when sugars <15 mmol/l
Continued management	• GCS, P, BP, RR, Temp • Test blood/urine ketones • Start fluid balance chart – urine output/fluid intake	• Blood sugars every 1 hour • Consider antibiotics • Look for cause—drugs, infection, other disease

WATCH FOR DETERIORATION
Seek medical advice and
arrange evacuation

Fig. 8.16 Diabetic emergencies.

Diabetic ketoacidosis

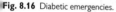

High blood sugars in a diabetic patient with poor glycaemic control may be secondary to infection or steroids. The classical clinical description of diabetic ketoacidosis (DKA) is of a comatose or pre-comatose patient who is dehydrated and hyperventilating.

History
- Tiredness, thirst, polyuria, frequency, dysuria, weight loss, vomiting, breathlessness, cough, sputum, fever, chest/abdominal pain, skin infections, teeth problems.
- Past history—diabetes, date of diagnosis, complications such as neuropathy, ulceration.
- Drugs—insulin dose, oral hypoglycaemics, steroids.
- Social/environmental—alcohol consumption, change in usual diet— often a problem on expeditions, particularly while travelling. Recent infection.

Examination
- Check blood glucose. Measure blood ketones if possible.
- Check observations: pulse, BP, RR, and temperature. BP may be low. GCS score. Record on chart.
- Look for facial flushing, dry mouth, and rapid breathing (Kussmaul respirations), 'pear-drop' smell of ketones on breath.
- Examine chest, abdomen, urine, and skin for signs of infection (➔ Fever, p. 280). Look for evidence of dental infection.
- Test the urine for ketonuria or evidence for infection.

Ongoing treatment
Mild hyperglycaemia (<20 mmol/L) will not necessitate evacuation from the field, provided that the patient is eating and drinking and blood sugars normalize with increased doses of insulin and rehydration. If the patient does not respond rapidly to treatment, evacuate urgently; limited amounts of IV fluids will be available on most expeditions. Change to usual insulin when eating and ketones <1.5mmol/L. Continue to monitor blood sugars regularly, preferably before each meal.

Gastrointestinal bleeding

History

- *Vomit*—colour, quantity, blood mixed in, frequency, onset, pain on vomiting.
- *Stools*—onset, quantity, colour (red, black, clots), pain on opening bowels, constipation, diarrhoea, change in bowel habit.
- *Other*—appetite, dysphagia, weight loss, dyspnoea, palpitations, tiredness, dizziness, fainting, sweating, abdominal/chest pain.
- *Past history*—previous bleeding, clotting problems, inflammatory bowel disease, liver disease (varices?), peptic ulceration, heartburn/indigestion.
- *Drugs*—aspirin, NSAIDs, steroids, warfarin, direct oral anticoagulants such as apixaban, rivaroxaban and dabigatran, clopidogrel. Iron, proton pump inhibitors (PPIs)/antacids.
- *Social/environmental*—alcohol/drugs, smoking status, recent stressors.

Examination

- Temperature, pulse, BP, blood sugar, GCS score (➔ p. 223). NEWS score (➔ p. 254).
- Look for ongoing bleeding, evidence of shock, abdominal distension/tenderness/rebound/masses. Bowel sounds. PR examination for fresh blood/melaena/palpable mass/haemorrhoids.

Gastrointestinal bleeding—differential diagnosis

Upper GI

- Gastroduodenal ulceration (➔ p. 278).
- Mallory–Weiss tears (➔ p. 418).
- Oesophageal varices.
- GI malignancy.

Lower GI

- Haemorrhoids/anal fissure (➔ p. 419).
- Inflammatory bowel disease.
- Diverticular disease.

Treatment

- Keep nil by mouth for 24 h. Maintain BP >90 mmHg systolic by cautious use of IV fluids. Give analgesia as required (not NSAIDs or aspirin!). Monitor urine output. Consider PPI/antacids. Avoid spicy food. Observe regularly and evacuate for further investigation.
- See Fig. 8.17.

> **Urgent treatment**
> - Place the patient supine with legs elevated. If vomiting, place in the recovery position.
> - Give high-flow oxygen.
> - Check observations: pulse, BP, RR, and temperature.
> - Obtain venous access.
> - Consider cautious use of IV saline depending on pulse and BP.

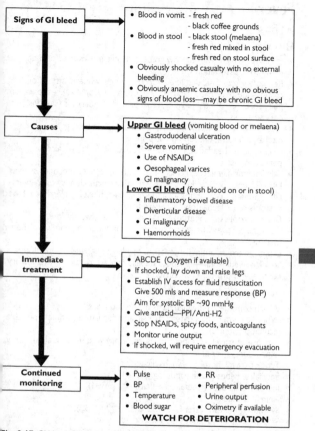

Signs of GI bleed
- Blood in vomit - fresh red
  - black coffee grounds
- Blood in stool - black stool (melaena)
  - fresh red mixed in stool
  - fresh red on stool surface
- Obviously shocked casualty with no external bleeding
- Obviously anaemic casualty with no obvious signs of blood loss—may be chronic GI bleed

Causes

Upper GI bleed (vomiting blood or melaena)
- Gastroduodenal ulceration
- Severe vomiting
- Use of NSAIDs
- Oesophageal varices
- GI malignancy

Lower GI bleed (fresh blood on or in stool)
- Inflammatory bowel disease
- Diverticular disease
- GI malignancy
- Haemorrhoids

Immediate treatment
- ABCDE (Oxygen if available)
- If shocked, lay down and raise legs
- Establish IV access for fluid resuscitation
  Give 500 mls and measure response (BP)
  Aim for systolic BP ~90 mmHg
- Give antacid—PPI/Anti-H2
- Stop NSAIDs, spicy foods, anticoagulants
- Monitor urine output
- If shocked, will require emergency evacuation

Continued monitoring
- Pulse
- BP
- Temperature
- Blood sugar
- RR
- Peripheral perfusion
- Urine output
- Oximetry if available

WATCH FOR DETERIORATION

Fig. 8.17 GI bleed algorithm.

Fever

See Fig. 8.18.

History

- *Fever type*—high swinging, low grade, periodic (i.e. every 2 or 3 days as in malaria), association with rigors.
- *Respiratory/ear, nose, and throat (ENT)*—cough, wheeze, stridor or croup, sputum or nasal catarrh, haemoptysis, dyspnoea, chest pain, ear pain, sore throat, hoarse voice, facial pain, or tenderness (sinusitis), coryzal illness.
- *Urinogenital*—frequency, dysuria, haematuria, loin pain, genital discharge/ulceration, suprapubic pain.
- *Neurological*—headache, photophobia, neck stiffness, impaired consciousness.
- *Skin/mucous membranes/joints*—rash, petechiae, skin infections such as bites/ulcers/sores, cellulitis, mucosal lesions, arthralgia, swollen joints.
- *GI*—vomiting, haematemesis, abdominal pain, bloating, diarrhoea, blood in stools or melaena, foul/excessive flatus.
- *Other*—changes in appetite, aching, night sweats, weight loss.
- *Past history*—previous similar symptoms, immunocompromise, diabetes mellitus.
- *Drugs*—steroids, antimalarials taken regularly, antipyretics, antibiotics.
- *Social/environmental*—infectious disease contact, detailed travel history, adequacy of pre-travel vaccinations.

Travel history

- Which countries and which parts of the countries?
- When? Length of trip, date of arrival, and departure (estimate possible incubation period).
- Purpose of travel—business, pleasure, family visit, military, airline crew, expedition, emigration?
- Type of travel, hotels, safari, backpacking.
- Special activities (climbing, diving, caving)?
- Insect bites/stings (tsetse, ticks, fleas) (➔ p. 304).
- Animal contact.
- Swimming in fresh water lakes (bilharzia) (➔ p. 530).
- Sexual or other infectious disease contact.
- Antimalarials taken/immunizations received pre-travel.
- Illness among other members of the family or party.

Examination

- Temperature (chart if possible), pulse/RR, BP, GCS score, urine output oxygen saturations.
- Warm or cool peripheries, CRT (➔ p. 192), sweating, rash, mucosal lesions, wounds, abscesses, insect bites, ulcers, eschar, buboes, cellulitis or other focal skin infection (examine the entire body surface, including the scalp, axillae, and perineum).
- Look up the nose and at throat, tonsils, tongue, and buccal mucous membrane. Look in the ears with an auriscope.

- Examine chest for breath sounds and heart murmurs; abdominal tenderness, bowel sounds, lymphadenopathy; joint pain or swelling, external genitalia (retained tampon) and rectal examination if relevant.

Investigations

Usually impossible in the field. The macroscopic appearance and odour of vomitus, stool, and urine may be helpful (e.g. obvious blood; cloudiness and foul, fishy smell of urine suggest infection). Consider dip testing urine, microscopic examination of blood, sputum, urine, stool (experience required). Rapid antigen tests for malaria (➔ Malaria, p. 512).

Possible diagnoses

- *URTI*—viral coryza, sinusitis, otitis media, tonsillitis, 'strep' throat.
- *Chest*—bronchitis, pneumonia, tuberculosis.
- *Gut*—gastroenteritis, dysentery.
- *Urinary*—UTI, pyelonephritis.
- *Neurological*—meningitis/encephalitis.
- *Tropical infections*—malaria, typhoid, legionella, leptospirosis, hepatitis, rabies, typhus/other rickettsiae, viral haemorrhagic fevers.

Treatment

- If reduced GCS, (see ➔ Coma, p. 267).
- Focal neurology or possibility of life-threatening sepsis: give oxygen, broad-spectrum antibiotics, evacuate urgently.
- If malaria is a possibility treat urgently (➔ p. 512).
- Reduce fever with regular paracetamol and/or ibuprofen.
- Encourage oral fluids and monitor urine output; start a fluid balance chart.
- Advise rest in a cool place. Observe closely, evacuate if not improving.
- Empirical antibiotic therapy:
  - *UTI*—trimethoprim 200 mg/12 h PO (or ciprofloxacin 250 mg/12 h PO), 5-day course.
  - *Cellulitis*—flucloxacillin 1 g/6 h IV + benzylpenicillin 1.2 g/6 h IV, 7-day courses.
  - *Wound infection*—flucloxacillin 500 mg/6 h PO, 7-day course.
  - *Meningitis*—ceftriaxone 2–4 g/12 h IV, 5-day course.
  - *Septic arthritis*—flucloxacillin 2 g/6 h IV, 7-day course.
  - *Pneumonia*—amoxicillin 500 mg/8 h PO or clarithromycin 500 mg/12 h PO, 7-day course.
  - *Intra-abdominal sepsis*—ceftriaxone 2g/12 h IV + metronidazole 500 mg/8 h IV, 7-day courses.

Penicillin allergy

For many infections a penicillin is a sensible first-line antibiotic of choice. If an expedition member is known to be allergic to penicillins, then the medical kit should contain additional quantities of a suitable alternative. Depending upon the nature of the infection, clarithromycin, metronidazole, or doxycycline may be appropriate; consult the *BNF* online.

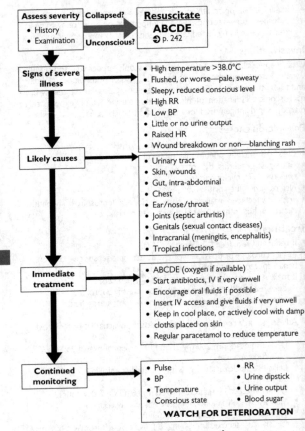

Fig. 8.18 Fever algorithm.

Chapter 9

Skin

Authors
Jon Dallimore
Roderick Hay
David A. Warrell (1st and 2nd editions)

Reviewer
Edi Albert

Solar skin damage

Introduction

Many travellers harbour the unstated aim of acquiring a 'good' tan. However, excessive exposure to solar radiation is damaging and may cause skin cancers:

- Basal cell carcinoma.
- Squamous cell carcinoma.
- Malignant melanoma.

In the UK, incidence of all skin cancers has increased—with >189,000 new cases reported in 2017. Chronic sun exposure is also associated with skin thickening, pigmentation, and increased wrinkles. A number of skin conditions are triggered by exposure to sunlight, sometimes as a reaction to medicines and some people are sensitive to the effects of sunlight, e.g. sufferers from polymorphic light eruption.

Solar radiation

Sunlight is the commonest source of ultraviolet radiation (UVR). UVR is subdivided into UVA (320–400 nm), UVB (280–320 nm), and UVC (100–280 nm). UVC is potentially very damaging to human skin but is normally absorbed by ozone in the earth's atmosphere. UVB plays an important role in sunburn, carcinogenesis, skin ageing, and vitamin D synthesis. UVA is responsible for tanning, ageing changes, and may be involved in carcinogenesis. Between 10 and 20 times more UVA reaches the earth's surface than UVB.

Intensity of sunlight increases nearer the equator, at increasing altitudes, and in polar regions where the protective atmospheric ozone layer may have thinned. It is also greatest when the sun is highest in the sky, between 10 am and 3 pm. UVR is reflected by water, white surfaces (such as snow and sand), and glass.

Sunburn

This follows acute, excessive exposure to UVR. It is an important risk factor for the development of malignant melanoma. Mild sunburn is characterized by skin redness, local heat, and pain. Severe sunburn may result in swelling, blistering, and generalized symptoms such as malaise, nausea, and rigors.

Treatment of sunburn

Sunburn is much easier to prevent than treat. Anti-inflammatories and paracetamol can be used for pain relief. Simple water-based emollient creams may relieve the symptoms. Hydrocortisone 1% cream also helps to reduce inflammation but should not be applied to large areas or to broken skin. Blisters should not be drained unless very large.

Susceptibility to solar damage

People with different skin types are more or less likely to burn in the sun. Generally, individuals with pale skin, red hair, blue or green eyes, and freckles are most susceptible to solar skin damage. Those with a personal or family history of skin cancer or polymorphic light eruption should be particularly careful to avoid excessive sun exposure.

Prevention of sunburn
- Avoid mid-day sun.
- Beware of bright hazy weather, UV can penetrate cloud.
- Use natural shade.
- Cover up with hats and clothing (some have a sunlight protection factor rating).
- Use a sunscreen that protects against UVA and UVB, is water-resistant, and has a SPF >15.

Sunscreens

There are two main types of sunscreen:
- Physical.
- Chemical.

Physical sunscreens contain zinc oxide or titanium dioxide. They are highly visible on the skin and are very effective at blocking UVA and UVB but may be cosmetically unacceptable to some. However, over the past few years these have become available in Dayglo colours and as a result have become more widely used by younger people.

Chemical sunscreens contain para-aminobenzoic acid or cinnamates and protect against UVB. Some newer compounds also protect against UVA. Chemical sunscreens sometimes cause allergic or irritant reactions. Waterproof sunscreens are available for aquatic/marine use.

Sun protection factor

SPF is a guide to the ability of a sunscreen to protect the skin from UVR. A star system, 1–4, where 4 is the strongest, indicates the capacity to block out UVA. In theory, the SPF increases the amount of time that can be spent in the sun by the factor quoted. However, variables such as the time of day, the amount of cloud cover, time of year, and the amount of reflection all affect the protective ability of the sunscreen.

Wounds

Minor wounds are common on expeditions but some wounds are life-threatening. An ABC approach should be used (➔ p. 198). All wounds need careful assessment, thorough cleaning, then closure and dressing. Wounds that involve tendon, nerve, or blood vessel injuries cannot be managed in the field—the patient will need to be evacuated.

Immediate assessment and treatment

See ➔ p. 202.

Take a focused history
- How did the injury occur? (Mechanism is all important; was it an insect, mammal, or snake-bite?)
- Where did it occur (clean, contaminated, or marine environment)?
- When did it occur? Old wounds >12 h should not be sutured and are more likely to become infected.
- Was the wound caused by broken glass or other foreign body? (Will need careful examination or preferably X-ray.)
- Was the limb trapped or crushed? (Swelling and compartment syndrome are possible; see also ➔ Crush injuries, p. 295.)
- When was the last tetanus booster? (Particularly for deep, penetrating wounds.)
- Is the patient allergic to any medications or dressings?
- Does the patient take any medication?

Examine the wound
- Measure wounds and consider drawing, using a diagram (Fig. 9.1), or taking a digital photograph using camera or smartphone/tablet.
- Look for contamination and foreign bodies.
- Check for signs of infection (red, hot, swollen, blistering, painful, tenderness, crepitus, lymphangitis, enlarged regional lymph nodes, fever). The earliest signs may develop after 8–12 h (mammal bites), but there is usually a delay of 2–7 days post injury.
- Check for pulses and CRT (➔ p. 439).
- Re-examine carefully for signs of nerve damage—change in sensation, weakness, or paralysis.
- Look for evidence of damage to deep structures—examine the wound, preferably under local or regional anaesthetic.

General wound care

All wounds should be managed using the following principles:
- Stop bleeding.
- Clean carefully to reduce the risk of infection.
- Dress the injury to keep it clean.
- Promote healing and restore function.

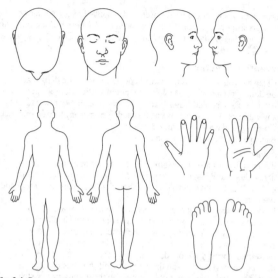

Fig. 9.1 Diagram of body for noting injury or skin feature.

Stopping bleeding

All wounds bleed to a greater or lesser extent; sometimes bleeding may be life-threatening:

- Apply direct pressure over the wound with a clean dressing.
- Lay the casualty down.
- Raise the wounded limb above the level of the heart (but not excessively).
- Apply a further dressing to control the bleeding on top of any original pad. If bleeding persists, remove the dressing, open the wound, and apply pressure deep in the wound (**⤳** p. 214).
- Bandage firmly to hold the dressing in place.

All wounds swell to some extent; watch for tourniquet effect.

When there are very deep wounds it may not be possible to control bleeding by applying pressure on the surface of the skin. The only way to stop severe, persistent bleeding from deep inside a wound may be to remove the dressings, open the wound, remove clots and debris, and to pack the wound open with sterile gauze or by placing haemostatic sutures using an absorbable suture material. The use of artery forceps should be avoided as they may damage important structures that follow the line of blood vessels such as tendons and nerves.

In torrential haemorrhage, e.g. following a landmine injury or traumatic amputation, it may be necessary to use other techniques such as a tourniquet (which should be released and reapplied every 30 min) or the use of pressure points. For those working in areas where ballistic trauma is a possibility, haemostatic agents such as QuikClot® or Celox® may be life-saving (→ p. 214).

Preventing infection

- Clean all wounds. This is the most important and useful thing that can be done. Purified water, sterile saline, or antiseptic solution can be used—boiled, cooled water is acceptable in an expedition setting but any water of drinking quality can be used. Remove any foreign material.
- Cover wound with a non-stick dressing.
- Bandage to hold the dressing in place.

Consider:

- If foreign bodies are deeply embedded and cannot be removed easily, they should be left and removed surgically. If an object remains embedded, the surrounding wound should still be cleaned carefully and then dressed.
- During an expedition it may be necessary to care for wounds for days or even weeks. Infection rates vary considerably in different environments from rare in polar or high mountain areas to very common in wet tropical areas. The threshold for antibiotic treatment will vary accordingly. Wounds should be inspected daily (maybe twice daily in the jungle) and clean dressings applied. Any pus or exudate should be gently removed but do not scrub the wound or use strong antiseptics which may damage healing tissues. If dressings stick, soaking in warm clean water will allow easier removal. Deep, contaminated, penetrating wounds are prone to tetanus infection.[1] If the casualty has definitely been immunized against tetanus in the past, give a booster of toxoid. If prior immunity is uncertain, consider giving tetanus immunoglobulin. (→ Immunization, p. 28).

Dressings and bandaging

Wounds should be dressed in layers:

- Use non-stick sterile dressing on the wound (such as non-adherent tulle dressings (e.g. Melolin®) or paraffin gauze).
- Sterile gauze swabs to absorb any pus or exudate from the wound.
- Next, apply a crepe bandage or other elasticated bandage to hold dressings in place.
- The bandage should hold the dressing in place without producing pressure or constriction.

Promoting healing and restoration of function

Wound healing is aided by a healthy diet and rest. Substantial wounds will heal more quickly in the higher ambient oxygen tensions at altitudes <3000 m. Rest is needed initially, but prolonged splinting leads to stiffness and muscle wasting. Joints adjacent to a wound or burn should be kept mobile. See → Physiotherapy, p. 478.

1 https://assets.publishing.service.gov.uk/government/uploads/system/uploads/attachment_data/file/849460/Tetanus_quick_guide_poster.pdf

Wound types and management

Lacerations are caused by a blunt injury and the skin is torn with irregular wound edges. There is often evidence of bruising in the surrounding tissues.

Cuts or incised wounds are a result of sharp edges such as knives or glass. They have clean-cut edges. Stab wounds are deep and slash wounds are long and superficial.

Closing cuts and lacerations

Gaping wounds will heal more quickly and result in a better scar if the skin edges are brought together.

Steri-Strips™

Steri-Strips™ are paper stitches that come in a variety of lengths and widths (Fig. 9.2). They are placed across a laceration and, if left in place for a week or so, result in a clean, neat scar. Steri-Strips™ do not stick near moving joints, on the palms of the hands and soles of the feet, or on the scalp. However, they are excellent for finger lacerations and facial wounds. In humid or wet environments, such as the jungle or at sea, consider applying tincture of benzoin (Friar's Balsam) to the skin—this helps the Steri-Strips™ to adhere to the skin. SkinLink® reinforced paper sutures are also useful.

(a)

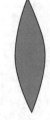

Superficial wound

(b)

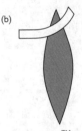

Apply Steri-Strip™ to one side of the wound

(c)

Pull edges together and apply to other side

(d)

Complete closure with strips as required

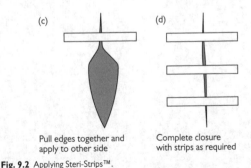

Fig. 9.2 Applying Steri-Strips™.

Suturing
(See Fig. 9.4.)

Steri-Strips™ should be used where possible. If Steri-Strips™ will not close the wound, suturing or staples should be considered, using local anaesthetic. Only clean wounds that are <12 h old are suitable for suturing. Deep wounds should be closed in layers by an experienced surgeon in an operating theatre because of the risk of wound infection. If this is not possible, clean the wound, pack with sterile gauze soaked in saline, and re-dress daily until definitive care is reached. Sutures should never be used to close deep or dirty wounds, particularly animal or human bites. Suturing should only be attempted by those who are adequately trained. Tissue staples are quick and easy to apply but also require some training—see Fig. 9.3.

> **Important points when suturing a wound**
> * Most inexperienced people use too many stitches, too tight, too close.
> * Lay the wound edges together to allow healing to occur—do not use tension.
> * Use toothed forceps to hold the skin edges and pass the needle close to the part of the skin which is being held with forceps.
> * Match up wound edges with strategically placed sutures along irregular wounds then close the gaps.
> * Do not be afraid to remove sutures and try again.

Choice of suture material: the skin should be closed with non-absorbable suture material such as Prolene® or nylon on a curved reverse cutting needle. Experienced operators may consider carrying absorbable suture material (such as Vicryl®) to close deep tissue layers and this will help to reduce the risk of haematoma formation and subsequent infection. Vicryl® can also be used to close wounds inside the mouth. Use 4/0 sutures for most parts of the body, 5/0 on fingers, and preferably 6/0 for the face.

Removal of sutures: sutures should be removed after 7–10 days except on the face where earlier removal results in better healing with less scarring when the foreign material is removed. Sutures can be replaced by Steri-Strips™ after 3–4 days.

Staples
These are easy to use with minimal training (Fig. 9.3) and may be used particularly to close scalp wounds rapidly. If carried, a staple remover must also be available.

Tissue glue
May be useful for superficial face and scalp wounds, particularly in children. When bleeding is controlled, clean and dry the wound edges and place glue on the skin edges, not in the wound. Hold the wound edges together for 1 min to let the glue set.

Histoacryl® tissue glue is used commonly for closing small lacerations and is particularly useful on the head and other areas where there is little skin movement during normal activities. On an expedition, the 'super glue' in a repair kit can be used quite safely. Ensure the wound edges are dry, gently bring the edges of the wound together, squeeze a bead of glue along the

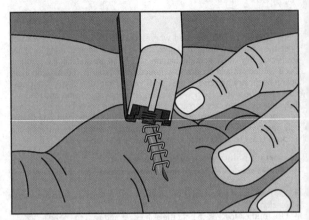

Fig. 9.3 Inserting staples.

surface of the wound and wait for 20 s before releasing. Make sure the part of the body with the wound on it is horizontal as glue has a tendency to run, and you don't want it to end up in the patient's eyes or gluing the medic's fingers to the patient!

Abrasions

Abrasions are grazing injuries where the top surface of the skin is removed. They should be cleaned carefully and a non-adherent dressing applied. Ingrained dirt, if not removed, will result in tattooing and makes wound infection more likely. Dressings may require changing once or twice daily in some environments such as the jungle. If dressings stick, they can be soaked off with warm, clean water or saline.

Puncture wounds

Infection may occur at the base of deep, penetrating wounds. Tetanus is a significant risk in the anaerobic conditions found deep in puncture wounds, and all expedition team members should be immunized before travel (Table 2.1, p. 30). Clean puncture wounds by encouraging bleeding, irrigate the wound with clean water using a syringe, and prevent the skin surface sealing over by placing a small sterile gauze wick into the wound. The wick encourages healing to occur from the bottom of the puncture wound upwards, otherwise abscess formation may occur. If deep infection in a puncture wound develops, evacuate the casualty for surgical exploration and cleaning.

Bites (animal and human)

Human bites carry a high risk of bacterial infections such as *Staphylococcus aureus* and *Eikenella corrodens*. Mammal bites should always raise the question of rabies, including the rabies-related bat lyssa viruses (p. 500) and

1

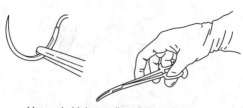

How to hold the needle and surgical instrument

2

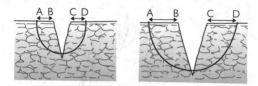

Distance from needle entry/exit points to wound edge. The greater the distance from the wound edge to the needle entry point, the deeper the bite of the needle. AB must equal CD, otherwise a step will occur

3

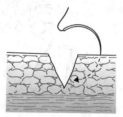

Depth of suture. Aim to close the wound fully by placing the suture to the deepest part of the wound

4

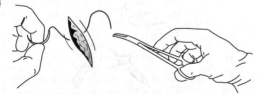

Instrument tie knot. Starting position, needle in left hand, needle-holder in right hand

5

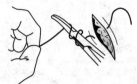

Wrapping the suture around the needle-holder.
Do this TWICE

6

The first throw: take the loose end of the suture in the
jaws of the needle-holder

7

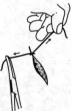

To tighten the first throw, cross the hands, needle-holder
going to the left, and the left hand going to the right

8

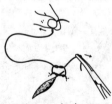

The second throw: the suture has been wrapped over the
needle-holder in the opposite direction and this time the
hand does not cross when tying the suture. Repeat this stage
to complete the surgical knot.

Fig. 9.4 Skin suturing technique.

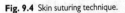

there are a range of other special pathogens such as *Pasteurella multocida* (dog and cat bites), *Capnocytophaga canimorsus* (dogs), *Bartonella henselae* (cats), and *Streptobacillus moniliformis* and *Spirillum minus* (rodents). Bites should be cleaned as a matter of urgency with liberal amounts of soap and water followed by an antiseptic such as povidone-iodine or alcohol. Consider whether tetanus immunization is required and whether an antibiotic such as co-amoxiclav should be prescribed. (See also ⮁ Chapter 17.)

Bruises

Contusions or bruises are caused by a blunt force applied to the tissues. Bleeding under the skin gives the bruise its characteristic coloured appearance. Large muscle haematomas may cause hypovolaemic shock. Rest, ice, compression, and elevation (RICE) all help to reduce swelling and pain. Compression may be achieved by applying a crepe bandage firmly around the affected area. Anti-inflammatory drugs such as ibuprofen or aspirin may also help but are not good for haemostasis. After a day or two the affected part should be mobilized to reduce stiffness (⮁ Physiotherapy, p. 478.) Avoid incising haematomas because of the risk of infection.

Blisters

Blisters are best prevented. Ideally, stop walking and cover any 'hot spots' before they develop into blisters. If a blister does form, the fluid may be drained using a clean (sterile) fine needle and the area covered with an adhesive plaster but never 'de-roof' the blister unless pus is accumulating. Moleskin®, Compeed®, and Spenco Second Skin® are dressings designed to relieve the discomfort. Simple zinc oxide tape may be effective. Blisters may become de-roofed; in this case treat with a non-adherent or hydrocolloid dressing. A thin application of Friar's Balsam at the edge of a blister or swathes of zinc oxide tape over the dressings may help to keep protective coverings in place. Healing is rapid if friction at the blister site can be eliminated. Try to correct the cause (faulty footwear). Where possible, leaving the blister uncovered will assist healing by allowing the area to dry out.

Crush injuries

(See also Crush injury, ⮁ p. 837.) Large amounts of tissue may be damaged in crushing injuries and the potential for infection is high. The crushed part should be carefully cleaned and then elevated. Swelling of muscles in the affected part may cut off the blood supply to the limb beyond the injury, a condition known as compartment syndrome. If the injury is severe, there may be a risk of losing the limb and acute kidney injury. Evacuate the casualty urgently for expert assessment; try to ensure the casualty maintains a good urine output during the evacuation. Under surgical operating conditions, the pressure may be released and circulation restored by splitting the sheath around the damaged muscles, a fasciotomy, but this is not a procedure to attempt in the field.

Amputation

A digit or limb may be replaced by microsurgery if the patient and the amputated part can be delivered to a surgeon in <6 h. The amputated part should be kept cool, preferably in a container with ice, but not in direct contact with the ice. In an expedition setting, it is highly unlikely that such surgical facilities will be available; in this case, treat the bleeding with direct pressure and elevation. The stump should be cleaned gently and then covered with a non-adherent dressing such as paraffin gauze. People with these injuries need to be evacuated to allow surgical treatment to shorten any bone ends and cover the stump with a flap of skin so that healing can take place (terminalization). Knife injuries that remove a chunk of palmar tissue such as the finger pulp are best treated by re-applying the excised tissue to the wound under a firm dressing or taking the tissue with the casualty.

Splinters

Splinters can usually be removed using a fine pair of tweezers (the ones on Swiss Army knives are good) or a sterile needle. For more stubborn splinters, soaking may help. Spines from sea urchins are easier to remove after a couple of days when the wound becomes inflamed, or after softening the skin by soaking or applying salicylic acid ointment (2% w/w) (→ Sea urchin and starfish injuries (echinoderms), p. 600).

Wound infections

Any wound can become infected; bites, dirty wounds, and deep wounds are more likely to become infected. Infections typically appear from 2–7 days after the injury but, in the case of mammal bite wounds (*Pasteurella multocida*), all the signs of inflammation may develop in as little as 8–12 h. Signs and symptoms of a wound infection are pain, redness, heat, swelling, and loss of function. In the later stages, red lines may be seen running from a limb wound up towards the trunk (lymphangitis). Lymph nodes in the armpit, groin, or neck may become enlarged and fever may develop.

Abscesses

An abscess is a collection of pus or a 'boil' and is usually caused by a bacterial infection. As pus accumulates, the skin over the abscess thins ('pointing'). Once the pus discharges through the skin, the throbbing pain rapidly resolves. If an abscess develops during an expedition, applying local heat and oral antibiotics (e.g. flucloxacillin) may help. However, once pus is present it is quicker and kinder to drain it. Exceptions include those affecting the face, genital and anal areas, and breast—abscesses in these areas should be referred for specialist treatment. Local anaesthetic is less effective in the presence of infection because of localized high tissue acidity. Regional nerve blocks such as a digital nerve block may provide good analgesia (➔ p. 627). An elliptical cut over the abscess must be large enough to let the pus drain. A small piece of gauze soaked in saline inserted into the incision will act as a wick and stop the roof of the abscess healing over before all the pus has drained. In this way the abscess cavity will heal from the bottom upwards. The wick should be changed daily until the abscess has healed. If there is evidence of spreading infection, antibiotics should be used.

Cellulitis

Cellulitis refers to a bacterial infection of the skin (usually staphylococcal or streptococcal). Small lesions on the feet or athlete's foot between the toes may provide the portal of entry, but there may not be an obvious source of infection. The signs are the same as for a wound infection; that is, circumscribed redness with a raised edge, heat, pain, swelling, tenderness, and fever with rigors which may precede the appearance of the skin lesion. Look for lymphangitis and lymphadenopathy. Treat with oral antibiotics initially (flucloxacillin or clarithromycin). Consider IV antibiotics if the infection is spreading or there are blisters or features of generalized infection such as fever and rigors. Necrotizing fasciitis is rare but can occur after trauma. Spreading infection with signs of shock would mandate urgent assessment in secondary care.

Burns

Burns may be caused by dry heat, chemicals, electricity, friction, or hot liquids. On expeditions, open fires and fuel stoves commonly cause injuries, particularly when people refuel lighted stoves or burn rubbish with petrol.

Assessing the severely burned patient

Use an ABC approach:

- Ensure a safe approach for rescuers. Disconnect the electricity supply in electrical burns. Smother flames with a blanket or roll the victim on the ground. Remove any source of heat and remove any clothing that is not adherent to the skin.
- *Airway*—look for signs of potential problems—hoarse voice, burning or soot around mouth and nose, difficulty swallowing, singed nasal hair. A surgical airway may be necessary (❷ p. 207) but the outlook on an expedition is likely to be very poor if evacuation times are long.
- *Cervical spine*—there may be other injuries, particularly if the patient jumped from a building to escape the fire. Immobilize the neck and spine if injury is suspected.
- *Breathing*—severe circumferential burns on the chest may require rapid surgical treatment (escharotomy) and are likely to be fatal in a very remote area.
- *Circulation*—shock is a feature of severe burns and large quantities of fluids may be needed. For fluid resuscitation see following section on assessing burns (see also ❷ Shock, p. 250).

History

Establish:

- Did the fire occur in an enclosed space?
- What was the burning material, if known?
- Was the patient unconscious at any time?
- Was there an explosion?

Examination

Assessing burns

The severity and extent of burns is often underestimated, even by doctors and nurses, and extensive burns need specialist assessment and treatment. The 'rule of nines', which divides the surface area of the body into areas of approximately 9%, is one method used to calculate the proportion of the body which is burned and so helps determine treatment (Fig. 9.5). It may be easier to remember that the patient's palm (excluding the fingers and thumb) represents ~1% of the body surface area. Mobile phone apps can also be used to help with assessment of burn areas.

Burns may be divided into superficial and full-thickness burns:

- Superficial burns: characterized by redness, swelling, and pain (first degree). Deep partial-thickness (second-degree) burns are blistered and do not blanch on pressure.
- Full-thickness (third-degree) burns: characterized by pale, leathery, and sometimes charred skin with a loss of sensation. There are no blisters.
- Photographs taken at the time of the initial assessment provide an effective record and may be very helpful to those providing definitive care.

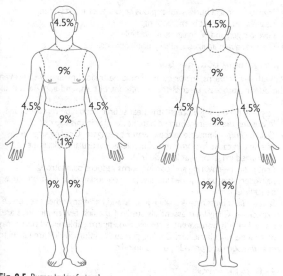

Fig. 9.5 Burns: 'rule of nines'.

Consider:
- On an expedition, it is important to differentiate between deep partial-thickness and full-thickness burns, although this may be difficult initially. Full-thickness burns need skin grafting, so evacuation to specialist medical help will be necessary.
- Fluid resuscitation for patients with >15% burns.
- Insert a cannula away from the burned areas and give 2–4 mL 0.9% saline/kg per % body surface area burned (excluding areas of erythema). This is the total volume to be given in the first 24 h; half of this volume should be given in the first 8 h. For example:
  - For a 70-kg man with 30% burns: 2 × 70 × 30 = 4200 mL/24 h. Give 2100 mL in the first 8 h.
  - Cover burned areas with clingfilm.
  - Monitor pulse, BP, RR, conscious level oxygen saturation (if possible) and body temperature.
  - Measure urine output.
  - Arrange urgent evacuation to hospital.

Treatment of severe burns and scalds

Ensure scene safety to prevent other people becoming burn victims. Remove the patient from the burning environment.
Halt the burning process and relieve pain by applying cold water for at least 10 min and cover burned areas with clingfilm or clean sheets.

- Irrigate chemical burns with copious amounts of tepid water.
- Leave any adherent burnt clothing.
- Give oxygen and IV analgesia if available.
- Give adequate analgesia, ideally using opioids.

Management of minor burns

As with severe burns, minor burns should be treated promptly to prevent the burning process, to cool the burn, control pain, and apply a suitable dressing.

- *Stopping the burning process*—the heat source should be removed. See 'Assessing the severely burned patient', earlier in this topic.
- *Cool the burn*—immerse in tepid water or irrigate. Cooling large areas of skin can cause hypothermia. Chemicals, particularly alkalis, need prolonged irrigation—at least 30 min.
- *Control pain*—covering and cooling burns reduces pain. Strong painkillers may be required initially; later co-codamol or ibuprofen may be sufficient.
- *Suitable burn dressings*—clingfilm is ideal and has many other uses on an expedition. Clingfilm is essentially sterile if the first few centimetres are discarded. It is transparent, stretchy, and impermeable. Hand burns may be treated in a plastic bag. Cooling gels such as Burnshield® are useful to cool the burn and provide good pain relief.

Key facts for burns

- Burns to significant areas such as hands, feet, face, and genitalia should be assessed by a specialist.
- Burns >10% body surface area need evacuation as many burns become infected.
- Full-thickness burns will almost certainly require skin grafting and should be evacuated early.
- Blistered burns: do not de-roof; however, large blisters may be aspirated with a sterile needle and syringe.
- In general, avoid prophylactic antibiotics.
- Mupirocin cream helps to prevent infection during evacuation and can be placed under clingfilm or inside a plastic bag in the case of hand burns. Paraffin gauze is very useful to dress burns as it is less likely to adhere to the burn.
- Granuflex® (a hydrocolloid dressing) is adhesive and waterproof and may be used for awkward areas which are difficult to dress. Change every 3–5 days.
- Elevate limb burns to reduce swelling.
- Early physiotherapy helps to maintain mobility (➲ p. 478).
- Regular ibuprofen is usually sufficient analgesia for a dressed burn.
- On an expedition, burns should be re-dressed every 24–48 h. Look for signs of infection (➲ p. 286). Healed burns should be protected from the sun for 6–12 months.

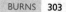

Insect bites

Bites by blood-feeding insects such as mosquitoes, midges, black flies, sand flies, tabanid flies (horse, deer, and stable flies), tsetse flies, and triatomine 'kissing' bugs pose a common irritation and nuisance during expeditions. These 'micro-predators' make brief blood-sucking attacks on humans and animals which can result in persisting medical problems.

Clinical features

Consequences of bites:
- Allergic reactions.
- Secondary infection of the bite site.
- Acquisition of systemic infections transmitted by the insect.

Bites may be immediately painful and traumatic (horse flies) but the commonest problem is delayed local swelling and itching from hypersensitivity to insects' salivary allergens incurred by previous exposure. A small, intensely itchy, reddish lump with a central (haemorrhagic) punctum develops immediately or after a delay of 24–48 h. A papule, urticarial weal, blister, or bulla may develop even after bites by tiny blackflies (*Simulium*), or bites may provoke a more generalized erythema multiforme or, especially in children, papular urticaria. Systemic anaphylaxis may be provoked (➲ p. 56). Scratching may lead to secondary infection, an inflamed, painful pustule or carbuncle (e.g. Lord Carnarvon's fatal septicaemia from an infected mosquito bite on his cheek near the tomb of Tutankhamun), or a demarcated, hot, bright red, raised area of erysipelas or cellulitis. Causative bacteria include *Staphylococcus aureus* and *Streptococcus pyogenes*. The risk of secondary infection seems to be higher under humid tropical conditions. Triatomine bug bites are usually multiple, often near the eye or angle of the mouth, and are painful, swollen, ooze blood, and may be surrounded by black staining from the bug's faeces (➲ Chagas' disease, p. 524).

Treatment

- Apply a cooling antiseptic solution, cream, or ointment to soothe irritation and prevent secondary infection. Reduce itch with counter irritants such as crotamiton cream/lotion, with or without hydrocortisone.
- Topical corticosteroids (e.g. hydrocortisone 0.5–1% can be purchased over the counter in the UK as creams or ointments) can be tried but topical antihistamines are not recommended as they may be sensitizing and are ineffective.
- For severe pruritus use oral antihistamines. Try full dose, non-sedating anti-H$_1$ drugs such as cetirizine (adult dose up to 10 mg twice a day) during the day and chlorphenamine 4 mg at night.
- Early systemic symptoms of anaphylaxis should be treated with adrenaline (epinephrine) 0.1% (1:1000) 0.5 mL by IM injection (adult dose). This dose may be repeated after 5–10 min if there is no response (➲ p. 256).
- If inflamed pustules develop, apply a topical antibacterial such as mupirocin. Multiple infected bites may warrant a course of oral antibiotic such as flucloxacillin or clarithromycin.

Prevention

Be prepared for insect bites, not only in tropical rain forests and beaches but also in the arctic and in cool mountainous terrain such as the Californian Sierra Nevada, Italian Dolomites, and Scottish Highlands. The risk of getting bitten varies geographically, seasonally, and diurnally. Seek specific advice.

- Clothing should be as ample and protective as comfort allows.
- Long sleeves and long trousers should be worn after dusk.
- Light colours are less attractive to mosquitoes than dark ones. Blue colour attracts African tsetse flies (⮕ Sleeping sickness, p. 523).
- Hats and face veils may protect against assaults on face and scalp by swarms of Scottish midges (*Culicoides*), tropical black flies (*Simulium*), or sand flies (*Phlebotomus, Lutzomyia*).
- Effective repellents include diethyltoluamide (DEET) and *p*-menthane-diol (Mosi-guard®)-containing preparations applied to exposed skin or impregnated into cotton clothing or forehead, wrist, and ankle bands. Beware that some preparations of DEET can dissolve plastics and synthetic fibres, causing damage to spectacles and synthetic clothing.
- Clothes can be impregnated with pyrethroid insecticides at the expense of waterproofing.
- Protect sleeping quarters. Mosquito-proofing of sleeping quarters and insecticide spraying at dusk reduces the risk. Night bites by mosquitoes that transmit malaria (⮕ p. 512), cone-nosed (triatomine) 'kissing' bugs (Central and South America) that transmit Chagas' disease (⮕ p. 524), bed bugs, ticks that transmit tick-borne encephalitis and tick-borne relapsing fever (⮕ p. 849), and even vampire and other bats that transmit rabies (⮕ p. 490) and venomous snakes can be prevented by sleeping under a pyrethroid-impregnated mosquito net. Burn pyrethroid releasing mosquito coils or, if there is electricity, plug-in insecticide vaporizers. Ceiling fans deter mosquitoes from biting.

Ectoparasitic infestations

Fleas, lice, mites, ticks, invasive flies (myiasis), and leeches

Some blood-feeding invertebrates take up temporary or long-term residence on the surface of humans' bodies or clothing. Tropical climate, poor socioeconomic conditions, and poor hygiene increase the risk of acquiring ectoparasites from other humans or from the environment. The very thought of these 'bugs' may induce psychosis and their presence, visible or palpable, is irritating, distressing, and embarrassing, but it is only in the past century that westerners have grown less accustomed to being flea-ridden and lousy. For example, Marie Curie was awoken by a myriad of bed bugs falling off her back as she rolled over in her poor Paris attic bedroom.

The biting and burrowing of these ectoparasites causes pain and irritation, and may lead to hypersensitivity, secondary local infection, or transmission of systemic diseases such as:

- Rickettsioses (typhus) and plague by fleas.
- Viral encephalitides and haemorrhagic fevers, spirochaetoses, rickettsioses, and bartonelloses by ticks.
- Spirochaetoses and rickettsioses by lice.
- Scrub typhus by trombiculid mites.
- Local streptococcal infection leading to acute glomerulonephritis by scabies mites.

Fleas

Humans can be infested and bitten by human fleas (*Pulex irritans*) and by dog, cat, rat, pigeon, and other animal fleas. Direct contact with an infested person or animal is not necessary. Tropical rodent fleas (*Xenopsylla* spp.) transmit plague and murine typhus. The first evidence of fleas is the appearance of small groups of intensely itchy bites (red macule with a central punctum), often in a line a few centimetres apart, especially on the trunk or buttocks. Fleas may not remain on the body after feeding but retreat to bedding or crevices and cracks in the bed or room. Examination of under clothing or quickly turning back the bedclothes may reveal the jumping fleas.

- *Treatment*: itching bites are treated with counter-irritants, topical corticosteroid, or systemic antihistamines (➲ Insect bites, p. 304). Domestic animals and the infested environment should be kept as clean as is practicable and treated with pyrethroid or other pesticides.

Lice

Human head lice (*Pediculus capitis*), body (clothing) lice (*P. humanus*), and pubic lice (*Pthirus pubis*) are obligate human parasitic insects that spread through close physical contact.

Head lice

Flourish in the human scalp even in hygienic, affluent conditions, especially among teenage children. Eggs ('nits') stuck to head hairs are recovered using a fine comb. Itching and scratching may cause secondary infection with occipital lymphadenopathy.

- *Treatment*: repeated application of insecticide lotion (pyrethroid or malathion) and combing.
- *Prevention*: avoid head-to-head contact.

Body lice

Infestation is promoted by poor hygiene (unwashed clothes and bodies) and crowding, common accompaniments of disasters, imprisonment, wars, forced immigration, and cold, wet seasons as in the highlands of Ethiopia. Lice and their eggs may be discovered on skin, body hair, or in clothing, especially in the seams. More than 21,500 lice have been found on one person. Individual bites look like flea bites but there is no linearity and only mild local irritation.

* Treatment: burn clothing or heat-sterilize and impregnate with pyrethroids. Bathe infested people with soap and 1% Lysol®.

Pubic (crab) lice

Sexually transmitted infestation of the pubic hair and also body hair, eyebrows, and eyelashes. They provoke itching, scratching, secondary infection, and curious bluish staining (maculae caeruliae). Eggs are stuck to the hairs.
Treatment: apply insecticides (see above) to affected areas and leave on for 1–2 days then repeat after a week. Treat sexual contacts.

Mites

Scabies mites (Sarcoptes scabei)

Burrow under the skin, creating linear papulo-vesicular tracks, typically in the interdigital clefts and skin creases. There is intense itching, especially at night, provoking scratching, excoriation, and secondary infection. Transmitted by close physical contact. Exuberant crusting (crusted scabies) develops in immuno-compromised patients.
Treatment: two treatments a week apart of aqueous lotion—5% permethrin or 0.5% malathion; benzyl benzoate is an alternative. Apply lotion to the whole body surface of all affected people and leave on for 24 h before being washing off. Itching may persist for several weeks and requires topical counter-irritant and corticosteroid (e.g. crotamiton and hydrocortisone) and sedating antihistamine (chlorphenamine at night). Ivermectin (200 micrograms/kg single dose) is used for crusted scabies and in patients whose severe excoriations make topical treatment intolerably irritating and painful.

Trombiculid (harvest) mites

Sometimes known very misleadingly as 'chiggers' (→ Tungiasis, p. 308), can infest in large numbers, especially under tight underpants, causing multiple, persisting, painful, itchy, blistering bites.
Prevention: use DEET-containing repellents, tuck trousers into boots, and avoid notorious 'mite islands' densely infested with trombiculids in cleared areas of jungle.

Bed bugs (Cimex)

At night, bed bugs emerge from cracks and crevices in the bedroom to bite sleeping humans. Insomnia and painful, red papules result.
Prevention: discourage bites by keeping the light on all night, by sleeping under a permethrin-impregnated mosquito net, and putting newspaper under the under-sheet. Eradication is by thorough cleaning of the environment and application of the usual residual insecticides. Sleeping bags should be exposed to the sun (including both outside and inside)

and treated with insecticide. However, insecticide-resistance has developed and bed bugs are becoming more abundant.

Ticks

- *Soft (argasid) ticks*: live in animal burrows and human dwellings. They attach briefly at night, engorge rapidly with blood, and then drop off and hide in cracks and crevices. Ticks of the genus *Ornithodoros* transmit relapsing fever.
- *Hard (ixodid) ticks* or their tiny nymphs may be picked up from vegetation or brought into gardens by deer or indoors by dogs. They find a secluded area (groin, perineum, waist, umbilicus, axilla, scalp, even external auditory meatus) and feed for days until they are spherical and engorged. Some species transmit Lyme disease (➔ p. 504), Rocky Mountain spotted fever (➔ p. 510), African tick fevers (➔ p. 510), European tick-borne encephalitis (➔ p. 488), Crimean–Congo haemorrhagic fever (➔ p. 496), Colorado tick fever, louping ill, babesiosis, ehrlichiosis, and other human infections. Some ticks in North America and Australia inject a paralysing neurotoxin (➔ p. 595).

Prevention of tick-transmitted infections

- Examine yourself at likely tick attachment sites (see previous section and use a mirror or a friend) when undressing at night while on the expedition. A prominent eschar may form at the site of a bite infected by rickettsiae. Watch for any subsequent widespread macular rash or fever that might indicate tick-related rickettsiosis.
- Avoid contact with tick-infested domestic animals.
- Wear light-coloured trousers against which ticks are more visible.
- Tuck trouser bottoms into boots.
- Apply DEET-containing repellents.
- Specific antibiotic chemoprophylaxis against tick-transmitted infections is not justified.

Removing ticks

'Tick forceps' (Fig. 9.6a) and 'tick removing cards' can be purchased at most outdoor leisure shops. Grasp the tick as close to the skin as possible with fine curved forceps (avoid squeezing the engorged body) and pull it out gently *without twisting* (Fig. 9.6b). If the mouth parts break off, remove them separately with forceps or a needle. The aim is not to leave the barbed hypostome in the wound as it may provoke inflammation and granuloma formation. Keep the tick for later expert examination in case you become

Invasive fly larvae (myiasis) and fleas (tungiasis)

Larvae (maggots) of some tropical flies hatch from eggs contaminating human skin and burrow into tissues, creating an uncomfortable, inflamed boil which wriggles, exudes blood-stained pus, and has a definite head through which the larval spiracles may protrude ('myiasis'). Secondary infection may cause fever and lymphadenopathy.

The *human bot fly* (*Dermatobia hominis*) of Central and South America is also known as ver macaque, berne, el torsalo, or beefworm. Eggs are laid on mosquitoes which deposit them on human skin. The larvae grow in 10 weeks.

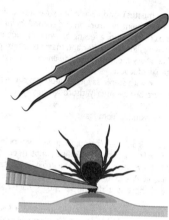

Fig. 9.6 Tick forceps and removal technique.

The *tumbu fly* (*Cordylobia anthropophaga*) of sub-Saharan Africa and southern Spain is also known as putsi fly or ver du cayor. Eggs are laid on land, stick to clothes (e.g. washing laid out on the ground to dry), and hatch on the skin. Larvae penetrate and grow for 10 days.

Treatment: folk remedies such as raw steak or bacon fat, and occlusion of the maggot's breathing hole in the skin with paraffin, petroleum gel, and candle wax occlusion sometimes work. However, attempts to squeeze them out like giant blackheads make matters worse. Injecting local anaesthetic into the base of the lesion may force the maggot out. The final solution is removal through a small scalpel incision.

Prevention: hang washing to dry on a clothes line in strong sunlight; do not lay clothing on the ground. Iron washing to kill the tumbu fly ova.

Congo floor maggots

Congo floor maggots larvae of the fly *Auchmeromyia luteola*, live in earthen floors of huts throughout tropical Africa between latitudes 18°N and 26°S. They suck blood from those sleeping on the ground, causing local swelling and itching. Fumigate the hut and treat the bites symptomatically, making sure that no secondary infection is introduced (wipe the skin with antiseptic and give systemic antimicrobials if there are signs of infection).

Prevention: if possible, don't sleep on the ground (there are several other good reasons for this advice—see snake-bites!).

Invasive myiasis

This involves wounds, body orifices, and cavities: aggressive larvae of screw worm flies, such as *Cochliomyia* (*Callitroga*) *hominivorax* in Latin America and *Chrysomyia bessania* in eastern Europe, Africa, and Asia, hatch from eggs laid in wounds or on healthy mucosae (especially of the eye, orbit, nasal cavity, or external auditory meatus), and invade body cavities, orifices, and living tissue, causing life-threatening destruction and secondary infection.

- *Clinical*: there is pain, irritation, a feeling of wriggling movement, discharge of serosanguineous matter and maggots, obstruction (e.g. of the external auditory meatus causing deafness), and symptoms of secondary bacterial infection.
- *Treatment*: irrigation with sterile saline solution and dilute antiseptic is a first aid measure but eventually, thorough surgical debridement is essential.
- *Prevention*: protect wounds from flies.

Tungiasis

Tungiasis ('jigger' or 'chigoe' flea) (*Tunga penetrans*) occurs in Latin America and Africa. After fertilization, the female flea jumps (feebly) and burrows alongside the nail fold or into the skin of the groin, loses its legs, and produces eggs each night. A painful swelling develops on the foot, typically under a toenail, and there is a risk of secondary bacterial infection and ulceration.

- *Treatment*: the encapsulated flea must be curetted out (excised, ideally with a small surgical spoon with sharpened edge) and antiseptic such as iodine applied. Complete enucleation is required.
- *Prevention*: wear proper shoes; do not walk around bare-footed.

'Creeping eruption' (cutaneous larva migrans)

Arthropod infestations must be distinguished from creeping eruption (➔ Colour plate 2) which occurs in tropical countries worldwide. It is caused by larvae of cat and dog hookworms, such as *Ancylostoma braziliense*, *Uncinaria stenocephala*, and *Ancylostoma caninum*. Contact with contaminated ground (especially from sleeping rough on beaches in Central/Southern America) allows filariform larvae to penetrate the skin. They crawl under the skin a few millimetres each day, causing severe itching. Feet, buttocks, knees, hands, and back are commonly affected, sometimes by dozens of worms. The best treatment is oral albendazole 400 mg daily for 3 days or a single 200 micrograms/kg dose of ivermectin (adult doses). But the condition will resolve in most without treatment.

Leeches

Leeches are blood-sucking ectoparasites that live in the water or on moist land surfaces. Usually those encountered are small, 7–40 mm, but the largest ones are 45 cm long.

Aquatic leeches cause bleeding after entering the nose, mouth, nostrils, ears, eyes, vulva, urethra, or anus of swimmers or being swallowed in water from natural sources. They tend to remain attached for longer than terrestrial leeches.

Land leeches frequent game paths in moist vegetation and may drop onto upper limbs from trees or bushes, or rapidly climb up from the ground, fastening onto the legs. Usually, they are far more upsetting than harmful.

Attachment is via a three- or two-jaw bite giving a Y- or V-shaped incision. There may be a tickling sensation or sharpness as they bite but, as they inject local anaesthetic as well as anticoagulants, bites often go undetected until bleeding is noticed. Bites may ooze for hours, but blood loss from a single bite is insignificant.

- *Prevention:* leeches can squeeze through small gaps such as shoelace eyes, and so boots, socks, or trousers offer little protection. Application of DEET to boots, socks, and skin or coarse tobacco rolled into the top of socks and kept moist is repellent. Take care when swimming and drink only filtered sterilized water. British troops in Malaya wore condoms at night to prevent urethral invasion by leeches while they were asleep in the jungle.
- *Treatment:* if detected before attachment flick or pull off.

Once attached: ripping off can leave the mouth parts behind and predispose to infection. Apply salt (kept dry in a screw top plastic container), iodine tincture, alcohol, lighted cigarette, tobacco, or other irritant to persuade them to release. This may precipitate regurgitation of ingested blood into the wound and, to avoid secondary infection, treat as an open wound; clean, apply antiseptic, and compression dressing.

If a leech has attached inside the mouth, gargle with strong salt solution but don't swallow the salt solution as it may induce vomiting.

Leeches will spontaneously release after feeding. Their gut contains symbiotic *Aeromonas hydrophila* which are potentially pathogenic.

Tropical ulcers

Tropical (phagedenic) ulcer

In tropical climates, even trivial wounds seem to heal slowly or persist. Classical tropical ulcers usually affect the shins and occur in 30% of some indigenous communities. They start as minor abrasions (thorn prick, scratch, insect bite, existing skin lesion, pressure blister) that become infected with saprophytic bacteria (e.g. *Fusobacterium ulcerans*, and spiral bacteria) in mud or stagnant water. Another very similar form of tropical ulcer caused by non-venereal *Haemophilus ducreyi* has been described in children in the tropics.

Clinical

A pustule appears and after 5–6 days discharges foul-smelling pus. A painful, circular ulcer develops with a defined, raised, undermined edge and floor of granulation tissue covered with purulent discharge. Over subsequent months and years the ulcer becomes painless but the infection penetrates to deeper tissue, tendon sheaths, periosteum, and bone, becomes gangrenous, and may show malignant transformation.

Treatment

In the early stages, high-dose penicillin or azithromycin may promote healing. Later, surgical debridement and reconstruction or even amputation may be needed.

Prevention

In tropical environments, especially in wet conditions, protect legs and ankles from scratches and pricks, and treat any new injury, however trivial, by washing with sterile (drinking) water, applying antiseptic or topical antibacterial (e.g. mupirocin), and protecting with a dry dressing.

Other types of tropical ulcer

(For genital ulcers, see ➜ p. 541.)

Ulcerating skin lesions can be caused by many different tropical pathogens:
- Pyogenic bacteria (*Staphylococcus*, *Streptococcus*, *Burkholderia pseudomallei*—melioidosis).
- Cutaneous diphtheria ('desert' or 'veldt' sore).
- Spirochaetes (yaws).
- Mycobacteria (TB, *Mycobacterium ulcerans*, 'Buruli ulcer').
- Protozoa (leishmaniasis).
- Fungi (histoplasmosis, cryptococcosis, and deep fungal infections).
- Non-infectious diseases such as sickle cell disease, varicose veins, and other vascular problems.

Other infective skin lesions

Pustules, furuncles, boils, styes, abscesses, paronychias, whitlows (felons), cellulitis, erysipelas, ecthyma, and other painful, inflamed, and obviously infected skin and soft tissue lesions should be treated promptly. Depending on their stage of development and severity, they may require only topical antiseptic or antibiotic treatment, but systemic antibiotics and drainage are often needed.

Marine wound infections

Swimmers, SCUBA divers, fishermen, sailors, wind-surfers, and anyone in contact with marine or brackish water or sea animals are susceptible to wound infections and otitis externa caused by unusual pathogens acquired from salt water. Infective otitis externa should be distinguished from swimmer's ear. Heatwaves associated with higher sea temperatures, even in the Baltic and North Seas, increase the risk. Infections complicate injuries such as coral cuts (➔ p. 599), skin penetration by fish or sea urchin spines and stings (➔ p. 600), and fish hooks, merely handling fish (erysipeloid) and other traumas associated with fishing and boating.

Marine pathogens

- Vibrios: *Vibrio vulnificus* infection starts with local erythema round the wound, followed by swelling, haemorrhagic blisters, necrotic ulceration, and severe systemic symptoms (fever, rigors, septic shock). Case fatality is high, especially in people with chronic debility (immunocompromise, chronic alcoholism, diabetes mellitus). *V. parahaemolyticus* (see also ➔ Traveller's diarrhoea, p. 420), *V. cholera*, and *V. alginolyticus* can also cause inflammation, sometimes within 8 h of injury, with the risk of deep, severe wound infections and bacteraemia in immunocompromised people.
- *Aeromonas hydrophila*: (brackish and fresh water) can cause muscle damage—myonecrosis and pyomyositis.
- *Erysipelothrix rhusiopathiae* (erysipeloid, 'seal finger', 'whale finger'): demarcated red/violaceous plaques appear on the hands after handling fish. The rash spreads proximally and may be associated with arthritis.
- *Plesiomonas shigelloides*, *Acinetobacter* spp., *Chromobacterium violaceum*, *Flavobacterium* spp., and *Pseudomonas aeruginosa* are commonly cultured from marine wounds.
- *Mycobacterium marinum* causes chronic granulomatous lesions in aquarium keepers and others who are exposed to sea water or fish farms.
- *Staphylococcus aureus*, pyogenic *Streptococcus*, and enteric pathogens derived from the patient rather than the marine environment. However, the sea water near some popular beaches (e.g. Waikiki Beach, Honolulu) is heavily contaminated with *Staph. aureus*, including methicillin-resistant *Staph. aureus* (MRSA).
- Achlorous algae (*Prototheca* spp.): cause a chronic papule, plaque or ulcer, or olecranon bursitis, and may become disseminated in immunocompromised people.
- Free-living amoebae (*Acanthamoeba*, *Naegleria*, *Balamuthia mandrillaris*): a hazard of tropical ponds, swimming pools, saunas or spas can cause keratitis in contact lens wearers and encephalitis.

Diagnosis

Clinical suspicion based on history of marine exposure and underlying illness is crucial for early antibiotic treatment. Expert microbiology involves special cultures in 3% saline media or PCR. Biopsy and histopathology may yield the diagnosis.

Treatment

Urgent surgical debridement is needed together with IV fluids if there is any suggestion of necrotizing fasciitis or myositis.

Blind antibiotic treatment:
- For mild lesions: oral doxycycline or co-trimoxazole.
- For severe lesions with systemic illness: combination treatment—tetracycline + aminoglycoside (e.g. gentamicin) + cefotaxime *or* tetracycline + aminoglycoside + a fluoroquinolone.

Specific treatment
- Marine vibrios: doxycycline, co-trimoxazole, fluoroquinolone, gentamicin, cefotaxime, or co-amoxiclav.
- *Aeromonas hydrophila*: doxycycline, fluoroquinolone, gentamicin, or cefotaxime.
- Erysipeloid: penicillin or erythromycin or tetracycline.
- *M. marinum*: doxycycline or co-trimoxazole for trivial lesions; rifampicin and clarithromycin for larger or destructive lesions.
- Others: as directed by laboratory sensitivities.

Prevention

Sensible behaviour, acquisition of technical skills, and appropriate protective clothing may reduce the risk of marine injuries. Beachcombers should not expose open wounds to sea water and should avoid eating undercooked or raw shellfish. Wounds contaminated by sea water should be cleaned immediately with drinking water (not rinsed in the brine). Foreign bodies should be removed and the wound watched carefully for early signs of infection. Start blind antibiotic treatment at the first hint of infection. For those at high risk of invasive marine vibrio infection (see earlier in this topic), prophylaxis with doxycycline or co-trimoxazole is recommended.

Minor skin conditions

Superficial fungal infections (dermatophytosis, ringworm, tinea)

Infection of the skin by *Trichophyton*, *Microsporum*, and *Epidermophyton* spp. is spread by direct contact with infected humans or animals or from soil saprophytes. It is common in tropical climates.

- *Clinical*: the classic lesion is a circumscribed round or oval scaly patch with vesicles around its border and central clearing. Scalp, face, body, beard area, hands, nails, intertriginous areas (groins, axillae, 'dhobie itch'), and feet ('athlete's foot'; ➜ p. 318) may be affected. Hyperkeratosis caused by scratching, and follicular and granulomatous lesions may be present.
- *Diagnosis*: direct microscopic examination of scrapings incubated for 20 min in 5–20% potassium hydroxide may reveal hyphae and spores.
- *Treatment*: topical creams or ointments containing imidazoles or terbinafine are usually effective (➜ Athlete's foot, p. 318), but *nail and scalp infections require systemic treatment* with triazoles (e.g. itraconazole 200 mg each day), or terbinafine (250 mg each day) for many months (adult doses).

Pityriasis versicolor

Skin infection with the yeast *Malassezia globosa* is an endogenous infection spread from oneself, affecting many in some tropical communities. Scaly macular rashes coalesce over large areas usually of the trunk. They appear hyperpigmented or hypopigmented, or yellowish or brownish. Fine scales can be scraped off these lesions.

- *Treatment*: topical imidazoles, 20% sodium thiosulfate solution, Whitfield's ointment, or selenium sulfide, or ketoconazole shampoos are applied overnight repeatedly. Relapses are common.

Skin conditions of the hands and feet

Ingrowing toenails

An edge of a big toenail is forced into the nail fold either by pressure of tight footwear or abnormal growth. This causes trauma, pain, bleeding, or serosanguineous discharge and infection of the nail fold (inflammation, swelling, pus formation; paronychia—see following section) that can make walking very painful.

- *Treatment*: soak in saline, clean with antiseptic, apply antiseptic cream, and relieve compressing footwear. Trimming the nail may make matters worse. Curative treatment of intractable in growing toenails: under digital block (➜ p. 457) incise the side of the nail back to and including the nail bed (Fig. 9.7).
- *Prevention*: cut toenails straight across and avoid wearing tight footwear, especially brand-new boots that have not been worn and thoroughly broken in before the expedition.

Paronychia

Frequent immersion of the hands in infected water may result in chronic *Candida* and acute staphylococcal nail fold infections. There is painful redness and swelling of the nail fold. Pus may be trapped under the nail.

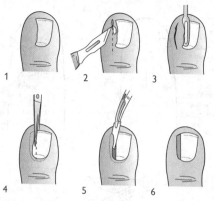

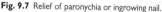

Fig. 9.7 Relief of paronychia or ingrowing nail.

Pseudomonas aeruginosa infection causes greenish discoloration of the nail and sometimes, foul-smelling greenish pus.

- *Treatment:* initially, warm saline soaks, topical antiseptic or antibacterial cream, and drainage of abscesses may be curative. Otherwise, consider systemic antibiotics or removal of the nail edge(s) under digital block (➔ p. 457) as for ingrowing toe nails.

Whitlow (felon)

Acute swelling, redness, inflammation, and throbbing pain of the pulp space of finger or toe is usually caused by *Staphylococcus* or *Streptococcus* from a splinter or spread from paronychia. Contact with herpes simplex virus causes a whitlow with painful vesicles. Orf, a sheep virus, causes pustular whitlow. Inflammatory swelling in the pulp space may compress the digital artery, causing necrosis. The terminal phalanx may be infected. Nail biters, especially diabetics, may self-inoculate oral *Eikenella corrodens*.

- *Treatment:* initially try warm saline soaks and antibiotics for suspected pyogenic infection (flucloxacillin or clarithromycin) and aciclovir for herpetic whitlow. If tense, painful swelling persists, a relieving incision (Fig. 9.8) may be needed under digital block (➔ p. 318). Herpetic whitlows should not be incised as this may spread the infection.

Fungal infection of nails (onychomycosis)

Initially there is white, yellow, or brown discoloration of the free edge of the nail and later hyperkeratotic thickening of the nail bed, and ridging and crumbling of the nail surface and separation from the nail bed (onycholysis). There is no inflammation of the nail fold (paronychia). Not all the nails are involved but there is usually superficial fungal infection elsewhere.

- *Treatment:* early infection responds to topical amorolfine nail lacquer or tioconazole cutaneous solution. Established infection requires systemic terbinafine 250 mg each day for 3 months or itraconazole 400 mg every day for 1 week each month for 3 months.

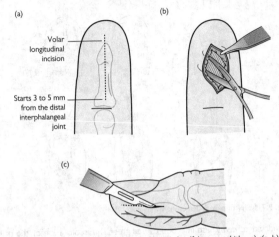

Fig. 9.8 Incisions for draining abscesses in finger pulps (felons or whitlows). (a, b) Incisions for abscesses pointing in central area. (c) Incision for those pointing laterally.

Athlete's foot (tinea pedis)

In shoe and sock wearers, skin of the interdigital spaces between the toes, especially the third and fourth, may become greyish white, fissured, dehiscent, itchy, and sore. An associated vesicular eruption is common. Lesions may become secondarily infected, causing cellulitis of the lower leg.

- *Treatment:* wear sandals at least in camp and keep the interdigital spaces dry and clean. Terbinafine cream applied twice daily for 1 week is the most effective antifungal, but a wide range of cheaper preparations is also effective such as compound benzoic acid (Whitfield's) ointment and azole creams (e.g. clotrimazole).

Other foot infections

In hot and humid environments, where the feet become wet in enclosed footwear, Gram-negative bacterial infection (e.g. *Pseudomonas*) can cause erosive and painful lesions between the toes and undersurface of the foot. In milder lesions, the toe webs are macerated and sore. This area needs to be dried carefully and an antiseptic such as povidone applied; more severe infections require oral ciprofloxacin.

Chapter 10

Head and neck

Chapter editor
Chris Johnson

Contributors
Alistair R. M. Cobb
Paul Cooper
Jon Dallimore
Daniel S. Morris
David Geddes (1st edition)
Stephen Hearns (1st edition)
Annabel H. Nickol (1st and 2nd editions)

Anatomy

The head can be thought of in terms of the neurocranium—the brain box—and the face (viscerocranium). The face acts as a protection to the brain in large impacts—rather like an airbag in a car. The two structures are intimately related to each other (at the skull base) and to the neck, which is forcibly extended following a frontal blow to the face. In any head injury, including any major facial trauma, it is essential to start head injury observations and to look for signs of cervical spine injury. About 10% of midface fractures will have a concomitant cervical spine fracture, while spinal injuries are especially likely if the trauma was the result of a vehicle accident (➲ p. 158).

Areas of the head are described according to their underlying bony parts (Fig. 10.1). The eyes lie protected within the orbit, while the prominent nose is susceptible to injury.

The breathing and digestive passages cross in the oropharynx, requiring complex mechanisms to ensure correct routing (Fig. 10.2). The nose and upper airway form a humidification and filtering mechanism. The opening to the lower airway is the larynx, a complex cartilaginous structure hung from the hyoid bone, which in turn is slung from the base of the skull. When foods or fluids are swallowed, the epiglottis, a roof-like flap, closes over the glottis and protects the trachea. Inside the lower end of the larynx are the vocal cords, used both to provide a watertight seal to the airways and to phonate. The two prominent thyroid cartilages form the anterior border, the 'Adam's apple' of the larynx. Just below these cartilages is an obvious groove, the cricothyroid membrane—the safest location for emergency surgical access to the airway.

The swallowing mechanism primarily involves the tongue and oropharynx. Movement of a food or fluid bolus to the back of the mouth causes reflex closure of the larynx and a peristaltic wave to pass down the oesophagus. Tongue swelling or a sore throat will disrupt swallowing.

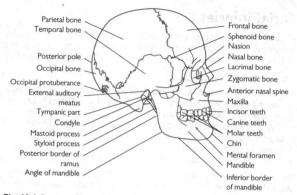

Fig. 10.1 Bony structures of the head.

Parietal bone
Temporal bone
Posterior pole
Occipital bone
Occipital protuberance
External auditory meatus
Tympanic part
Condyle
Mastoid process
Styloid process
Posterior border of ramus
Angle of mandible

Frontal bone
Sphenoid bone
Nasion
Nasal bone
Lacrimal bone
Zygomatic bone
Anterior nasal spine
Maxilla
Incisor teeth
Canine teeth
Molar teeth
Chin
Mental foramen
Mandible
Inferior border of mandible

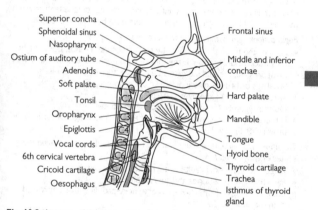

Fig. 10.2 Anatomy of the airway.

Superior concha
Sphenoidal sinus
Nasopharynx
Ostium of auditory tube
Adenoids
Soft palate
Tonsil
Oropharynx
Epiglottis
Vocal cords
6th cervical vertebra
Cricoid cartilage
Oesophagus

Frontal sinus
Middle and inferior conchae
Hard palate
Mandible
Tongue
Hyoid bone
Thyroid cartilage
Trachea
Isthmus of thyroid gland

Facial injuries

Whatever the outdoor pursuit, the face is an easy target for injuries as it is left uncovered by most protective helmets so that we can see, breathe, and talk. Facial injuries may affect bones, soft tissues, and teeth (➲ Chapter 11).

Maxillofacial examination

Consider the face as divided into equal thirds, plus the inside of the mouth:
- Upper 1/3 is from the eyebrows up to the hairline and when examining we look right over the cranium too.
- Middle 1/3 runs from under the supraorbital rims to the tip of the upper front teeth.
- Lower 1/3 is the mandible.
- The inside of the mouth is the fourth area to examine.

In each area, check the bony tissues for tenderness, mobility, or unexpected steps; the soft tissues for lacerations, bruising, and foreign bodies; and nerve function. Sensation is conveniently conveyed by a branch of the trigeminal nerve for each of the thirds of the face. Motor function is via the five branches of the facial nerve. Any lacerations which cross the path of these nerves may cause a nerve injury. Finally, each area has unique features summarized in Table 10.1 and which you should note have been checked.

Begin by looking at symmetry of the face and any injuries
- Each of the three thirds should be equal height and if not, there might be a fracture dislocation. If the middle third of the face looks elongated or depressed, it could indicate a Le Fort fracture of the maxilla.
- Swellings or bruises may indicate an underlying injury.
- Assess the level of the eyes—are they equal?
- Do the zygomas (cheek bones) look symmetrical?
- Is there any subconjunctival, or sub-scleral haemorrhage, or periorbital bruising of the eye?

The upper 1/3 and cranium are best examined from above and behind the seated or lying patient
- Check over the skull vault for depressions and bruising.
- Palpate the frontal bones and supraorbital rims.
- Look at the eyes from above—is one more prominent or depressed than the other?
- Curl your index fingers to lie over the zygomatic bones as you look from above down: if asymmetrical, the depressed one may be fractured and you may palpate a dent at the fracture site.
- Ask the casualty to open and close their mouth while your fingers feel the temporomandibular joints (TMJs) in front of the tragus of the ear—pain may indicate a mandibular condyle fracture.
- Look for leakage of clear CSF fluid from the ear or bruising behind the ear (Battle's sign): both signs of possible skull base fracture.
- If any laceration passes over the path of the parotid duct (the middle third of the line from the tragus of the ear to the middle of the upper lip philtrum) check that saliva is milkable from Stensen's duct which opens opposite the upper second molar tooth and is not evident through the laceration.

Table 10.1 Assessment of facial injuries

	Nerves	Special features
Upper 1/3 and cranium	Va	Battle's sign (Mastoid bruising)
	VII temporal	External ear
Middle 1/3	Vb	Eye movements
	VII temporal	Visual acuity
	VII zygomatic	CSF rhinorrhoea
	VII buccal	CSF otorrhoea
		Parotid duct
Lower 1/3	Vc	Temporomandibular joint
	VII marginal	
	VII mandibular	
Intraoral	XII lingual	Dental occlusion
		Salivary flow from parotid duct

In each of the four zones assess:

Soft tissues—lacerations, bruising, and foreign bodies

Hard tissues—palpate for fractures and broken teeth

Nerve injuries:
* Sensory (i.e. V cranial nerve branch region)
* Motor function (i.e. mostly VII cranial nerve branch regions)

(Continued)

Table 10.1 (*Contd.*)

Special features (unique to a specific area)
- Signs of skull base fracture
- Eye examination including visual acuity and range of movement
- CSF leak from nose or ear
- Temporomandibular joint movement
- Dental occlusion
- Parotid duct

Now stand in front of the patient

- Grasp the front of the maxilla between finger and thumb placed above the incisors in the mouth. Gently see if the maxilla moves.
- Assess the sensation and muscles movement (i.e. V and VII cranial nerve functions). Does part of the face droop, can the patient smile evenly and close eyes tightly?
- Examine visual acuity (eye sight), pupil reactions, and check for double vision especially in upward gaze—characteristic of an orbital blowout fracture.
- Check the symmetry of the nose and look for blood or clear CSF fluid from the nostrils.

Now look in the mouth

- Ask the patient to bite their teeth together and if it feels different from normal (changed dental occlusion). Do the teeth close properly and look even, or are there any step defects or gaps?
- Check for lacerations, bleeding, bruising, or broken teeth.

Minor injuries to head and neck

Head injuries such as bruises, black eyes, or lacerations are relatively common; more serious head injuries are fortunately rare, but are an ever-present risk during outdoor activities.

Lacerations

(See ➋ Wound types and management, p. 286.)

Scalp lacerations tend to bleed a lot initially and can look a lot worse than they really are. Apply firm pressure until the bleeding stops. Small wounds can be closed using cyanoacrylate tissue glue; if available, larger wounds should be closed using skin staples (➋ p. 291). Conventional superglue has been used for this purpose but can provoke tissue reactions and is not recommended.[1] Shaving the hair around large lacerations may make wound closure easier.

Simple facial lacerations usually heal well, but it is important to minimize scarring. Clean the wounds carefully and, where possible, use glue or skin fixers (Steri-Strips™, etc.) to bring the edges together. If wounds are deep, try to remove tension from the surface by placing resorbable subcutaneous sutures (e.g.4/0 Vicryl® Rapide) to approximate the edges and then suture the skin itself using a fine suture material (e.g. 5/0 Novafil® on face; 6/0 for lips and eyelids) to finish the job. Ensure that tension is even throughout the wound and that the edges are aligned. When a lip has been cut, make every effort to realign the vermilion edges as even small deviations are very obvious and may require subsequent corrective surgery. Remove sutures after 5 days. Most facial lacerations do not require antibiotics.

Complex or heavily contaminated lacerations will require specialist surgical management. Cover exposed bone with saline-soaked dressing, begin an IV antibiotic such as co-amoxiclav 1.2 g IV three times daily (if no penicillin allergy), and evacuate the casualty urgently for specialist surgical treatment. *Intraoral lacerations* are closed with resorbable 3/0 or 4/0 sutures. Explore them well using suction if available. If the labial mucosa is involved ask for help from a colleague to pull the lip tightly away from the teeth to give you a flat surface to suture.

Nasal injuries

(See ➋ Nasal fracture, p. 329 and ➋ Epistaxis (nose bleed), p. 357.)

Injured noses tend to bleed a lot. Apply cool compresses. Almost all nose bleeds can be controlled by pinching the soft tissues together across the tip of the nostrils, although rarely it may be necessary to pack a nostril using either a nasal tampon (e.g. Rapid Rhino®), or ribbon gauze lubricated with paraffin ointment or a suitable antibiotic ointment.

Tongue

Bitten tongues and burnt tongues are usually made worse by attempting surgical treatment. Provide pain relief, rest, and keep the patient head-up if there is significant airway swelling. Sucking ice, if available, can relieve pain and swelling.

---

1 Cascarini L, Kumar A. Case of the month: honey I glued the kids: tissue adhesives are not the same as 'superglue'. *Emerg Med J.* 2007;24:228–231.

Tongue suturing should be limited to really deep lacerations involving the muscles or if the wound is bleeding really badly. Even in these situations intervention will normally prove unnecessary as bleeding almost always stops and sutures may result in a residual lump within the tongue.

Acute neck sprains

Neck sprains most commonly result from low-velocity, rear-end RTCs but may also occur in other circumstances such as being rolled by a wave while surfing. Initial assessment should attempt to eliminate the possibility of a fracture or dislocation of the neck, which can be indicated by the mechanism of injury, usually severe pain, and localized midline tenderness of the cervical spine. Assessment and exclusion without the aid of X-rays is difficult, especially for the inexperienced. If in doubt, immobilize and evacuate for specialist assessment (see the NEXUS criteria shown in ➜ Neck and other spinal injuries, p. 219).

However, if muscular pain predominates without bony tenderness or neurological symptoms, then it is probably that the neck has been sprained with damage to trapezius and sternomastoid muscles. Neck sprains are managed with analgesia and early mobilization. Immobilization with neck collars causes stiffness and should be avoided.

Fractured facial bones

Detailed diagnosis of facial bone fractures is impossible and irrelevant in a remote environment. Fractures to both the mandible and maxilla will cause pain and swelling, limit diet, and may threaten the airway. The best advice is to arrange early evacuation to specialist care. However, this may take time and in the interim the following can help, assuming there are no other life-threatening injuries:

- Reduce and stabilize the fracture.
- Apply comfortable and supportive bandaging.
- Arrange for a soft food or liquid diet.
- Provide details of the circumstances of the accident, treatment to date, and medication.
- Arrange for a carer to accompany the casualty to specialist care.

Mandibular fractures

The bottom jaw is typically fractured following a fall or punch. Patients complain of sensory loss of the lower lip, pain, and teeth not meeting properly ('malocclusion'). There may be blood and/ or gaps around individual teeth and step defects along the plane of the tops of the teeth. It may be possible to elicit movement of the mandible between teeth—passive and active on examination.

Broadly speaking we can consider the fractures as being in the tooth-bearing area (Fig. 10.3a–d) or in the ramus and condyle of the mandible (Fig. 10.3e–h).

Treatment

- In the tooth-bearing area, the fracture is at risk of infection and amoxicillin and metronidazole together or co-amoxiclav should be started (assuming no penicillin allergy; see ➔ Penicillin allergy, p. 281, if allergic).
- If there is a lot of movement at the fracture site, the jaw may be very painful. Consider placing a wire or a thick nylon suture around the two teeth either side of the fracture to close and stabilize the

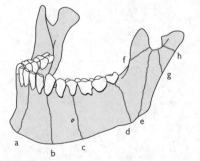

a Symphysis
b Para symphysis
c Body
d Angle
e Ramus
f Coronoid process
g Low condylar
h High condylar

Fig. 10.3 Mandibular fracture sites. Adapted from O'Connor, Isobel, and Urdanq, Michael, *Handbook of Surgical Cross-Cover* (2008), with permission from Oxford University Press.

fracture. These fractures require surgical fixation with miniplates, ideally within 24 h.

- If undisplaced, ramus or condylar fractures are treated conservatively. There may be swelling and difficulty opening and closing the mouth. They are reassessed at a week after the injury. If displaced they may require surgical reduction.
- Give simple analgesics and a soft diet. Arrange evacuation for surgical management.

Maxillary fracture

There are many categories—don't worry about them. Once you have identified the presence of a fracture of the maxilla, check the airway, eyes, and cervical spine (especially in falls from height) and arrange for evacuation. The type of fracture can be determined by the receiving medical team by CT scan. Typically, the window for operating is 2 weeks.

Treatment

The airway is very rarely a problem. An awake patient will naturally sit forward to keep their airway open. In an unconscious patient with a high fracture, the facial bones may be pushed down and back along the skull base, causing the soft palate to snag on the tongue and so closing the airway. A Guedel airway, laryngeal mask, or endotracheal tube may be required, or, if there is extreme airway swelling or bleeding, a cricothyroidotomy (➔ Maintaining an open airway, p. 207) could be life-saving. Fortunately, such situations are very unusual. Deal with epistaxis if present using pressure or nasal packs.

Zygomatic fractures

Cheek bone fractures can involve either the arch of the zygoma causing a dimple in the skin over the arch and possibly entrapment of the coronoid process of the mandible limiting jaw movement, or the zygomatic body. There may be bruising and swelling in the region with flattening deformity if displaced. Look for bloody injection of the white of eye lateral to pupil—subconjunctival haemorrhage and paraesthesia of the face below the eye (infraorbital nerve).

Examine for signs of eye involvement (diplopia, visual acuity loss, or an injury to the globe), a blow-out fracture of the orbit, or even retrobulbar haemorrhage (➔ Examination of the eye, p. 347; ➔ Orbital compartment syndrome, p. 354).

Treatment

- Give antibiotics against sinus bacteria—oral amoxicillin 500 mg three times a day for 1 week (if not penicillin allergic).
- The patient should not blow their nose for 2 weeks to prevent periorbital surgical emphysema.
- There is a 2-week window for surgical reduction.

Nasal fracture

- If the casualty is conscious and not seriously injured, sit them up with head well forward to allow secretions to drain.
- Exclude associated head or cervical spine injury.

- The diagnosis of a nasal fracture is a clinical one. X-rays are not routinely required. Swelling, tenderness, and possibly deformity of the bridge of the nose are visible. Consider whether the nasal injury could be part of a more complicated fracture—involving the orbit, ethmoids, or frontal bones. If it is an isolated injury it may be possible to straighten a deformed nasal bone fracture soon after the injury, although the casualty may be reluctant to permit this.
- It is essential to look for and exclude a septal haematoma—a smooth swelling of the midline of the nose that can develop into septal necrosis. In the wilderness a septal haematoma should be incised under local anaesthetic, and then the nostrils packed to prevent recurrence.
- Swelling often prevents an early assessment of the degree of nasal deformity. Between 5 and 7 days after injury, the nose should be re-examined; if there is evidence of deformity or septal deviation, the patient requires evacuation for specialist surgical assessment and management. Deformities should be corrected operatively within 10 days of injury.
- Open fractures of the nose require prophylactic antibiotics such as co-amoxiclav or clarithromycin.

Blow-out fracture of orbit

Blunt trauma to the globe of the eye (e.g. from a fall or a punch) can cause the weak bony orbital floor to fracture. This may cause prolapse of orbital fat into the maxillary sinus below. Double vision can occur from the swelling, which may be intolerable and require patching of the damaged eye. Surgical repair, if required, is possible for up to 2 weeks following injury.

In children, the inferior rectus muscle can become trapped and be the cause of diplopia. A simple test to check is to get them to look up and if the globe cannot move, there is entrapment (Fig. 10.4). This can cause malaise, vomiting, and headache, and be confused with a head injury. These children need urgent surgical release—ideally within 24 h—to prevent permanent visual impairment.

Diagnosis is made on the basis of:
- History.
- Pain on eye movement.
- Double vision (diplopia).
- Sunken eye (enophthalmos).

If you suspect this injury
- Check visual acuity in both eyes ('Can you read this?').
- Feel around the bony margins of the eye socket.
- Make sure that the whole of the globe of the eye is intact.
- If the double vision is intolerable, cover the damaged eye with a patch (see ➔ Fig. 10.8, p. 352).

Injuries of this type may also lead to:
- Corneal abrasion.
- Hyphaema (blood in the anterior chamber of the eye).
- Subluxed lens.
- Vitreous haemorrhage.
- Retinal detachment.
- Posterior globe rupture.

- Surgical emphysema periorbitally—the patient should not blow their nose for 2 weeks.
- Orbital compartment syndrome (➔ Orbital compartment syndrome, p. 353).

If visual acuity is reduced after a blunt trauma, evacuation is essential.

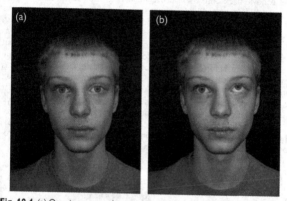

Fig. 10.4 (a) On primary gaze, the entrapment of the right inferior orbital soft tissues may be missed. (b) Limitation of right globe movement on upward gaze; entrapment of the right inferior rectus was confirmed at subsequent surgical exploration. Published with the consent of the patient's parents.

Dislocated jaw joints

The TMJ may dislocate, typically when yawning too wide. The individual may well have a history of this. If dislocation occurs in association with trauma, be wary—fracture dislocations require specialist surgical management.

The TMJ consists of the mandibular condyle (the finer projection up from the mandible) and the glenoid fossa—the dished surface on the temporal bone skull base, in which the condyle articulates. During small movements the condyle just pivots in a fixed position, but when the jaw opens wide it slides forward, down, and out of the glenoid fossa. It soon meets a physical block—the articular eminence, which stops it moving further—but in extremely wide opening it can flip over this eminence and get stuck leaving the mouth fixed open, the lower jaw jutting forward and the chin very prominent.

A *closed* fixed mouth is not a dislocated jaw, by definition.

Just pushing the mandible backwards will not reduce the dislocation—it simply pushes the condyle straight back into the articular eminence, so the mandibular condyle has to be pushed *down* and over the articular eminence. Attempt relocation as soon as you can before the jaw muscles go into spasm and prevent further movement. Lie the patient flat in a quiet environment. The process is not painful but it can be uncomfortable.

Stand in front of the patient. With gloved hands insert your index finger into the mouth behind the most posterior lower tooth onto the mucosa overlying the bone behind the molar teeth (Fig. 10.5). Do this on both sides if both condyles are dislocated. Make sure that your fingers lie *around* the cheek side of the back teeth and not over them or you will get bitten when the jaw goes back into place! Then curl the thumbs under the chin on each side. Your aim is not to push the mandible straight back as this just pushes the condyle back onto the articular eminence. Instead, you have to push the condyle down and back, *over* the articular eminence before it returns to the glenoid fossa. Press down and back with the index fingers and push the chin up with the thumbs. This rotates the mandible making the condyle move down and back more easily. It is not a sudden relocation but instead is a slow sustained pressure for up to several minutes. Usually one condyle returns before the other. Obviously in unilateral dislocation that is enough, but most are bilateral and will require a little more effort. However, once one side is in the other usually swiftly follows. Then advise the patient to rest the jaw joint for a few weeks by stifling yawns by preventing wide mouth opening with a hand underneath the chin and having a soft diet.

Cases which cannot be relocated easily may need sedation, local anaesthetic injections to the muscles around the joint, or evacuation to be relocated under a short general anaesthetic.

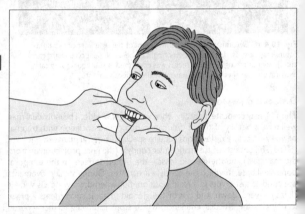

Fig. 10.5 Relocating a dislocated jaw.

Cervical spine

For discussion of the assessment and management of suspected cervical spine trauma, see ➲ Neck and other spinal injuries, p. 219.

Head injury

A person should be considered to have a traumatic brain injury if they have suffered any trauma to the head, apart from superficial lacerations to the face. Traumatic brain injury can be:

- Direct or indirect.
- Closed or open.

It may result in primary or secondary brain damage.

Epidemiology

It is best to avoid a head injury! About 60% of adults with moderate traumatic brain injuries and 85% with severe traumatic brain injuries remain disabled 1 year after their accident. Even a minor head injury can ruin a trip: 3 months later, 80% have persistent headaches and 60% have memory problems. Wear a suitable helmet if at risk of head injury.

Causes

- Direct head injuries are caused by a blow to the head of some form; this can result in a closed injury, without penetration of the skull, or an open injury, where the skull is penetrated.
- Indirect injury is caused by a 'whiplash' effect of the brain moving within the skull, though without a direct blow to the head; this can result in brief concussion, but in a young adult is unlikely to cause significant damage.

History and examination

- Ask about amnesia for events before and after the injury. Brief amnesia of <1 min is common with even mild concussion, but any significant amnesia should be a cause for concern. Post-traumatic amnesia may be a more reliable marker of severity, and should be taken to end at the point when the victim regains continuous memory, rather than just islands of recollection. Significant head injuries are usually associated with post-traumatic amnesia of >30 min.
- Care is particularly needed for high-energy injuries, e.g. a pedestrian struck by a vehicle, any high-speed RTC, or any accident involving motorized off-road vehicles such as snowmobiles, jet skis, or quad bikes. High-energy injuries also include any significant fall from a height, or being struck by falling objects such as a rock.
- Assess level of consciousness, using the GCS and the derived score (→ Table 7.2, p. 223). This is easily and reliably administered with minimal experience and is particularly useful to monitor progress. Failure of the GCS score to improve and, in particular, a fall in GCS score is of significant concern. The score has a range of 3–15. A score of 8 or less indicates a very severe head injury, one that, if it were available, would prompt immediate critical care. A score of 12 or less at any point after a closed head injury indicates possible significant injury, but secondary intracranial bleeding can develop even in someone who was fully conscious initially.

- Carry out *careful inspection* of the head, looking particularly for signs of any skull fracture. Classically, basal skull fracture may be associated with:
  - Fluid leaking from ear (otorrhoea) or nose (rhinorrhoea).
  - Blood behind tympanic membrane ('haemotympanum').
  - 'Battle's sign' (bruising and tenderness over mastoid).
  - 'Panda eyes' (black eye(s) without orbital injury).
  - However, these signs are often absent.
- Carry out and document a *simple neurological examination*. As a minimum this should include:
  - Examination of pupil size and reaction.
  - Check of visual acuity.
  - Eye movements.
  - Assess hearing and examine tympanic membranes if possible.
  - Assess gag reflex if not fully conscious.
  - Examine for any focal motor deficit, including plantar responses.
  - Check for any sensory loss.
  - Ask about paraesthesia.
  - Look for clumsiness or unsteadiness. Unsteadiness might be due to vertigo, in which case the person typically describes a sensation of spinning, like having been on a roundabout: this can be less significant.
- Other features may include irritability and/or altered behaviour, persistent headaches, or vomiting. A short-lived convulsion at the moment of impact is a well-recognized feature of concussion, often seen in contact sports, and need not be of great significance. Any subsequent seizure is of great concern.
- Do not attribute a depressed conscious level and/or altered behaviour to intoxication with alcohol or drugs unless you are sure that there has been no significant brain injury. Any intoxicated person with a suspected head injury needs close observation.
- Always carefully examine the spine, especially the cervical spine in any significant head injury, particularly those with a dangerous mechanism of injury. Around 10% of those knocked out with a head injury have an associated neck injury (in urban trauma) (➔ Neck and other spinal injuries, p. 218).
- Document any findings and repeat examination; judgement is needed to determine the frequency and extent of repeat examination, but if you are concerned about a possible significant head injury it would be reasonable to repeat the GCS every 30 min for 2 h; by then the GCS score should be 13 or better. Continue to repeat hourly for 4 h, then 2-hourly thereafter until the GCS is normal, and do not leave the person alone for 24 h.

Clinical features

Closed head injury

Results from falls, RTCs, etc.

Typically high-energy injury.

No penetration of the skull.

Primary damage tends to be diffuse, and can have serious long-term consequences; with the possibility of damage to important brain functions.

Open head injury
- Penetrating injury to the skull.
- *Primary* damage may be to just one part of the brain, but the effects can be just as serious.

Secondary deterioration is usually due to:
- *Oedema* (swelling) of damaged tissue, resulting in increased intracranial pressure (ICP) and possible brain herniation.
- Intracranial *haemorrhage* (bleeding) from torn vessels, which can be:
  - *Subdural:* between the dura and the brain.
  - *Extradural:* outside the dura, beneath the skull vault.

Swelling inside the closed cranium interferes with blood flow into the brain. Cerebral perfusion pressure (CPP) is the balance of mean arterial pressure (MAP) minus ICP:

$$CPP = MAP - ICP$$

It is therefore important to maintain BP, with fluid replacement, and minimize ICP. Factors that increase ICP that can be correctable in the wilderness include pain and hypoxia due to altitude.

Management

Management options for a significant head injury in a remote environment are limited:
- Maintain airway and breathing, and replace fluids when possible.
- Assess and manage cervical spine.
- Give adequate analgesia to control pain, and try to be calm and provide reassurance. Opiates, if available, may be needed to control severe pain, but can mask signs of deteriorating cerebral function.
- Elevation of the head to 20° improves venous outflow from the brain and may reduce ICP. This should be attempted only after any hypovolaemia has been corrected.
- If the casualty is at altitude sufficient to cause hypoxia then, if possible, bring them to a lower altitude, and give oxygen when available.
- Steroids should not be given; they have been shown to increase mortality rates.
- Secondary deterioration owing to cerebral oedema may respond to diuretics. Mannitol is preferred because it causes less electrolyte disturbance than loop diuretics, but it is unlikely to be available. Furosemide and other diuretics should be used with care; give sufficient to induce diuresis but ensure that BP is maintained.
- The major issue is whether to arrange evacuation. This decision depends on the situation and the severity of the injury. Most head injuries do not require neurosurgery, but there are many factors following any significant injury that are better managed in hospital, and secondary deterioration because of intracranial bleeding is potentially correctable. If evacuation is realistically possible, following anything other than a minor head injury it should be arranged.

Complications
- *Infection:* meningitis is a recognized complication of any skull fracture where the integrity of the blood–brain barrier may be breached. If

transfer to hospital may be delayed, it is appropriate to give a broad-spectrum antibiotic. There is particular risk if there is a CSF leak, a common presentation of which is the loss of clear, slightly salty, watery fluid coming from the nose or ear.

- *Seizures*: epileptic seizures can occur early or late. Early seizures, within 24 h, may not require long-term treatment, but in the wilderness any seizure is best treated until definitive care is available. A seizure should be considered a sign of possible intracranial deterioration. Medication available is likely to be limited to a benzodiazepine such as lorazepam or diazepam. The risk of sedation is outweighed by the need to control seizures (and further hypoxia developing during a convulsion).
- *Neurological symptoms*: these can be divided into minor symptoms that can follow any concussion, and more significant deficits. Headaches, unsteadiness, and poor concentration are common after minor head injury; they are likely to last for up to 3 months and possibly longer. Benign positional vertigo can follow any blow to the head; it results in intense vertigo with a sensation of spinning precipitated by movement of the head. Give prochlorperazine or cyclizine and arrange an ENT assessment.

Severe head injuries have many consequences and may require long-term rehabilitation.

Resource

NICE. *Head Injury: Assessment and Early Management.* 2014 (updated Sept 2019). ℞ http://www.nice.org.uk/Guidance/CG176

Blackouts, syncope, and epilepsy

An episode of transient loss of consciousness is often referred to as a 'blackout'. Blackouts commonly result from:

- A disorder of the circulation—e.g. syncope (fainting).
- A disorder of the brain—e.g. epilepsy.
- A disorder of the psyche—e.g. psychogenic blackouts.

It may prove difficult, if not impossible, to determine the cause of some blackouts in the wilderness. Any previous diagnosis in an expedition member should be treated with caution, particularly if there are unusual features about the new attack.

Treatment

- Turn patient onto their side in the recovery position (◑ Recovery position, p. 248 (Fig. 8.5 and Fig. 8.6)).
- Take the pulse; it is quicker and easier to compare the patient's pulse to your own, rather than to try and count it. If the pulse is weak, thready, and particularly if it is slow, it may well be that the person has fainted, and had associated muscle twitching.
- Give oxygen if available, particularly if the seizure is prolonged.
- Do not attempt to force anything into their mouth.
- Your choice of available antiepileptic drugs is likely to be limited. Most seizures are self-limiting, and a single seizure does not require treatment unless the seizure is prolonged (>5 min).
- If the seizure is prolonged, then give any available benzodiazepine buccally, IV, IM or PR. It is safest to titrate lorazepam or diazepam IV.
- An alcoholic withdrawal seizure may be complicated by low blood sugar levels. If possible, measure the blood glucose level and correct with sugar or GlucoGel®.

Management

- Question the patient carefully for any prior history. If they are confused, or you doubt their medical history, consider contacting their family or GP if communications are available.
- Carry out as comprehensive a neurological examination as you can, looking carefully for papilloedema if possible, and checking for any persisting focal neurological deficit.
- If you believe that a team member has developed epilepsy for the first time in a wilderness environment, particularly if the patient is unwell, if there are any focal features to the seizure, or focal neurological deficit, then evacuate as soon as possible.
- Consider cerebral malaria (◑ Malaria, p. 512) and give therapeutic doses of antimalarials if in doubt.
- Consider meningitis (◑ Meningitis, p. 505) and give suitable antibiotics.

Seizures may occasionally complicate HACE (◑ High-altitude cerebral oedema, p. 698).

Syncope (fainting)

Incidence

Cardiac syncope accounts for most blackouts, and of these most cases are due to reflex syncope, with up to 30% of people suffering reflex syncope during their lives. In contrast, epilepsy only affects 0.5% of the population at any one time, with a lifetime incidence of 2%, and many of these will develop at one or other extreme of age. Blackouts are also often seen in the absence of organic physical disease; such attacks may be accompanied by apparent convulsive movements, but their origin could be psychological rather than physical, particularly in very stressful circumstances.

The cause of syncope may be either *cardiac* or *vascular*:

- *Cardiac causes* could be due to structural heart disease or an arrhythmia. Sudden death in young people is occasionally associated with a structural cardiomyopathy. An arrhythmia in the wilderness could be a marker of myocardial infarction, although otherwise very fit middle-aged individuals can develop atrial fibrillation and feel awful. Syncope *during* (as opposed to *after*) exercise is potentially serious and may presage sudden cardiac death owing to a familial arrhythmia such as long QT syndrome.
- *Vascular causes* are more likely, and include:
  - Reflex causes, such as vasovagal syncope.
  - Situational causes, such as cough and micturition syncope.
  - Postural causes, such as orthostatic hypotension which may reflect dehydration.
  - PE.

In hot environments, consider heatstroke (➋ Heat-related illnesses (HRIs), p. 790).

Clinical diagnosis

Diagnosis is made from the history, particularly the circumstances around the blackout. Syncope results in transient self-limited loss of consciousness owing to transient reduction in blood flow to the brain, typically leading to collapse; most attacks, particularly those with vascular causes, therefore occur when patient is standing, although fainting can occur while sitting.

- The patient may recall a brief lightheadedness, when voices sounded distant, and vision faded.
- Onset is rapid; recovery is spontaneous, complete, and usually prompt, particularly if a person lies down.
- During the episode the pulse may be slow and BP low, but often the episode is too brief and the bystanders too panicked for either to be reliably measured.
- The patient characteristically appears limp and pale.
- Limb jerks (myoclonus) commonly occur. These are usually brief, but complex movements resembling epilepsy can be seen. This 'convulsive syncope' often results in panic in bystanders and may be reported as an 'epileptic fit' by even medically trained observers unfamiliar with the phenomenon.
- During recovery there may be brief bewilderment, but prolonged confusion is rare.

- If the person gets up too quickly, they may collapse again. If someone feels they are going to faint, lie them down and keep them horizontal for several minutes.

Epilepsy

Epilepsy is most simply classified as idiopathic, a condition in isolation, or symptomatic, resulting from some underlying disease, although current academic classifications are more complex. The resulting seizures are either generalized, involving the whole brain from onset, or focal, starting in one area but then affecting all areas.

- *Idiopathic epilepsy* usually starts in childhood, so is unlikely to be a diagnostic issue in the wilderness; however, some syndromes first appear during adolescence, and could therefore present in a teenager. Idiopathic epilepsies usually cause generalized seizures, tonic–clonic convulsions, myoclonus, and absences; most probably have a genetic basis.
- *Symptomatic epilepsy*, particularly in the context of wilderness medicine, is more likely to result in focal or secondarily generalized seizures. The seizure may indicate an underlying localized brain disorder, and in this circumstance, concern should be raised about infection, including cerebral malaria, encephalitis, and meningitis.

A separate classification describes the resultant seizures: these are *partial* or *generalized*.

Partial (or 'focal') seizures

- More likely to be caused by a symptomatic epilepsy, i.e. where pathology has developed in part of the brain, causing the seizures—this is potentially of more concern in the wilderness.
- Begin in one part of the body and may then spread—'Jacksonian marching'.
- Signs are variable: the patient may or may not lose awareness, and may or may not collapse.
- If the attack is witnessed, record its details, which may include automatic behaviour, asymmetrical limb jerking, or a forced turn of the head.
- Afterwards the patient may recall a strong unpleasant smell, bright lights, changes in hearing, or a brief but intense sense of déjà vu.

Generalized seizures

- Involve the whole of the brain.
- Best recognized form is a tonic–clonic convulsion.
- Onset is sudden with an initial tonic phase: all muscles stiffen, the limbs become rigid, and there may be a strangled cry. The person falls to the ground and may become cyanosed.
- The subsequent clonic phase involves rhythmic jerking of the limbs; initially this may be vigorous, but the movements slow and become irregular.
- Victim is then usually unconscious for a period.
- When they come round, they may be confused, muscles may ache, and they will usually complain of headache.
- They may have bitten their tongue (usually the side).
- The tonic–clonic seizure itself rarely lasts >1–2 min, but post-ictal drowsiness and confusion can be prolonged, with general malaise lasting several hours.

- A generalized tonic–clonic convulsion can also develop from an initial partial seizure, the seizure activity starting focally and then spreading to the whole brain; these are secondarily generalized convulsions.

Other types of generalized seizures include collapse with rigidity (tonic seizure) or without change in muscle tone (atonic seizures). These usually only occur in the context of a complex epilepsy associated with learning disability. Generalized seizures also include absences, with preserved posture, and daytime myoclonus, both of which may be seen in previously diagnosed idiopathic childhood and juvenile epilepsies.

Psychogenic blackouts and disturbances

These range from simple panic attacks with hyperventilation, which rarely cause blackout and are usually readily recognized, to a wide spectrum of non-epileptic seizures. Typically occurring in adolescents or young adults, they can be frequent and without apparent cause. Assessment is very difficult, and it is essential to exclude organic disease. Such behaviour is disruptive, especially in a hazardous environment, so evacuation or repatriation may be required.

Differential diagnosis of blackouts and seizures

If you consider that the blackout was due to syncope, then check for any predisposing systemic illness:

- Anaemia is likely, particularly in young people who faint; check for blood loss—acute or chronic, including heavy periods in a woman.
- Dehydration or heat exhaustion.
- Salt deficiency.
- Excess alcohol can predispose to fainting, possibly due to dehydration, but can also be associated with epileptic seizures.
- Hypoxia and HACE (see ➋ High-altitude cerebral oedema, p. 698) may cause fitting.
- An initial epileptic seizure may be the first indication of an underlying neurological disease, especially if the seizure was focal. Possible causes include:
  - *Neurocysticercosis:* the most common cause of new adult-onset epilepsy in rural countries with poor hygiene, where pigs are allowed to roam freely. It results from human ingestion of the eggs from the pork tape worm. Visitors are vulnerable, the condition usually presenting some months after exposure.
  - *Schistosomiasis:* may present with epilepsy.
  - *Bacterial meningitis:* can cause seizures. The individual is likely to be very unwell with associated fever, photophobia, and a stiff neck.
  - *Cerebral malaria:* should always be considered in malarial zones.

Investigations

Few investigations are possible in the wilderness. Check pulse and temperature to check for systemic illness, and check blood glucose if possible. Measure oxygen saturation if a pulse oximeter is available.[2]

NICE guideline on blackouts: ✍ http://www.nice.org/guidance/cg109 ✍ https://www.epilepsydiagnosis.org

Migraine

Migraine is a disorder characterized by recurrent, usually unilateral, moderate to severe headaches that may be accompanied by dizziness, nausea, vomiting, or extreme sensitivity to light and sound. Migraine is common in young adults. Most migraine sufferers know they have the condition, so a first attack would be unusual but could be precipitated by, for instance, high altitude. The cause of migraine is unknown.[3]

Risk factors

Women may be more prone to migraine if on the combined oral contraceptive pill. Focal migraine is a contraindication to the use of the oestrogen-containing contraceptive pill—it may increase the risk of stroke. Triggering factors include:

- Stress, tiredness, exertion, and menstruation.
- Alcohol, especially red wine.
- Citrus fruits.
- Cheese.
- Chocolate.
- Caffeine.

History and examination

Migraine often develops in a predictable way, but some will not experience these features:

- *Prodromal*: change in mood, depression or restlessness, tiredness, or listlessness.
- *Aura*: including visual flashes, shimmering, and other hallucinations.
- *Headache*: typically one-sided but may affect both sides of the head. It is usually gradual in onset, moderate to severe in pain intensity, throbbing, and worse with physical exertion, and it can last anywhere from 2 h to 2 days in children and 4 h to 3 days in adults. The headache stage is often accompanied by loss of appetite, nausea, vomiting, sensitivity to light and sound, blurred vision, tenderness of the scalp or neck, lightheadedness, sweating, and pallor. In severe cases there may be visual field defects and unilateral limb weakness; these are very frightening symptoms which should be treated seriously unless the patient knows that they are regularly associated with their migraines.

Treatment

Rest, hydration, and adequate analgesia. If the individual is known to have migraine, they may have brought their medication with them. Otherwise give 900 mg soluble aspirin, which should be given with a glass of milk if available, to protect the stomach, and ideally also with an antiemetic. Metoclopramide or domperidone are particularly useful as they promote gastric emptying, but avoid metoclopramide in adolescents and young adults, as it can precipitate an extrapyramidal reaction. Prochlorperazine is a suitable alternative.

3 https://cks.nice.org.uk/topics/migraine/

Complications

Complications are unlikely. If migraine develops for first time in women on oral contraception then this should be stopped, particularly if migraine has focal features. Be aware that migraine can develop for the first time during pregnancy.

Sleep disturbances

On an expedition many factors may disturb sleep, including time zone shifts, unfamiliar harsh living conditions, physical discomfort, environmental extremes including high altitude, sport-specific disturbances (night watches sailing, pre-dawn starts climbing), and psychological factors such as anxiety about the venture ahead or homesickness. Few things erode team morale and daytime performance as much as disturbed sleep; however, forward planning and simple measures can improve things considerably.

General measures to improve sleep

- Comfortable bed—careful choice of tent site, padded sleeping mat.
- Temperature control—fan, hot water bottle (e.g. tomorrow's boiled drinking water wrapped in a fleece), appropriate sleeping bag and mat.
- Mosquito deterrents—nets and repellents.
- Earplugs.
- Safe environment—away from rock fall, avalanche run out zones, flood pathways, or marauding animals.

Jet lag

Many body functions are under circadian control, including hormone secretion, body temperature, cellular and enzymatic function, and sleep. The natural circadian rhythm approximates 24 h. Rapid travel across time zones is associated with desynchronization between the body's circadian clock and the actual local time, resulting in jet lag. This is experienced as difficulty getting to sleep following an eastward flight, wakening early following a westward flight, disturbed sleep, daytime sleepiness, difficulty concentrating, irritability, depressed mood, anorexia, and nocturia. These symptoms usually only pose a minor inconvenience for travellers; however, performance, including decision-making, may be impaired in the first few days following arrival in a new time zone, and this should be allowed for in the travel schedule.

Decreasing jet lag

- Obtain adequate sleep. Use daytime flights in preference or sleep as much as possible during overnight flights. Use short naps terminated by an alarm clock to improve daytime alertness and concentration. Avoid napping late in the day as this will decrease the ability to sleep at night.
- Adopt the new time frame in the country you are leaving and in transit, including bed and get up times, and meal times.
- Optimize light exposure. The light–dark cycle is the principal time cue for resetting human circadian rhythms. Bright light exposure during the daytime for the new time zone and avoidance of bright light at other times of day may have a beneficial effect on the circadian clock and jet lag. This usually means maximizing the exposure to light early in the day after flying eastwards and late in the day after flying westwards.
- Take exercise. Exercise both improves sleep quality and has a minor effect on entraining circadian rhythms, with night-time exercise delaying the circadian clock.
- Avoid excess caffeine and alcohol as these can have a deleterious effect on sleep quality.

- Short-acting hypnotic drugs used on overnight flights and for a few nights after arrival may help. Drug-induced sleepiness carrying over into the next day must be taken into account, particularly after short flights followed by driving.
- Melatonin is a hormone that is secreted by the pineal gland and linked to the circadian rhythm. Melatonin requires a prescription in the UK, but can be purchased without prescription in many countries, although the stated strengths may be unreliable. A Cochrane analysis suggests that taken in doses of 0.5–5 mg at the right time of day, it can be effective at preventing and reducing jet lag. However incorrect timing of doses can cause drowsiness and failure to adapt to the new time zone, and exact dosages are as yet uncertain. Low mood, and even frank depression, is a fairly common side effect of melatonin, and it may therefore exacerbate homesickness. Patients taking warfarin and those with epilepsy should avoid melatonin.[4]

Obstructive sleep apnoea syndrome

Obstructive sleep apnoea (OSA) is a condition in which repeated blockage of the upper airway fragments sleep. It presents with snoring, pauses in breathing, and daytime sleepiness. People with this pre-existing condition should consult their physician prior to travel.

OSA may be treated using nasal continuous positive airway pressure (CPAP) during sleep. If CPAP has to be discontinued briefly, there is some carry forward benefit for 1–2 nights before symptoms return. An alternative to CPAP for patients with milder OSA is a jaw advancement device, which has the merits of being small, readily portable, and requiring no electrical power. Interestingly mild OSA improves somewhat on ascent to high altitude, presumably as tone in the upper airway is increased by the additional respiratory effort driven by hypoxia.

⅍ http://www.cochrane.org/CD001520/DEPRESSN_melatonin-for-the-prevention-and-treatment-of-jet-lag

The eye

Ophthalmology is viewed by the general physician with anything from mild boredom to abject fear. Unfortunately, eye problems may occur while travelling and this section is designed to help you assess and treat them. An expedition medic should have some experience of using a magnifying loupe and ophthalmoscope as well as administering eye drops and applying a double eye pad.

Ocular anatomy

It is important to have a basic understanding of ocular anatomy to assess the severity of an injury. Fig. 10.6 shows an external and internal view of the eye; note that the cornea is continuous with the sclera and that the conjunctiva lines both the inside of the eyelids and covers the sclera up to the cornea.

Pre-expedition ocular history

Relevant ocular information can be obtained from the pre-departure health questionnaire (Box 10.1; also see ➲ Box 2.3, p. 49).

> **Box 10.1 Ocular history taking**
> - Do you wear contact lenses?
>   - If yes, what type are they (e.g. hard/soft, monthlies/dailies)?
> - Have you ever been treated by a doctor for an eye problem?
> - Have you ever had any type of operation on your eyes including laser refraction correction? If so, what and when?
> - Does anyone in your family suffer from glaucoma or other eye disease?
> - Are you diabetic?

Travellers with chronic eye conditions may need to take other precautions and should ensure that they have ample supplies of regular medications.

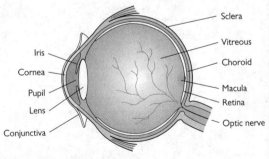

Fig. 10.6 Anatomy of the eye.

Contact lenses

In the wilderness, contact lens users are vulnerable to dry eyes and serious corneal infections, so should be advised on sensible contact lens use (no more than 8 h a day) and strict hygiene when handling lenses. Remind them to bring spectacles as well as plenty of spare contact lenses.

Any potential infection, even an apparently simple conjunctivitis, should be taken very seriously. Contact lens wear should be stopped and intensive broad-spectrum antibiotic drops should be started (e.g. ofloxacin hourly). If there is no improvement within 5 days, evacuate the patient for specialist review.

Refractive surgery and high altitude

Refractive surgery is becoming increasingly popular among outdoor enthusiasts to decrease dependence on spectacles or contact lenses. During this type of surgery, the refractive power of the cornea is changed either through surgical incisions or laser ablation. However, high altitude can affect the surgical results, causing blurred vision that usually resolves upon descent. Radial keratotomy (RK) has now been superseded by laser *in situ* keratomileusis (LASIK), laser epithelial keratomileusis (LASEK), and photorefractive keratectomy (PRK).

RK tends to cause long-sightedness (hypermetropia) at altitude whereas LASIK, LASEK, and PRK may cause short-sightedness (myopia) at altitude. This phenomenon is not predictable and can severely affect vision. Avoid elective refractive surgery within 3 months of an expedition as refraction can be unstable and infection a risk.

Another form of refractive surgery is to have the natural lens removed and replaced with an intraocular lens in a procedure similar to cataract surgery. There is a risk of dry eye and a small chance of intraocular infection after clear lens extraction, but vision is unlikely to change at high altitude.

Any decreased vision, redness, or pain in the eyes of someone who has had refractive surgery should be taken seriously, as they are more vulnerable to infection. If necessary, consider descent and evacuation.

Examination of the eye

- *Visual acuity* is the single most important sign when examining the eye and you do not need a Snellen chart to test it; either compare it with the other eye or simply ask the patient if their vision has changed.
- Do not be afraid to *dilate* the pupil to obtain a reasonable view of the retina. If tropicamide alone is used, it can be easily reversed with pilocarpine in the extremely unlikely event of an acute rise in intraocular pressure owing to angle closure.
- Measurement of *intraocular pressure* does not require specialist equipment. Ask the patient to close their eyes and, with your thumbs, simply press gently on the globe, comparing one eye with the other. This will easily reveal the 'marble' of high pressure from the 'avocado' of normal pressure.
- *Fluorescein* is useful to assess the integrity of the corneal epithelium and the globe. It should only be administered after topical anaesthetic (e.g. tetracaine (amethocaine)). It is best viewed with a blue light in the dark.

Drops or ointment?

Drops are easy to administer but are short lived. Ointments sooth and lubricate, but blur the vision. It is therefore worth having antibiotics in both preparations depending on the patient's needs.

Loss of vision

Loss of vision, even if it is transient, whether or not associated with pain, should be of great concern to the expedition medic especially if no obvious cause such as snow blindness can be found. Always consider evacuating the patient for specialist evaluation.

- Take a full history.
- Evaluate optic nerve function (Box 10.2).
- Digital intraocular pressure (as described in ⊃ Examination of the eye, p. 347).
- Eye movements.
- Ophthalmoscopy.

Box 10.2 Tests of optic nerve function in the wilderness

- Visual acuity: compare with the other eye reading any text at distance (beyond 2 m) and at reading distance.
- Colour vision: 'How red is my hat compared with the other eye?'
- Visual fields: simple confrontational visual fields.
- Pupils: check for a relative afferent pupillary defect by swinging a torch from one pupil to the other. If the pupil dilates instead of constricts it suggests a weakness of that optic nerve.
- Ophthalmoscopy: look for optic disc pallor compared to the other eye with a direct ophthalmoscope if available.

Causes of painful loss of vision

- Snow blindness.
- Orbital cellulitis.
- Bacterial keratitis.
- Acute angle-closure glaucoma.
- Optic neuritis.
- Giant cell arteritis.
- Endophthalmitis.

Causes of painless loss of vision

- Migraine.
- Amaurosis fugax (transient ischaemic loss of vision).
- Cerebral hypoxia.
- High-altitude retinopathy (HAR).
- Hypertensive retinopathy.
- Ischaemic optic neuropathy.
- Retinal artery occlusion.
- Retinal vein occlusion.
- Vitreous haemorrhage.
- Retinal detachment.

Conjunctivitis

Conjunctivitis is the most common eye problem likely to be encountered in the wilderness setting.

Symptoms and signs

One or both eyes are red and painful with pus (bacterial), profuse watering (viral), or itch (allergic) depending on aetiology. Visual acuity is usually unaffected, the conjunctiva red and inflamed, and the cornea clear.

Treatment

Bacterial conjunctivitis should respond rapidly to topical antibiotics, whereas viral conjunctivitis can persist for many days but is eventually self-limiting. If the patient is a contact lens wearer then follow the specific advice earlier in the chapter (→ Contact lenses, p. 347). Allergic conjunctivitis may respond to sodium cromoglicate. Bacterial and especially viral conjunctivitis are extremely contagious so enforce strict hygiene measures.

Dry eyes

Dry eyes can be exacerbated by the dry, windy, bright conditions found at high altitude or in polar regions. Contact lens wearers are particularly vulnerable. The eyes are red, painful, and gritty.

Treatment

- Symptoms are relieved by topical anaesthetic; subsequent fluorescein reveals punctuate staining.
- Use an ocular lubricant frequently.
- Minimize contact lens wear.
- Goggles can decrease tear evaporation.
- Although usually just a nuisance, severely dry eyes can be very painful, vision blurred, and the eyes susceptible to infection.

Corneal abrasion

A tear in the corneal epithelium, usually through mild trauma such as removing a contact lens or perhaps even while asleep.

Symptoms and signs

An acute and exquisitely painful eye. Topical anaesthetic will provide immediate relief, but should not be used as a treatment. Fluorescein will confirm the diagnosis.

Treatment

Prescribe an antibiotic ointment. An eye pad is not usually necessary and can encourage infection.

Snow blindness

Snow blindness is caused by unprotected exposure of the cornea and conjunctiva to ultraviolet light (UVB). Like sunburn, by the time you realize there is a problem, it is too late, and it can be extremely painful. Prevention and treatment are discussed in → Snow blindness (photokeratitis), p. 349.

Corneal foreign body

Occasionally the protective blink reflex fails and allows a foreign body to embed itself into the cornea. This can be metallic or organic; a metallic foreign body will often leave a rust ring.

Symptoms and signs

Red, painful, gritty eye, and foreign body sensation. The foreign body is usually very small, but fluorescein and a magnifying loupe can assist identification and removal. Always evert the eyelid to exclude a subtarsal foreign body (Fig. 10.7).

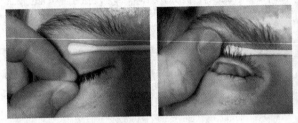

Fig. 10.7 Technique for eyelid inversion.

Treatment

- The foreign body should be removed either with a moistened cotton bud or a needle. Irrigation with sterile saline may assist removal.
- Antibiotic ointment.
- An eye pad is not usually necessary and can encourage infection.
- Remember to ask about the mechanism of injury, as a high-velocity foreign body, such as a shard of metal from an ice-axe, is more likely to penetrate the globe.

Chemical eye injury

Immediately irrigate a chemical injury before any further assessment. A chemical splash can be sight-threatening. It is important to identify the chemical because alkali penetrates the ocular tissues much faster than acid and therefore has a worse prognosis.

Symptoms and signs

- A red irritable eye following chemical splash.
- Visual acuity may be impaired.
- If severe, there may be blepharospasm.

Treatment

- Immediate profuse irrigation, preferably with sterile normal saline and a giving set. If unavailable, use the cleanest water available.
- Irrigate for a minimum of 30 min.
- Antibiotic ointment (e.g. chloramphenicol three times a day).
- Ocular lubrication (e.g. artificial tears hourly).
- Cycloplegic drops for pain relief (e.g. cyclopentolate three times a day).
- A white eye following chemical injury can indicate severe ischaemia.
- If there is any concern regarding a chemical injury, especially if visual acuity is affected or there was any delay initiating irrigation, evacuate for specialist treatment.

Eyelid laceration

The eyelids play an important role in protecting the eye and preventing corneal desiccation. If they are damaged, the eye can be rendered vulnerable.

Assessment

- Check visual acuity.
- Assess globe integrity.
- Examine the eyelid carefully for any embedded foreign body.
- Decide whether the eyelid margin is interrupted.

Management

- Remove any foreign body from the eyelid.
- Clean the wound thoroughly.
- If skilled, consider primary repair using a 6/0 non-absorbable suture if the eyelid margin is interrupted and the ends are not opposed. This is especially important for the upper eyelid.
- Antibiotic ointment.
- Broad-spectrum oral antibiotics to prevent orbital cellulitis.
- Patch the eye if there is concern about corneal exposure and to control bleeding.

Complications

- Corneal exposure is a problem, especially after upper eyelid laceration. This can affect visual acuity and encourage infection.
- Lacerations near the medial canthus may involve the tear duct and, if left unrepaired, may cause a permanent watery eye (epiphora).
- A patient with an eyelid laceration with the eyelid margin severed should be evacuated—a primary repair needs to be done properly by an ophthalmic surgeon under magnification. A poor repair performed in the field is likely to result in a permanent defect in the lid margin, which will require revision at a later date.
- Always check that there is no underlying penetrating injury to the globe, especially if the mechanism of eyelid injury was high velocity.

Penetrating eye injury

A penetrating eye injury involves disruption of the globe integrity and is a serious, sight-threatening problem. The mechanism of injury is important in determining whether there could be an intraocular foreign body or a perforating injury (entry and exit).

Symptoms and signs

- Pain.
- Decreased vision.
- Soft watery eye.
- Peaked pupil.
- Expulsion of ocular contents.

Siedel's test involves a drop of fluorescein (after topical anaesthetic) on a suspected corneal penetrating injury. The leak of aqueous fluid out of the wound will dilute the dye, showing up easily with a blue light and loupe. Beware of false negatives, however, as some wounds will seal themselves quickly, potentially leaving an undiscovered intraocular foreign body.

Management
- A casualty with a suspected penetrating eye injury should be evacuated as soon as practical.
- Do not touch any expulsed ocular contents.
- If available, use a topical antibiotic eye ointment.
- Start broad-spectrum systemic antibiotics.
- Both eyes should move as little as possible.
- Protect the injured eye using a double pad and eye shield (Fig. 10.8).
- An increased suspicion of penetrating injury should be maintained in any high-velocity eye injury, such as those involving firearms or hammering.

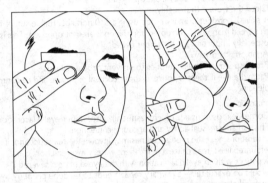

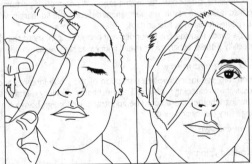

Fig. 10.8 The correct technique to pad an eye.

Orbital cellulitis

Orbital cellulitis is a sight-threatening condition that can also be life-threatening if it spreads to form a brain abscess. The infection may originate from an adjacent ethmoid sinus or from mild trauma to the orbital region.

Symptoms and signs
- Pain.
- Reduced and painful eye movements.
- Conjunctival redness.
- Possible visual loss.
- General malaise.
- Pyrexia.

Treatment
- Broad-spectrum antibiotics, preferably IV.
- Optic nerve function should be closely monitored (➲ Box 10.2, p. 348).
- Immediate evacuation for hospitalization.

Complications
- Decreased vision owing to optic nerve compression. This can be permanent without rapid orbital decompression.
- Orbital abscess requiring surgical drainage.
- Brain abscess which can be fatal.

Preseptal cellulitis

Preseptal cellulitis involves only the eyelid tissue. There is periorbital inflammation and swelling but none of the other features mentioned previously for orbital cellulitis. However, preseptal cellulitis can progress to orbital cellulitis so should be treated with broad-spectrum oral antibiotics and closely watched.

Orbital compartment syndrome

The orbit is a relatively closed compartment with limited ability to expand, so orbital pressure can rise rapidly when an acute rise in orbital volume occurs. This is an emergency where prompt simple treatment can prevent blindness.

The most common cause of orbital compartment syndrome, especially in the wilderness, is retrobulbar haemorrhage from trauma, but spontaneous retrobulbar haemorrhage can also occur due to venous anomalies, intraorbital aneurysms, or malignant hypertension. Severe orbital cellulitis with an abscess can also cause an orbital compartment syndrome. Patients with increased orbital pressure present with pain causing vomiting, proptosis, red and swollen conjunctiva, limited eye movements, and decreased optic nerve function (decreased vision and an afferent pupillary defect).

Treatment is with a surgical lateral canthotomy and cantholysis to release the pressure. This is a relatively straightforward procedure that can be performed as an emergency procedure under local anaesthesia if evacuation is not possible (Fig. 10.9).

Following infiltration with local anaesthesia (e.g. lidocaine with adrenaline) the lower eyelid is completely detached from the lateral orbital rim using sharp sterile scissors, first horizontally to cut through the lateral canthal angle (canthotomy) and then vertically to cut the lateral canthal tendon (cantholysis). This may be followed by a gush of blood from behind the eye as pressure is relieved. If the lid is held with forceps it is possible to feel when the tendon has been severed. The patient should then be evacuated for specialist evaluation and treatment.

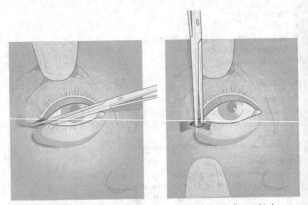

Fig. 10.9 Technique for lateral canthotomy and cantholysis to relieve orbital compartment pressure caused by retro-orbital haematoma. Illustration: Janice Sharp, Snr Med artist, University Hospital of Wales.

High-altitude retinopathy

(See also ⊃ High-altitude retinal haemorrhages, p. 701; ⊃ Colour plate 3.)

HAR is defined as 'one or more haemorrhages in either eye of a person ascending above 2500 m'. It is normally asymptomatic but affects ~30% of lowlanders ascending to 5000 m and can cause sudden painless loss of central vision.

Signs
- Retinal haemorrhages (flame, pre-retinal, dot, and blot).
- Cotton wool spots.
- Optic disc hyperaemia.
- Decreased visual acuity (only if the macula is affected).

Aetiology

The pathophysiology of HAR is not entirely clear; extreme altitudes are proposed to alter the integrity of the blood–brain barrier, injure retinal neurons, increase release of inflammatory mediators and cytokines, and cause retinal blood vessel dysfunction. The altitude attained, rate of ascent, and exertion levels en route appear to be risk factors.

There is only anecdotal evidence to suggest a relationship between HAR, acute mountain sickness (AMS), HACE, and HAPE. However retinal vascular dysregulation could herald similar problems in other organs and should not be taken lightly. Optic disc swelling may indicate early HACE so should be monitored and taken in context of the patient's general condition.

Any visual disturbance at altitude is an indication for descent.

Ocular first-aid kit

Appropriate drugs and equipment for an easily transportable lightweight ocular first-aid kit are listed in ⊃ Ocular first-aid kit, p. 864.

Ear problems

Ear problems are relatively common, particularly on diving expeditions (→ Barotrauma, p. 778; → Otitis externa, p. 782), owing to pressure changes and prolonged exposure to salt water.

Otitis externa

An infection of the outer ear often associated with constant moisture due to diving, or living in tropical environments. The ear canal itches, hurts, and may discharge; moving the pinna causes pain. The external canal looks swollen and red debris is usually obvious. In severe cases, hearing loss develops if the external canal becomes blocked by debris and swelling. Systemic upset with lymphadenopathy can occur.

Treat by gently cleaning the external canal with saline or clean water. Use a combination preparation of antibiotic and steroid such as gentamicin with hydrocortisone drops four times a day or Otomize® spray, and in severe cases prescribe an oral antibiotic such as co-amoxiclav. Avoid further exposure to water until the condition resolves.

Otitis media

A viral or bacterial infection of the middle ear, often associated with a URTI. It presents as pain and decreased hearing. The pain is made worse by changes in pressure.

Through an otoscope, the eardrum will usually appear red, but if pus collects behind the drum it can look yellow. Sometimes the drum perforates and pus discharges, with loss of hearing but relief of pain.

Prescribe painkillers and a basic antibiotic such as amoxicillin or erythromycin. A decongestant such as oral pseudoephedrine or nasal drops may help to relieve eustachian tube obstruction.

Very occasionally, severe cases of otitis media can be complicated by *mastoiditis*, which causes pain, tenderness, and inflammation over the mastoid process, the bony prominence immediately behind and below the pinna. High-dose PO or, ideally, IV antibiotics should be commenced and the patient evacuated for specialist care because there is a small risk that meningitis or cerebral abscess could develop.

Tympanic membrane rupture and barotrauma

Tympanic membrane rupture may be caused by direct trauma or associated with a base of skull fracture. Leakage of blood or clear fluid from the ear may indicate a serious injury (→ Facial injuries, p. 322). The eardrum may also rupture as a result of barotrauma—especially during diving (see → Barotrauma, p. 778). Most eardrum perforations heal spontaneously and do not require specific management. Avoid swimming until the hole has healed.

Inner ear barotrauma is unpleasant. It results from inner ear haemorrhage or a rupture of the oval window. Patients experience vertigo, hearing loss, and tinnitus. Evacuate for examination by an ENT surgeon.

Foreign bodies in the ear canal

On expeditions, these are most commonly insects that have crawled into the external canal. Insects should be drowned in oil and will usually float out. Other foreign bodies may require removal with suitable hooks. If difficulty is experienced in foreign body removal, do not persist at the expense of damage to the tympanic membrane or external canal.

Nasal problems

Epistaxis (nose bleed)

Nose bleeds are quite common in expedition situations and may be precipitated by the low humidity found at high altitude, in cold climates, or aircraft cabin atmospheres. Other associations include direct trauma to the nose, URTIs, and hayfever. Ninety per cent are anterior and 10% are posterior.

First-aid measures are usually effective in controlling haemorrhage. Press on the soft part of the nose with a finger and thumb for 15 min. If simple pressure is unsuccessful, try cauterizing off any identified anterior bleeding points with a silver nitrate stick. Before cauterizing the vessel you should apply a topical local anaesthetic such as lidocaine and adrenaline (epinephrine). Look up the nose using a head torch and apply the cauterization stick to the bleeding point for no longer than 5s.

If cautery is not possible or is unsuccessful, then insert a commercially available nasal tampon. Such tampons should be lubricated before insertion. Once correctly positioned, expand the device by dropping saline from a syringe or, with some devices, inflating with air. Often both nostrils have to be packed. They are uncomfortable so prescribe painkillers. If nasal tampons are unavailable, then the nose can be packed with lubricated gauze or a small vaginal tampon.

Nasal packs can precipitate sinusitis and in the expedition setting amoxicillin should be prescribed. Leave the packs in place overnight and then remove them.

If bleeding continues despite insertion of a nasal tampon, it is probable that the bleeding point is in the posterior part of the nose. Remove the tampon and insert a deflated urinary catheter along the floor of the nose. Gently inflate the balloon with air and pull the catheter forward until resistance is felt. The pack or tampon should then be re-inserted.

A patient with a persistent nose bleed that does not respond to the measures described will have to be evacuated for further treatment and investigation which must include a blood count and clotting studies. Rarely, transfusion is required.

Nasal fracture

See Nasal fracture, p. 329.

Nasal foreign bodies

Foreign bodies in the nose need to be removed as they may lead to infection or aspiration. Anterior foreign bodies can be removed with hooked implements or forceps using a head torch to look up the nose.

Upper respiratory tract

Coryza (common cold)

URTIs are very common and often originate before departure. The condition is usually self-limiting and requires only symptomatic treatment. Catarrh may block sinus openings and Eustachian tubes. Pressure differences during flight or ascent may cause ear or sinus pain, which may be severe. Nasal decongestants such as phenylephrine can help. Antibiotics may help if persistent sinus pain and tenderness suggests secondary bacterial infection.

Pharyngitis/tonsillitis

Sore throats with painful swallowing are common in travellers, especially following air travel. The throat infection may be associated with fever and systemic upset. Most are viral in origin. Pus around the tonsils suggests bacterial infection but it is not usually possible to differentiate the two clinically.

Most cases of tonsillitis settle with time and analgesia. In the remote setting, if symptoms fail to improve after a few days then antibiotics should be prescribed. A suitable antibiotic for the most common bacterial pathogen, beta haemolytic *Streptococcus*, is co-amoxiclav 250/125 mg three times a day for 7 days. This dose can be doubled if infection severe. Clarithromycin is an alternative in penicillin-allergic patients.

Peritonsillar abscess (quinsy)

Quinsy causes severe unilateral throat pain and dysphagia, with associated pyrexia and systemic upset. Trismus (an inability to open the mouth due to pain) and drooling occur. The tonsil is swollen, inflamed, and deviated medially; the uvula is usually displaced away from the affected side. IV antibiotics are required. In the remote setting the abscess should be drained by needle aspiration rather than incision and drainage.

Throat foreign bodies

These are most commonly fish or chicken bones. The patient complains of pain, especially on swallowing. Foreign bodies stuck in the tonsil or base of the tongue can usually be seen and removed with forceps. If no foreign body is visible it is possible that it may simply have scratched the pharyngeal mucosa on passing. A foreign body stuck out of sight in the pharynx may become infected and abscesses can develop, so if symptoms persist the patient must be evacuated.

Equipment

A list of additional drugs and equipment that may assist with ENT problems is given in ➔ Useful equipment and drugs for ENT problems, p. 864.

Chapter 11

Dental

Chapter editor
Burjor K. Langdana

Contributors
Alistair Cobb
Ben Molyneux
Burjor K. Langdana
Penelope B. Granger
David Geddes (1st edition)

Tooth, gum, and mouth problems are common especially on longer expeditions. This chapter offers advice on the prevention, diagnosis, and practical management of dental problems in the field.

On shorter journeys travellers may experience:
• Chips or damage to dental enamel and dentine.
• Broken or lost crowns or fillings.
• Acute oral infections or dental abscesses.

On lengthy expeditions, the risk of dental problems increases due to:
• Changes in diet, especially increased sugar intake.
• Decreased fluid intake, resulting in dry mouth.
• Exposure to extreme temperatures resulting in dental sensitivity.
• Problems with maintaining good oral hygiene.

Dental terminology

Naming teeth

Complete adult dentition consists of 32 teeth, eight per quadrant with the quadrants termed upper and lower, left and right, *looking at* the patient, with individual teeth named and numbered (using a two-digit numbering system) as in Fig. 11.1. Key dental structures are shown in Fig. 11.2.

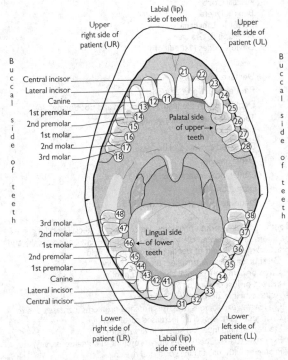

Fig. 11.1 Naming teeth.

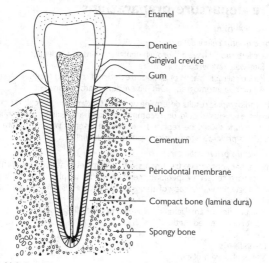

Fig. 11.2 Dental anatomy.

Pre-departure preparations

The traveller

Three months before departure

Travellers should have a thorough dental examination including:

- Bite-wing radiographs.
- Periapical radiographs of all root treated and crowned teeth.
- An orthopantomogram (OPG) if wisdom teeth are present.

The radiographic results determine whether third molar extractions or root canal treatments should be recommended and any existing poor quality dental work should be replaced electively. Preventative care before departure is preferable to treating problems in the field.

Two months before departure

Ensure that appropriate treatments will be completed at least 1 month before departure. Each expedition member should supply a detailed dental chart, together with a copy of their dental radiographs. This should accurately tell you:

- The position of amalgam and white composite fillings.
- Root canal-treated teeth.
- Crowns.
- Deep fillings.
- Status of third molars.
- Teeth with cause for concern.

One month before departure

The dentist should ideally meet with expedition members to:

- Ensure that appropriate dental treatments have been completed.
- Explain causes of tooth and gum problems, including dental decay.
- Plan and encourage a sensible diet avoiding too many fermentable carbohydrates, the 'hidden' sugars in processed food, and natural sugars in fruit.
- Reinforce good oral hygiene, interdental brushing, and flossing.
- Recommend brushing twice daily using a fluoride toothpaste for 2 min, spit but don't rinse after brushing.
- If the traveller has sensitive teeth, supply an anti-sensitivity toothpaste and encourage patient to use the same brand. Usually a month is needed to develop a sufficient barrier.

During the expedition

- Cold conditions: continuing use of the same anti-sensitivity toothpaste.
- Hot conditions: supply a high-fluoride toothpaste such as Colgate Duraphat 5000™.
- Altered diet: a high-frequency, high-carbohydrate diet will inherently increase risk of dental and gum problems. This will need to be balanced with an aggressive oral hygiene protocol.

Preparations by the medic

The commonest presentation in field dentistry is dental pain. The expedition medic should possess sufficient knowledge, skills, and experience to deal with this problem.

Other key skills include:
- Being able to diagnose dental problems.
- Being capable of giving an effective dental local anaesthetic (LA).
- Being able to manage dental injuries, especially those that are time dependent such as avulsed teeth.
- Being able to deal with lost dental fillings or displaced crowns.

Treatments typically involve the mixing of dental materials to provide a temporary fix. As a medic, it is likely you will be limited to using traditional materials that set by means of a chemical reaction. You should practise the mixing technique. There are two distinct timings:

1. *Mixing time* during which the material is workable and will not set and must be placed in the mouth.
2. *Setting time* during which the material needs to be undisturbed, kept dry, and adjusted so that it does not interfere with other teeth or the chewing function.

It is sensible to learn and practise these techniques under supervision. Medics accompanying prolonged expeditions may additionally need to familiarize themselves with the techniques of dental extraction (➔ p. 386).

Resource

Faculty of Pre-Hospital Care, Royal College of Surgeons of Edinburgh. *Updated Guidance for Medical Provision for Wilderness Medicine.* ℛ https://wildernessmedicaltraining.co.uk/wp-content/uploads/2020/03/Updated-guidance-for-medical-provision-for-wilderness-medicine-2019.pdf

Dental work in the field: Preparation and positioning

Effective dentistry requires good lighting and a dry field of work. On expedition, the necessary equipment may need to be improvised:

- Face sunlight or good artificial light—a head torch is helpful.
- Provide a good backrest for the patient, and ensure that yourself, your assistant, and the patient are comfortable and that you can work without strain.
- Protect area from wind and insects.
- Familiarize yourself with the dental charting and keep the patient's dental records to hand.
- Use an assistant to support the patient's head, retract their lips and tongue, and help light the clinical area.
- In certain circumstances, for instance in a small tent, the patient can assist with the procedure.

The patient should be appropriately positioned:

- If the lower teeth require examination, seat patient with the lower teeth parallel to the floor and upper teeth at 45° to the floor.
- For the upper teeth, the patient lies on their back with their head rotated back for additional direct vision.

It is essential to control saliva so that you work in a dry field:

- Parotid duct—place cotton rolls on cheek side of upper second molars.
- Submandibular duct—place cotton rolls on tongue side of the front bottom teeth.
- Tilt the head to the opposite side so that saliva pools away from working area.

Toothache and dental swellings

Toothache and dental swellings

Dental pain is caused either through direct trauma to the pulp (pulpitis) or by the swelling and pressure affecting the proprioceptors and connective tissues surrounding the tooth, induced by infection (Fig. 11.3). Whether it originates from the tooth, gingiva, or third molar infections, the aim of treatment in field dentistry is to reduce this pressure swiftly. Pragmatically, the field medic will be treating the effects of dental disease and not its cause.

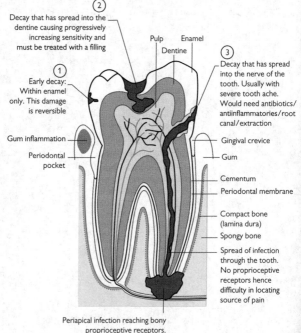

Fig. 11.3 Diagram indicating areas of a tooth at risk of dental decay.

Diagnosing dental pain

Use Table 11.1 to make a diagnosis and decide upon the appropriate treatment.

Table 11.1 Dental diagnosis and treatment

Level	Problem	Symptoms	Objective	Treatment
0	No fracture but concussion	Tender to touch, bite on, or tap	Concussed tooth management	NSAIDs for pain control
1	Enamel fracture	Asymptomatic or sharpness or sensitivity	Control further discomfort	Asymptomatic: do nothing Sharpness: if available, use a nail file to smooth sharp edge or place glass ionomer over sharp edge
2	Enamel + dentine fracture	Sensitivity but not tender to percussion, or mobile	Reduce sensitivity	(a) Use adhesive dental filling material (glass ionomer) to cover exposed enamel and dentine (b) Use surgical or wound glue to cover exposed part of tooth (c) Use IRM® or Cavit® to cover exposed tooth surface. These are non-adhesive. Retention can be improved by tucking the dressing between teeth
3	Enamel + dentine + pulp fracture (pulp exposure <1 mm)	Exposed pulp may be bleeding and sensitive to stimuli but not tender to percussion, or mobile	Preserve tooth vitality, stop pulpal bleeding, and seal root canal system to prevent ingress of bacteria	(a) Place LA. Use saline or chlorhexidine or hydrogen peroxide with cotton wool to stop the bleeding from the pulp and clean tooth surface. Attempt to dry tooth. Cover exposed nerve with calcium hydroxide cement (Dycal®). This material is tricky to use and rarely available. Seal over with glass ionomer Or (b) Cover exposed nerve with Cavit® or Ledermix® paste and seal it over with adhesive glass ionomer Or (c) Cover exposed nerve and tooth structure with IRM® or Cavit®. Due to poor mechanical retention these may not last for long

(Continued)

Table 11.1 (Contd.)

Level	Problem	Symptoms	Objective	Treatment
4	Enamel + dentine + pulp fracture (pulp exposure >1 mm)	Exposed pulp may be bleeding and sensitive to stimuli but not tender to percussion or mobile	Management of painful bleeding pulp. This tooth will gradually die	(a) Arrest pulpal bleeding with pressure/LA + adrenaline (epinephrine)/hydrogen peroxide (b) Cover with sedative dressing. Ledermix® or Cavit® sealed over by glass ionomer or IRM®
5	Root fracture	Tooth mobile, tender to touch and bite on, may be interfering with bite	Eliminate any other injury and stabilize	(a) Coronal portion of fracture loose and interfering in bite—place LA buccally and palatally. Extract loose section of tooth. May have to place temporary cover over exposed root surface if clot does not fill in (b) Minimal mobility—splint with adjacent teeth. Will need dental review as soon as possible

All patients should be followed up with a general dental practitioner on return.

Treatment of dental pain

Local measures

- *Anti-sensitivity toothpastes* help if hot, cold, or sweet stimuli are causing uncomfortable twinges of pain in an area of tooth where placing a temporary filling is impossible. To reduce sensitivity, retain the paste in the affected area for as long as practical.
- *Oil of cloves (eugenol)* is a traditional topical agent that may temporarily relieve pain and reduce sensitivity.
- *Duraphat® high-fluoride varnish* applied to dry tooth surfaces reduces sensitivity.
- *LA*, either as a nerve block or infiltration around the tooth, can provide temporary respite (➲ p. 380).
- *Temporary adhesive fillings like glass ionomer* designed to cover exposed, sharp, or sensitive dentine, keeping the filling clear of the gingivae and free of the bite.
- *Ledermix® paste*, a mix of antibiotics with an anti-inflammatory agent, can treat an unremitting, pulsating toothache, e.g. resulting from a large, deep cavity or loose filling. Remove the loose filling and soft debris from the tooth. Apply the paste with a small pellet of cotton wool to the depth of the cavity (Fig. 11.4), which can then be sealed with a temporary dressing such as Cavit™, Coltosol™, or IRM™.

Painkillers

- Paracetamol up to 1000 mg four times daily.
- Ibuprofen (NSAID) 400 mg four times daily.
- Diclofenac sodium (NSAID) tablets 50 mg three times daily; also available as rectal suppositories—useful when a patient has difficulty swallowing.
- Codeine phosphate 30–60 mg four times daily.

Avoid NSAIDs in extreme endurance athletes (potential for kidney injury in association with dehydration) or if the patient has contraindications to their use such as asthma, a history of peptic problems, a bleeding tendency, renal problems, or is taking an anticoagulant drug. Avoid diclofenac in elderly travellers with heart problems.

Combining paracetamol with ibuprofen, and alternating doses every 2 h, controls ongoing pain and pyrexia without exceeding the maximum recommended doses. Codeine and paracetamol singly or in combination, are an alternative to NSAIDs, and all three may be used in combination in very severe pain.

When pain is very severe, a NSAID such as ibuprofen 400 mg may be given up to six times per day but this high dose should be reduced after 36–48 h as symptoms decrease.

Pain, loss of sleep, and the stronger painkillers including codeine can slow reflexes and cause drowsiness. Anyone so affected should avoid high-risk activities including climbing and driving. Opiate painkillers are not very effective in dentistry other than for the relief of pain from an unreduced facial or mandibular fracture. Pain should settle within a few days, if it does not, the condition should be reviewed by an expert as soon as practical.

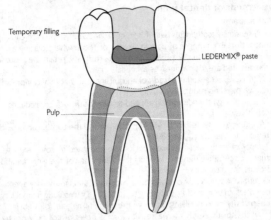

Fig. 11.4 Ledermix® cement placement.

Antibiotics

Dental infections are typically caused by anaerobic bacteria and require treatment with a broad-spectrum antibiotic. For treatment in remote locations, it is often appropriate to use more aggressive antibiotic therapy than that used in general dental practice. Antibiotics will generally reduce swelling and associated pain in 2–3 days.

The principles of controlling dental infection are:

1. Removal of pus (incise and drain either through tooth or by means of gum line incision).
2. Removal of source of infection (extract infected tooth if adequately trained).
3. Antibiotic therapy.

If objectives (1) or (2) cannot be achieved (many medics in the field will be reluctant to attempt drainage or extraction), or there is evidence of cellulitis, spreading infection, or systemic involvement, then begin antibiotic therapy immediately.

If the patient is not penicillin allergic:

• Co-amoxiclav 500/125 mg tablet (adult dose) three times daily for 5 days. If unavailable, a combination of amoxicillin 500 mg and metronidazole 400 mg three times daily for 5 days can be used.

If the patient is penicillin allergic:
- Metronidazole 400 mg three times daily for 5 days. The patient must avoid alcohol as its interaction with metronidazole is very unpleasant.
- Clarithromycin 500 mg twice daily for 5 days. May cause nausea or vomiting, and many organisms are nowadays resistant.

Second-line antibiotics should be used if there is no response to the first-line antibiotics, in the case of severe infections with spreading cellulitis, or if the patient cannot tolerate metronidazole:
- Clindamycin 150 mg four times daily for 5 days.

Mouthwashes

Dental pain can be caused by infections of the gums including:
- Gingivitis.
- Periodontitis.
- Acute ulcerative gingivitis (very destructive).
- Third molar infections (pericoronitis).

Gum disease (gingivitis) is typically associated with poor oral hygiene but may also originate around buried or partly erupted third molars. The gums look swollen, reddish-purple in colour, may bleed spontaneously or on touch with an instrument, and may smell foul. Having diagnosed periodontal infection, it is essential to minimize bacteria between the teeth and along the gum margins.

Treatment involves improving dental hygiene with better brushing and flossing and mouthwashes used as an adjunct:
- The patient should be encouraged to brush and floss the painful area. A case of being cruel to be kind!
- Warm salty water mouthwash: mix a half-teaspoon of salt in a half a cup of tea-temperature water.
- Or chlorhexidine 0.2% mouthwash: 1 min twice daily.
- Encourage smoking patients to stop, as gum problems are exacerbated.

Acute ulcerative gingivitis/pericoronitis

These local gum diseases can be treated by debridement and irrigation with mouthwash together with:
Metronidazole 400 mg three times daily for 3 days *or/and*
Amoxicillin 500 mg three times daily for 3 days.

Fillings

Temporary filling materials are used to insulate the pulp from temperature, hypertonic solutions, chemicals, or irritating foods. If a tooth is damaged—due to a lost or broken filling, decayed dentine, or cracked or broken enamel—but is not giving symptoms, then a temporary filling may be a helpful preventive measure.

Premixed filling materials

Supplied in a sealed tube; squeeze out and apply.
- Premixed materials such as Cavit™ or Coltosol™ are easy to use but have less structural strength.
- Composition is usually a variation on zinc oxide powder and some include fluoride, it sets in contact with saliva and can be easily removed.
- Require a mechanically retentive cavity to stay put.
- Erode and may require replacing as often as every few days.
- Cavity can be damp but not wet.
- Will soothe exposed dentine and reversible dental pulpitis.

Materials that require mixing

Examples include intermediate restorative material or any glass ionomer filling material. These materials are more difficult to use; however, they are also very sticky and retentive. Before starting, consider the following:
- Isolating and drying the cavity—the cavity must be protected on either side with absorbent pads or cotton wool.
- A small dry-air aerosol such as that used to clean cameras can be used to dry the cavity or a pledget of cotton wool.
- The exact ratio of powder to liquid is critical.
- The mixing time is about 1 min and the setting time is similar.
- Mix on a glass slab with a flat spatula into a dough-like consistency.
- Apply and compress into a dry cavity, immediately removing all excess material from the biting surface. A petroleum jelly-coated finger can help to smooth and shape the filling.
- Get the patient to bite together to ensure filling is not high.
- Intermediate restorative material may be colour-coded: white for a clean cavity, blue for decay present, red for pulpal symptoms.
- The same glass ionomer filling materials, if mixed into a 'double cream-like' consistency, are excellent for reseating and cementing crowns. For greater effectiveness, after removing excess cement, seal the margins of the cement around the crown, while setting, with petroleum gel to protect from saliva erosion.

If filling materials are unavailable

Improvisation can be attempted. Dip cotton pellet into oil of cloves or eugenol. Swab the depth of the cavity. Then seal the cavity with candle wax, ski wax, or sugarless chewing gum. Expect limited success of a very short duration.

Dislodged crowns and bridges

Crowns (also often called 'caps') are made of porcelain, sometimes with an inner metal core, used to restore the outer structure of a badly damaged tooth.

Bridges are a series of joined crowns used to support and replace a missing tooth.

Normal crowns rarely dislodge, but you may encounter the following types of dental loss:

- A crown retained by a metal post that inserts into an existing prepared root may displace. The underlying tooth will have already been root-treated (the root tip sealed to prevent bacterial colonization).
- A crown where the cementation has failed or been removed by trauma. In the case of trauma, the crown may hold the original, but now fractured, tooth structure.
- An implant-retained crown. The porcelain cap is normally attached to a titanium root surgically implanted into the underlying bone. Implants are a specialist area and you should avoid offering any treatment that tampers with the prosthetics.
- An adhesive bridge fixed onto the hidden surfaces of teeth by metal wings and strong adhesives. The techniques required to restore such bridges are impossible in the field.

Re-cementing a crown with post

Check by carefully flexing the root with a long probe to ensure that the root has not split vertically. If split, then do not re-cement the crown as a gingival abscess may ensue. If the root is intact then:

- Use an aerosol camera cleaner to clean and dry the inside of the root canal. Maintain moisture control.
- Test, by rehearsing the positioning, the ease of replacing the post inside the root canal.
- Have someone else mix the glass ionomer cement into a thick creamy consistency.
- Apply a little inside the root canal and most to the clean post.
- Reposition and hold in the correct place until set (2–3 min).
- Remove excess when still soft with the probe and seal the cement margins with petroleum gel.

Re-cementing a crown with broken core

A problem arises if the core of the tooth breaks off inside the crown.

Tooth previously root treated

If the tooth has already been root treated, the crown can safely be left out as the nerves have already been removed. The root treatment is typically seen as pink rubbery material running up the long axis of the centre of the root. Root-treated teeth are brittle and damage of this type is quite common. Temporary filling material like adhesive glass ionomer placed over the sharp stump, will act as an intraoral bandage and avoid soft tissue trauma.

No previous root treatment

If the dental stump has not been root treated and the exposed nervous tissue is very sensitive, you are duty bound to try to cover the sensitive area. If there is no damaged tooth core inside the dislodged crown, re-cement the crown using a glass ionomer mixed into cement consistency. The steps are the same as for the post crown. If the core of the tooth bleeds, prescribe antibiotics and NSAIDs to reduce nerve and blood vessel inflammation that could lead to dental pain.

If the tooth has not been root treated, and the original tooth structure has fractured and remains inside the crown, then attempt the following:
* Remove the fractured tooth substance from inside the crown as best you can.
* Clean and dry the fitting surface of the crown.
* Clean and dry the remains of the tooth.
* Have someone else mix a glass ionomer cement into a wet dough-like consistency.
* Place a slight excess of cement into the crown.
* Press home onto the remaining tooth, seating it down fully.
* Check the patient can bite correctly without impediment from the crown.
* Hold in this position for 2–3 min until the cement begins to set.
* Reduce any excess cement, when still soft, gently with the probe, and seal the margins with petroleum gel. Slight excess cement helps in retention.

Alternatively, preserve the root for future treatment options by sealing the post hole with a temporary filling material. Make sure the patient retains the crown for possible re-use.

It is possible to mistakenly place some crowns back to front. Check the orientation before cementation. A porcelain crown made on a metal base will usually have a shiny metal margin on the palatal/lingual aspect of the tooth.

Dental injuries

Dental injuries may be isolated, or be associated with other facial injuries (➲ Facial injuries, p. 322).

Traumatic injuries to front teeth

Management will depend upon:
1. The level at which the tooth has fractured and which structures (enamel/dentine/pulp/root/alveolar bone) have been involved in the trauma.
2. The severity of any associated injuries such as alveolar fracture, dental intrusion, extrusion or luxation, root fracture, or an inability unable to bite together.
3. The distance to the nearest dentist.
4. The availability locally of suitable instruments and materials.

If part of tooth fractured, try to find out what has happened to the broken fragment which could be on the floor, swallowed, impacted into the soft tissues of the mouth or, most worryingly, inhaled.

Dental trauma guide based on level of tooth fracture
See Fig. 11.5.

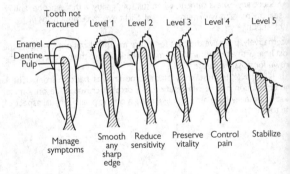

Fig. 11.5 Levels of dental trauma.

Reduction of tooth luxation

Repositioning a tooth that has been moved by trauma involves the reduction of the fractured alveolar bone immediately surrounding the affected dental roots. This is not difficult and usually not too uncomfortable for the patient but must be done quickly after an accident to stand much chance of success—certainly within an hour and preferably within 20 min of the injury. One of three situations can occur:
1. The tooth or teeth and bone have been moved a short distance but are reasonably solid. There is a good chance the teeth have retained a functioning blood supply and will survive. The patient, with encouragement, may be able to bite these teeth the short distance back into the correct relationship.

2. The tooth or teeth are very loose, independent of what has happened to the bone structure. If the blood supply has been severed—and there is no way of being sure other than speculating on the looseness—then root treatment will be required soon, and splinting will be required now. Reduce all malpositioned teeth, supporting the teeth by wire and/ or glass ionomer cement splinting if you can, and consider evacuation to specialist care.

3. The tooth or teeth are mobile because their roots have fractured. Remove the fractured teeth and leave the roots to be removed by an expert; consider evacuation to specialist care.

n all cases, prescribe antibiotics and NSAIDs.

Teeth lying loose in fractured bone can usually be moved quite easily. Typically, frontal trauma will cause upper incisors to be displaced towards he palate. The patient will be unable to close their mouth properly as the ront teeth will collide. To reduce the cross-bite:

- Numb the affected area with LA if possible.
- Place yourself above and behind the patient.
- Exert slow but very firm forward pressure from your thumb placed on the palatal aspect of the pre-maxilla and palatal aspect of the loose teeth.
- Maintain the firm pressure until the bone and teeth move back into a normal occlusion.
- The patient will tell you when they can bite together naturally.
- You now need to consider whether the reduction will hold naturally or will need a splint of some type (⊃ p. 379) (Fig. 11.6).
- With the best intentions and correct technique, most intrusive luxation will still have a poor prognosis and extrusive/lateral luxation may only have a 50% dental survival rate.

Dental avulsion

he repositioning and fixation by splinting of any totally avulsed tooth is etting into the realms of dental heroics, especially in the field. Consider:

- Are there bigger clinical issues that take precedence for triage?
- If the patient requires or may require airway intubation then do not reposition.
- If a dental root is fractured, do not attempt to reimplant the tooth.

eimplantation stands a worthwhile chance of success if the accident oc- urred within the past hour. Teeth displaced for more than an hour are uch less likely to recover.

Transport of tooth

- Tooth and root must both be clean.
- The best way to carry the tooth after avulsion is in the mouth—saliva is reasonably isotonic, is at body temperature, and the presence of friendly commensal bacteria and protein matrices will help control the risk of infection. Otherwise use milk.
- Never handle the avulsed tooth by touching the root, always handle using the enamel.

Repositioning technique

ee Fig. 11.6.)

Consider whether you have the necessary equipment and whether the teeth adjacent to the avulsed tooth are solid enough to act as supports. There are several ways to help support a tooth:
- Ideally the affected tooth is splinted to the teeth on either side of it by means of a wire stuck on with white filling material. One or more teeth on each side are used to splint the damaged tooth.
- An alternative is a temporary measure—use cyanoacrylic tissue adhesive, with supplementary paper sutures (e.g. Steri-Strips™) if needed.
- Thermoplastic beads, melted in hot water to a pliable plastic, can be moulded around the teeth and used as a temporary splint.
- Alternative temporary splints can be made of Blu Tack®, aluminium foil, or Compeed®.

Process
- Numb the affected area with LA if practical.
- Create a splint by cutting a suitable metallic material (e.g. the nasal clip from a face mask or wire cut from a paperclip) to an appropriate length. Its length could equate to one or more teeth on either side of the recently avulsed tooth. If several teeth are loose, use a longer splint Bend the splint to a suitable curve.
- Remove the displaced tooth from the saliva.
- Rinse the tooth briefly in sterile water, to remove visible debris. Avoid touching root surface or taking >10 s.
- Normal haemostasis in a tooth socket occurs within 8 min. This blood clot will have to be removed with a sterile instrument to make way for the root to be firmly embedded full depth into the socket. As the clot is removed, gently stimulate the periodontium to bleed again as this will improve the chances of healing.
- Re-insert tooth to its full depth within its socket so that it stands level height with the adjacent teeth.
- Hold in position until haemostasis is re-achieved—typically 4–8 min. This can be achieved by patient biting on a wooden spatula (or ice cream stick).
- Attach the splint wire to the displaced tooth and its neighbours ideally using glass ionomer cement or composite resin white filling materials. Cavit™ will not work.
- If you have no dental filling materials, an alternative but weaker bond can be made by sticking the tooth to its neighbours with cyanoacrylate tissue adhesive.
- Prescribe NSAIDs and a broad-spectrum antibiotic for at least 5 days (◑ Antibiotics, p. 370).
- Ensure diligent oral hygiene after every meal even though it will be difficult and uncomfortable. No biting on the tooth for a week.

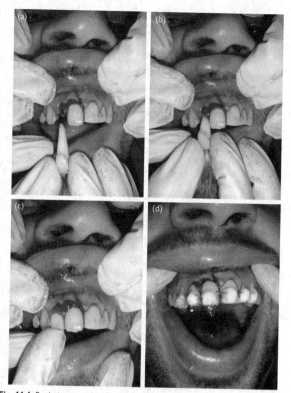

Fig. 11.6 Replacing an avulsed tooth. Adapted from O'Connor, Isobel, and Urdanq, Michael, *Handbook of Surgical Cross-Cover* (2008), with permission from Oxford University Press.

Dental local anaesthesia

Being able to apply dental LA accurately is a great advantage in many circumstances:

- To enable treatment for painful teeth.
- To permit practical procedures such as dental fillings and fixing dislodged crowns.
- To enable reduction of fractures and splinting.
- To permit dental extractions.
- To give immediate relief from intractable chronic toothache and allow sleep.

Almost all dental LA drugs are premixed in 1.8–2.2 mL cartridges and include a vasoconstrictor that prolongs their duration of action. A well-placed mandibular block will give pain relief for up to 3 h. Check that the syringes you take match the cartridges! The needle gauge will be either 27 or 30, with a length of at least 3 cm.

LAs commonly used in dentistry include:

- *Lignospan®*: 2% lidocaine with 1:80,000 adrenaline (epinephrine) injection solution, used for regional blocks and infiltration. Onset 2–3 min, duration 60 min.
- *Citanest®*: 3% prilocaine hydrochloride with 0.03 IU/mL octapressin (adrenaline free), used for regional blocks and infiltration. Onset 2–3 min, duration 60 min. Used on patients where lidocaine or adrenaline are contraindicated.

Metal dental syringes are slightly heavier but much simpler to use; disposable syringes are an alternative, although less easy to handle. If dental LA cartridges are unavailable, other LAs may be used but take care to avoid toxicity from excessive volumes, or accidental intravascular injection.

Three main methods are used to numb the mouth cavity:

- Regional nerve blockade.
- Local infiltration.
- Intraligamentary injections.

Different techniques are used to block the upper and lower jaws.

Blocking teeth in the lower jaw

A well-placed inferior dental nerve block will provide pain relief along the whole mandible for up to 3 h and, owing to the density of mandibular bone, is the only effective way to numb the area from the second pre-molar to the third molar teeth at the back of the lower jaw (35–38 and 45–48). Infiltration techniques in which LA is injected into the gum margins below the roots of mandibular teeth can be used for the front teeth as far back as the first premolar (31–34 and 41–44 ➲ Fig. 11.1, p. 360).

Regional nerve blockade (inferior dental block)

The mandibular branch of the trigeminal nerve runs down the inside of the mandible and supplies sensation to all the teeth in that half of the mandible. Halfway down the vertical part of the bone the nerve divides into two, with the inferior dental nerve entering a canal within the mandible, and the long buccal nerve continuing outside the bone (Fig. 11.7). You must place the LA drug just above the canal entrance (the lingula):

1. Ask the patient to open their mouth as wide as possible. Stand in such a way that you can see clearly where you need to inject. If right-handed, position yourself behind the patient to anaesthetize the lower left quadrant, and in front of the patient for the lower right. If left-handed, reverse these instructions (Fig. 11.8).

2. Aim the needle point at the mucous membrane on the medial border of the mandibular ramus. The target is the intersection of a horizontal line (the height of injection) with a vertical line (the anteroposterior plane).
   • Height of injection: put your thumb beside the last molar tooth. Feel the jaw bone as it turns upwards to the head. Rest your thumb in the depression there, the coronoid notch. It is about 6–10 mm above the occlusal table of the mandibular teeth. That defines your horizontal plane.
   • Anteroposterior plane: lies just lateral to the pterygomandibular raphe—defined as the muscular pillar that connects the lower third molar region to the upper third molar region.

3. Approach the area of injection from the opposite premolar region using your non-dominant hand to retract the patient's buccal soft tissue (your thumb is in the coronoid notch of the mandible and index finger on the posterior border of extraoral mandible). See Fig. 11.9.

4. Angle the needle backwards towards and just above the lingula.
   • The needle should touch bone at 3 cm deep; a shallower touch indicates you are in front of the lingula and in the wrong place. If you don't touch bone once 3 cm of needle have been inserted, your needle point is probably deep to the lingula. See Fig. 11.10.

5. Aspirate the syringe to check you are not in a blood vessel. Reposition if necessary. Deliver a full cartridge of LA slowly over 1 min.

6. Continue to inject slowly on withdrawing from injection site to anaesthetize the lingual branch.

7. Inject another cartridge into the coronoid notch region of the mandible in the mucous membrane distal and buccal to most distal molar to perform a long buccal nerve block.

8. Wait for a clear indication of anaesthetic effect to the midline of the mandible and full length on the side of the tongue. This may take seconds or minutes. Work should commence only when there is a clear sensory distinction across the mandibular midline.

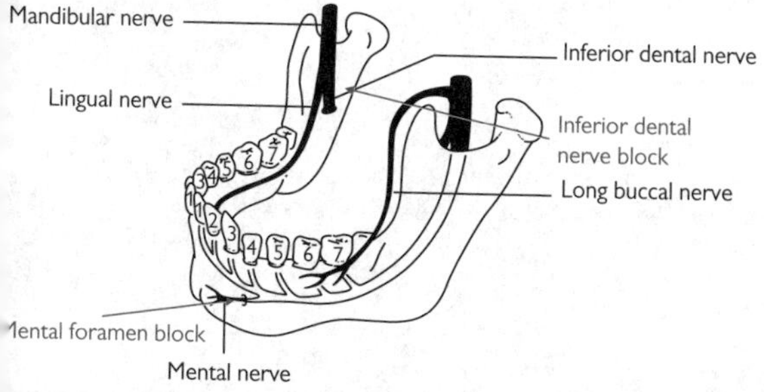

Fig. 11.7 Lower jaw anatomy and nerve supply.

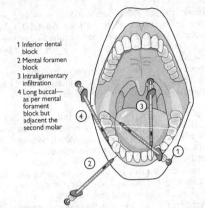

1 Inferior dental block
2 Mental foramen block
3 Intraligamentary infiltration
4 Long buccal— as per mental foramen block but adjacent the second molar

Fig. 11.8 Mandibular dental blocks.

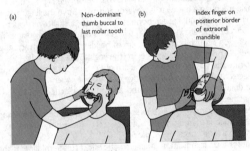

(a) Non-dominant thumb buccal to last molar tooth

(b) Index finger on posterior border of extraoral mandible

Fig. 11.9 Inferior dental block—position.

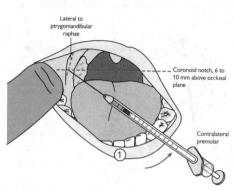

Fig. 11.10 Inferior dental block—landmarks.

Blocking teeth in the upper jaw

Maxillary alveolar bone is significantly less dense than mandibular bone. This facilitates rapid penetration of anaesthetic around teeth, allowing anaesthesia by simple infiltration injection into the buccal/labial sulcus adjacent to the affected tooth or teeth. The anaesthetic is placed slightly above the apices of the dental roots. (Figs. 11.11–11.13). Most roots can be considered to be about 20 mm from the occlusal surface of the tooth. Upper canines can occasionally be up to 30 mm long.

- Insert the needle into the buccal or labial sulcus and slightly angled towards the facial bone structure.
- Place the needle tip above the level of the root apices.
- Deliver a full cartridge.

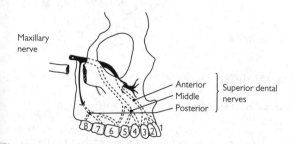

Fig. 11.11 Maxillary division of trigeminal nerve.

- When delivering LA for incisors and canines, place the needle slowly and inject very slowly. The tissue is tight and the nerve plexus considerable. This is a very painful injection if rushed.
- If attempting an extraction, a very small infiltration must also be placed on the palatal side of the tooth until visible blanching is seen.

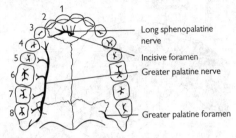

Long sphenopalatine nerve

Incisive foramen

Greater palatine nerve

Greater palatine foramen

Fig. 11.12 Palatal nerves.

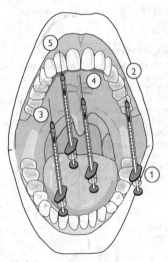

1 Buccal/labial infiltration
2 As per no 1 but go to the level of the lower orbit—suborbital block
3 Sphenopalatine block
4 Incisal papilla block
5 Intraligamentary infiltration

Fig. 11.13 Maxillary dental nerve blocks.

Buccal/labial intraligamentary injection

(See Fig. 11.14.)

The objective is to place a small amount of LA directly into the periodontal ligament with a very fine gauge and preferably short needle. The intention is to use the vascularity of the narrow periodontal attachment between root and bone to deliver the LA to the apical nerve fibres. This approach, when in practised hands, is sufficient even for extractions. In the context of fieldwork, it should be considered as an adjunct to block or infiltration to gain profound LA. It is particularly useful when attempting to anaesthetize an area that has been heavily infected or luxated. When infection has been present for some time, there is often buffering of the LA which reduces its effectiveness. The intraligamentary approach is sufficiently direct to overcome this problem.

- Select a fine short needle.
- Place the needle tip between tooth and bone by sliding the needle along the tooth surface and inserting 2–3 mm into the periodontal ligament.
- The needle will always follow the long axis of the root of the tooth.
- Using considerable pressure, place about 0.2 mL of LA.
- Repeat for each root—molars have three roots, premolars can be considered to have two, while incisors and canines have one root.

If, after your best efforts, there is inadequate anaesthesia, then repeat all the stages—LA block, infiltration, and intraligamentary injection—again and again. Six or seven full cartridges might be considered a maximum dose for a fit young person. Then wait patiently for the anaesthetic to take effect.

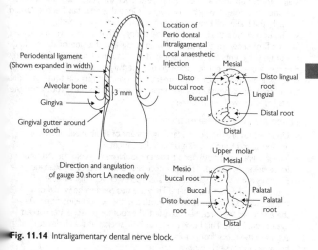

Fig. 11.14 Intraligamentary dental nerve block.

What if you don't have a dental syringe?

A standard needle and syringe can be used. Blocks towards the back of the mouth will be more difficult than if a dental needle is available. The standard short 25 G orange needle is too short for an inferior alveolar block but a blue 23 G needle, while more painful and slightly more likely to cause direct damage to the nerve, should enable you to place LA close to the nerves.

Extractions

It is essential that you seek appropriate training before departure if intending to offer extractions as a treatment. Do not attempt dental extractions for the first time in the wilderness.

There are situations where a successful extraction might mean otherwise inevitable evacuation is avoided. Reasons for attempting an extraction in a remote location might be as follows:

- Loose teeth either side of a bone fracture.
- A tooth fractured with the live neurovascular pulp exposed—you will see bleeding from the pulp.
- Intractable toothache which does not respond to antibiotics and NSAIDs, and when the patient is a long distance from expert help.

Principles of tooth extraction

Establish effective LA (➔ Dental local anaesthesia, p. 380) before attempting dental extraction.

During the extraction process you need to both expand and enlarge the socket, thus separating the tooth from its ligament, to the point where it is free to come out. If you have ever tried to remove a tent stake that has been driven deeply into the ground, you know that you can't just pull the stake straight up. Instead, you first have to rock the stake back and forth so to widen the hole in which it is lodged. Once the hole has been enlarged enough, the stake will come out easily. It's the same with teeth.

The bone inside the jaw is relatively spongy. That means, when a dentist applies firm pressure to a tooth (forcing it against the side of the socket), the bone will compress. After repeated application of pressure from many different angles, the entire socket gradually enlarges, and eventually enough space will be created for the ligament to separate from the tooth and the tooth itself can emerge. You are aiming to extract both the tooth and the roots together, without fracturing.

Procedure for dental extraction

- Upper teeth are extracted standing in front of the patient; lower teeth are extracted from a stance behind the patient.
- The jaw and head both need to be immobilized to avoid the extraction force being dissipated. This may necessitate the help of a colleague.
- *Elevators* are levers that look like small screwdrivers. If available it is a good idea to start with them. They are designed to be wedged in the ligament space between the tooth and the surrounding bone. As the elevators are forced and twisted, the tooth is pressed and rocked against the bone. This helps to expand the socket. It also helps to separate the tooth from its ligament. As this work continues, the tooth becomes increasingly mobile.
- You can then switch to *forceps*, which should grip the tooth as far below the gum level as possible—force is never applied in any other way than very precisely along the long axis of the roots. If instead, force is applied tangentially to the root long axis it is likely that the tooth will break leaving its roots in the jaw.

- Never pull a tooth. A great deal of very focused force is slowly and relentlessly applied up or down the long axis of the root. The tooth is then pushed and slowly rotated out using a figure-of-eight movement and following the line of least resistance, which can be increasingly sensed.
- Once the tooth has been removed, check carefully to ensure that all roots have been removed intact.
- Using your finger each side of the dental socket, squeeze the soft tissue together, thereby also reducing fractured and displaced socket bone.

Extraction aftercare

Once the tooth is out, the bone and periosteum remain exposed and painful infections can develop that last up to 14 days. You should aim for complete coverage of the bone by a solid blood clot. Place a small firm pack of cotton wool roll or absorbent paper over the socket and tell the patient to bite hard onto this. Continual pressure will almost always achieve haemostasis within 5 min. The pack should then be rotated out to avoid lifting the clot. Antibiotics are not usually necessary unless the socket was already badly infected, painkillers (➋ p. 369) may be needed for the first 12 h. Sometimes the wound requires suturing using 3/0 black silk or Vicryl sutures on a small curved needle. Black silk sutures can be removed after a minimum of 5 days. Though uncomfortable, thorough oral hygiene is essential.

Advice to patient after extractions

The objective is to avoid further bleeding, returning for further treatment, and infection. The patient should be advised as follows:
- No hot drinks, alcohol, or heavy lifting for 12 h.
- Use a pressure pack to control any subsequent bleeding. Bite hard on this for at least 15 min and then gently rotate out.
- Avoid vigorous rinsing and spitting for 24 h.
- Advise the patient not to smoke for at least 24 h.
- Red-coloured saliva is not a bleed and can be expected; a bleed looks like a substantial mass of 'jelly-like' blood clot.
- Mouth washing and gentle brushing after every meal is essential to limit the food source of damaging bacteria that cause infection.

Final consideration

The extraction of a tooth is irreversible and may have significant long-term health, aesthetic, and financial consequences. Subsequent treatment may be complex, unpredictable, and expensive. So avoid dental extractions if at all possible.

Medevac for dental problems

Indications

Evacuating casualties can be difficult, expensive, and may be dangerous. It is not a decision to be taken lightly, but certain circumstances demand it as a precaution. Medevac is indicated for:

- Possibility of airway obstruction from trauma or infection.
- Uncontrolled pain causing severe distress.
- Uncontrollable oral or nasal bleeding.
- Facial fractures (◑ Fractured facial bones p. 328).
- Sepsis not responding to antibiotics.
- Post-septal extension of maxillary abscess (i.e. into eye socket).
- Suspected mediastinal extension of parapharyngeal infection.
- Suspected Ludwig's angina.

Dental pain may result from trauma or infection; individual ability to cope with dental pain varies considerably. Irreversible pulpitis is agony and the only definitive treatment is removal of the pulp (root canal therapy), or extraction of the tooth itself. Pulpal pain is little affected by painkillers, wakes the patient at night, and recedes only after 1–2 weeks when the pulp finally becomes necrotic. The pain may then cease for several days because of pulpal necrosis, but if infection develops and extends through the apical foramen the tooth becomes exquisitely sensitive to pressure and percussion. This secondary pain is now of inflammatory origin and can be controlled with antibiotics and NSAIDs.

Ludwig's angina

An acute severe diffuse infective cellulitis typically caused by dental or tonsillar infection that spreads rapidly, bilaterally affecting submandibular, sublingual, and submental spaces. Airway compromise is likely. It may be associated with:

- Painful neck swelling.
- Dental pain.
- Dysphagia.
- Dyspnoea.
- Fever and malaise.
- Protruding or elevated tongue.
- 'Hot potato' voice.
- When advanced: oedema and induration of the anterior neck often with cellulitis.

Management

Evacuate the patient as an emergency to a base hospital. Definitive dental and supportive medical therapies are required urgently as the condition rapidly becomes life-threatening.

- Airway management is of paramount importance. If swelling compromises the airway, give supplementary oxygen whenever possible. In medical facilities high-flow oxygen or Heliox mixtures are desirable, but such treatments are impractical in the field.

- Initially IV amoxicillin and metronidazole, or co-amoxiclav (➲ p. 370), definitive treatment requires specialist microbiological input.
- Consider IV corticosteroids if swelling compromises airway. At the time of writing there is no clear evidence for or against their use in the pre-hospital setting. Individual case reports from hospitals suggest that steroids may reduce the risk of airway obstruction and need for intubation, provided that they are used in association with high-dose antibiotics, but the literature is very limited.
- Extract the tooth or drain the tonsillar abscess as soon as possible. The patient will require operative drainage under general anaesthetic by a specialist team if pus is present or intubation on an intensive care unit with medical management if no focal sepsis.

Medical supplies

Suggestions for suitable equipment for field dentistry are given elsewhere (➲ p. 864). The quantity and extent of this equipment will depend upon the size and duration of the expedition and accessibility of dental help in the local area.

Resources

Atraumatic restorative techniques (ARTs): internet search recommended for variety of helpful websites.
Dental Directory: ℘ www.dental-directory.co.uk
Dental Trauma Guide: ℘ www.dentaltraumaguide.org
Scottish Dental Clinical Effectiveness Programme: ℘ www.sdcep.org.uk

Further reading

Andreasen JO, Andreasen FM. *Essentials of Traumatic Injuries to the Teeth*, 2nd ed. Oxford: Blackwell; 2010.
Wray D, Stonehouse D, Lee D, Clark AJE. *Textbook of General and Oral Surgery*. Edinburgh: Churchill Livingstone; 2003.

Chapter 12

Chest

Chapter editor
Jon Dallimore

Contributors
Nicholas Chilvers
Jonathan Ferguson
Julian Thompson
Annabel H. Nickol (1st and 2nd editions)
Andrew Thurgood (1st and 2nd editions)
David A. Warrell (1st and 2nd editions)

Introduction

The chest is the region of the body between the neck and the abdomen, along with its internal organs and other contents. It is mostly protected and supported by the ribcage, spine, and shoulder girdle. The chest contains:
• Heart and major blood vessels.
• Trachea, lungs, and pleura.
• Diaphragm.
• Oesophagus.

Also protected by the lower ribs are:
• Liver and gallbladder.
• Spleen.
• Upper part of stomach.
• Upper poles of kidneys.

Injuries to the ribcage may damage the underlying organs. Chest pain may originate from thoracic or intra-abdominal organs.

Chest pain

Chest pain is a relatively common complaint on expeditions. Most chest pain is musculoskeletal in origin and may be treated by analgesics and, where possible, rest. However, severe central chest pains and pleuritic pain made worse by deep inspiration may signal more serious conditions that might require urgent treatment or evacuation. Diagnosis of these conditions is covered on p. 260 and the algorithm in Fig. 8.10, p. 261.

Myocardial infarction

An MI or 'heart attack' results from blockage of a coronary artery that distributes blood to the heart muscle. Although this may, especially in those with diabetes, go almost unnoticed, the symptoms and signs are usually obvious. The vascular obstruction can result in failure of the heart to pump properly (cardiac failure) or the development of irregular heart rhythms that can be fatal. MI is more likely to develop in middle- and older-aged people with known risk factors such as previous angina, heart attack, diabetes, high BP, raised cholesterol levels, or history of smoking but can occasionally affect young adults.

Symptoms

- Central, crushing retrosternal pain.
- Pain may radiate to shoulder and neck.
- May mimic severe heartburn, but discomfort not relieved by antacids, and may be helped by GTN or oxygen.
- Palpitations.
- Breathlessness.
- Nausea.

Differential diagnosis

Causes of chest pain are discussed in ➲ Differential diagnosis, p. 261.

Signs

Patient is anxious, distressed, and often pale, cold, and clammy.

Monitoring

If facilities are available, monitor BP and pulse (by palpation or oximeter). Portable fully automated defibrillators (AEDs) are becoming cheaper and more widely available; they are located in many transport terminals and large stores. Apply electrode pads and listen to instructions. AEDs are unlikely to contribute to outcome when parties are travelling alone in remote areas, but medics associated with major endurance sporting challenges and those supporting groups of elderly travellers should consider whether having an AED available would be appropriate if support helicopters or land transport could facilitate rapid transfer to tertiary care.

In the wilderness, options are limited:

- Give supplementary oxygen if available.
- Give aspirin 300 mg if no contraindication.
- Obtain IV access.
- Give analgesia—opiates are valuable both for treating pain and relieving breathlessness. Consider use of GTN as spray or sublingual tablets.
- Inform rescue services of possible diagnosis; in remote areas many paramedics are able to administer thrombolytic ('clot-busting') drugs.
- Evacuate as soon as possible to tertiary care hospital.

Rib fractures

Isolated rib fractures are not dangerous in themselves but are extremely painful. The pain will probably impede further participation in the expedition as sleep will be disturbed and carrying a rucksack very painful. Morbidity correlates with the degree of injury to underlying structures.

The pain from a fractured rib can severely restrict breathing and can predispose to reduced movement and infection of the underlying lung. Basic treatment involves managing the pain and monitoring for more serious injuries. When there is evidence of significant injury or multiple rib fractures (as opposed to just chest wall bruising), the patient should be evacuated to definitive medical care as soon as possible.

Signs and symptoms

Suspect a simple fractured rib if any of the following are present:
- Chest wall bruising or swelling.
- Tenderness over a specific bony point on the chest.
- Sharp pain when coughing or breathing in deeply.
- Rarely, deformity of the chest.

Treatment
- Assess ABCD (➜ p. 198).
- Reassure, and try to keep the patient calm to reduce effort of breathing.
- Deal with the identified rib fractures once you are sure there are no other life-threatening problems such as an obstructed airway or bleeding.
- If the patient is compromised with possible underlying organ damage, administer oxygen if it is available.
- Administer ibuprofen 400–800 mg stat (with food) then 400 mg four times daily for pain. If additional pain relief is required, add paracetamol 1 g four times daily.
- Encourage exercises that facilitate lung expansion and prevent pooling of secretions, which could cause chest infection:
  - Breathe deeply in an upright position at least every hour.
  - Mobilize frequently as tolerated, aiming for at least 30 min in total of exercise per day.
  - Cough frequently.
  - Support the chest during these manoeuvres by applying gentle pressure over the injured area with a small cushion or a rolled and taped towel.

Serious chest injuries including multiple fractures

Look for signs that may suggest injury to the lungs:
- Rapid and shallow breathing.
- Elevated HR.
- Increased difficulty breathing.
- Coughing up blood.

The mechanism of injury may indicate serious underlying chest injury; fo instance, fall from height, crushing forces, or rapid deceleration injuries i a RTC.

- Place one hand on each side of the injured person's chest and observe the way the chest moves with inhalations. If one side of the chest rises during inhalation while the other falls, at least two adjacent ribs have been broken in two or more places on the falling side of the chest—a 'flail chest.' This is best visualized by looking from the patient's feet along the patient's body towards their head, meanwhile watching the chest rise and fall—the 'sunset view' of the chest wall.
- Place the casualty into a position that is comfortable for them but also allows easy access to both sides of the chest for ongoing assessment and, if required, intervention.
- If stable, sitting the patient up can often improve their breathing.
- Continually monitor for breathing difficulties and consider the possibility of a tension pneumothorax (● p. 210).
- Evacuate immediately to a hospital for even the simplest of rib fractures. The injured person must be flown or carried out if there are any signs of respiratory distress (consider chest drain if risk of pneumothorax) but may be able to walk out with simple fractures.
- Morphine or other analgesics: the pain of the fractures may hinder breathing sufficiently for it to be necessary to administer small amounts of an opiate painkiller to enable more effective breathing. If available, morphine should be administered, ideally IV. Give 1 mg doses every 1–2 min and monitor closely the effects of the analgesia while taking care to avoid respiratory depression. Any dose of opiate can cause nausea, reduced awareness, and confusion, and can make evacuation more difficult.
- Strapping should not be used as, by restricting expansion, it encourages infection. Counter-pressure over the affected area before coughing may help reduce pain, as described above.

Tips and warnings

- Examine the patient's left and right, front, back, and sides for hidden rib injuries.
- Serious rib fractures will very likely have underlying lung bruising (contusions) accompanying the condition and this injured lung reduces lung function. Although often initially stable, these patients must be monitored closely for deterioration and evacuated as soon as possible.
- Older persons are more prone to rib fractures than younger adults owing to weaker bones.
- Position of the fractured rib in the thorax helps identify potential injury to specific underlying organs. Fracture of the lower ribs is usually associated with injury to abdominal organs rather than to lung tissue.
- Fracture of the left lower ribs is associated with splenic injuries.
- Fracture of the right lower ribs is associated with liver injuries.
- Fracture of the floating ribs (ribs 11, 12) is often associated with kidney injuries.
- Assessment should therefore also include examination of the abdomen and monitoring for relevant signs and symptoms.

Spontaneous pneumothorax

A pneumothorax is a collection of air or gas within the pleural cavity (see also ➔ Pneumothorax, p. 210). Spontaneous pneumothoraces occur more commonly in tall, thin, young males, in conditions where airway pressure is increased (such as during SCUBA diving or during acute asthma attacks) and in people with underlying lung conditions such as chronic obstructive pulmonary disease (COPD).

Symptoms and signs

- Shortness of breath.
- Increased RR.
- Lateral sharp chest pain on breathing in.
- If massive: reduced chest movement and air entry on the affected side.
- Hyper-resonant to percussion on the affected side (can be subtle).

Treatment

- Oxygen, if available.
- Pain relief.
- All patients with a pneumothorax require hospital assessment.
- Regularly reassess the patient for the development of a tension pneumothorax.
- Unless the patient is compromised with increasing breathless and signs of shock or must be evacuated by aircraft, avoid insertion of needles or drains into the chest. Note that the pneumothorax will expand with gain in altitude. See also Heimlich valve and chest drainage (➔ p. 211).
- If immediate decompression is required then this can be achieved with a large-bore cannula or needle, simple decompression adjuncts such as the Air Release System® (ARS®), more complex devices such as the ThoraQuik® or Rocket Pleural Vent™ or thoracostomy and traditional chest drain. Relevant training for these devices should be undertaken before performing these procedures.

Chest infections

Respiratory infections are a common medical problem on expeditions. Chest infections often follow an initial URTI. Coryza, sore throat, tonsillitis, quinsy, and sinusitis, are covered in ➲ Chapter 10.

Acute lower respiratory tract infections (LRTIs) can be caused by a wide range of pathogens. Those likely to affect members of expeditions include:

- Viruses:
  - Influenza viruses.
  - Measles—rare if immunized.
  - Respiratory syncytial virus.
  - COVID, MERS, and other coronaviruses.
- Bacteria:
  - *Streptococcus pneumoniae*.
  - *Haemophilus influenzae*.
  - *Mycoplasma pneumoniae*.
  - *Chlamydia* spp.
  - Q fever—*Coxiella burnetii*.
  - *Legionella*.
  - *Mycobacterium tuberculosis*.
- Fungi:
  - *Pneumocystis (carinii) jirovecii*.
  - *Histoplasma capsulatum*.
  - *Cryptococcus neoformans*.

Immunocompromise and underlying chronic illness determines special vulnerabilities, e.g. to *P. jirovecii* pneumonia in HIV-positive patients, to *Strep. pneumoniae* in alcoholics, and to a range of pathogens in smokers and those with chronic bronchitis.

Transmission is usually by inhaled aerosol from infected people, including asymptomatic carriers and, in the case of some pathogens, from animals (e.g. *Chlamydia psittaci*) and from the environment (e.g. Q fever, fungal pneumonias). Crowded and enclosed areas such as buses, hostels, travel terminals, aircraft, and underground trains increase the risk of transmission. Wearing of face masks and social distancing have become standard during the COVID-19 pandemic as means of reducing viral transmission.

Symptoms

- Cough with or without sputum production developing after URTI or influenza.
- Fever (sometimes with rigors).
- Breathlessness.
- Wheeze.
- Exacerbation of underlying asthma.
- Pleuritic chest pain.
- Myalgia.
- Other 'flu-like' symptoms.

Examination

- Temperature.
- Cold sores.
- Upper respiratory tract—catarrh and post-nasal drip from sinusitis.
- Rashes (e.g. measles, *Mycoplasma pneumoniae*).
- Auscultation:
  - Added sounds.
  - Reduced air entry.
  - Pleural friction rub.
- Pleural effusion—suggested by reduced air entry and dullness on percussion.

Lower lobe pneumonia can cause misleading upper abdominal tenderness. Look at the sputum! Yellowish, greenish purulent sputum, sometimes 'rusty' or streaked with frank blood, is a typical sign of infection.

Complications include respiratory failure, sepsis, haematogenous spread such as meningitis and infective endocarditis, pericarditis and pericardial effusion, pneumothorax, pneumomediastinum, empyema, and lung abscess.

Diagnosis

In the field, diagnosis is made on clinical grounds and can be confirmed later by chest radiography/CT, sputum microscopy, blood cultures, leucocyte count, serology, and antigen detection in urine (*Legionella*).

Antibiotic treatment

Clinically convincing acute respiratory infection during an expedition in a remote location deserves immediate antibiotic treatment.

If classic pneumococcal lobar pneumonia is suspected, treatment with oral amoxicillin 500 mg three times a day for 7 days (clarithromycin 500 mg twice a day for penicillin-hypersensitive patients). In severe cases, or if oral treatment is impossible, start ceftriaxone IV or IM, 2 g once a day.

For broader-spectrum empirical treatment (also covering *H. influenzae*, *Legionella* spp., *Mycoplasma*, *Chlamydia*, Q fever), use oral doxycycline 100 mg twice each day, or clarithromycin 500 mg twice daily.

Supportive treatment

Cough suppressants (cough mixture, linctus) have limited effect but can be soothing, especially if sleep is disturbed. Codeine or pholcodine linctus or sedating antihistamines such as chlorphenamine may be helpful provided they do not cause respiratory depression.

Asthma exacerbations should be treated with bronchodilators and, in some cases, a short course of oral corticosteroid (Asthma, p. 402).

Severe pleuritic pain warrants strong analgesia. Start with NSAIDs and add regular paracetamol.

Oxygen (if available, e.g. on climbing or diving expeditions) may relieve severe dyspnoea and hypoxaemia. Affected mountaineers should be moved to lower altitudes as a LRTI may predispose to/or be hard to distinguish from HAPE. Oxygen may be needed for air evacuation of patients with acute respiratory infections.

Prevention

Vaccination against *Strep. pneumoniae* and influenza viruses (➥ p. 35) is appropriate if a high risk of exposure is anticipated; this depends on the expedition's programme, the influenza epidemic status, and the medical history of the expedition member.

Provision of antiviral treatment or prophylaxis (ribavirin for respiratory syncytial virus; amantadine for influenza A, zanamivir or oseltamivir for influenza B) would be appropriate only in exceptional circumstances such as unavoidable travel to an area where an epidemic was predicted.

Asthma

Asthma affects 10–15% of the population and is becoming increasingly common, especially in the young. It is characterized by recurrent episodes of shortness of breath, cough, and wheeze caused by reversible airway obstruction, often worse in the night and mornings, and sometimes associated with an atopic history with eczema, hayfever or rhinitis. In 2017 1484 people died from asthma in the UK, with most deaths occurring outside hospital. Risk factors for death include chronic severe disease, inadequate medical treatment, and those with adverse behavioural and psychosocial factors.

Asthma on expeditions

A person with well-controlled asthma should be able to participate in most expeditions, although any obstructive airways condition except very mild asthma is a contraindication to diving (→ p. 767). Remote environments restrict the treatment available for severe asthma attacks. Severe or unstable asthma may preclude an individual from joining a trip to a remote area (see → Pre-existing disease, p. 52). Any new environment can alter symptoms either worsening or improving the condition. Emphasis must be placed on the prevention of asthma attacks, and plans made for early evacuation if symptoms develop.

Asthmatics should be identified at the pre-expedition planning stage and efforts made to optimize the condition, assess medication requirements, formulate a plan for an exacerbation, and, if necessary, modify medevac plans. If space permits, they should bring a peak flow meter. For normal peak flow values, see Fig. 12.1 (you can download an asthma action plan from www.asthma.org.uk).

During an expedition, an asthmatic person should note symptoms and, if worsening, record their peak flows regularly. This will identify exacerbations early and prompt the use of pre-arranged medication increases. Spares of essential medications should be packed separately from regular supplies and a bronchodilator included in the expedition medical kit.

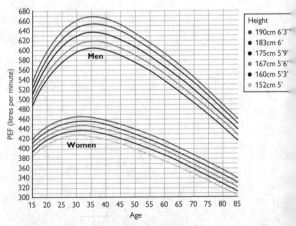

Fig. 12.1 Peak expiratory flow (PEF)—normal values, EU scale.

Altitude

Symptoms may improve in some people at altitude owing to reduced airway resistance and fewer allergens. In others, cold air and exercise may exacerbate it. Peak flow meters may marginally under-read at altitude because of reduced air density.

Prevention of acute asthma attacks

Provoking factors

Cold air, exercise, emotion, allergens (house dust mite, pollen, animal fur), infection, drugs (aspirin, NSAIDs, beta-blockers).

Ensure:

- Medication compliance and good inhaler technique.
- Written asthma action plan for deteriorating symptoms and reduced peak expiratory flow.
- Appropriate preventative treatment, e.g. with an inhaled steroid ± long-acting beta agonist, montelukast tablets.

Avoid

- Triggering allergens.
- Smoking.

Symptoms

- Shortness of breath, wheeze, cough, and sputum, especially at night or first thing in the morning.

Signs

- Rapid RR.
- Widespread, polyphonic wheeze.
- Hyperinflated and hyper-resonant chest.
- Diminished air entry.
- Severe life-threatening asthma may have no wheeze and a silent chest.

Assess and record

- Peak expiratory flow rate (see Fig. 12.1 for normal values).
- Symptoms and response to self-treatment.
- HR and RR.
- Oxygen saturation (by pulse oximetry if available). See ➜ Fig. 8.7, p. 254.

Severity of acute asthma—SIGN British guideline 2019

Moderate asthma

- Peak expiratory flow 50–75% best or predicted.
- Speech normal.
- RR <25 breaths/min.
- Pulse <110 beats/min.
- Saturations >92%.

Acute severe asthma

- Peak expiratory flow 33–50% best or predicted.
- Unable to complete sentences.
- RR >25 breaths/min.
- Pulse >110 beats/min.
- Saturations >92%.

Life-threatening asthma
- Peak expiratory flow <33% best or predicted.
- Silent chest, cyanosis, or feeble respiratory effort.
- Bradycardia, dysrhythmia, or hypotension.
- Exhaustion, confusion, or coma.
- SpO_2 <92% (caution: saturation may be maintained in severe disease, particularly when supplementary oxygen administered).

Differential diagnosis
- Upper airway obstruction.
- Pneumonia/LRTI.
- Hyperventilation.
- Anaphylaxis (➔ p. 256).
- Pulmonary oedema.
- Congestive cardiac failure.
- HAPE (➔ p. 695).
- COPD.
- Pneumothorax.

Immediate management
- High-flow oxygen for severe attacks (if available).
- B_2 bronchodilator—e.g. salbutamol.
- 4–6 puffs repeated at intervals of 10–20 min (via spacer or nebulizer if available).
- Hydrocortisone 100–200 mg IV.
- Prednisolone 40–50 mg orally.

If there is acute severe asthma, life-threatening asthma, or a poor response to initial treatment, medevac to hospital.

If moderate asthma and good response to initial treatment (reduced symptoms, RR, and HR, peak expiratory flow >75%), consider increasing usual treatment and continue oral prednisolone 40 mg for 5 days. Evacuate if any further deterioration.

Life-threatening asthma in a remote environment
- Death results from cardiac arrest secondary to hypoxia and acidosis. Give high-flow oxygen if available.
- Consider tension pneumothorax (➔ p. 211).
- Epinephrine (adrenaline) 1:1000 solution 0.5 mL IM may be used to relieve bronchospasm if peri-arrest. An adrenaline auto-injector can be used.
- In a resource-poor environment, a paper bag or empty water bottle can be used as an improvised spacer for inhalers. Caffeine, a methylxanthine in coffee, tea, and chocolate, is a bronchodilator. Caffeine is readily absorbed from the buccal mucosa and instant coffee granules may be administered in this way.

Reference
The British Thoracic Society publishes comprehensive guidelines for the assessment and management of asthma: ℘ https://www.sign.ac.uk/media/1383/qrg158.pdf

Chapter 13

Abdomen

Chapter editor
Chris Imray

Contributors
Tim Campbell-Smith
Jane Wilson-Howarth
Sarah R. Anderson (1st and 2nd editions)

Acute abdominal pain

Mild or moderate abdominal pain or colic is relatively common when exposed to new cultures, diets, and living conditions overseas. Acute abdominal pain can cause great anxiety in a wilderness setting. Often the first thought is of appendicitis; indeed, historically, acute appendicitis gave rise to such concern that doctors venturing to the Antarctic with the British Antarctic Survey were offered a prophylactic appendicectomy, and the Australian Antarctic programme still offers this on a voluntary basis. In reality, acute surgical emergencies account for only 0.7% of medical problems during an expedition.[1] Abdominal pain tends to be more common in women, although abdominal pain in men is more likely to require surgical intervention.

When a patient in a remote location presents with acute abdominal pain, the specific diagnosis is less important than the need to decide whether their condition justifies evacuation. Assess on the basis of history, general condition, and examine the abdomen looking for abdominal tenderness and guarding or localization (see 'Examination' later in this topic). Peritoneal inflammation suggests a significant surgical problem; resuscitate, provide pain relief, and, if appropriate, give antibiotics while evacuation is considered and or organized.

Managing acute abdominal pain

History
- Age and sex, including menstrual history in women.
- Pain: its onset, location, character, severity, and radiation together with any exacerbating or relieving factors.
- Associated symptoms: vomiting, diarrhoea, fever, melaena, frequency, volume, and any pain on passing urine, etc.
- Past medical, surgical, or gynaecological history.

Examination
- General condition including conscious level. Is the patient in pain or distressed, lying still or rolling in pain?
- Flushed or cold, and clammy?
- Cardiovascular system—look for signs of shock—tachycardia, and hypotension.
- Dehydration—assess capillary return, strength of pulse, lips/mucous membranes, skin turgor, and the colour and quantity of urine.
- Respiratory system—cyanosis, RR, and breath sounds (lower lobe pneumonia can cause abdominal pain).
- Abdomen—note any scars, distension, or tenderness. Is there guarding, a reflex contraction of the abdominal wall muscles on palpation? If present:
  - Is the guarding localized or generalized?
  - Is the guarding distractible (i.e. could it be voluntary)?

1 Anderson SR, Johnson CJH. Expedition health and safety: a risk assessment. *J R Soc Med* 2000;93:557–562. https://doi.org/10.1177/014107680009301102

- Is there 'rebound tenderness'?
- 'Percussion tenderness' is more sensitive than rebound. Percuss gently over the abdomen and watch the patient's face for signs of discomfort.
- Listen for bowel sounds (useful if obstructed).
- Signs of chronic liver disease, such as enlarged liver, plethora, spider naevi.
- Rectal and vaginal examinations are rarely of value in evaluating abdominal pain on an expedition.

Always document: consultation findings, differential diagnoses, and your management plan. Begin a chart of regular observations which should include pulse rate, BP, RR, temperature, fluid balance, and arterial saturations if a pulse oximeter is available (→ Fig. 8.7, p. 254). The chart trends can provide valuable information about whether the patient is improving or deteriorating and may also be medico-legally important.

Management of patient with an acute abdomen

Care will depend upon available equipment, facilities, and skills:
- Good analgesia. Patient may require opiates, if possible IV, particularly if vomiting. Opiates will not mask the signs of peritonitis.
- Antiemetic such as cyclizine.
- Oxygen, if available.
- IV fluid resuscitation.
- Nasogastric tube if evidence of obstruction or persistent vomiting. This can be difficult in the wilderness with risk of misplacement, and uncertainty about position. It should only be attempted in a patient who is fully conscious.
- Consider urinary catheterization if equipment and skills available. Continued urine output gives a good indication of adequate fluid resuscitation. Not appropriate if patient is to make an ambulatory evacuation.
- Consider diabetic ketoacidosis, check blood glucose.
- Start broad-spectrum antibiotics, i.e. co-amoxiclav or metronidazole and a cephalosporin. Check for allergies.
- If available prescribe PPI or H_2 blocker—now available as sublingual preparations.

If the patient has signs of shock or peritonitis, evacuate urgently.

Upper abdominal pain

Common causes of severe upper abdominal pain include:
- Peptic ulcer disease.
- Indigestion and GORD.
- Gallstone disease.

Peptic ulcer disease

Risk factors for peptic ulcer disease include smoking, stress, NSAIDs, steroids, and alcohol. Presentation can be insidious: initially with aching upper abdominal discomfort and irritability, but possibly leading on to severe abdominal pain, bleeding, or perforation.

Symptoms
- Gnawing upper abdominal pain.
- Occurs 1–4 h after eating.
- Relieved by bland foods such as milk and yoghurts which buffer stomach acids.

Examination findings
- Often none, sometimes mild epigastric tenderness.

Management
- Avoid risk factors such as smoking and alcohol—especially binge drinking, and spicy foods.
- Antacids.
- H_2 antagonists—ranitidine or famotidine.
- PPI—e.g. omeprazole, lansoprazole, etc.

Indigestion and gastro-oesophageal reflux disease

Symptoms
- Upper abdominal fullness.
- Belching.
- Regurgitation of food or stomach acid.
- 'Heartburn'—usually worse after eating and on lying.
- Improves about an hour or so later.
- If intermittent, think of gallstones.

Examination findings
- Usually none, patient commonly overweight.

Management
- Avoid smoking.
- Eat smaller meals.
- Antacids and PPI.
- Try low-fat meals (to minimize gallstone colic).

Gallstone disease

Gallstones are common. They are more common with obesity, increasing age, and in women, but patients are presenting younger and younger with them even in their late teens and early 20s. Gallstones are often asymptomatic, but once symptoms develop, they are commonly recurrent. Conditions caused by gallstones range from intolerance to fatty foods to life-threatening acute pancreatitis and cholangitis. If a prospective member of an expedition to a remote area has recurrent symptomatic gallstones, serious consideration should be given to having a laparoscopic cholecystectomy well in advance of departure. See Table 13.1.

Table 13.1 Differential diagnosis of gallstone disease

	Symptoms	Signs	Management
Biliary colic	Colicky or constant RUQ or epigastric pain Radiates to shoulders, some nausea or vomiting	Mild RUQ tenderness No guarding	Analgesia, rest Avoid fatty foods
Acute cholecystitis	RUQ pain, radiates to right shoulder tip Pain worse on deep breath Nausea and vomiting	RUQ tenderness, localized guarding, fever	Analgesia, antibiotics: such as IV ceftriaxone 2 g od plus: Metronidazole 500 mg tds, or Piperacillin/ tazobactam 4 g qds, or Ticarcillin/ clavulanate 4 g qds. *Evacuate*
Acute pancreatitis	Epigastric or central abdominal pain, radiates through to the back Nausea and vomiting	Central or generalized tenderness and guarding Hypotension and tachycardia, sometimes fever, occasional jaundice	Analgesia, fluid resuscitation, catheter, omeprazole 40 mg and antibiotics* (to treat other possible causes) *Evacuate*
Ascending cholangitis	RUQ or epigastric pain, rigors	RUQ tenderness, fever, jaundice	Analgesia, resuscitation, broad-spectrum antibiotics (co-amoxiclav 375–625 mg tds or ciprofloxacin 500– 750 mg bd) *Evacuate*

(Continued)

Table 13.1   (Contd.)

	Symptoms	Signs	Management
Obstructive jaundice	May be associated with any biliary condition, itching	Jaundice Pale stools Dark urine	Analgesia if required, broad-spectrum antibiotics (if febrile), i.e. co-amoxiclav 375–625 mg tds or ciprofloxacin 500–750 mg bd *Evacuate*

bd, twice daily; od, once daily; qds, four times daily; RUQ, right upper quadrant; tds, three times daily.

*Acute pancreatitis: antibiotics are not usually part of the acute treatment of mild pancreatitis, but without the ability to confirm the diagnosis, treat as for a perforated viscus.

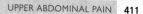

Lower abdominal pain

Differential diagnosis of lower abdominal pain includes:
- Acute appendicitis.
- Acute diverticulitis.
- GI obstruction.
- Hernias.
- Obstetric and gynaecological problems.

Acute appendicitis

Acute appendicitis is a feared condition to diagnose in the wilderness, and often a cause of anxiety for those going even before the expedition leaves home shores. Appendicitis can occur at any age but is more common in the young. The diagnosis, even in hospital, is primarily a clinical one, but there is increasing use of imaging (CT and ultrasound scanning). Clinical review after an interval can be very useful. *A patient diagnosed with signs of peritonitis requires urgent evacuation.*

Classically, pain begins as a vague central visceral aching. Over 12–48 h the pain migrates to settle in the right iliac fossa (RIF), becoming a more focal sharp pain, made worse by moving, coughing, or straining. Anorexia is common, and the most reliable associated symptom. Nausea is common, vomiting less so. Occasionally, patients have diarrhoea (pelvic appendicitis) but this is not profuse as in gastroenteritis. With children, watch them walk; if they limp or bend forward slightly, holding the RIF this is an indicator of significant pain. Get patients to jump up and down; if they can do this without pain, it is unlikely that they have peritoneal inflammation. Examine them supine. Before even laying a hand, ask them to blow their abdomen up like a balloon and then suck it in. Percuss with your fingers gently throughout the abdomen while distracting them with chat, i.e. about the expedition. Both of these manoeuvres will hurt if there is peritonitis.

Symptoms
- Central abdominal pain that migrates to the RIF or solely RIF pain.
- Worse on movement, coughing.
- Occasional loin pain (retrocaecal appendicitis).
- Anorexia (very common).
- Nausea and occasional vomiting.
- Occasional loose stool.

Clinical findings
- Flushed, feverish, tachycardic.
- Furred tongue, fetor oris.
- Tenderness in the RIF with guarding.
- Percussion tenderness (as above).
- Pain in RIF when palpating the *left* iliac fossa (LIF) (Rovsing's sign).
- Pain in RIF when extending or rotating the right hip (psoas irritation).

Management
- Analgesia.
- IV fluids (if available; if not, sip clear fluids slowly).
- Start broad-spectrum antibiotics if >6 h from definitive medical care: cephalosporin and metronidazole, or co-amoxiclav 1.2 g three times daily (preferably IV, or PR metronidazole 1 g twice daily. Check for penicillin allergy).
- Evacuate urgently to base hospital if possible.

If evacuation is impossible, or is likely to be significantly delayed (e.g. over-wintering in polar regions, off-shore sailing, prolonged bad weather), then conservative management may need to be considered. When access to safe hospital care is not possible, this approach offers a long-recognized alternative approach and consists of the first three steps: pain-relief, fluids, and ideally IV antibiotics, listed at the start of this section. Meta analyses on the non-operative management of uncomplicated appendicitis with antibiotics was associated with fewer complications, better pain control, and shorter sick leave, but overall had inferior efficacy because of the high rate of recurrence in comparison with appendicectomy.[2,3] Approximately 27% require surgery within 1 year.

Differential diagnoses
- Gastroenteritis.
- Mesenteric adenitis (children).
- Mittelschmerz (mid-cycle ovulation pain).
- Ovarian cyst (➲ p. 434–435).
- Ectopic pregnancy (➲ p. 416–417, 434–435).
- Pelvic inflammatory disease (PID; ➲ p. 417).
- Endometriosis.
- Sigmoid diverticulitis (➲ p. 413–414).
- Crohn's ileitis or ulcerative colitis (usually has preceding GI history; loose stools/pain) (➲ p. 56–57).
- Typhoid (➲ p. 424–425, 510).
- Torsion of testis (➲ p. 430).

If in doubt, treat as acute appendicitis and evacuate.

Acute diverticulitis

Diverticulosis is common in developed countries and increases with age (unusual in those <40 years), affecting 5% of 50-year-olds and up to 70% of 85-year-olds. Acute diverticulitis is caused by a microscopic perforation of a diverticulum with a resultant surrounding inflammation. This may cause mild systemic upset, which resolves with antibiotics, or can progress to a pericolic abscess, or free perforation and generalized peritonitis.

2 Mason RJ, Moazzez A, Sohn H, et al. Meta-analysis of randomized trials comparing antibiotic therapy with appendectomy for acute uncomplicated (no abscess or phlegmon) appendicitis. *Surg Infect (Larchmt)*. 2012;13(2):74–84. https://doi.org/10.1089/sur.2011.058

3 Di Saverio S, Podda M, De Simone B, et al. Diagnosis and treatment of acute appendicitis: 2020 update of the WSES Jerusalem guidelines. *World J Emerg Surg*. 2020;15:27. https://doi.org/10.1186/s13017-020-00306-3

Symptoms
- Lethargy and anorexia.
- Lower abdominal pain, often localizing to LIF.
- Diarrhoea.
- Nausea, vomiting (occasional).

Examination findings
- Pyrexia.
- Tachycardia.
- Tenderness in the LIF ± localized guarding.

Management
- Analgesia.
- Rest.
- Fluid diet for 24–48 h.
- Broad-spectrum antibiotics.
- If signs of peritonitis are present, *evacuate*.

Gastrointestinal obstruction

GI obstruction is a serious condition requiring fluid resuscitation, evacuation, and treatment of the underlying cause. The commonest causes in the UK are adhesional obstruction from previous surgery and strangulated hernias. In the wilderness, making a specific diagnosis is less important than recognizing the problem and initiating fluid resuscitation and evacuation. Fluid losses into the obstructed bowel can be considerable (several litres) and patients can rapidly become dehydrated and shocked.

Symptoms
- Abdominal pain (initially colicky then constant).
- Vomiting, may be bile-stained (early with proximal obstructions).
- Absolute constipation (no passage of flatus or faeces).
- Abdominal distension.
- Painful swelling (i.e. groin, umbilicus).

Examination findings
- Dehydration (mucous membranes, skin turgor).
- Tachycardia.
- Hypotension.
- Poor urine output.
- Distended abdomen.
- High-pitched (tinkling) bowel sounds.
- Hernia (inguinal, femoral, or umbilical are most common).
- Evidence of abdominal scars.
- Abdominal tenderness (a very worrying sign of possible perforation).

Management
- Analgesia.
- Rest.
- IV fluids.
- Nasogastric tube if vomiting.
- Consider urinary catheter.
- Correct fluid and electrolyte imbalances.
- *Evacuate*.

Hernias

Hernias should be diagnosed and repaired well before departure. The commonest sites are groin and umbilical. Most hernias will cause discomfort and limit activity, particularly heavy work. If strangulation occurs, urgent evacuation is required. If a hernia becomes apparent on an expedition but is not strangulated, it does not require evacuation. Limit the patient to light activities which are comfortable to perform and avoid lifting (particularly rucksacks). Improvised trusses are of little or no value.

Symptoms

- Swelling in the groin, around the umbilicus, or associated with scars.
- Discomfort.
- Incarceration: irreducible but not tender ('imprisoned').
- With strangulation:
  - Lump that 'won't go down'.
  - Constant severe pain.
  - Vomiting.
  - Distension.
  - Absolute constipation.

Examination findings

- Uncomplicated hernia:
  - Soft, non-tender swelling.
  - *Groin* (may extend into the scrotum).
  - *Umbilical*.
  - *Femoral* (higher risk of strangulation).
  - *Incisional* (associated with previous surgery).
  - Reducible.
- Strangulated hernia:
  - Tender swelling.
  - Hot, erythematous overlying skin.
  - Signs of obstruction.

Management—if uncomplicated

- Avoid heavy lifting/work/carrying bags.
- Simple pain relief.

Management—if strangulated

- If presentation is early, it is worth attempting to reduce the hernia using a combination of analgesia, bed rest, mild Trendelenberg position, and gentle, firm pressure along the axis of the sac (this is obliquely for an indirect inguinal hernia). Even if it reduces, the patient should be evacuated for full assessment and urgent repair.
- As for GI obstruction: *evacuate*.
- IV antibiotics.

Acute ovarian conditions

Acute ovarian problems include haemorrhage, rupture of a cyst, and torsion. All these conditions are associated with pain. The time of pain can help distinguish the various diagnoses. Mittelschmerz pain is mid-cycle from ovulatory bleeding and is usually unilateral. Pain from a ruptured ovarian cyst can occur at any time in the cycle. There may be signs of peritonism or the patient may complain of shoulder tip pain if blood tracks up to the diaphragm. Torsion presents as sudden onset of unilateral severe lower abdominal pain and may be accompanied by nausea, vomiting, and diarrhoea. In hospital, these conditions are often thought initially to be appendicitis and are diagnosed at laparoscopy or appendicectomy. These patients, therefore, will commonly be evacuated.

Symptoms
- Lower abdominal/pelvic pain.
- Nausea, vomiting, diarrhoea.
- Shoulder tip pain.
- Examination findings:
  - Low iliac fossa tenderness and guarding.
  - Tachycardia but apyrexial.

Management
- Check pregnancy test if possible.
- Analgesia.
- Rest.
- Reassurance with Mittelschmerz.
- If there are signs of peritonism: *evacuate*.

Ectopic pregnancy

All women of childbearing age with abdominal pain should have a pregnancy test performed. The site and onset of pain depends on site of implantation. Pain is usually preceded by a period of amenorrhoea for 6–8 weeks, but patients can still have what appear to be regular periods. Pain is usually unilateral. If there is enough internal bleeding, pain is more generalized or may give shoulder tip pain. Vaginal bleeding is scant or absent and usually dark brown and appears a few hours after the onset of the pain. Risk factors include previous ectopic, progesterone-only pill, *in vitro* fertilization, IUCDs, and previous pelvic sepsis, i.e. appendicitis or PID. Once suspected *evacuate urgently*, as these patients can deteriorate very rapidly.

Symptoms
- Amenorrhoea and breast tenderness. 'When was your last period which was normal for you?'
- Previous period atypical.
- Lower abdominal pain.
- Shoulder tip pain.
- Vaginal bleeding (scant and often dark) in <50%.

Examination findings
- Lower abdominal tenderness ± guarding.
- Signs of shock.
- Vaginal bleeding.
- Positive pregnancy test.

Management
- Analgesia.
- Resuscitate.
- IV fluids.
- *Evacuate*.

Pelvic inflammatory disease

PID is almost always caused by ascending infection from the genital tract. It is acquired as a sexually transmitted infection (STI). The condition used to be commonly gonococcal; now, up to half of cases are due to *Chlamydia*. Infection usually involves the endometrium and both fallopian tubes. Risk factors include age at first sexual intercourse, number of partners, and presence of an IUCD. The severity is variable, and it may be mistaken for appendicitis.

Symptoms
- Pelvic pain.
- Fever.
- Deep pelvic pain on intercourse.
- Dysmenorrhoea.
- GI upset.

Examination findings
- Pyrexia.
- Signs of systemic sepsis (● p. 250).
- Bilateral iliac fossa tenderness and guarding.
- Cervical tenderness on vaginal examination.
- Speculum examination may reveal pus from the cervical os.
- Occasional pelvic mass.

Management
- Analgesia.
- Combination antibiotics.
- Ceftriaxone 500 mg IM once plus metronidazole 400 mg twice daily and doxycycline 100 mg twice daily for 14 days.
- *Evacuate if there are signs of systemic sepsis.*

Gastrointestinal bleeding

Upper gastrointestinal bleeding

GI bleeding is a serious problem that even in hospital is associated with significant mortality. Haematemesis (vomit of fresh blood), coffee ground vomiting, or the passage of melaena (black, sticky, offensive smelling, tar-like stools) are true emergencies requiring prompt treatment and evacuation. Even if bleeding stops and the patient appears better, they should still be evacuated urgently, as re-bleeding is common and carries a high mortality.

If the expedition is in a very remote location, attempts to carry-out a casualty who is actively bleeding are not recommended. Evacuate by mechanical transport (vehicle, boat, or helicopter) if possible.

Following prolonged, vigorous vomiting, minor streaks of blood may be seen in the vomitus. These are caused by small tears in the oesophageal mucosa (Mallory–Weiss tear) and, unlike true haematemesis, are not serious.

History
- There is often a history of peptic ulcer disease.
- NSAID use, smoking, alcohol.

Symptoms
- Haematemesis.
- 'Coffee grounds' vomiting.
- Passage of melaena or dark blood PR.

Examination findings
- Pale.
- Tachycardia.
- Hypotension (a very ominous sign in the young).
- Confusion and agitation.
- Decreased urine output.
- Concentrated urine.
- Melaena on examining stool or on digital rectal examination.
- Fresh blood per rectum; if from a bleeding peptic ulcer, indicates rapid, life-threatening haemorrhage.

Management
- Rest.
- Place the patient supine with legs elevated.
- IV access and fluids if available.
- PPI or H_2 blockers (sublingual preparations are available, e.g. Fastab®).
- Avoid NSAIDs, smoking, alcohol, caffeine.
- Catheterize if possible or measure urine output.
- *Evacuate.*

Lower gastrointestinal (rectal) bleeding

The passage of small amounts of fresh blood PR following defecation is common and is usually due to haemorrhoids (piles). On expeditions, constipation can be a problem, particularly with dehydration, change in diet, and being confined to a tent in a storm.

Causes of lower GI bleeding
- Haemorrhoids.
- Anal fissure.
- Diverticular disease (age generally >60 years when bleeding can be profuse and alarming).

- Acute colitis (stool also contains pus and mucus, usually there is previous history).
- Dysentery (diarrhoea and fever) (➔ p. 420–425).

Haemorrhoids (piles)

Haemorrhoids are caused by abnormal swelling of anorectal tissue, which may become traumatized and bleed during defecation. Piles occasionally prolapse, strangulate, or thrombose. This requires pain relief and ice packs and topical analgesia to reduce the swelling, and laxatives to soften the stools.

Symptoms

- Fresh red rectal bleeding following bowel motion (often painless and only seen on toilet paper).
- Perianal itching.
- Prolapsing piles (very painful, if thrombosed).

Examination findings

- Unless prolapsed, haemorrhoids are impalpable.

Management

- Soften stools—high-fibre diet and good hydration, ± laxatives.
- Avoid straining at stool.
- Proctosedyl® or Xyloproct® ointment or suppositories can help.
- Use water or baby wipes instead of toilet paper.
- If thrombosed, use analgesia and ice packs (not directly on the skin).

Perianal haematoma

A painful small purple swelling at the anal margin, usually developing after straining at stool. Perianal haematoma usually settles with conservative treatment, but this takes time (2–3 weeks usually).

Management

- Anaesthetize the area with a topical LA or ice.
- Soften stools.

Anal fissure

An acute, painful condition where there is a tear/split in the skin lining the anus. It is usually precipitated by an episode of constipation.

Symptoms

- Severe anal pain on defecation.
- Small amount of fresh, red, rectal bleeding.

Examination findings

- Soft, non-tender abdomen.
- Rectal examination is usually impossible due to pain and sphincter spasm.

Management

- Soften the stools—high-fibre diet, good hydration, laxative (e.g. lactulose).
- Pain relief—LA gel (Proctosedyl® or Xyloproct® ointment).
- Relax the sphincter spasm with Rectogesic® (0.4% GTN ointment—shelf-life 3 months). Use a pea-size amount rubbed on to the perianal skin twice daily for 6 weeks. Can cause headache and postural hypotension.

Diarrhoea and vomiting

Acute diarrhoea is defined as three unformed stools in 24 h plus one of the following symptoms—nausea, vomiting, abdominal pain/cramps, faecal urgency, or moderate–severe flatulence. *Dysentery* is acute diarrhoea with blood mixed in the motions, and there is often fever.

Diarrhoeal illness causes more than a billion episodes of illness a year worldwide, and in the low-income settings is a major cause of death in the young and elderly. Up to a third of medical problems encountered on an expedition are related to GI 'upset' or diarrhoea. The conditions may arise as a result of:

• Changes in diet.
• Changes in water supplies.
• Altered schedules.
• Stress of foreign travel.
• Infections.

If diarrhoea has continued for <3 weeks, then infection is the most likely cause.

The commonest route of infection is faecal–oral, caused by poor hygiene or contaminated water (Table 13.2). Scrupulous hygiene precautions (➔ p. 100–101, 742–743) should be maintained throughout the expedition, without this, diarrhoea can be the cause of an expedition failing and/or everyone on it having a miserable time.

History
• Duration.
• Stools: colour, consistency, frequency, blood, or pus.
• Vomiting.
• Fever.
• Abdominal pain.
• Thirst (a late symptom).
• Recent eating and drinking habits.
• Others affected?

Examination
• General condition.
• Signs of dehydration:
  • Reduced volume of concentrated urine.
  • Dry lips and mucous membranes.
  • Reduced skin turgor.
  • Sunken eyes.
  • Raised pulse (late sign).
  • ↓ BP—including postural drop (very late sign).
• Temperature.

Usually diarrhoeal illnesses will settle. Some will require specific treatments but the most important factor in minimizing morbidity and mortality is hydration. Most patients can maintain their hydration with rest and oral rehydration, although occasionally IV fluids are necessary.

Table 13.2 Common causes of diarrhoea

Condition	Diarrhoea no blood	Diarrhoea with blood
No fever	Food poisoning (bacteria or toxins)	Amoebic dysentery
	Traveller's diarrhoea	
	Viruses	
	Giardia	
Fever	*Salmonella*	*Shigella*
		Campylobacter
		Salmonella

General treatment guidelines and rehydration

See Table 13.3.
- Rehydration is fundamental.
- Antibiotics are not first-line treatment for diarrhoea. Most episodes are self-limiting and usually settle within 2 days.
- However, a single dose of azithromycin (1 g) at the onset of diarrhoea (plus plenty of fluids) should shorten the duration.
- Basic treatment is similar regardless of the cause.
  - Rest.
  - Replace fluids, orally if possible, with oral rehydration fluids—frequent sips if vomiting.
  - Aim for good volumes (>0.5–1.0 mL/kg body weight/h) of clear urine.
  - Antiemetics may help (suppositories or buccal prochlorperazine, or IM/IV injection).
  - Paracetamol if febrile or abdominal pain.
  - Avoid dairy products, but don't fast.
  - Avoid loperamide unless absolutely necessary.
  - Loperamide (4 mg initially, then 2 mg after each loose stool) may be useful to limit symptoms if travel is essential or if tent-bound by a storm.
  - IV fluids if unable to manage oral fluids (if IV fluids are required the patient should be evacuated).
  - If diarrhoea persists, it could be protozoal; give metronidazole or tinidazole.

When to seek external medical attention:
- Temperature >40°C or significant fever for >48 h.
- Diarrhoea lasting >4 days.
- Difficulty keeping fluid down.
- Diarrhoea with blood.
- Severe non-colicky abdominal pain (>2 h) not relieved by passing flatus or stool.

Table 13.3 Diagnosis and treatment of diarrhoea and vomiting

Category of Diarrhoea	Organisms	Foods	Incubation	Symptoms	Treatment
Diarrhoea—no blood—no fever	Staph aureus (toxin)	Meat, poultry, dairy produce, particularly, if eaten cold	Usual: 2–4 h Range: 1–7 h	V, AP, (D) short-lived, abrupt Onset	Antibiotics ineffective, as due to toxins
	Bacillus cereus (toxin)	Fried rice, raw or dried foods particularly, if inadequate reheating	Usual: vomiting syndrome 1–6 h Usual: diarrhoea syndrome 6–16 h	V and nausea—lasts <12 h, D (short lived), AP—lasts <24 h	Antibiotics ineffective, as due to toxins
	E.coli (toxin) (known as traveller's diarrhoea)	Faecal contamination of water or food	Usual: 12–48 h	D (watery), AP (cramps) Duration: 2–5 days	Usually self-limiting but single dose of azithromycin 500mg
	Clostridium perfringens	Cooked meat, poultry, particularly, if inadequate re-heating	Usual: 8–12 h Range: 4–24 h	D (watery, often violent), AP, V (rarely)	Supportive only
	Cryptosporidium	Faecal contamination of food or water	Usual: 7–10 days Range: 1–28 days	D (watery), AP, bloating	Self-limiting but severe disease in immunocompromised
	Viral-norovirus, rotavirus	Usually person–person or environmental contamination	Usual: 24–72 h Duration: 1–2 days	Norovirus—projectile vomiting, mild D, AP Rotavirus—watery D, V,	No antibiotics
	Giardia lamblia protozoal infection	Contaminated water, often from mountain streams	Incubation: 7–10 days Duration: 2–6 weeks	D (often pale and persistent) AP (cramps), bloating Flatulence—'eggy burps'	Metronidazole 500 mg tds for 5 days or tinidazole single dose 2 g

Category	Organism	Source	Incubation/Duration	Symptoms	Treatment
Diarrhoea—no blood—FEVER	Salmonella	Undercooked or raw meat, poultry, dairy produce, eggs	Usual: 12–36 h, Range: 6–72 h	D (& blood/mucus) V, AP (cramps), fever. Duration: 2–5 days	Usually self-limiting ciprofloxacin 500 mg bd or cefotaxime if needed
	Cholera	Contaminated water, shellfish, or raw food	Incubation: 1–3 days	D (profuse and watery = 'rice water') Rapid dehydration leading to shock	Fluids +++ (IV) Doxycycline or azithromycin Evacuate
Diarrhoea—BLOOD—no fever	Entamoeba (amoebic dysentery; protozoal infection)	Raw or undercooked food. Waterborne	Incubation: >7 days Duration: until successfully treated	D (bloody/gradual onset), AP (cramps), weight loss	Metronidazole 800 mg tds for 5 days Followed by diloxanide 500 mg tds for 10 days
	E. coli O157	Meat, poultry, dairy produce. Contaminated water	Usual: 3–4 days Range: 1–9 days	D or D with blood, AP (severe), HUS (2–7%)	Antibiotics contraindicated
Diarrhoea—BLOOD—AND FEVER	Shigella	Faecal contamination of water or food	Usual: 24–72 h Range: 1–7 days	D (explosive and bloody), AP (cramps), fever, anorexia	Azithromycin usually
	Campylobacter	Poultry, raw milk, eggs. Contaminated water	Usual: 2–5 days Range: 1–10 days	D (often bloody and profuse), AP (severe cramps) ± fever Duration 2–7 days	Usually self-limiting, clarithromycin or azithromycin or erythromycin

Symptom definitions: AP, abdominal pain; D, diarrhoea; V, vomiting; HUS, haemolytic uraemic syndrome.

Hawker J et al. (2005). Communicable Disease Control Handbook. Oxford: Blackwell.

Prevention of diarrhoeal illness

Prevention is better than treatment of diarrhoeal illness on an expedition which, once present, can spread rapidly through the group, disrupting plans, and at worst putting the group at risk. It is possible to prevent it entirely with education and care.

- Meticulous hand hygiene is essential for all expedition members and cooking staff.
- Ensure that there are facilities to wash hands at the latrine, preferably with soap and water; alcohol gel is less effective.
- Hands must be washed before entering a mess tent. A wash basin (or alcohol gel) at the entrance to the mess tent is a good reminder.
- Boil or sterilize water (◐ p. 108–114) before drinking.
- Avoid ice in drinks.
- Check seals on bottled water.
- Take care with salads, unpeelable fruit, shellfish, and avoid raw or undercooked meat (particularly chicken).
- Carefully clean plates and cooking equipment.

Cholera

Most people ingesting the bacterium *Vibrio cholerae* remain asymptomatic. Infection is through contaminated water. Cholera can reach epidemic proportions where there is malnutrition and sanitation systems have broken down (natural disasters or in war). Profuse watery diarrhoea and rapid dehydration kill. Incubation is 1–3 days.

Symptoms and signs
- Mild diarrhoea initially.
- Profuse watery diarrhoea ('rice water stools').
- Vomiting.
- Prostration.
- Fever.
- Dehydration.
- Signs of shock.

Treatment
- Rest.
- Fluids +++.
- IV fluids.
- Doxycycline used in most countries, or azithromycin in children and in pregnancy.
- Evacuate.

Typhoid

This is a generalized infection, which later in its course can cause diarrhoea. Initially there may be constipation. Incubation is 7–14 days.

Symptoms and signs
- Fever.
- Headache.
- Abdominal pain.
- Rash (50% of cases may have rose spots—2 mm pink papules on torso, which fade with pressure).

- After >7 days:
  - General deterioration.
  - High swinging fever.
  - Low pulse (= relative bradycardia).
- After 20 days:
  - Confusion or encephalitis.
  - Gravely ill.
  - 'Pea soup' diarrhoea.
  - Perforation of the terminal ileum.

Treatment

- Rest.
- Fluids—oral or IV.
- Ceftriaxone IV or azithromycin.
- Evacuate.

Other gastrointestinal problems

These less serious but common problems can, in the wilderness, lead to the sufferer having a miserable time and possibly having to leave the expedition.

Constipation

Normal bowel habit varies enormously, from three stools per day to one stool every 3–4 days. Alterations of bowel habit are common on expeditions, with many people developing diarrhoea (⮕ p. 67, 420–425), but constipation can be equally uncomfortable and inconvenient.

Causes
- Dehydration from exertion.
- High altitude.
- Confinement to a tent during a storm.
- Low-fibre diet.

Symptoms
- Cramping abdominal pains.
- Reduced stool frequency with difficult passage of hard stools.

Examination findings
- Soft abdomen.
- Mild tenderness occasionally.
- May be able to palpate stools in the descending colon—LIF.

Management
Ensure that expedition food includes adequate dietary fibre. Encourage good hydration, aiming for the regular passing of dilute urine. Simple laxatives (macrogol or bisacodyl) may be required if a person is symptomatic but taking laxatives prophylactically is unwise.

Perianal abscess

An acute condition of the anus, presenting with pain and swelling in the perianal skin. It develops over a few days and if caught early may resolve with a course of antibiotics.

Symptoms
- Perianal pain and swelling.
- Fever.
- Chills and rigors.

Examination findings
- Pyrexia.
- Tender, erythematous perianal swelling.

Management
- Antibiotics (co-amoxiclav or erythromycin + metronidazole).
- Analgesia.
- If very remote, some form of drainage will probably be required to enable ambulatory evacuation.
- An abscess generally requires surgical incision and drainage, but some abscesses can also be treated with needle aspiration and antibiotics.
- It is reasonable to attempt to drain the abscess with a large needle through the most fluctuant area.

- LA does not work well in inflamed tissue—try oral analgesia, ice packs, and LA to the more normal-looking skin surrounding the abscess.
- Evacuate for formal drainage.

Pilonidal abscess

An infection most commonly found in the natal cleft, the area over the sacrum between the buttocks. It is caused by infected ingrown hair and can occur in any hair-bearing area. Most common in males aged 15–35 years old.

Symptoms

- Pain and swelling over the sacrum between the buttocks (there may be a previous history of this or even of previous surgery).
- Discharge (from minimal serum to large amounts of pus).

Examination findings

- Swelling in the natal cleft (usually slightly to one side).
- The swelling maybe hot, red, and tender.
- On close inspection of the cleft, tiny black pits may be visible in the midline (pilonidal pits).

Management

- Antibiotics (flucloxacillin, or erythromycin).
- If not settling, drain the abscess under LA:
  - Infiltrate a wide area around the abscess with LA (preferably non-inflamed tissue; LA works better here).
  - Make a longitudinal linear incision off the midline into the most fluctuant part of the abscess.
  - Break down any loculations with a gloved little finger and irrigate with sterile saline.
  - Cover with a dressing.
- If this then fails to settle: *evacuate*.
- If the situation makes draining the abscess inappropriate, *evacuate* for surgical drainage.

Urological problems

Urinary tract infection

A common problem, particularly among women. Symptoms include urinary frequency, a burning sensation during micturition (dysuria), which is maximal as flow stops (terminal dysuria). Fever is rare unless associated with pyelonephritis. *Urethritis* is the term given to a collection of symptoms resulting from inflammation of the urethra, most commonly the result of infection, which may sometimes be associated with a STI (→ p. 417, 536–543).

Examination
- Often clinically normal.
- Blood, leucocytes, nitrites, and protein on urine dipstick.

Treatment
- Increase oral fluids.
- Co-amoxiclav, trimethoprim, or ciprofloxacin.

Pyelonephritis

An infection of one or both kidneys, usually resulting from an ascending infection from the bladder, but more rarely secondary to ureteric obstruction. Differential diagnosis includes possible retro-caecal appendicitis.

Symptoms
- Sudden onset of fever, sweats, rigors.
- Flank and/or back pain.
- Patient feels 'terrible'.
- Dysuria, urinary frequency, and urgency.

Examination findings
- High fever.
- Loin tenderness.
- Blood, leucocytes, nitrites, and protein on urine dipstick.

Treatment
- Ensure good hydration.
- Ciprofloxacin, co-amoxiclav, or a cephalosporin for 10 days.

Indications for evacuation
- Failure to respond to treatment.
- Systemic sepsis (→ p. 250).

Acute urinary retention

An acute, painful inability to void urine despite a desperate need to do so. It almost invariably affects men from middle age onwards. The symptoms are incapacitating and require prompt relief.

Symptoms
- Lower abdominal/suprapubic pain.
- Intense desire to void.
- Dribbling of urine.
- Suprapubic distension.
- History of previous hesitancy, poor stream, and nocturia.

Examination findings
- Distressed patient.
- Distended lower abdomen.
- Palpable bladder, dull to percussion, tender.
- Examination of the prostate may reveal enlargement, but this does not correlate with prostatic symptoms, and does not alter management.

Treatment
- Decompress bladder using a Foley urethral catheter if available. Smaller catheters (12–14 F) may be more difficult to pass than larger ones (16–18 F).
- If unsuccessful, suprapubic needle decompression is required:
  - Aseptic technique using a specialized suprapubic needle.
  - Infiltrate 1% lidocaine two finger breadths above the symphysis pubis.
  - Direct the needle towards the anus while aspirating.
  - Aspirate as much urine as possible.
  - May require repeating but will enable ambulatory evacuation.
- Watch for excessive diuresis, although this situation is more common following chronic urinary obstruction.
- Evacuate.

Renal (ureteric) colic

A collection of symptoms resulting from ureteric obstruction secondary to a kidney stone (calculus).

Symptoms
- Severe unrelieved flank pain that causes patient to writhe around, possibly clutching side of abdomen. Pain radiates around along the course of the ureter into the groin, to the testicle or the labia.
- Nausea and vomiting are common.

Examination findings
- Mild loin tenderness.
- Haematuria often present: on dipstick and occasionally frank.

Treatment
- Pain control:
  - NSAIDs are very effective if no contraindications: diclofenac PR (if vomiting).
  - Additional opiates may be required.
- Forced diuresis is of no benefit but maintain adequate hydration.
- Most calculi pass within a few hours, but some become stuck in the ureter and require surgical intervention.
- Evacuate if anuric, signs of sepsis, or pain uncontrollable.

Acute scrotal pain

Acute scrotal pain with swelling is a true surgical emergency requiring urgent assessment and treatment. Differential diagnosis includes strangulated hernia (➔ p. 415) and testicular torsion, both conditions that must be diagnosed and the patient evacuated.

Testicular torsion

- Any age, commoner near puberty.
- Sudden onset of severe scrotal pain.
- Associated with vomiting.
- Pain on walking.

Examination findings

- Oedematous scrotal skin.
- Discoloured with a blue tinge.
- No relief when elevated (negative Prehn's sign).
- Sometimes there are no physical signs other than pain.

Treatment

Scrotal exploration is inappropriate and unrealistic in the wilderness, but i may be worth attempting manual detorsion:

- Lie the patient supine.
- Elevate the testis. Most commonly the testis has rotated medially (inwards or towards the midline). Non-surgical correction or de-rotation has been described and could be attempted if evacuation is difficult. If successful, relief is swift.

  If unable to untwist:
- Provide strong analgesia and evacuate as quickly as possible. The testis will become non-viable in 4–6 h and the other testis needs to be fixed to prevent recurrence and possible infertility.

Epididymitis

An inflammation or pain in the epididymis (which lies on the superior aspec of the testis). In acute epididymitis the pain is often accompanied by inflammation, redness, swelling, and/or warmth.

- More gradual onset than torsion.
- Associated with fever and dysuria.
- Relieved by gentle elevation.
- Careful palpation reveals a tender, swollen epididymis.
- Often caused by an infection. In sexually active men, *Chlamydia trachomatis* or *Neisseria gonorrhoea* are the most common organisms.
- Treatment is with azithromycin or ciprofloxacin.

Prostatitis

An acute infection of the prostate gland by viral or bacterial pathogen Though uncommon, it can be associated with severe sepsis. Of the ba terial causes, 80% are due to *Escherichia coli*.

Symptoms

- Fever, sweats, rigors.
- Perineal pain.

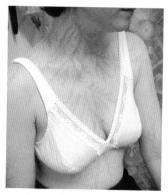

Plate 1 Cutaneous manifestation of phone electrocution from lightning.

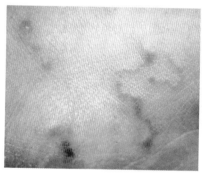

Plate 2 Cutaneous larva migrans.

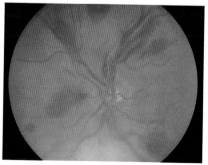

Plate 3 High altitude retinal haemorrhage.

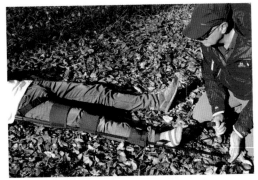

Plate 4 Commercial thigh traction splint for mid-shaft femoral fracture.

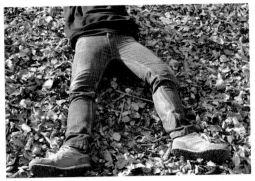

Plate 5 Typical posture seen with pelvic injury—abduction and external rotation of both legs.

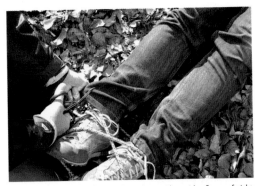

Plate 6 Improvised pelvic binder. Legs brought together with a figure-of-eight binding.

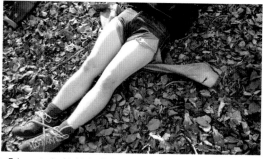

Plate 7 Improvised pelvic binder. Both trouser legs cut to level of greater trochanters.

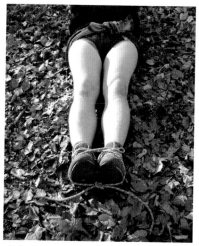

Plate 8 Improvised pelvic binder. Cut trouser legs tied across front of the pelvis .

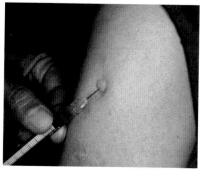

Plate 9 Intradermal injection technique.

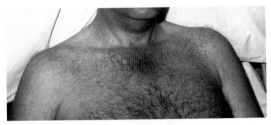

Plate 10 Dengue fever rash in a European traveller.

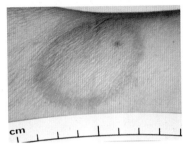

Plate 11 Lyme disease—erythema chronicum migrans.

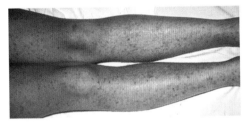

Plate 12 African tick typhus: generalised rash.

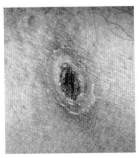

Plate 13 Scrub typhus: eschar and lymphangitic lines.

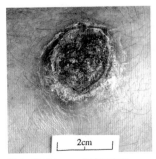

2cm

Plate 14 Cutaneous leishmaniasis.

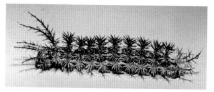

Plate 15 Caterpillar of giant silkworm moth (*Lonomia Achelous-Saturniidae*) 4.4–5.5cm long from northern Brazil. Also occurs in Ecuador, Guyana, and Columbia. Its stinging bristles inject haemorrhagic toxins.

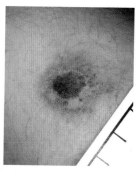

Plate 16 Recluse spider (*Loxosceles*) bite: red-white-and-blue sign 18hr after the bite. Scale in cm.

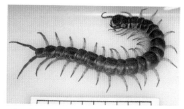

Plate 17 Giant yellow-legged centipede (*Scolopendra dehaani*) from Thailand (scale in cm). May exceed 25cm in length. Extensively distributed in southern Asia and introduced elsewhere.

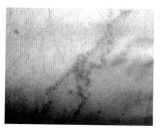

late 18 Portuguese Man o' War (*Physalia*) sting.

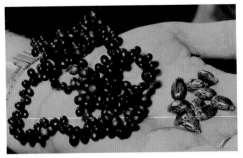

Plate 19 Toxic beans. LEFT—jequirity bean or rosary pea (*Abrus precatorius*) made into jewellery. Its toxin, abrin, is 75 times deadlier than ricin from castor oil bean (*Ricinus communis*) RIGHT.

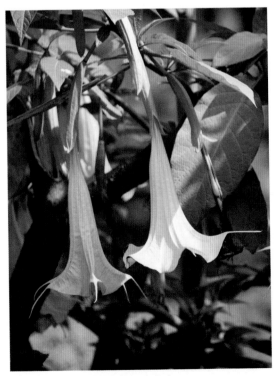

Plate 20 Angel's Trumpet (*Brugmansia sauveolens*).

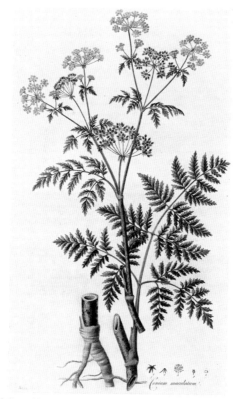

Plate 21 Spotted hemlock (*conium maculatum*). Grows to 1-3.6m tall. There are purple spots on the stem, especially near the base.

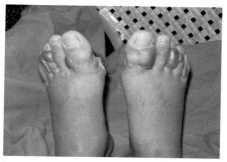

Plate 22 Frostbite—early.

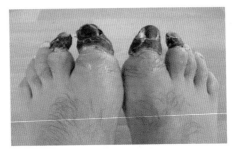

Plate 23 Frostbite—late.

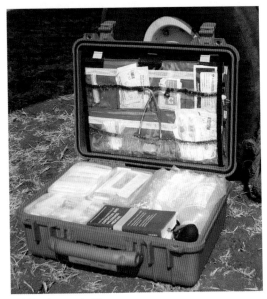

Plate 24 Expedition medical kit.

- Dysuria, frequency, urgency.
- Urinary retention uncommon.

Examination findings
- Pyrexia.
- Tachycardia.
- Boggy, tender prostate on rectal examination.

Treatment
In absence of laboratory findings, treat as a bacterial infection. Prolonged courses of ciprofloxacin or co-amoxiclav may be required.

Indications for evacuation
- Systemic sepsis (p. 250).
- Poor response to treatment.

Gynaecological problems

Gynaecological problems may occur in women who venture into remote regions, even among those who have made careful preparations.

Menstrual issues

On average, a woman loses about 40 mL of blood with each menstruation. Although this amounts to only eight teaspoonfuls over 4 or 5 days, coping with this can be surprisingly challenging. There may be no privacy to change sanitary protection and no easy access to water. Some medical advisers encourage young women to start the combined oral contraceptive pill to control menstruation, but a study of young women on expeditions suggested that this intervention was unhelpful, particularly in light of the fact that DVT risk is highest in the first few months of beginning to take the pill. Furthermore, periods often lighten or even stop during the physical demands of an expedition so periods may become less problematic. Introducing the pill can complicate matters if traveller's diarrhoea interferes with its absorption, thus allowing unpredictable and inconvenient breakthrough bleeding; erratic bleeding is also common in those who have newly started taking the pill as well as occurring in those whose periods are usually regulated by it.

Planning

Ideally, each adventurer will have considered her gynaecological needs long before setting out. One option that is often overlooked is to suppress menstruation by arranging 12-weekly Depo-Provera® injections. This will stop monthly bleeds in most women by the second or third injection. Lack of periods then persist beyond the 3 months between injections, although the woman is, of course, at risk of pregnancy beyond 13 weeks. This contraceptive method has a lot to recommend it among travelling women, not least because, being a progesterone-only method, it barely increases the risk of DVT, whereas women taking the combined oral contraceptive pill have a significantly increased risk; this adds to any risk arising from a long-haul flight, or from ascending to extreme altitude. A progestogen implant (e.g. Nexplanon®) has similar advantages, although it can increase menses in some women; to avoid this troublesome side effect, women can be trialled on desogestrel progestogen-only contraceptive pill. Women who bleed on desogestrel are likely to have unwanted bleeding with an implant. Both Depo-Provera® and implants need to be organized some time—preferably 4–6 months—before departure.

Contraceptive types

- *Depo injections* can cause spotting in the first months but thereafter usually suppress menstruation; does not significantly increase DVT risk.
- *Implants* can cause spotting in the first months but thereafter usually suppress menstruation; does not significantly increase DVT risk.
- *Combined pill* increases DVT risk compared to non-pill-takers by at least three times so these are not good for women ascending to extreme altitude; breakthrough bleeding is often a problem after diarrhoea and in the first 3 months after starting. Clot risk is also greatest in the first few months of starting or restarting the pill.

- *Progestogen-only pill* can cause spotting, especially in the first month or two; does not significantly increase DVT risk.
- *IUCDs* (copper 'coils') tend to increase dysmenorrhoea, the amount and duration of blood flow; they do not increase risk of DVT.
- *Intrauterine contraceptive* hormonal systems (e.g. Mirena™) can cause spotting in the first months but thereafter usually suppress menstruation; does not significantly increase DVT risk.
- *Barrier methods* are always worth packing as a back-up and for safer sex.

Dysmenorrhoea

Pain during the first day or two of a menstrual period is often due to blood clots at the neck of the womb and implies a heavier loss than usual. Those with recurrent and distressing pain on menstruation will be helped by taking a NSAID preparation regularly for a few days starting a day or two before the onset of bleeding. If a woman complains about her periods, ask whether there is any odour or coloured discharge, which suggests a STI (➔ p. 417, 536–543).

Heavy periods in themselves can be debilitating but when combined with a poor diet can lead to anaemia. Anaemia then tends to exacerbate heavy menstrual loss and in turn contributes further to anaemia. Iron tablets can often be purchased cheaply overseas.

Logistics

Plenty of sanitary products need to be packed in waterproof containers (zip-lock bags are ideal) and consideration given to responsible disposal. Burying tampons and sanitary towels in desert environments, for example, can allow retrieval by village dogs or exposure by wind. Some sanitary items compost but some towels contain a lot of plastic and do not. Washable products are available. Alternatively, there are devices to collect blood such as the Mooncup® (➔ http://www.mooncup.co.uk). This is a small soft cup with a stalk, which sits in the vagina and collects menstrual blood. It removes the need to carry disposables where they might be difficult to obtain, but clean hands are required to take it out and empty it. The user also needs somewhere to dispose of the still-liquid blood and access to water to clean the Mooncup® before reinserting it. The solution is perhaps to use both reusable and some conventional disposable supplies.

Vaginal irritation/discharge

Normal vaginal discharge is colourless and its consistency changes with the menstrual cycle. A woman might complain of a *change* in discharge:
  Yellow or green or foul-smelling discharge implies infection (➔ Table 15.2, p. 539).
  Vaginal/vulval thrush (➔ Table 15.2, p. 539); usually causes itch and can be treated with miconazole pessaries (ideally 200 mg on three consecutive nights) or oral fluconazole 150 mg stat. Recurrent thrush may be cleared with oral fluconazole 50 mg daily for a week.
  A fishy odour suggests bacterial vaginosis which is cleared with vaginal clindamycin cream inserted for 7 nights or oral metronidazole.
  Foul-smelling black discharge suggests a forgotten tampon; the discharge settles once the tampon is removed, but clearly there would be a risk of toxic shock syndrome in this case.

- Pregnancy also changes the quality of discharge.
- Finally, mid-cycle bleeding might indicate *Chlamydia* infection and must be investigated or treated with doxycycline 100 mg twice a day for 10 days; make diplomatic enquires about possible contacts.

Urinary tract infections

Ascending infections within the female urinary tract are not uncommon in women of all ages (➜ p. 428–429); they are more frequent in those who are sexually active. Mild dehydration of the kind experienced in warm climates seems to predispose to UTIs. Sufferers need to continue to drink in quantity, and take 3 days of oral broad-spectrum antibiotic (e.g. co-amoxiclav). If antibiotics are not available, substances which alter urinary pH will help; a teaspoonful of baking soda in a large glass of water is ideal; alternatives are ascorbic acid (vitamin C) or cranberry juice.

Abdominal pain

A woman who complains of significant abdominal pain should be examined especially if the pain is on one side; lateralized lower abdomen pain is often gynaecological in origin but left-sided pain may be caused by GI unease, while right-sided pain may be due to appendicitis. A soft abdomen will be reassuring, but vaginal examination is required to exclude problems within the pelvis. An ovarian cyst or fibroid may be palpable during bimanual examination. During vaginal examination, position a finger either side of the cervix so that it can be moved from side to side; if movement of the cervix is painless there is unlikely to be any problem within the pelvis. Equally, pain-free love-making suggests a benign cause for low abdominal pain.

Abdominal pain predominantly in right or left lower quadrants

Causes of lateralized abdominal pain that usually require evacuation:
- Right-sided pain may be appendicitis (➜ p. 406–407, 412–413), ectopic pregnancy, or ovarian torsion (➜ p. 434–435): all are serious.
- Ectopic pregnancy—pain on left or right then often erratic menstrual bleeding sometimes described as 'prune juice' appearance; most often 6–8 weeks (or more) from last period. There may be a tense abdomen (guarding); shock will soon follow, and death is a significant risk.
- Twisted ovarian cyst—management depends upon the severity of the pain and size of the cyst; it needs to be assessed in hospital if the cyst is >5 cm in diameter.
- Hernias (➜ p. 415).

Causes of left- or right-sided abdominal pain that don't usually require evacuation:
- Cystitis—causes malaise and pain on passing urine and sometimes low abdominal pain; blood may be seen in the urine (➜ p. 434–435).
- Ovulation pain—mid-cycle pain located on one side; tender but no guarding; settles in 36–48 h; treat with pain relief. In the longer term, the contraceptive pill will stop the pain.
- Gastroenteritis—often left lower abdominal pain associated with passage of stool or flatus; a bland diet reduces symptoms (➜ p. 434–435).
- Constipation.
- Irritable bowel disease.

- Kidney stones.
- Endometriosis (anti-inflammatory tablets are helpful).
- Salpingitis—pain may be on both sides, but one side is often worse than the other; it may be accompanied by nausea, vomiting, and often fever. Treat with ceftriaxone 500 mg IM plus metronidazole 400 mg three times daily and doxycycline 100 mg twice daily for 14 days. Patients should be investigated on reaching HOME.

Further reading

Wilson-Howarth J (2020). *How to Shit Around the World*. Palo Alto, CA: Travelers Tales.

Wilson-Howarth J. *Staying Healthy on Your Travels: Avoiding Bugs, Bites, Bellyaches and More*. Mount Joy, PA: Fox Chapel; 2020.

Chapter 14

Limbs and back

Chapter editor
Jon Dallimore

Contributors
Jules Blackham
Jon Dallimore
Carey M. McClellan
Harvey Pynn
James Calder (1st edition)
James Watson (1st edition)

Limb injuries

Limb injuries may be life-threatening and an initial ABC evaluation should be performed, with respiratory and circulation status regularly re-evaluated (➲ p. 236–237). Consider the possibility of associated head, spine, chest, abdominal, or pelvic injuries, particularly if the patient is unconscious.

Initial assessment and treatment

- Approach the casualty when safe to do so.
- Ensure that the airway is open, assess the breathing rate, and look for signs of shock (➲ p. 250). Remember the possibility of cervical spine injury with any significant injury above the collarbones, with multiple injuries, and with head injuries resulting in unconsciousness.
- Control any external bleeding with direct pressure. If the bleeding is catastrophic (traumatic amputation), apply a tourniquet (➲ p. 214).
- Consider the use of tranexamic acid, if available.
- Anticipate and treat shock, particularly with thigh fractures. Where appropriate use a suitable traction splint. See ➲ Colour plate 4.
- Remember that painful limb injuries may distract attention from less painful but more significant trunk injuries.
- Expose the affected part and cut off clothing only if absolutely necessary given that in some circumstances clothing, footwear, and waterproofs will be needed to protect the patient from the environment.
- Look for signs of an interrupted blood supply: pale, pulseless, painful, perishingly cold.
- With fractures/dislocations, attempt manipulation early in an attempt to restore distal circulation. Check and document pulses or CRT and sensation before and after any manipulation.
- Look for nerve damage affecting movement and/or sensation.
- Give painkillers.
- Splint fractures using commercially available or improvised materials.
- Transfer to suitable shelter.

Improvised splinting materials on an expedition

- Sleeping mat.
- Paddles.
- Skis or ski poles.
- Slings and karabiners.
- Tree branches.
- Sleeping bags and clothing.
- Ropes.

When applying splints, remember that they must be well padded and must immobilize the joints above and below the injury (Fig. 14.1). Where possible, splint with the limb in the anatomical position.

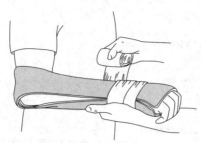

Fig. 14.1 Diagram of a field splint.

Detailed assessment of limb injuries

History

- How did the injury occur? The mechanism is significant; for instance, twisting injuries tend to produce spiral fractures, while a fall onto the heels may produce fractures of the, knees, hips, spine, or base of skull.
- Did the accident occur in a clean or contaminated environment? Consider IV antibiotics for open wounds.
- What time did the injury happen?
- Was the limb trapped or crushed? (Swelling and compartment syndrome are possible; see also ➲ Crush injuries, p. 295, 837–838.)
- When was the last tetanus booster? This is very important for open fractures.
- Is the patient allergic to anything?
- Does the patient take any medication?

Examination

- Look for contamination and foreign bodies.
- Check for pulses and CRT—it is useful to compare with the uninjured side.
- Examine carefully for signs of nerve damage: change in sensation, weakness, or paralysis.
- In a wilderness situation, a fracture should be assumed until further investigations confirm otherwise.

Capillary refill time

To check for capillary refill, press firmly over a fingernail or a bony prominence such as the sternum, forehead, or a malleolus for 5 s to produce blanching. When the pressure is released, the colour should begin to return quickly (in <2 s). Slow filling indicates that the patient is extremely cold, shocked, or that the blood supply to the limb is interrupted.

Fractures

Features of a fracture
- Pain/tenderness.
- Loss of function.
- Swelling/bruising.
- Deformity.
- Crepitus.

Fracture classification
A fracture is a soft tissue injury with an underlying break in the bone. Fractures are closed or open if the skin is broken. They are *comminuted* if there are more than two fragments. Children's bones may bend, leading to *greenstick* fractures. *Complicated* fractures involve damage to blood vessels, nerves, tendons, or organs.

Management of fractures in the field
- Stop bleeding (may require a tourniquet or haemostatic agents; ⊃ p. 214).
- Treat shock.
- Monitor pulse, BP, and urine output. See ⊃ Fig. 8.7, p. 254.
- Give adequate analgesia.
- Remove rings distal to injury on upper limb fractures.
- Take a digital photo of open fractures or significant soft tissue injuries.
- Clean with clean water and cover exposed bone ends, e.g. with saline-soaked gauze, and consider using antibiotics.
- Consider reducing and then immobilize in an appropriate sling/splint.
- Evacuate for X-ray and definitive fracture management.

Dislocations

Dislocations

A dislocation is an injury in which the normal relationships of a joint are disrupted. In some dislocations, the bone end may be forced out of a socket (shoulder, hip, and elbow dislocations); in others, the joint surfaces may simply be displaced (finger dislocations). Fractures, nerve injuries, and blood vessel injuries may also be present with a dislocation.

Management of dislocations in the field

Correction of dislocations can be technically difficult. Attempts to correct the deformity are justified in certain circumstances, particularly in remote areas. If the blood supply to the distal part of the limb is obstructed by a dislocation, reduction must be attempted. Steady, firm traction along the limb's long axis may correct the deformity or at least relieve the obstruction temporarily. Reduction should be attempted as soon as possible because of increasing muscle spasm with delay. After reduction, splint the limb as for a fracture.

Upper limb supports and slings

Collar and cuff

(See Fig. 14.2.) In the wilderness, this may be improvised by passing a long sock around the patient's neck and wrist on the affected side. This can then be secured using a cable tie or piece of cord. This uses the weight of the arm to apply slight traction to the upper arm and should be used for fractures of the humerus.

High arm sling

(See Fig. 14.3.) This is mainly used to reduce hand swelling with hand injuries. Avoid excessive flexion of the elbow as this reduces venous drainage of the forearm.

Broad arm sling

(See Fig. 14.4.) This is commonly used to support the weight of the arm and reduce movement in shoulder and clavicle injuries, dislocations/fractures of the elbow, forearm, and wrist. If used during evacuation of a walking casualty, a swathe around the chest placed on top of the broad arm sling further reduces movement. A broad arm sling may be improvised by pulling the lower edge of a jacket over the arm and then securing with a safety pin.

Arm slings and splints should be worn inside clothing to keep the hand and arm warm.

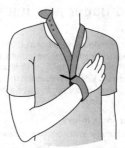

Fig. 14.2 Collar and cuff sling.

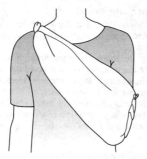

Fig. 14.3 High arm sling.

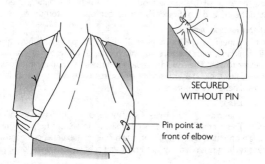

SECURED
WITHOUT PIN

Pin point at
front of elbow

Fig. 14.4 Broad arm sling.

Shoulder and upper arm injuries

Fractured clavicle

This is a common injury following a fall onto the outstretched arm. The clavicle is palpable along its length and there is often obvious deformity and localized tenderness. If the skin over the fracture is tented, then gentle traction with the arm out to the side will reduce the risk of developing an open fracture. Check movement, circulation, and sensation carefully. Treat with analgesia and a broad arm sling.

Acromioclavicular joint injury

Injury to the acromioclavicular joint commonly follows a fall onto the point of the shoulder. There is usually a characteristic step together with point tenderness at the joint. Treat with analgesia and a broad arm sling. X-rays will show the grade of injury, and the most severe may require surgical treatment.

Anterior shoulder dislocation

The shoulder joint may be dislocated after violent injury (particularly forced abduction/external rotation) or after minimal injury in those with previous shoulder dislocations.

Most dislocations are anterior and are straightforward to diagnose as there is 'squaring' of the shoulder on the affected side and reduced movement, particularly abduction and forward flexion. The humeral head may be palpated anteroinferiorly to the glenoid fossa.

After any shoulder injury examine the area carefully for complications such as damage to the axillary nerve (loss of sensation over the insertion of deltoid—the 'regimental badge area'). Axillary nerve damage merits expert assessment.

Reduction of shoulder dislocations

On an expedition, it is reasonable to attempt reduction in the field, preferably with strong analgesia such as methoxyflurane (Penthrox®). Reduce using the external rotation method or Spaso method. A clunk is often seen felt, or heard, and the shoulder's normal contour is restored.

External rotation method

Sit the patient as upright as possible. Hold the patient's elbow next to the trunk and, with the forearm mid-prone, slowly externally rotate the shoulder to 90°. The shoulder usually reduces at this point; if it does not forward flex the upper arm slowly. An assistant may help to manipulate the humeral head into position.

Spaso method

Spaso Miljesic and Anne-Maree Kelly first reported the Spaso technique in 1998.[1] This method is simple, needs minimal force, can be performed by a single operator, and is highly effective even in inexperienced hands. The Spaso technique is relatively atraumatic and countertraction is not required

---

1 Miljesic S, Kelly AM. Reduction of anterior dislocation of the shoulder: the Spaso technique. *Emer Med*. 1998;10:173–175. https://doi.org/10.1111/j.1442-2026.1998.tb00676.x

Lay the patient on their back and give sedation/analgesia as available. Grasp the affected arm around the wrist and slowly lift vertically to 90° shoulder flexion, applying gentle vertical traction as well as external rotation of the shoulder at the elbow. If difficulty is experienced, it may be helpful to use one hand to palpate the head of the humerus and gently push it to assist reduction, while maintaining traction with the other hand.

Stimson's method

Lie the patient prone with the arm hanging down with a 5-kg weight attached to the wrist/hand. This method may take half an hour or more to achieve reduction.

After reduction of any shoulder dislocation

Re-examine for axillary and radial nerve movement/sensation. Check pulses. Rest in a broad arm sling or Polysling®. Evacuate for X-rays and orthopaedic follow-up/physiotherapy. Recurrent dislocations of the shoulder may not require an X-ray and can be managed with a broad arm sling and early mobilization.

Posterior dislocation of the shoulder

This injury is rare and may follow electric shock or convulsions. It is easy to miss. It results from force applied to the anterior shoulder. The shoulder is internally rotated and there is marked loss of movement. Attempt reduction by applying traction and external rotation with the arm at 90° to the body. Manipulation under anaesthesia may be required.

Inferior dislocation of the shoulder (luxatio erecta)

The patient presents with the arm held above the head. Examine carefully for neurovascular deficits. Attempt reduction by applying traction along the abducted arm, then adduction. If it is not possible to reduce in the field, give strong analgesia, support the arm using padding with sleeping bags or similar, and evacuate for reduction under anaesthesia/sedation.

Fracture–dislocation of the shoulder

If crepitus is felt during manipulation of a shoulder dislocation, suspect an associated fracture and desist from further attempts at reduction in the field until the fracture has been identified or excluded by an X-ray. Support in a broad arm sling, give analgesia, and evacuate.

Supraspinatus tendinitis, subacromial bursitis, and rotator cuff injuries

All these conditions are caused by acute injury or soft tissue degenerative changes and may be provoked by unaccustomed activity as may occur on wilderness trips. The main symptom is of pain, often following lifting or a fall, and onset may be sudden or gradual. Abduction and forward flexion in particular are restricted (unable to upturn a drinks can with arms outstretched in front of patient). There may be a painful arc of movement. Treatment with rest, NSAIDs, and a broad arm sling will usually reduce symptoms. Further assessment will be required if pain and restricted movements persist. Significant loss of range of motion in the absence of pain may indicate a complete rotator cuff tear. Avoid prolonged periods of immobilization in a sling.

Fractures of the humerus

These are caused by a fall onto the outstretched arm or onto the elbow. Midshaft fractures can involve the radial nerve as it runs through the spiral groove and injury results in a wrist drop.

Treatment for proximal injuries is with a collar and cuff sling. Midshaft injuries may benefit from a splint or broad arm sling and strapping arm against the body. Any involvement of neurovascular structures, particularly the radial nerve or brachial artery, should prompt urgent evacuation for definitive care.

Ruptured long head of biceps

This can be torn during lifting and may not require large forces. It is seen more commonly in elderly males. There is a characteristic bulge of biceps muscle above the elbow but often little pain; bruising may, however, be extensive. Surgical repair may be considered if the arm is not fully functional.

Elbow and forearm injuries

The elbow may be injured by a direct blow or transmitted forces such as a fall onto the outstretched hand. Full extension without pain makes the presence of fracture or serious injury very unlikely.

Elbow dislocation

This requires considerable force and may be associated with fractures. The radius and ulna are usually dislocated posteriorly. Damage to the brachial artery or radial/ulnar/median nerves may occur. Attempted reduction is justified in a wilderness environment, particularly if evacuation to definitive care will take more than a few hours.

Treatment

After suitable analgesia, apply steady traction to the limb by pulling at the wrist. The elbow is usually flexed at around 30°. Counter-traction above the elbow with concurrent pushing of the protruding olecranon forwards is essential. Rest in a broad arm sling and evacuate for X-ray and further assessment/rehabilitation. If reduction proves impossible, place in a broad arm sling and give analgesia. Monitor radial pulse and assess for nerve damage.

Epicondylitis—golfer's and tennis elbow

Golfer's elbow refers to inflammation around the common flexor origin at the elbow; tennis elbow involves the same process at the common extensor origin. Both conditions are caused by repetitive hand and wrist movements, particularly rowing and paddling on expeditions. On examination there is tenderness at the medial (golfer's) or lateral (tennis) epicondyles of the humerus and pain on gripping.

Treatment

Rest, anti-inflammatory drugs, and, where possible, avoidance of the provoking activity and gentle stretching after 3–4 days.

Olecranon bursitis

The olecranon bursa may become inflamed and painful, sometimes after minor trauma. The lump over the elbow is fluctuant and may be very tender if it becomes infected. Markedly reduced movements at the elbow and circumferential redness may indicate septic arthritis.

Treatment

This condition may take weeks to resolve but usually only requires rest in a broad arm sling and anti-inflammatory drugs. If there is evidence of spreading infection or fever then give antibiotics. Avoid aspiration in the field because of the danger of introducing infection.

Fractures around the elbow

Displaced fractures around the elbow may be associated with neurovascular injury, particularly the brachial artery. Check distal pulses and seek evidence of neurological deficit. Such fractures usually require orthopaedic assessment and often need internal fixation. With the forearm midprone, splint either in the position found, or with the elbow at 90°. Evacuate for X-ray and further management.

Fractured radial head

This injury can only be diagnosed with the help of radiographs but clinically is suggested by a history of a fall onto the outstretched hand and then pain and tenderness on palpating the radial head. Pronation/supination is often very painful. Support the forearm in a broad arm sling and evacuate for assessment.

Fractures of the forearm

These tend to be unstable fractures and may affect the radius and ulna at the same level, at different levels with spiral fractures, or involve a fracture of one bone with associated dislocation at one of the radioulnar joints. Check carefully for neurovascular compromise. Treat with analgesia, splinting, imaging, and evacuate for definitive care. If there is evidence of an open fracture, clean and dress the wound and give antibiotics.

Wrist injuries

Fractures of the distal radius

These fractures are commonly caused by a fall onto the outstretched hand. There is often obvious deformity together with pain and swelling. Dorsal displacement of the distal fragment is most common—Colles' fracture. For those familiar with a haematoma block, 10 mL of lidocaine 1% can be injected into the fracture site before reduction—a haematoma block. All potential wrist fractures on an expedition should be supported in a suitably padded splint and rested in a broad arm sling. Imaging and definitive treatment will be required after evacuation from the field.

Scaphoid fracture

A fall onto the outstretched hand may lead to pain and swelling, together with difficulty gripping. If there is tenderness in the anatomical snuffbox, pain when 'telescoping' the thumb (pushing the straight thumb towards the wrist), or palpating over the scaphoid tubercle, a scaphoid injury must be considered. Avascular necrosis, non-union, and osteoarthritis may complicate scaphoid fractures. On an expedition, immobilize in a below-elbow splint, and evacuate for X-rays and follow-up as long-term disability may result from undiagnosed scaphoid injury.

Wrist sprains

If the mechanism of injury makes a fracture unlikely and if findings on examination are non-specific, it is reasonable on an expedition to treat a tender wrist as for a sprain using a support bandage, anti-inflammatories, and early mobilization. If there is any uncertainty or if symptoms are not settling, it is safer to assume that there is a fracture and arrangements should be made to image the wrist in a suitable facility.

Tenosynovitis

Inflammation of tendon sheaths may follow repetitive strain injuries. Characteristically there is pain on moving the wrist or thumb and a 'creaking' or 'buzzing' sensation may be felt over the affected tendons, usually on the dorsum of the wrist. Treatment consists of rest in a suitable splint for up to 3 weeks and anti-inflammatories.

Hand injuries

Initial management of hand injuries

- Stop major bleeding using direct pressure and elevation. Consider the use of a temporary tourniquet (a BP cuff can be used).
- Establish the exact mechanism of injury.
- Remove rings early before swelling develops.
- Hand injuries are very painful and adequate analgesia should be given promptly. After neurological assessment, consider early use of LA, particularly ring blocks for finger injuries (➔ Fig. 14.6, p. 457). Clean hand wounds carefully (the patient may be able to clean the surrounding area first).
- Open fractures should be treated with careful cleaning and antibiotics.
- Punching injuries with a break in the skin (usually at the knuckles) should be considered to be a bite wound (➔ p. 292).
- To avoid later disability, all hand injuries must be carefully assessed and managed.

Examination of the hand

- Record whether the injury affects the patient's dominant hand.
- Compare both hands.
- Look for swelling, deformity, redness, and wounds.
- In the relaxed hand there is increasing flexion from the index to the little finger. A finger which is out of line should raise the possibility of a tendon or nerve injury. Rotation of the digit points to a fracture.
- Ask the patient to make a fist and then fully extend fingers. Look for any obvious motor deficit and crossing of fingers.
- Assess flexor digitorum profundus by holding the proximal interphalangeal joint (PIPJ) extended and asking the patient to flex the finger.
- Assess flexor digitorum superficialis by holding the fingers not being assessed in extension. Ask the patient to flex the finger at the PIPJ.
- Assess the lumbricals by flexing the fingers in turn at the metacarpophalangeal joints (MCPJs).
- Finger extensors can be tested by placing the patient's PIPJs level with a table edge then asking the patient to straighten the finger.
- Test movements at the interphalangeal joint (IPJ), MCPJ, and carpometacarpal joint of the thumb.
- Assess median nerve power by asking the patient to oppose the little finger and the thumb.
- The ulnar nerve may be assessed by abducting or adducting the fingers.
- Check sensation on each side of the digit (digital nerves), in the first web space dorsally (radial nerve), middle finger (median nerve), and little finger (ulnar nerve).

Hand fractures and dislocations

Fractures may be suggested by the mechanism of injury, swelling, bruising, deformity, and loss of normal function. In all cases, check for neurovascular deficit. If suspected, immobilize the hand in a boxing glove dressing (Fig. 14.5) and broad high arm sling. Evacuate for imaging and further treatment.

Finger dislocations

Dislocations can occur at the MCPJs or IPJs. After assessing for obvious fractures (small avulsion fractures cannot be diagnosed without imaging), check for any neurovascular damage. It is worth attempting reduction with in-line traction under LA (ring block). If successful, apply buddy strapping or use a boxing glove dressing (Fig. 14.5).

Thumb dislocations

Attempt reduction, then immobilize in a suitable splint or 'boxing glove' (Fig. 14.5). Evacuate for definitive care as internal fixation may be required if there is an associated fracture.

Ligament injuries

These can occur at the MCPJs or IPJs. If the joint is grossly unstable when gently stressing the collateral ligaments, surgical treatment may be required. For most ligament injuries, rest with neighbour strapping will allow healing to occur. Warn patients that swelling may take weeks to settle. This occurs in particular with injuries to the volar plate at the PIPJs. If the mechanism of injury involves a forced abduction at the thumb MCPJ (gamekeeper's/skier's thumb), test for laxity of the ulnar collateral ligament of the thumb MCPJ and compare with the uninjured thumb. If there is no end point on stressing, surgical repair will be required.

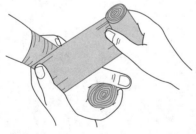

Fig. 14.5 'Boxing glove' dressing.

Tendon injuries

Small cuts or lacerations may damage tendons and these injuries may easily be missed unless hand injuries are carefully assessed. (Beware of any injuries caused by broken glass—evacuation for X-ray is recommended.)

Loss of function is the only reliable sign that a tendon has been damaged but pain out of proportion to the injury should suggest damage to underlying structures. Ensure that you examine the wound with the fingers moving through their range of movement as tendons move with the finger so the injury may not initially be visible.

Extensor tendon injury

This injury is usually obvious. Partial tendon ruptures are easily overlooked—explore wounds under LA or evacuate for full assessment in a bloodless field.

Flexor tendon injuries

Flexor digitorum superficialis flexes the PIPJ. Flexor digitorum profundus flexes the distal interphalangeal joint (DIPJ).

To test these tendons, see ➍ Examination of the hand, p. 452.

Tendon injuries should be repaired in a suitably equipped hospital, not in the field, because of the danger of infection of the flexor sheath that can cause long-term disability.

Finger injuries

On an expedition, fingers can be injured in many ways; they may be crushed in vehicle doors or under heavy weights or during the use of tools/machinery. After release, the digits should be carefully examined (under LA if possible), cleaned, and elevated. Open fractures should be given an antibiotic such as co-amoxiclav and evacuated for X-ray and further management. Always remember to remove rings.

Mallet finger

Rupture of the central slip of the extensor tendon to the distal phalanx results in loss of extension at the DIPJ. This may be associated with an avulsion fracture of the base of the distal phalanx. On an expedition, splint the DIPJ in extension for 6 weeks and arrange for orthopaedic review on return. Do not remove the splint as movement will disrupt the healing tendon.

Finger tip amputation

Provided the bone is not exposed and the area of skin loss is <1 cm² it may be possible to treat these injuries in the field. After assessment, clean and dress (using Vaseline® gauze or similar). Re-examine every 2 days. If the wound is not healing, evacuate for imaging and possible terminalization of bone or skin grafting.

Nail injuries

Finger entrapment or crushing injuries may result in partial or complete avulsion of a nail. The finger should be anaesthetized (Fig. 14.6) and cleaned. The patient may be able to help to clean the finger by immersing in warm, clean water. If the nail is displaced it should be removed under LA, any defect should be repaired, the nail should be replaced for protection, and the finger dressed and splinted.

Subungual haematoma

Crush injuries to the nail may result in bleeding under the finger nail. The pressure results in throbbing pain which may be relieved by heating a paper clip to red heat and burning a hole in the centre of the nail, using minimal pressure. On an expedition a needle holder or multi-tool can be used to hold the heated wire paper clip. It may be necessary to reheat the wire on several occasions. Alternatively, a 21 G hypodermic needle can be used to drill a hole in the nail by gentle twisting motion. Once the blood has drained the pain is significantly reduced.

Foreign body under the nail

Splinters of metal or wood under the fingernail are common. A ring block may allow removal with splinter forceps or trimming of part of the nail to allow removal.

Paronychia

See ➲ Paronychia, p. 316–317.

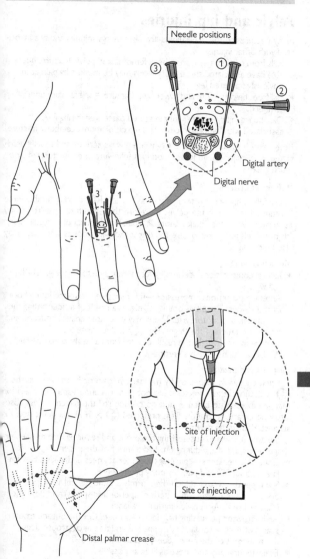

Needle positions

① ③ ②

Digital artery

Digital nerve

3 1

Site of injection

Site of injection

Distal palmar crease

Fig. 14.6 Local anaesthesia of hand.

Pelvic and hip injuries

Many fractures to the lower limbs are high-energy injuries and are associated with other injuries:

- Falls from heights may lead to heel, femoral, and pelvic fracture, but 10% have associated spinal injury—this may be masked by pain at the obviously fractured leg.
- Fall from heights >2 m and lower limb fracture = spinal injury until excluded.
- Dashboard injury—knee injury in seated passenger during RTC associated with femoral fracture and hip dislocation/acetabular fracture.

Bony injuries to the pelvis and thighs are always serious and usually associated with major blood loss. Blood loss following open fractures may be much greater.

Pelvic fractures

These follow high-energy trauma such as falls and RTCs. Considerable force is required to disrupt the pelvis, therefore these fractures are frequently associated with other major thoracic/spinal/abdominal or skeletal injury. Major vessels and pelvic organs lie adjacent to pelvic bones, and these may also be damaged.

Mechanism of injury

- Lateral compression—deforming force from side to side, e.g. vehicle rollover.
- Anterior–posterior compression—this may give rise to the 'open book' fracture where the pelvis opens up; e.g. as a result of a rider hitting the petrol tank of a motorcycle. There may be characteristic abduction and external rotation of the thighs/legs (→ Colour plate 5).
- Vertical shear—usually the result of a fall from a height onto one leg, displacing the hemi-pelvis vertically.

Diagnosis and treatment

If a pelvic injury is suspected by mechanism, pain or hypovolaemic shock (→ p. 250) treat as a fracture. Do not perform unnecessary examination that will exacerbate bleeding and do not log roll the patient unless absolutely necessary. A straddle lift is preferred (→ p. 162) If a pelvic injury is suspected, bind the pelvis.

Treatment is aimed at stabilizing the pelvis and reducing further haemorrhage/visceral damage during onward transfer of the patient.

- Control lower limbs—splint legs together at knees and ankles. Flex the knees about 20° and pad any bony prominences.
- Splint pelvis—wrap a folded sheet firmly around the pelvis (upper border of sheet level with anterior superior iliac spines) and tie at the front or use a SAM pelvic sling® if available.
- An improvised pelvic sling has been described. Cut the outside trouser seams of each leg as far as the hip joint and tie the cut trouser legs firmly in front of the pelvis. See → Colour plates 6–8.
- Evacuate urgently and move as little as possible.

Hip fractures

The elderly and those with osteoporotic bones may fracture the neck of the femur with relatively minor trauma; however, the same fracture in younger patients indicates high-energy trauma such as a climbing fall or a RTC.

Diagnosis and treatment

Often there is a history of a fall onto the lateral aspect of the hip. Pain may radiate to the knee and the affected leg may be shortened and externally rotated. Give analgesia; look for and treat shock. A traction splint may improve comfort during evacuation (see following section on 'Femoral fracture'). If experienced, consider a fascia-iliaca nerve block (➋ p. 630–631).

Hip dislocation

These usually follow a fall from a height or dashboard injury in RTCs. The hip joint usually dislocates posteriorly with or without fracture of the acetabulum. Travellers with hip replacements are at greater risk of dislocation with minimal trauma.

Diagnosis and treatment

There is pain and deformity of the leg, which is shortened and rotated (internally if posterior dislocation). Assess neurological status and distal pulses—hip dislocations may be associated with injury to the femoral or sciatic nerve. If immediate evacuation is possible then splint legs in position and give strong analgesia. If >6 h before evacuation to hospital, then blood supply to the femoral head may become compromised and an attempt at reduction is justified but will require adequate analgesia such as methoxyflurane (Penthrox®).

Reduction of hip dislocations

The 'Captain Morgan technique' (Fig. 14.7) has been described. Place the patient on their back and apply a strap across the pelvis to prevent movement of the pelvis. Flex the patient's knee to 90° on the injured side and place the operator's knee behind the patient's upper calf. Stabilize the patient's foot and then the operator should lift their knee while maintaining downward pressure on the foot. If this is not successful, try internal and external rotation movements of the hip.

Check neurovascular status after reduction. The hip may re-dislocate owing to an unstable acetabular fracture. Repeated attempts at reduction are not justified—evacuation is required ASAP for operative intervention.

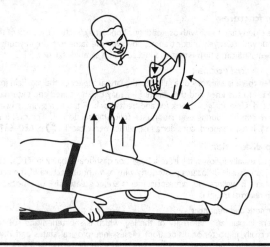

Fig. 14.7 Captain Morgan technique.

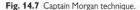

Femoral fracture

A great deal of force is required to fracture the femur—usually following a fall from a height or RTC. It can be associated with other head, spinal, chest, or abdominal/pelvic trauma.

Diagnosis and treatment

There is pain and deformity of the thigh, together with swelling and fracture crepitus. Assess neurological status and distal pulses. Anticipate and whenever possible treat hypovolaemia (the patient may lose 20% of blood volume rapidly even in closed injury). Splint legs in position (splint to uninjured leg); apply traction through a splint if available to maintain alignment and to reduce bleeding into the thigh compartment. Cover any open wounds with sterile dressings (e.g. saline-soaked gauze).

Traction is contraindicated for femoral fractures at or just proximal to the knee—the distal fragment may be displaced posteriorly into the popliteal artery.

Strongly consider a fascia-iliaca block if suitably experienced (➡ p. 630–631).

Knee injuries

Knee injuries on expeditions are relatively common. In all cases take a careful history which may give clues to the diagnosis. Ask about previous knee problems such as swelling, clicking, locking, or 'giving way'.

Examination of the injured knee:

- Look for bruising, swelling, redness, deformity, and compare with the uninjured side.
- Feel for an effusion, warmth, or crepitus. Identify any tender areas—joint line or origin/insertion of collateral ligaments.
- Observe straight leg raising (which assesses the extensor mechanism, below).
- Assess movement—extension (0°), flexion (135°).
- Palpate along the medial and lateral joint lines, and over the fibular head for tenderness.
- Test the joint stability—in 30° flexion support the lower leg and apply valgus stress (medial collateral) and in extension a varus stress (lateral collateral) at the knee. With the knee flexed at 90°, place the thumbs on the tibial tubercle and rest index fingers behind the knee. With the hamstrings relaxed, gently draw the lower leg forward, looking for any abnormal shift (anterior draw test).
- McMurray's test for meniscal injury—place thumb and index finger on medial and lateral joint lines, flex the knee, and externally rotate the foot followed by abduction and extension of the knee. Pain and a click suggest a medial meniscal injury. In the acute knee McMurray's test can be difficult and medial or lateral joint line tenderness can be as useful in identifying meniscus injuries.

Treatment
RICE, analgesia, and evacuate for further assessment.

Bursitis

There will be good range of movement at the knee. Inflammation of the fluid-filled bursa in front of or below the patella may result from unaccustomed, frequent minor trauma such as kneeling. Rest and NSAIDs usually relieve symptoms. If there are features of spreading cellulitis and a fever, antibiotics should be given (e.g. co-amoxiclav).

Patellar fracture

Sudden knee flexion or a direct blow may result in a fracture of the patella. There is usually pain, swelling (sometimes from a haemarthrosis), and inability to straight leg raise. If suspected, splint the leg almost straight (with 5° of flexion at the knee) and evacuate for imaging and definitive treatment.

Other fractures around the knee

Suspected fractures around the knee should be treated with adequate analgesia and splint, as for patellar fracture. Avoid traction splints if there is a possible fracture in the supracondylar region of the distal femur. Traction may displace the distal part of the fracture posteriorly and damage the popliteal artery.

Patellar dislocation

This is not uncommon and may be a recurrent problem (more common in females). The patella dislocates laterally and, typically, the patient's knee is held flexed with obvious displacement of the patella. Give analgesia and reduce the patella by pressing with the thumbs on the lateral aspect of the patella as the knee is straightened. Once reduced it may be possible to re-habilitate this injury in the field without evacuation.

Dislocation of the knee

This is a rare injury and huge forces are required to produce disruption of the knee ligaments. There is a high likelihood of nerve and blood vessel damage—check distal pulses and sensation carefully. These are limb-threatening injuries. Treat with strong analgesia and aim to restore normal alignment to optimize circulation and immobilize as for patellar fracture be-fore evacuation. Keep monitoring foot pulses, as popliteal artery injury may not be apparent initially. If there are signs of vascular compromise, evacuate urgently for vascular surgery.

Ligament injuries to knee

Medial collateral ligament

The medial collateral ligament runs from the medial epicondyle of the femur to 4 cm distal to the knee joint on the medial aspect of the tibia. An isolated rupture usually results from a direct blow to the lateral aspect of the knee in slight flexion. If there is a rotational component, such as a fall when skiing, there may also be injury to the cruciate ligament.

Diagnosis and treatment

- On examination there is tenderness over the medial collateral ligament ± knee swelling. Test valgus stability with knee flexed 20–30° (in full extension the cruciate ligaments stabilize the knee).
- Mild–moderate (<10 mm opening of joint)—rest, ice, compression, and then early mobilization/strengthening with physiotherapy (➔ p. 478–481).
- Severe (>10 mm opening of joint)—may require hinged brace for 3–6 weeks after initial management and so will benefit from evacuation for definitive care.

Lateral collateral ligament

The lateral collateral ligament runs from the lateral epicondyle of the femur to the head of the fibula. Isolated injuries are rare but are more usually associated with injury to all the lateral capsular ligamentous structures. Telemark skiing can result in significant knee injuries due to the forces on the knee when turning.

Diagnosis and treatment

Tenderness ± knee swelling. Test varus stability. An isolated lateral collateral ligament injury may be treated as for medial collateral ligament, but more common complex injury may require evacuation for surgery.

Cruciate ligaments

Anterior cruciate ligament (ACL) injuries account for 50% of documented knee ligament injuries. Posterior cruciate ligament (PCL) injury is rare (10% knee ligament injuries). Usually, injuries are caused by non-contact twisting injury, occasionally following hyper-extension. There is pain and difficulty in weight-bearing. Swelling usually develops immediately with an ACL rupture. A PCL rupture will have no swelling and a dull posterior knee ache.

Diagnosis and treatment
- There is an acute haemarthrosis following typical history. Examination is often difficult during the acute phase due to pain and swelling. A subjective description of a 'popping' sensation is often noted.
- The Lachman test will usually be positive in an ACL rupture—grip the tibia at 30° flexion and pull it anteriorly over the distal femur. There will be no firm end point. There may also be anterior draw and pivot shift. If suspected, evacuate for X-rays and further imaging (MRI) or arthroscopy. Younger active individuals may have continuing joint instability and may require reconstruction of the cruciate ligament. The PCL will have a positive posterior draw at 90°.

Meniscal injuries

The menisci act as stabilizers for the knee and distribute forces across the articular surfaces. There is usually a history of an axial load with a twisting injury to the knee. 'Degenerative' tears may occur in patients >35 years with very little history of injury.

Diagnosis and treatment
- Patients may complain of the knee 'locking' or 'giving way'. Pain and intermittent swelling may occur. Squatting particularly may aggravate posterior horn tears.
- Acute tears may cause gradual swelling of the knee over 4–6 h and occasionally haemarthrosis. Degenerative tears may settle with physiotherapy.
- If the knee is acutely locked, from a loose body, do not attempt to unlock the knee (painful and usually futile). Splint in a comfortable position and evacuate for definitive care.

Knee extensor mechanism injuries

Disruption to any one of these may prevent straight leg raising or active extension of the knee. (NB. Tense knee effusion and pain may also prevent straight leg raise without disruption of extensor mechanism.)

Quadriceps tendon rupture
- 80% occur in individuals >40 years. Normally a gap is palpable close to the superior pole of the patella (defect at insertion of vastus medialis).

Patellar tendon rupture
- Usually occurs in those >40 years. Tender inferior pole patella.

Patellar and tibial tuberosity fractures
- Usually occur as result of direct trauma.
- Manage with rest, support, and splinting in extension. Tendons usually require operative repair if the extensor mechanism is disrupted. Fractures often require reduction and fixation if displaced.

Lower leg injuries

Tibial fracture

This can occur as a result of a fall, RTC, or twisting injury (particularly when skiing). There is often an associated fibula fracture. Because there is little soft tissue cover, tibial fractures are commonly open.

There is a significant risk of compartment syndrome whether an open or closed injury.

Splint legs in position (splint to the other uninjured leg); apply traction through a splint, if available, to maintain alignment. Cover open wounds with a sterile dressing (take a photo first) and give antibiotics during evacuation (e.g. co-amoxiclav).

Compartment syndrome

This refers to increased soft tissue pressure within an enclosed soft tissue compartment which can lead to devastating muscle necrosis and nerve damage.

The soft tissues swell but the surrounding envelope does not allow expansion, causing pressure to rise above the capillary pressure. It usually follows fractures or crush injuries (particularly to the lower leg, thigh, forearm, and foot/hand), and is most common following closed fractures to the tibial shaft. Occasionally it occurs as a chronic exercise-induced condition ('shin splints').

Diagnosis and treatment

Try to prevent occurrence in the field with elevation of the affected limb above the level of the heart. The soft tissue compartment looks swollen and tense. The most reliable sign is pain on passive stretching of a muscle group within the compartment, e.g. great toe or fingers. Remember the 5Ps—Pain, Pallor, Paraesthesia, Paralysis, and Pulseless, reflecting tissue ischaemia. Pain 'out of proportion to the injury' and local tenderness are the earliest features and are difficult to control with even opiate analgesics. Loss of pulse is a very late sign.

Acute compartment syndrome is an emergency requiring urgent evacuation and surgical decompression.

Achilles tendon disorders

Achilles tendinopathy

This refers to micro-tears in the Achilles tendon. It usually affects those aged 35–55 years and follows unaccustomed activity such as running, trekking, and jumping, or direct trauma to the tendon.

This occurs in two areas:

- Non-insertional—4–8 cm proximal to Achilles insertion into calcaneum. It is probably a result of reduced blood supply and a point of high tension in the tendon. A tender fusiform swelling develops.
- Insertional—occurs at the insertion of the Achilles into the calcaneum. A hardened bony lump develops, causing painful rubbing and difficulty with shoes/boots. A bony prominence on the posterior–superior aspect of the calcaneus (Haglund's spur deformity) may be present along with an inflamed bursa (retrocalcaneal bursitis).

Treatment

Conservative measures improve symptoms in 90%. In the acute stage, RICE and regular NSAIDs are required. Modify activity to reduce strain on heels.

After the acute phase has settled consider Achilles stretching exercises (eccentric loading) and removal of heel tabs in training shoes. A heel-raise to reduce stretching of the tendons can also be considered. There is a small risk of complete rupture.

Acute Achilles tendon rupture

There is a relatively poor vascular supply and high tension ~4–8 cm proximal to the insertion into the calcaneum. Age is usually 35–55 years. The injury occurs during sudden contraction during 'push-off' or an injury with forced dorsiflexion of the ankle.

The patient complains of sudden pain and weakness of plantar flexion at the ankle. A 'gun shot' may be felt/heard as the tendon ruptures. On examination there is tenderness and a palpable boggy gap in the tendon.

Simmonds' test-positive—lay the patient prone with foot over end of bed. Gently squeezing the calf causes plantar flexion at ankle in the unaffected side but no or minimal plantar flexion with rupture of Achilles tendon.

Treatment

Initial management is RICE and splint ankle in equinus position (foot plantar flexed), non-weight-bearing. Evacuate for expert assessment and management. There is considerable debate regarding non-operative treatment in equinus cast for 9 weeks (slow recovery and possibly higher re-rupture rate) versus operative repair (wound problems and sural nerve injuries).

Other causes of calf pain

- Shin splints—pain over the anterior shin muscles following running may be treated with rest and NSAIDs. Ice may help. The condition may be avoided by warming up before exercise and stretching afterwards.
- Gastrocnemius/soleus muscle tear. There may be delayed bruising and ongoing pain following a sudden shock load or stretch to the affected

muscles. Analgesia and early mobilization should allow a casualty to
continue walking after a day or two.
- Stress fracture of the tibia (see → Lower limb stress fractures, p. 470).
- DVT (→ p. 264).
- Cellulitis (→ p. 298).

Ankle injuries

Ankle ligament injuries

These commonly occur during a forced inversion injury of the hindfoot. Generally, the lateral ligaments are injured—anterior talofibular ligament and calcaneofibular ligament. Bruising and swelling may be severe, occurring within hours and is often disproportional to the degree of injury. Tenderness is usually maximal laterally.

Following a soft tissue ankle injury, it is normal to experience pain, swelling and bruising as inflammation starts the repair process. Over the first 2 weeks there is usually a gradual improvement in these symptoms as the body is designed to heal and produce new tissue.

You can do a lot to aid this process by using ice, elevation, and taking medication if needed. Use the 'POLICE' care plan (see following 'Treatment' section).

New scar tissue is weak and therefore it is important to protect the area to avoid re-injury and promote healing. Modify activity by reducing the activity or weight you place through the area. This is especially important in the first 10 days–2 weeks.

Tape or a semi-rigid brace might give you the confidence to start walking more normally or return to activity. However, it is important they do not stop you moving the ankle or completing exercise as these are an important part of recovery.

A fracture may be difficult to exclude clinically; however, the Ottawa rules suggest that X-rays should be arranged if the patient is unable to weight bear immediately after the injury (walk four steps) or if there is tenderness behind the medial or lateral malleolus, over the navicular (proximal to base of first metatarsal), or at the base of the fifth metatarsal. Palpate the fibula head as ankle injuries can cause fracture of the fibular head.

Treatment

'POLICE' (➔ p. 478):
- **P**rotect.
- **O**ptimal **L**oading.
- **I**ce.
- **C**ompression.
- **E**levation.

Following a bad ankle sprain, the ability to tolerate weight may be severely reduced for about a week—this is normal but makes assessment difficult. Strapping or taping may help support the ankle initially, while allowing some weight-bearing as tolerated. If pain allows, active exercises should begin immediately, with the aim of regaining full movement. Persistent or worsening pain on weight-bearing after 1 week may require further review.

Ankle fractures

Normally the talus sits in the mortise of the tibia and fibula; twisting may rupture the ligaments or fracture the malleoli. This occurs when the foot is anchored on the ground and the momentum of the body continues forwards. There is swelling, pain, and bruising, with deformity and tenderness along the bony landmarks of the medial and lateral malleoli.

Treatment

If the ankle is obviously dislocated, this may cause pressure necrosis on the soft tissues and neurovascular compromise. Reduction by traction and re-location is indicated urgently (with suitable analgesia). Raise the leg by lifting the big toe on the affected side and mould the ankle with the other hand while attempting to place at the ankle at 90° of flexion. After reduction, check pulses and sensation then immobilize in a suitable splint. Treat with RICE. X-rays are needed to confirm the nature of the fracture. Evacuate for definitive treatment; many displaced ankle fractures will require operative fixation.

Foot fractures and dislocations

Foot injuries can be devastating on trekking expeditions as the victim may require stretcher evacuation. The feet are particularly vulnerable when in-adequately protected by lightweight footwear in the tropics or jungle.

Talus and calcaneal fractures

Falls from a height onto the feet can result in fractures around the heel. These may be bilateral and are associated with other significant injuries such as to the spine, pelvis, hips, or knees.

Treatment

Give strong analgesia, elevate, and immobilize in a splint. Early definitive treatment is necessary to prevent long-term disability.

Metatarsal fractures

Heavy weights such as vehicle wheels or large machinery may break mul-tiple metatarsal bones. Ankle twisting may lead to fractures of the meta-tarsal bones.

Treatment

Check for pulses and evacuate for imaging and definitive care.

Lower limb stress fractures

These most commonly affect the metatarsals, but can occasionally occur in the tibia, the calcaneum, or talus. They follow repeated trauma such as occurs in over-training. There is an underlying biomechanical problem that may be resolved with a change in shoes/boots.

Diagnosis and treatment

- Metatarsals—there is gradual onset of pain ± swelling of the forefoot without specific trauma. Tenderness is specifically along the bone (usually second metatarsal neck). Early X-rays are often normal but may show callus formation at 3–6 weeks.
- Tibia—shin-splint pain on exercise. Pain may settle after a period of rest. May have tenderness along the medial border of the tibia.
- Calcaneum—exertional non-specific heel pain. Squeezing heel causes pain. (NB: plantar fasciitis may cause pain under the heel when walking, which is normally worse for the first few steps after rest, but there is tenderness specifically at the insertion of the plantar fascia under the heel.) X-rays are normal.

In all cases give analgesia and remove the cause, often necessitating a reduc-tion in training/exercise. Reduce weight-bearing with crutches until com-fortable and then start mobilization, as tolerated.

Toe fractures and dislocations

These rarely require any more than 'buddy strapping' to relieve pain for 2–3 weeks. If there is obvious deformity, this may be reduced under ring block (inject 1 mL of plain lidocaine 1% on each side of the base of the broken or dislocated digit).

Lacerations to sole of foot

These are painful, difficult to manage, and prone to infection. To anaesthetize the area, consider topical LA or regional anaesthesia by performing a nerve block of the posterior tibial nerve just posterior to the artery where it runs behind the medial malleolus. This will anaesthetize the majority of the sole of the foot. If the wound is on the lateral sole, consider a nerve block of the sural nerve as it runs behind the lateral malleolus. The tough skin of the sole makes local infiltration of LA painful and ineffective. There is a significant risk of infection—puncture wounds should be treated with antibiotics prophylactically. Ensure tetanus immunization is up to date.

Plantar fasciitis

This is inflammation of the connective tissue that forms the sole of the foot. There may be pain over the heel, under the arch of the foot forward to the metatarsal heads. It commonly occurs in individuals not accustomed to exercise who suddenly increase exercise intensity. Pain is common for the first few steps of the day or on dorsiflexion of the foot. The condition can be eased with calf stretching exercises and orthotics or cushioned footwear. The condition can become chronic.

Spinal injury

(See also ⊃ Chapters 7 and 15.)

Spinal cord injuries are relatively rare. However, it is vital that the possibility of spinal injuries is considered in all trauma patients especially:

- High-speed injuries.
- Patients with multiple injuries.
- Falls, or those who have been hit by a falling object such as a rock.
- Head-injured and unresponsive patients.

The implications of missing one of these injuries can be life-changing or life threatening for the patient. Excessive spinal movement can cause additional neurological damage and worsen outcome.

Injuries most frequently occur at junctions of mobile and fixed section of the spine (C6,7/T1, T12/L1). In patients with multiple injuries who have a spinal injury, over half will have a cervical spinal injury. Many patients with one spinal fracture will be found to have another, particularly with axia loading and increasing age of the patient.

Signs of a spinal injury

The patient may complain of:
- Neck or back pain. This may be masked by another more painful injury.
- Loss of movement and/or sensation in the limbs.
- Sensation of burning/electric shock in the trunk or limbs.

On examination the patient may have:
- Swelling or midline tenderness over the spinous processes.
  In the unconscious patient, a serious spinal injury may be indicated by:
- Hypotension with bradycardia (neurogenic shock).
- The skin may be warm below the level of the lesion.
- Diaphragmatic breathing.
- Flaccid tone.
- Priapism (involuntary erection of the penis) in spinal cord injuries above T6.
- Loss of sphincter control.

Management

The aim of spinal management is to prevent any secondary injury to th spinal cord. If a casualty with a spinal injury is moved carefully, they are u likely to come to further harm but do follow these precautions:

- Ensure that the airway is open. Use the jaw-thrust manoeuvre in preference to head tilt and chin lift. All airway manoeuvres should be performed in a controlled manner but an open airway always takes priority.
- Conscious patients should remain in a position which is comfortable fo them. Unconscious patients should be handled carefully and if possible transported using a vacuum mattress. Restraining an agitated patient is unhelpful and may cause harm.
- Assess breathing and look for and treat any life-threatening chest injury (⊃ p. 394–395). Give oxygen if available to keep sats >94%. Adequa

oxygenation and tissue perfusion must be maintained as the spinal cord is very sensitive to hypoxia and hypotension.

• Identify any signs of shock and treat cautiously with IV fluids. Ensure an adequate BP (systolic >90 mmHg).

• Rapidly assess the conscious level with the ACVPU scale or GCS, look at the pupils, and ask the patient if they can move and feel their fingers and toes.

• There is little benefit in palpating the spine or performing a rectal examination. Only examine the back if a penetrating injury is suspected. Log rolling should be avoided and a 'straddle lift' used instead (➔ p. 162).

If the patient must be moved, do so with caution but ensure that pressure areas are padded and if there is a spinal injury causing bowel and/or bladder dysfunction, ensure attention is paid to keeping the skin clean and dry.

Clearing the suspected spinal injury

Not all patients who are involved in trauma need to have full spinal precautions maintained. Box 14.1 indicates when a spinal injury can safely be excluded clinically.

If it is necessary to move the patient, they should be moved carefully, keeping the spine in alignment throughout (Fig. 14.8), and should be kept horizontal if at all possible. This is because blood vessels below the level of spinal cord injury may have lost their spinal reflexes and so cannot contract in response to hypotension. This can cause a precipitous drop in BP and hence further damage to the spinal cord.

Box 14.1 Excluding spinal injury ('clearing the spine')

No midline cervical tenderness.
No reduced conscious level.
No evidence of intoxication.
No neurological abnormality.
No distracting injury.

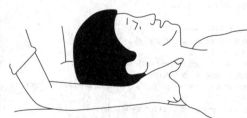

14.8 Manual immobilization of the neck.

Low back pain

Back pain is a common complaint and on expeditions may be provoked by unaccustomed activity or injuries such as lifting awkwardly, falls, or twisting injury. 80% will resolve within 2–8 weeks. Low back pain is very common and most require general self-management without the need for investigation of treatment.

Sort into:
- Mechanical back pain (most prevalent).
- Nerve root pain—only concerning if progressive or persistent.
- Serious spinal pathology—will need definitive care.
- Traumatic.
- Infectious.
- Visceral (~2%).
- Suspected cord compression—needs immediate evacuation.

Consider other systemic disease, such as back pain associated with weight loss, fever/rigors, cough/haemoptysis.

Remember to stratify patients by considering the following:
- <20 years where mechanical back pain is less likely; consider scoliosis, spondylolisthesis (vertebrae slip out of position), or structural bone injury, e.g. pars defect (stress fracture).
- 20–50 years where most likely non-specific lower back pain. Consider infection, cauda equina syndrome (CES; ➲ p. 476), or history of cancer.
- >50 years increased prevalence of visceral cause, fragility fracture, or serious spinal pathology.

History
- Recent back trauma—note the mechanism of any injury.
- Characterize the pain, noting particularly leg symptoms and aggravating and relieving factors.
- Ask if there is any disturbance of bladder/bowel function, in particular incontinence or reduced awareness.
- Ask about previous back injuries or surgery.
- Ask about history of cardiovascular disease (e.g. stroke).
- Presence of red flag signs.

Red flag signs
- Uncontrolled pain, worse at night.
- Bilateral sciatica.
- Fever and/or unexplained weight loss.
- Loss of bladder or bowel control.
- History of carcinoma—particularly thyroid, breast, lung, prostate, kidney.
- Ill health or presence of other medical illness.
- Significant motor weakness or sensory loss.
- Previous osteoporotic fractures.
- Disturbed gait, saddle anaesthesia.
- Age of onset <20 or >50 years.

Examination

'*Unwell*' *patient*—immediately assess ABCs and check for presence of pulsatile, expansile abdominal mass and presence/absence of femoral pulses (abdominal aortic aneurysm often presents with tearing back pain); this is very uncommon in patients <55 years old.

'*Well*' *patient*—look for signs of weight loss, scoliosis, and muscle spasm. Watch the patient walk, looking for limping or abnormal posture. Assess spinal movements and note any significant loss. With the patient supine, palpate for tenderness over lumbar spine and sacrum, ribs, and renal angles. Look for muscle wasting in the legs.

Perform on both legs:
- Straight leg raise—note angle at which patient detects pain (lumbar nerve root irritation). Normal 70° but compare with other side.
- Check for perineal and perianal sensation.

Neurological examination
See Table 14.1.

Table 14.1 Neurological examination

	Sensation	Motor	Reflex
L3/4	Medial lower leg	Quadriceps	Knee jerk
L5	Lateral lower leg	Extensor hallucis longus	Hamstring jerk
S1	Lateral foot and little toe	Foot plantar flexors	Ankle jerk

Management

- If any red flag signs are found, evacuate for specialist investigation of the cause of the back pain.
- In the absence of red flag signs, even with the presence of nerve root pain, conservative treatment should be effective.

Manage symptoms with:
- Reassurance and education that most back pains completely resolve in 2–8 weeks.
- Simple analgesics and NSAIDS, and a short course of a low dose of benzodiazepines (2–5 mg diazepam three times daily for 2 days). Consider opioids for a limited period if needed.
- Use heat, not ice.
- Avoid bed rest; encourage gentle, normal movements.
- Consider physiotherapy or manipulation if available.
- Always keep the diagnosis under review if symptoms change. Almost all back pain will benefit and resolve with good self-management. Clear advice, movement, analgesia, and monitoring.

Cauda equina syndrome

CES is a set of symptoms that are experienced as spinal nerves are compressed in the lower back. The compression can be caused by a structure close to these nerves, such as a disc, narrowing of the spinal canal, very rarely a tumour, or occasionally an injection. About 20% are as a result of an acute disc prolapse. Onset may be more insidious because of spinal stenosis.

CES is very rare but if not diagnosed quickly, can be serious and life-changing. Compression to the nerves of the cauda equina (below the level of the conus at the bottom of the spinal cord) inhibits the function of parts of the lower body, including the bladder, bowel, reproductive organs, as well as the legs. It can also cause pain and pins and needles in these areas, as well as a lack of light, sharp, or deep pressure sensation.

The symptoms of CES can be subtle and vague (Box 14.1). The symptoms do not necessarily develop in a recognized pattern and it can be a challenge to recognize them.

> **Box 14.1 Cauda equina syndrome warning signs**
> - Loss of feeling/pins and needles between inner thighs and genitals.
> - Numbness in or around back passage or buttocks.
> - Altered feeling when using toilet paper to wipe yourself.
> - Increasing difficulty starting to urinate.
> - Increasing difficulty when trying to stop or control the flow of urine.
> - Loss of sensation passing urine.
> - Leaking urine.
> - Not knowing when the bladder is full or empty.
> - Inability to stop a bowel movement or leaking faeces.
> - Loss of sensation when passing a bowel motion.
> - Change in ability to achieve an erection or ejaculate.
> - Loss of sensation in genitals during sexual intercourse.

Objective assessment

The presence of two or more of the symptoms/signs listed in Box 14.1 should warrant further assessment:
- Ascertain if patient is in urinary retention.
- Examine for any neurological deficit, in particular bilateral neurological symptoms, saddle anaesthesia, and loss of anal tone (subjective).

Management

Signs and symptoms such as urinary retention and perianal sensory loss indicate the need for urgent evacuation for imaging with MRI and surgery. Delays in surgery can result in long-term sensory and motor changes.

Physiotherapy

Most soft tissue injuries will benefit from a short period of rest/protection (splinting) followed by early mobilization to prevent stiffness and to regain full movements.

POLICE

It is important to *protect* and *ice* any injured area, as well as *modify* the patient's activity and routine.

'*POLICE*' stands for:
* **P**rotection.
* **O**ptimal **L**oading.
* **I**ce.
* **C**ompression.
* **E**levation.

Protection: protecting the area might involve using crutches to reduce weight through the leg, wearing a brace, or resting frequently throughout the day. This is especially important in the first 48–72 h.

Optimal loading: it is important to adjust and regulate your amount of activity as overdoing it can increase pain and slow your return to normal. For example: take a lift instead of the stairs, reduce unnecessary walking, or consider other alternatives.

Ice is very helpful in the first 2 days to reduce pain. Ice is better than a chemical pack as it cools more effectively but naturally this will not be available in all expedition areas. A packet of frozen peas wrapped in a tea towel works well. Place it on the area for up to *20 min* and repeat as often as possible. If ice is not available, cold packs would be a suitable alternative or even placing the injured limb in cold water.

Compression, such as an elastic bandage can be applied to the swollen area and has been reported to reduce pain and swelling. It is important the bandage is not too tight as this might restrict blood flow and increase swelling. Patients find Tubigrip® comfortable; it is therefore a useful tool but the evidence for its use is mixed.

Elevate the area of injury frequently throughout the day—ideally above the level of the heart if this is possible.

Advice for the patient

* 1–3 days: POLICE.
* 3–14 days: POLICE + gentle regular exercises building up activity, avoiding excessive discomfort or strain.
* 14 days onwards: can increase optimal load—injury requires less protection. Concentrate on getting the injured part back to full fitness with exercises. Gentle range of motion exercises should start after day 3. Aim for graded exercises which move joints slightly more each day. Avoid excessive stretching and try to normalize movement as early as possible within the limits of pain. Always provide adequate analgesia.
* By 8 weeks all usual activities should have been resumed.

Heat not ice?

ICE is beneficial for up to 2 weeks after an injury. After the acute phase, heat can be useful. Heat, in the form of a hot water bottle, wheat bag, or h packs, brings more blood to the area for healing. This is useful in the later stages of soft tissue healing but will increase swelling and pain if applied too early after an injury.

It is important that the temperature is not too hot, gentle heat is enough. Place a towel between the heat source and the skin to protect the area and avoid a burn. Check the skin regularly and avoid areas of the skin in poor condition (such as cuts, sores, or eczema), with poor blood supply or reduced sensation.

Sleep

Sleep is important to help aid recovery. Ensure the patient is as comfortable as possible. After an injury pain tends to be worse at the end of the day or first thing in the morning. Use suitable analgesia to allow sleep. Other strategies include placing a pillow under the knee for lower limb injuries. A slight bend makes the joint less compressed and can reduce pain. An improvised pillow between the knees or to support an arm may be used when sleeping on the side.

Guide to taping and strapping

Taping or strapping is simply the application of adhesive tape to provide extrinsic stability and/or to offload weakened structures. Its proprioceptive qualities play a significant part in protection and rehabilitation. The principal aim of applying tape is to prevent disability and thus improve otherwise impaired physical function. Techniques can be used for a multitude of musculoskeletal conditions, either following tissue injury or as a preventative measure when a history or risk of injury is present (Fig. 14.9).

Materials

The most commonly used types of taping material are the adhesive elastic type (such as Elastoplast®) and zinc oxide tape (a non-stretch, highly adhesive tape). The indications for each type depend on the aim of the technique being used, but often both types will be used concurrently; e.g. elastic adhesive tape is ideal for providing anchor strips as these are often circumferential strips of tape and must stretch to allow contraction of muscle from these anchor strips. Zinc oxide tape can be used to act as a non-stretchy stabilizer to prevent particular joint movements. Zinc oxide tape requires changing every day as after stretching it over a day, it will no longer be supportive.

In a number of techniques, a pre-taping under-wrap can be used to prevent direct contact of the tape with the skin. However, it is the traction of the skin–tape interface that is thought to give the techniques their effectiveness and therefore the use of under-wrap can be questioned.

Preparation and precautions

Prior to undertaking any taping technique, patients should have undergone a comprehensive assessment of the injury with particular reference to mechanism of injury, precise direction of any resultant instability/weakness, and the phase of healing that is likely to be ongoing. These factors will lead to a clinical decision being made regarding the selection of taping material as well as the technique that is to be applied. Patients should also be questioned as to whether any known allergy to the taping materials is known.

Adequate preparation of the contact area is vital to ensure ease of technique and a good skin–tape interface. The following can be used as a guide:

- The area to be taped should be clean and dry.
- Hairy areas should be shaved.
- Areas of broken skin should be covered with a suitable dressing such as Mepore®.
- The patient should be positioned to allow the therapist access to the taped area without having to reposition throughout the technique.
- Once the tape is applied, simple checks to observe circulation to the area should be performed.

Acute injuries

Acutely injured joints are at greater risk of further injury owing to the loss of proprioceptive input caused by painful stimuli. The use of taping as an adjunct to improving joint stability extrinsically is commonly used in the sports setting and is aimed at restoring function at an early stage while protecting structures from further injury. Adhesive tape has been found to provide compression to acute ankle sprains for up to 10 days post injury.[2] It should be noted, though, that applying tape for such prolonged periods can be counterproductive as it will limit venous flow from the injured area and thus prevent resolution of swelling.

In the presence of swelling around an acutely injured joint, it is often wise to ensure that the circumference of the joint and the surrounding muscular tissues are not completely covered. This allows for further swelling to take place without causing any vascular compromise.

In acute muscle strain, longitudinal taping crossing both the origin and insertion of the muscle can prevent further injury and reduce disability by limiting the muscle's potential to lengthen. This technique, known as physiological taping, can also be used during rehabilitation to offload the muscle at the point of stretch and, through the elastic quality of the tape, it can assist muscle contraction.

Preventative taping

The most common use of musculoskeletal taping is as a preventative measure when returning athletes to sporting activity. Taping itself has been compared to functional sports bracing as a means of providing effective joint stability. No difference was found between the overall effectiveness and practicality of taping versus a laced ankle support across a number of sporting activities, but taping has the advantage of being adaptable to the individual athlete or expedition team member.

2 Capasso G, Maffuli N, Testa V. Ankle taping: support given by different materials. *Br J Sports Med* 1989;23:239–240. https://doi.org/10.1136/bjsm.23.4.239

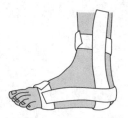
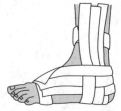

Ankle taping can provide excellent
support and allow use of a sprained ankle.

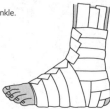

Fig. 14.9 Ankle strapping.

Further reading

MacDonald R. *Taping Techniques: Principles and Practice*, 2nd ed. London: Butterworth–
    Heinemann; 2004.

Chapter 15

Infectious diseases

Chapter editor
Matthew Dryden

Contributors
Matthew Dryden
Alastair Miller
Clare Warrell
David A. Warrell (1st and 2nd editions)

Reviewer
Kirsten MacGregor

Introduction

Infections are among the commonest medical problems encountered on expeditions. This chapter describes some infectious diseases that are common, potentially serious, or inspire great anxiety. Most involve skin, respiratory tract, conjunctivae, ears, gut (traveller's diarrhoea), and the genitourinary tract, and are readily diagnosed and treated even in a remote location. If a particular system is involved, refer to the appropriate section of this handbook:

- Superficial fungal infections and myiasis—see ⟳ Chapter 9.
- For bronchitis, pneumonia, and other respiratory tract infections—see ⟳ Chapter 12.
- Upper respiratory tract, ear, and eye infections—see ⟳ Chapter 10.
- Urinary tract and gut infections, diarrhoea, vomiting, and appendicitis—⟳ see Chapter 13.
- Sexually transmitted diseases are covered in this chapter (⟳ p. 536).
- If the patient is severely ill—see ⟳ Septic shock, p. 250.

The risk of catching a dangerous exotic infection while travelling overseas is small but worrying. Prevention is by far the best strategy.

Find out in advance which important health issues and diseases may be occurring in the areas where you are travelling. The best way to do this is via the NaTHNaC website: ℬ https://travelhealthpro.org.uk/

It is also important to check the UK Government travel advice website: ℬ https://www.gov.uk/foreign-travel-advice

A thorough medical history and risk assessment of all team members must be carried out before travel (⟳ p. 48). Reduce risk by:

- Basic hygiene and regular handwashing.
- Good food hygiene.
- Anti-bug-bite measures (clothing, repellents, nets, etc.).
- Vaccination (⟳ Immunizations, p. 28–40, 64).
- Malaria prophylaxis.
- Carrying antibiotics appropriate for treating common infections in case they are needed.
- Safe sex practices.

Diagnosis in the field

During the expedition, diagnosis will depend largely upon clinical assessment. Simple rapid point-of-care tests on blood and urine may be available, and it may be possible to get some investigations done at the base hospital. Consider in advance whether this may be feasible and reliable.

Some potential pathogens can be excluded:

- Geographically—e.g. yellow fever (YF) does not occur outside Latin America and Equatorial Africa.
- Local medical experience that the disease doesn't occur there.
- Because of assumed immunity from pre-expedition vaccinations.

- Because of the incubation period (e.g. fever starting <7 days after entering a malarious area cannot be due to malaria; fever starting >21 days after leaving West Africa cannot be Lassa fever).
- On clinical grounds (e.g. a fever with lymphadenopathy and rash is not compatible with malaria).
- By carrying out a therapeutic trial (e.g. of antimalarial or anti-rickettsial treatment).

Additional important considerations in the planning phase:
- There must be a plan for evacuation and repatriation of seriously ill team members.
- Suspicion of a serious infectious disease such as bacterial meningitis should prompt initiation of empirical antimicrobial treatment and urgent evacuation to the nearest base hospital (→ Crisis Management, Ch 5).
- Confirmation of diagnosis, using a wider range of laboratory and other investigations, may be possible after evacuation to the base hospital identified at the planning stage. Depending on the experience and attitude of local doctors and nurses, the expedition MO may still have a role and responsibility at this stage, hence the relevance of some of the information about diagnosis and more advanced treatment given in Box 15.1.
- Diagnostic testing in remote hospitals in many developing countries may be non-existent, limited, or inaccurate. Ensure that you know just what testing is available and how to access it.

Box 15.1 Some common patterns of infection and pragmatic empirical treatments

- *Fever ± headache without other signs*—treat for malaria (if exposure was possible). Influenza usually has respiratory signs and symptoms.
  - After 48 h still fever but no signs—treat for rickettsia.
  - Combination for fever of unknown origin: ceftriaxone IV + oral doxycycline *after* malaria treatment.
  - After 96 h still fever—evacuate.
- *Spreading skin inflammation ± pus*—treat with flucloxacillin + pus drainage.
- *Pain passing urine ± loin pain*—urinary tract infection—treat with trimethoprim. Ciprofloxacin if pyelonephritis suspected.
- *Coughing up yellow/green phlegm ± pleuritic pain*—chest infection—treat with doxycycline or clarithromycin.
- *Diarrhoea and vomiting*—traveller's diarrhoea—treat with fluids, rehydration salts, and ciprofloxacin or azithromycin.
- *Severe abdominal pain with rigid abdomen*—peritonitis—treat with fluids and co-amoxiclav and evacuate.
- *Headache, stiff neck, photophobia, impaired consciousness ± rash*—meningitis/encephalitis—treat with ceftriaxone and evacuate.

Viral infections

(See also ➔ Emerging infections, p. 532–534.)

Viral hepatitis

Many different viruses and some bacteria (➔ Leptospirosis, p. 503) are capable of producing the clinical and biochemical picture of acute hepatitis. These include some flaviviruses (➔ p. 488–489, 493–494), herpes viruses, such as Epstein–Barr virus (EBV) and cytomegalovirus (CMV), and the 'hepatitis viruses' (hepatitis A virus (HAV) to hepatitis G virus (HGV)) that specifically target the liver (➔ Figs. 2.2 and 2.3, p. 33, 34). Of the specific hepatitis viruses, HAV and HBV are of particular concern to the traveller who should have received appropriate vaccination. HCV is only a concern to those who inject drugs or who receive medical care overseas.

Transmission and incubation period

- *HAV* is transmitted faecal–orally and rarely by blood transfusion, needlestick, and sexually. Incubation is 4–6 weeks.
- *HBV*, sometimes associated with HDV ('delta agent'), is transmitted by transfusion, needlestick, from mother to baby at birth, or sexually. Incubation is 4–24 weeks.
- *HCV* is transmitted by needlestick, transfusion, rarely from mother to baby at birth, and sexually. Incubation is 2–26 weeks.
- *HEV* is transmitted faecal–orally and zoonotically via pork and other animal products. Incubation is about 6 weeks. Many epidemics attributed to HAV are thought to have been due to HEV. Pregnant women are susceptible to severe disease.

Clinical

Many infections are anicteric and some asymptomatic. In the rest, cholestatic jaundice appears after a few days of general malaise, anorexia, nausea, vomiting, fever with chills, weakness, fatigue, headache, aches and pains, and upper abdominal discomfort. Dark urine, pale stools, and pruritis are common. Signs include RUQ tenderness, tender hepatomegaly, spider naevi, and vasculitic or urticarial rashes. Splenomegaly is common with CMV and EBV but not with the specific hepatitis viruses. Fulminant, potentially fatal, hepatic failure may occur with HBV, HEV (during pregnancy), and rarely with HAV, presenting with hepatic encephalopathy. The acute illness, which may relapse, lasts days or weeks and in severe cases is complicated by persistent nausea, vomiting, ascites, oedema, or liver failure. Chronic viral infection (that may lead in time to chronic hepatitis, cirrhosis, and hepatoma) are complications of HBV and HCV infection.

Diagnosis

Urine dipstick testing reveals urobilinogen (early) and bilirubin (later). If laboratory services are available, rapidly rising serum aminotransferase concentrations (to thousands of units) suggest hepatitis and the diagnosis is confirmed by serology or antigen detection. High alkaline phosphatase suggests 'surgical' obstructive jaundice (e.g. gallstones).

Treatment

There is no specific treatment for acute viral hepatitis. Hepatotoxic drugs and alcohol must be avoided. Supportive management, including rest and low-fat diet improve comfort. Corticosteroids and A low-protein diet have no proven benefit. It is essential that the patient attends an infectious diseases unit on return, to screen for other blood-borne viruses and to exclude chronic HBV, HCV, and HDV infection, any of which may require specific treatment.

Prevention

(See ➲ p. 33–34.) Effective vaccines are available against HAV and HBV and are strongly recommended to all travellers to developing countries. HBV vaccine is mandatory for medical personnel. Avoidance of HAV and HEV involves food and water hygiene, especially in hyperendemic developing countries. For the parenterally/sexually transmitted viruses such as HBV and HBC, extreme caution is necessary with blood and blood products unless they have been properly screened. Surgical and dental procedures, ear piercing, tattooing, acupuncture, and injections in or out of hospital, unprotected sex, and intimate contact that risks inoculation of blood or tissue fluids, even sharing a toothbrush, are potentially hazardous.

Websites

℠ http://www.cdc.gov/ncidod/diseases/hepatitis/
℠ http://www.who.int/topics/hepatitis/factsheets/en/

Poliomyelitis

Poliomyelitis, caused by the polioviruses (enteroviruses), has been eliminated from the western hemisphere but wild poliovirus (WPV) infections still occur in a few African and Asian countries (Fig. 15.1). In 2019, 173 WPV cases were confirmed, only in Pakistan, and Afghanistan.

Transmission

Transmission is faecal–oral.

Clinical

Most infections are asymptomatic or cause only mild upper respiratory tract symptoms, but in ~1% of cases, there is aseptic meningitis or flaccid paralysis of one limb or more extensive quadriplegia or bulbar and respiratory paralysis due to infection of spinal anterior horn cells. Other viruses such as enterovirus 71, adenoviruses, and Japanese encephalitis virus can also cause polio-like flaccid paralysis.

Prevention

Everyone must be vaccinated or boosted if visiting an endemic area 10 years after their previous vaccination. Proof of polio vaccination within the previous 12 months is required for all visitors leaving Pakistan who have stayed for ≥4 weeks. Inactivated (Salk) vaccine is used increasingly. In the UK, it is combined with tetanus and diphtheria vaccine (DPT) (➲ p. 28). Oral (Sabin) vaccine (live, attenuated virus) can cause vaccine-related poliomyelitis (0.5–3.4 cases/1 million vaccines).

Website

℠ http://www.who.int/topics/poliomyelitis/en/

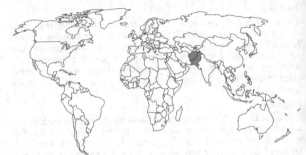

Fig. 15.1 Distribution of wild poliovirus (⅋ https://www.cdc.gov/polio/progress/index.htm).

Viral encephalitides

Japanese encephalitis

This is a common, dangerous, vaccine-preventable, mosquito-borne flavivirus encephalitis of Asia and parts of Oceania (➔ Fig. 2.4, p. 35). There are 30,000–50,000 cases reported annually with 10,000–15,000 deaths. 40 clinical cases in travellers have been reported over 30 years.

Prevention: IXIARO vaccine is recommended for those spending prolonged periods in rural areas (two doses 4 weeks apart followed by a booster after 1 year. Children >2 months but <3-year-olds receive half the adult dose).

Website

⅋ https://travelhealthpro.org.uk/disease/98/japanese-encephalitis

Tick-borne encephalitis (TBE)

TBE, caused by a flavivirus, occurs throughout a vast area from German and the whole of Scandinavia in the west, through eastern Europe, Baltic countries, Russia, and central Asia ('Russian spring–summer encephalitis see ➔ Fig. 2.6, p. 37). Each year, 3000 clinical cases are reported in Europe and >10,000 in Russia. The incidence is increasing in all countries except Austria where an aggressive vaccination policy has proved effective (for distribution, see ➔ Immunizations, p. 28).

Transmission: hard ticks (*Ixodes ricinus*, *I. persulcatus*) transmit three subtypes of TBE flaviviruses. Infection can also be acquired by drinking unpasteurized dairy products, especially goats' milk.

Clinical: a feverish illness (myalgia, headache, and fatigue) may appear 4–28 days after the tick bite; 1–33 days later about one-third will develop meningitis, meningo-encephalomyelitis, myelitis, or meningo-radiculitis.

Diagnosis: (at the base hospital): can be confirmed by detecting virus blood or CSF (early) or serologically.

Treatment: is supportive

Prevention: (➐ Immunizations, p. 28) vaccination (two doses 4–6 weeks apart followed by a booster at 1 year) is effective for those walking and camping in tick-infested coniferous forests of endemic areas, especially during the tick season (May–October and 'Russian spring–summer encephalitis'). In Austria, everyone is vaccinated. Avoid tick infestation (➐ p. 308–309) and unpasteurized (goats') milk products.

West Nile fever

West Nile fever, caused by a flavivirus, occurs in Africa, Europe, Asia, Australia, and the Americas. Kunjin virus is the Australian subtype.

Transmission: is by *Culex* mosquitoes, primarily among migratory birds but sometimes to humans, horses, and other mammals and also by blood transfusion.

Clinical: after an incubation period of 3–15 days, ~20% of infected people develop a dengue-like feverish illness. Fewer than 1% have meningitis or encephalitis, although these may prove fatal in elderly patients. Rashes and lymphadenopathy are uncommon.

Diagnosis: confirmation is by PCR/serology.

Prevention: there is no vaccine. Avoid mosquito bites (➐ p. 305), especially from dusk to dawn. Wear gloves when handling bird carcasses.

Website

🕮 http://www.cdc.gov/ncidod/dvbid/westnile/index.htm

Zika virus infection

Zika, an RNA flavivirus, originated in Africa and became prominent in 2014 when a large epidemic began in Brazil and spread to other South and Central America countries, the Caribbean, North America, Africa, and Southern Asia (Fig. 15.2). In Brazil alone there have been >131,000 confirmed cases with 2386 cases of congenital microcephaly and 11 deaths. In the UK, 295 imported cases have been diagnosed, seven in pregnant women. In 2020 there are no active outbreaks.

Transmission

Zika virus infection is a zoonosis of monkeys and other mammals, transmitted by bites of *Aedes* mosquitoes, and, in humans, to the fetus, sexually (vaginal, anal, oral), by blood transfusion, organ transplantation, and laboratory exposure.

Clinical

After an incubation period of 3–12 days, only one in five infected people develop symptoms which are usually mild and self-limiting, lasting 4–7 days. Commonly there is fever (65%), pruritic maculopapular rash starting on face (90%), headache (45%), non-purulent conjunctivitis or hyperaemia (55%), myalgia (48%), and arthralgia or arthritis (65%). Less frequently, there is fatigue, retro-orbital pain, GI symptoms, and haematospermia. The most important implications are for pregnant women and include microcephaly (1% of infected pregnancies) and more subtle neuromusculoskeletal, developmental, and cognitive abnormalities (one in five infected fetuses). In adults, Guillain–Barré syndrome may occur (2.4 cases/10,000 infections).

Depending upon where the infection was contracted, differential diagnoses include dengue, chikungunya, malaria, other viral exanthems such as parvovirus, measles, rubella, enteroviruses, etc., scarlet fever, and rickettsial infections.

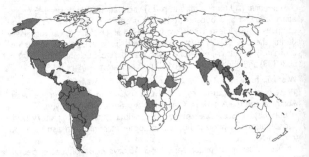

Fig. 15.2 World map of areas with current or previous Zika infection.

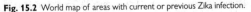

Laboratory diagnosis

At 3–5 days after first symptom: viral RNA is detectable by rT-PCR (urine up to 21 days, semen up to 131 days). From day 5 onwards: anti-Zika IgM and IgG are detectable by ELISA (but there is cross-reactivity with other flaviviruses, notably—Japanese encephalitis, West Nile virus, dengue, and YF).

Treatment

None is specific.

Prevention

No vaccine is available. The risk of fetal transmission is during the first two trimesters of pregnancy. Residents of endemic areas should endeavour to avoid mosquito bites. Women who are pregnant or planning pregnancy should carefully consider the risks of travel to Zika-endemic countries, Women returning from endemic areas should avoid conception for 2 months after return. Men returning from endemic areas should use condoms for 3 months after return, and, if their partner is pregnant, for the whole of the pregnancy.

Website

℘ https://www.gov.uk/government/collections/zika-virus-zikv-clinical-and-travel-guidance

Rabies

Rabies is a very serious disease that can be transmitted to humans by the bite of an infected animal. Most of the world is endemic for rabies (➔ Fig. 2.5, p. 36). Domestic dogs are by far the most important source of human rabies worldwide. Other vectors include cats, wolves, foxes, jackals, skunks, mongooses, raccoons, monkeys, vampire bats (Caribbean and Latin America only), flying foxes (fruit bats), and insectivorous bats. Bats are the only mammals which can harbour the virus long term, without succumbing to the disease, and are thus an important reservoir. Bites by rodents, by contrast, pose negligible risk, as due to their small size, they usually die before they get a chance to pass it on. All mammal bites and scratches should be taken seriously because rabies is such a fatal disease.

Rabies is especially common in parts of Africa, the Indian subcontinent, South-East Asia, and China causing >60,000 human deaths each year and untold fear and suffering.

Transmission

Virus-laden saliva is inoculated through the skin by a bite or scratch and the virus can also penetrate intact mucosae if airborne droplets of bat urine are inhaled or land in the eyes, e.g. in tropical caves infected by large numbers of bats.

Clinical

The virus spreads from the wound along nerves to reach the central nervous system (CNS), causing fatal encephalomyelitis. The incubation period is usually a few months but can vary from 4 days to many years. Rabies has the highest case fatality rate of any infectious disease and is almost always fatal once it reached the CNS (there has been only one documented human survivor who made a full recovery). However, rabies is readily preventable.

Prevention

Avoid all unnecessary and close contact with domestic, wild, or pet mammals, especially carnivores and bats. Beware of wild animals that appear unusually tame or aggressive: they may be rabid! Pre-exposure rabies vaccination is recommended by the WHO for all travellers to moderate or highly endemic countries, but is particularly important for expedition members, who may be some distance from a major or capital city with reliable access to rabies immunoglobulin or post-exposure vaccine.

In case of mammal bites licks or scratches

Irrespective of the risk of rabies, mammal bites, scratches, and licks on mucous membranes or broken skin should be thoroughly cleaned immediately.

Pre-exposure rabies vaccination (→ Rabies, p. 36) is strongly recommended for all travellers to rabies-endemic regions because optimal post-exposure prophylaxis may not be readily available and this is a deadly disease! Cost can be reduced if a group of two or more travellers are vaccinated together, using a recognized intradermal (ID) regimen (→ Colour plate 9).

- Scrub wound with soap and water, ideally under a running tap.
- Rinse and apply povidone–iodine *or* strong (40–70%) alcohol (gin and whisky contain >40% alcohol).
- Consider other mammal bite pathogens (e.g. *Pasteurella multocida*), and treat any bites that break the skin with an antibiotic (e.g. co-amoxiclav).
- In a rabies-endemic country, if the skin has been broken by the bite or scratch, or if a mucosal membrane or open wound, including a scratch, has been contaminated with the animal's saliva, start post-exposure prophylaxis (Box 15.2). The decision should be made as soon as possible by the expedition MO or, failing that, a doctor working in the area where the bite has occurred. On no account should it be delayed until the traveller's return to their own country. If in doubt, start prophylaxis!

Websites

℘ http://www.cdc.gov/ncidod/dvrd/rabies/

℘ http://www.who.int/rabies/en/

℘ https://assets.publishing.service.gov.uk/government/uploads/system/uploads/attachment_data/file/843017/Rabies_summary_risk_assessment_treatment.pdf

Box 15.2 Post-exposure prophylaxis of rabies

Modern tissue/cell culture vaccines, such as human diploid cell vaccine (Sanofi-Pasteur), vero cell vaccine (Sanofi-Pasteur Verorab®), and purified chick embryo cell vaccine (Novartis-Chiron Rabipur® and RabAvert®), are potent and safe. Consider including at least one dose of rabies vaccine in your medical kit as emergency ID post-exposure booster treatment.

For those who *have* received two or three doses of pre-exposure immunization in the past (or post-exposure prophylaxis):

- *Either* two IM post-exposure booster injections of vaccine should be given on days 0 and 3 but no rabies immune globulin (RIG) is necessary.
- *Or* give 0.1 mL of vaccine ID at each of four sites (deltoids, lateral thighs, or suprascapular area) on one occasion only.

For those who *have not* previously received a course of rabies vaccine *and* those who are immunosuppressed:

- *RIG* is infiltrated around the bite wound and any remaining is given IM (lateral thigh). Human RIG 20 units/kg body weight; equine RIG 40 units/kg.
  And:
- Rabies tissue culture vaccine (detailed in ➓ Rabies, p. 36):
  - *Either IM* (deltoid) injections of one vial, 1 mL (0.5 mL for Verorab®) of reconstituted vaccine on days 0, 3, 7, 14, and 28.
  - *Or ID* four-site injections (so that a small papule is produced—see ➓ Colour plate 9 just like with BCG vaccination):
    - On day 0: divide one ampoule of vaccine between *four* sites (both deltoids and both thighs or suprascapular regions).
    - On day 7: 0.2 mL (in the case of 1 mL vials) or 0.1 mL (in the case of 0.5 mL vials) at each of *two* sites (both deltoids).
    - On day 28: single site 0.2/0.1 mL.

Early, vigorous cleaning of the bite wound (➓ p. 294–295) combined with vaccination and use of RIG has proved very effective in preventing rabies. If no suitable vaccine is available where and when the exposure occurs, the traveller should be repatriated immediately to start post-exposure prophylaxis as a matter of urgency.

No case of rabies has been reported in anyone who was exposed to rabies after receiving pre-exposure prophylaxis and in whom post-exposure booster shots of vaccine were given. By contrast, there are at least 15 documented cases of people treated by post-exposure prophylaxis only who have gone on to get rabies and die.

See: ℘ https://assets.publishing.service.gov.uk/government/uploads/system/uploads/attachment_data/file/843017/Rabies_summary_risk_assessment_treatment.pdf

Yellow fever

YF is the classic flavivirus haemorrhagic fever. It occurs only in Africa and South America (➲ Fig. 2.7, p. 39); 90% of cases are reported from Africa. There have been as many as 200,000 cases of YF each year, with 30,000 deaths. Ten unvaccinated travellers were infected in the 2016 Brazilian YF outbreak, four of whom died.

Transmission

Transmission is by *Aedes* mosquitoes. Jungle (sylvatic) YF is transmitted between monkeys and occasionally humans by tree hole breeding mosquitoes in South America and Africa, while urban epidemics are transmitted between humans by peri-domestic *Aedes aegypti*.

Clinical

After an incubation period of 3–6 days, around 5% of those infected become feverish with chills, headache, photophobia, myalgia, back ache, pain in limbs and knees, nausea, vomiting, epigastric pain, and prostration. Heart rate may be slow relative to the temperature. After a temporary remission, jaundice, generalized bleeding (black vomit, melaena), acute kidney injury, shock, and coma may supervene.

Diagnosis (at the base hospital)

Leucopenia and thrombocytopenia are typical. Confirmation is by detecting virus in blood or liver tissue (postmortem) or serological.

Treatment

Treatment is supportive.

Prevention

(See ➲ Immunizations, p. 28.) Vaccination is recommended for all visitors to the endemic area and is a statutory requirement in many countries. For example, you will not be allowed to fly from Ecuador to Brazil without a valid vaccination certificate. The live, attenuated 17D vaccine is contraindicated before the age of 6 months, and in the immunosuppressed. The risk of giving the vaccine to a pregnant women is unknown and must be weighed against the risks of the disease.[1] There have been problems with vaccine supply (India), safety, fake vaccine, and fake certificates (India, West Africa). YF-associated neurotropic disease (YEL-AND) is an abnormal allergic response to the vaccine, as with other vaccines (e.g. flu) causing post-vaccinal encephalitis, Guillain–Barré syndrome, etc. It occurs more commonly in older people (1.0/100,000 doses in people aged 60–69 years and 2.3/100,000 doses in people aged ≥70 years). YF-associated viscerotropic disease (YEL-AVD) is a severe infection (case fatality >60%) caused by massive replication of the vaccine virus with multiple organ failure occurring only after primary vaccination in 0.4/100,000 doses. In those >60 years old, the combined incidence of YEL-AND and YEL-AVD increases to around 1/50,000, the highest risk for any vaccine currently in use. It is therefore critical to balance this risk against the real risk of being exposed to YF. Immunity from vaccination appears to be lifelong, but a small subset of people may need reimmunization.

1 ♒ https://nathnacyfzone.org.uk/factsheet/55/pre-conception-pregnant-women-and-breastfeeding

Websites

℘ http://www.nhs.uk/Conditions/Yellow-fever/Pages/Prevention.aspx
℘ http://www.travelhealthpro.org.uk/factsheet/18/yellow-fever
℘ http://wwwnc.cdc.gov/travel/yellowbook/2014/chapter-3-infecti
ous-diseases-related-to-travel/yellow-fever

Dengue fever ('break bone' fever)

Dengue viruses are flaviviruses. The global incidence of dengue has grown dramatically in recent decades. About half of the world's population is now at risk. There are an estimated 100–400 million infections each year, throughout the tropics, notably in South-East Asia, South America, and the Caribbean, and increasingly in urban areas (Fig. 15.3). There are four sero-types, DEN-1 to -4.

Transmission

Day-biting, peri-domestic mosquitoes such as *Aedes aegypti* and *Ae. albopictus* transmit the four types of dengue virus between humans.

Clinical

In most foreign travellers, dengue causes an acute fever associated with headache, backache, pains in the muscles and joints ('break bone' fever), and a rash. A reddish blotchy rash that may blanch on pressure often appears after a temporary lull in the fever. Petechial haemorrhages may be found in the skin and conjunctivae. See ➡ Colour plate 10.

Severe dengue

200,000–500,000 cases of severe, life-threatening dengue occur each year, with 5% case fatality, usually in children born and brought up in endemic areas who are suffering their second infection with a dengue virus type different from that causing their first attack. However, severe and even fatal, apparently primary, dengue infections have been seen in adults, including travellers. After 2–7 days of fever, spontaneous bleeding (nose, gums, GI) and increased capillary permeability leads to shock, haemoconcentration, and thrombocytopenia.

Diagnosis (at the base hospital)

Diagnosis is supported if the blood count shows leucopenia with relative lymphocytosis and thrombocytopenia often with raised liver enzymes and may be confirmed serologically and by PCR.

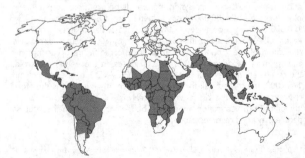

Fig. 15.3 Global distribution of dengue.

Treatment

Generally supportive treatment is needed (bed rest, control of fever and pain with paracetamol). Suspected severe dengue warrants immediate evacuation and correction of hypovolaemia, hypoglycaemia, and electrolyte and acid–base homeostasis but avoidance of corticosteroids, heparin, NSAIDs, and aspirin. Supportive treatment reduces case fatality to <1%.

Prevention

Wear sensible clothing (➲ Box 15.3, p. 305) during the daytime biting period and apply DEET-containing repellents to exposed skin surfaces. Dengvaxia® CYD-TDV vaccine is protective against severe dengue in individuals with serologically confirmed previous dengue and is licensed in the US and Europe. A child immunization programme in the Philippines has been controversial following reports of subsequent severe dengue in some immunized children. Several other vaccines are in phase III trials.

Websites

𝄞 https://travelhealthpro.org.uk/factsheet/13/dengue
𝄞 http://www.cdc.gov/Dengue/
𝄞 http://www.who.int/topics/dengue/en/

Arenaviruses: Lassa fever (West Africa) and Bolivian, Argentine, and Venezuelan haemorrhagic fevers

These Arenavirus zoonoses are acquired through contact with urine of peri-domestic or feral rodents. In West Africa there are thought to be 300,000–500,000 cases of Lassa fever, with 5000 deaths each year. In parts of Liberia and Sierra Leone, the prevalence of Lassa fever among hospital admissions is 10–16%. The overall case fatality rate is 1%, up to 15% among hospitalized patients. Pregnant women and their fetuses are at very high risk. Worldwide >30 cases of imported Lassa fever have been described, the most recent from Mali to UK.

Transmission

Transmission is by contact with urine of multimammate rat (*Mastomys natalensis*) and between humans by contamination with infected body fluids, needlesticks, and sexual contact.

Symptoms

After an incubation period of 6–21 days, Lassa fever presents with insidious fever, malaise, headache, and painful sore throat with visible exudative pharyngitis, conjunctivitis, backache, chest pain, cough, nausea, vomiting and diarrhoea, but no jaundice (despite hepatitis), bleeding, or rash. Hypovolaemic shock (associated with facial oedema) may supervene after ~1 week. Early antiviral treatment with ribavirin (tribavirin) reduces case fatality five- to tenfold.

Prevention

Avoid all contact with rodents (including not eating them) and rodent-contaminated accommodation and food in endemic areas. No vaccine is available.

Websites

𝄞 http://www.who.int/csr/disease/lassafever/en/
𝄞 https://www.cdc.gov/vhf/lassa/

Filoviruses: Marburg and Ebola viruses

In 2013–2014, these filoviruses caused epidemics of highly fatal haemorrhagic fever in Congo DR and Uganda. The first West African epidemic of Ebola virus disease broke out in Guinea in early February 2014, spreading to Sierra Leone and Liberia, with a few cases in adjoining countries.

By the end of the epidemic in early 2016, there had been a total of 28,652 cases (suspected, probable, and confirmed), 15,261 laboratory-confirmed cases, and 11,325 deaths (case fatality 40%). The natural reservoir is probably fruit bats, while other mammals, including higher primates can be infected. Epidemics probably start when infected wild animals ('bush meat') are killed and eaten.

Transmission

Contact with organs, blood, secretions, or other body fluids of infected patients.

Symptoms

After an incubation period of 2–21 days there is sudden fever, fatigue, headache, vomiting, diarrhoea, loss of appetite, weakness, myalgias, and sometimes, a generalized non-pruritic, papular, desquamating, erythematous rash without jaundice (despite hepatitis). In West African patients, hypovolaemia from severe vomiting and diarrhoea is a prominent feature, while bleeding, usually manifest as blood in the stools, is relatively uncommon. Case fatality is from 30% to 90%.

Prevention

By avoiding epidemic areas, especially bat caves and contact with patients blood, vomitus, stool, sputum, and other body fluids and secretions and risk of parenteral infection by needles and sharps. Novel Ebola vaccines are being evaluated in outbreak areas.

Websites

🏵 http://www.cdc.gov/vhf/ebola
🏵 https://travelhealthpro.org.uk/factsheet/68/viral-haemorrhagic-fever
🏵 https://www.gov.uk/government/collections/viral-haemorrhagic-fevers-epidemiology-characteristics-diagnosis-and-management
🏵 https://www.who.int/health-topics/ebola/

Crimean–Congo haemorrhagic fever (CCHF)

This Bunyavirus occurs in Eastern Europe, the Middle East, Africa, and Asia in 2013 in Russia, Kosovo, India, Bulgaria, and South Africa. In 2012, a man, infected in rural Afghanistan, died in UK. It is transmitted by ticks or in infected animal blood (abattoirs, ritual sacrifice). After 3–7 days' incubation period there is sudden fever, headache, photophobia, nausea, vomiting, generalized body pains, thrombocytopenia, leucopenia, and severe bleeding with a case fatality of 15–80%. Treatment with ribavirin may be helpful. No vaccine is available. Avoid tick bites (⟱ p. 308–309) and parenteral exposure.

Hantavirus haemorrhagic fever with renal syndrome (HHFRS or Korean haemorrhagic fever)

A bunyavirus found in Europe, especially Scandinavia, Germany and the Balkans, and Asia. Its symptoms closely resemble leptospirosis. Hantavirus pulmonary syndrome (HPS) occurs in the Americas. In 2012, deer mic

(*Peromys cusmaniculatus*) transmitted hantavirus to ten campers in Yosemite National Park, US, three of whom died.

HHFRS is spread by aerosol from rodent urine or bites. After a long incubation period (12–16 days, up to 2 months), fever, facial flushing, and subconjunctival haemorrhages develop, followed by shock and pulmonary oedema. The case fatality is up to 15% (50% in HPS). Avoid rodent contact and human-to-human spread in HPS. No vaccines are generally available.

Website

℥ http://www.cdc.gov/hantavirus/

Rift valley fever (RVF)

In Africa and the Middle East, RVF is a bunyavirus spread from camels and domestic ruminants by mosquitoes and contamination by infected blood in abattoirs. The largest epizootics since 2006 have been in Kenya, Tanzania, and Sudan. 684 cases with 234 deaths were reported in Kenya (case fatality 34%), 264 cases with 109 deaths in Tanzania (41%), and 738 cases with 230 deaths in Sudan (31%). After 3–6 days' incubation, there is acute fever, mucocutaneous haemorrhages, conjunctivitis, photophobia, eye pains, blinding retinitis, and lymphadenopathy, with occasional progression to disseminated intravascular coagulation (DIC), severe bleeding, encephalopathy, hepatorenal failure, and death. Veterinary vaccines are marketed. Avoid mosquito bites and contact with infected animal blood.

Website

℥ https://www.who.int/news-room/fact-sheets/detail/rift-valley-fever

Chikungunya fever

Chikungunya is a dengue-like *Aedes* mosquito-transmitted alphavirus infection that has caused massive epidemics in Indian Ocean islands, Comoros, Mauritius, Seychelles, Madagascar, Mayotte and Réunion, Africa, Latin America, and Caribbean and Pacific islands (>1.3 million cases) since 2006. Hundreds of cases were imported into France and other European countries from Réunion and the other islands popular with tourists. Local (autochthonous) transmission of Chikungunya by indigenous *Aedes albopictus* mosquitoes was established around Ravenna, Italy, causing thousands of cases. More than 200 imported cases have been identified in UK, mainly from the Caribbean and Latin America.

Clinical

After 2–4 days' incubation there is sudden fever, headache, malaise, conjunctivitis, arthralgia, arthritis (ankles and small joints), myalgia, and low back pain with rash in half the cases. Rashes are very variable: erythematous (blanching), vesicular, bullous, dyshidrotic, keratolytic, purpuric, and hyperpigmented, associated with facial oedema, erythema nodosum, and aphthous ulcers. Joints may be severely and persistently involved with effusions and bursitis. A useful sign is pain on squeezing the wrists (tenosynovitis). Severe and occasionally fatal features are meningoencephalitis, Guillain–Barré polyradiculopathy, myocarditis, hepatic dysfunction, and acute kidney injury.

Prevention

An effective vaccine has been developed in the US but is not generally available. Anti-mosquito measures are the only protection.

Website

🕭 http://www.who.int/mediacentre/factsheets/fs327/en/

Measles, mumps, and rubella (MMR)

There is still widespread global transmission of these predominantly childhood viral illnesses, exacerbated by vaccine hesitancy. Not all travellers will be appropriately immunized and so will be at risk of acquiring these infections on trips.

Transmission

Airborne droplet spread.

Measles

Measles is a highly contagious paramyxovirus illness that is a leading cause of death in young children globally. An infected person can transmit the virus to >90% of unprotected close contacts. Following inhalation of virus-containing droplets, measles replicates in the cells of the nose and throat, and 5–7 days after exposure infection is spread through the blood to the skin, the eye, and the respiratory tract. Patients develop high fever, cold-like symptoms, and conjunctivitis. A typical rash appears after another 3–4 days, spreading from the face and neck to the trunk and extremities. Severe disease is frequently complicated by middle-ear infection or bronchopneumonia. Encephalitis occurs in approximately one in every 2000 reported cases; survivors often have permanent brain damage and intellectual disability. Death, predominantly from respiratory and neurological causes, occurs in one of every 3000 reported measles cases, and is highest in infants and adults compared to children and adolescents. In 2018 there were >140,000 deaths worldwide, predominantly of children aged <5 years in low-income families.

Mumps

Mumps is an acute disease of children and young adults, caused by a paramyxovirus of which there is only a single serotype. Mumps virus is asymptomatic in one-third of infected people. The most common presentation is a few days of fever, headache, anorexia, and myalgia, often followed by swelling of the parotid glands within 48 h. Complications, which may appear simultaneously with these signs or in any sequence, are epididymo-orchitis (frequently in young adults), meningoencephalitis (commonest in children), cranial nerve involvement (especially eighth cranial nerve damage leading to hearing impairment), pancreatitis, oophoritis, mastitis, and myocarditis. Most complications due to mumps infection resolve without permanent damage, in some instances, one or more may be present in the absence of parotitis. Death following mumps is rare and mostly due to encephalitis.

Rubella

Rubella (German measles) gives rise to a mild exanthematous illness, accompanied by few constitutional symptoms, and occurs most commonly in childhood. If the infection occurs in a woman in early pregnancy however the virus may cross the placenta to reach the fetus, in which the infection can induce birth defects. These defects may be serious and permanent and include congenital heart disease, cataract formation, deafness, and intellectual disability.

Prevention

Travellers should ensure that they are adequately immunized with the combined MMR vaccine.

Websites

Measles: 🔗 https://travelhealthpro.org.uk/disease/116/measles
Mumps: 🔗 https://www.cdc.gov/mumps
Rubella: 🔗 https://www.who.int/news-room/fact-sheets/detail/rubella

Middle East respiratory syndrome coronavirus (MERS-CoV)

This coronavirus disease emerged from Saudi Arabia in September 2012. As of January 2020, >2519 cases including 866 deaths have been reported (case fatality 34%). Deaths are mainly in people with chronic comorbidities. Although currently confined to the Arabian Peninsula including Madinah, site of the annual Hajj in the Kingdom of Saudi Arabia, and adjacent countries (Iran, Jordan, etc.), it has been exported to several Western countries in travellers. Possible mammalian reservoirs include camels, cats, and various species of bats. The infection presents as a severe acute pneumonia with respiratory distress and acute kidney injury. It can spread between humans (e.g. to hospital staff). The virus is thought to have pandemic potential. Recent travellers returning from the Middle East who develop severe acute respiratory infections (SARIs) should be tested for MERS-CoV.

Website

🔗 https://www.who.int/csr/don/24-february-2020-mers-saudi-arabia/en/

Avian influenza H5N1

Avian flu is caused by H5N1 influenza virus which naturally infects wild birds and has caused large outbreaks in domestic poultry. The first human cases were identified in Hong Kong in 1997 and it re-emerged in 2003. By 2013, 633 infections with 377 deaths (case fatality 60%) had been reported in Asia, Europe, the Near East, and Africa, the highest burden was in Indonesia and Vietnam. Over 90% of cases have been <40 years old.

Transmission

Transmission is by close contact (aerosol) with infected birds (usually poultry) and eating their uncooked blood or meat.

Clinical

Typical 'flu-like' symptoms such as fever, cough, sore throat, myalgia, conjunctivitis, and pneumonia with acute respiratory distress requiring mechanical ventilation.

Treatment

Oseltamivir and zanamivir may be effective for treatment and prevention of H5N1 viruses, but resistant strains have already evolved.

Prevention
Candidate vaccines have been approved. Watch the epidemic news (see 'Websites') and avoid contact with poultry and wild birds as far as possible, especially commercial or backyard poultry farms and live poultry markets. Do not eat uncooked or undercooked poultry or poultry products, including dishes made with uncooked poultry blood. H5N1 vaccines are being developed. If there is an epidemic, prophylactic/therapeutic oseltamivir will be distributed by WHO and perhaps by some embassies in affected countries. Face mask (preferably N-95) are recommended for high-risk environments by some authorities.

Websites
℧ http://www.cdc.gov/flu/avian/
℧ http://www.who.int/csr/disease/avian_influenza/en/
℧ https://www.gov.uk/government/publications/avian-influenza-guidance-and-algorithms-for-managing-human-cases

Avian influenza H7N9

This strain of avian influenza emerged from China in April 2013 causing >140 confirmed cases with a case fatality of >30%. New cases were reported in Hong Kong in late 2013. A principal risk factor was exposure to poultry in contaminated environments, especially live poultry markets (chickens, ducks, pigeons; not migratory birds). Compared to H5N1 victims the patients were older and more likely to be males. It causes rapidly progressive pneumonia, respiratory failure, acute respiratory distress syndrome (ARDS), and death. Patients had been exposed to poultry and contaminated environments, especially live poultry markets, where H7N9 was found in chickens, ducks, and pigeons. Migratory birds do not seem to be affected.

H1N1 pandemic swine flu

This new H1N1 'triple-reassortant' swine virus, with avian and human flu virus components, arose in Mexico, spreading worldwide via air-travel routes. Between April 2009 and August 2010, it caused 284,500–570,000 estimated deaths (18,500 lab confirmed). Seasonal flu vaccines were ineffective, but those born before the 1950s were protected. The disease was usually mild, sometimes with diarrhoea and vomiting. Case fatality 0.03%. Severe cases (ARDS) were associated with pregnancy, asthma, pulmonary, cardiovascular, neurological, and autoimmune diseases, diabetes, and obesity. Chemotherapy and the WHO's vaccine tender process proved highly contentious.

Other emerging viruses

Australian bat lyssavirus

Closely related to classic rabies virus, was discovered in 1996 in flying foxes (fruit bats) and other bats. It has caused three known human deaths in people who handled bats.

New paramyxoviruses (Henipaviruses)

These are a group of viruses associated with flying foxes and other bats in South Asia and Australia. They include the Nipah virus that caused an epidemic of encephalitis, mainly among pig farmers in Malaysia and Singapore in 1999. In 2018 there was an outbreak resulting in at least 17 deaths in Kerala, South India. As of May 2018, an estimated 700 people have died of Nipah virus, with 50–75% mortality.

Human bocavirus

This is a newly recognized parvovirus associated with lower respiratory tract infection in children in Europe, Thailand, China, Japan, and Australia.

Monkeypox virus

This is an endemic smallpox-like disease in equatorial Africa, which caused a multistate outbreak of >70 human cases in the US in 2003. Pet prairie ('dogs') marmots had been infected by rodents imported from West Africa.

Bacterial infections

Brucellosis

This globally prevalent zoonosis of goats, sheep, and camels (*Brucella melitensis*), cattle (*B. abortus*), and dogs (*B. canis*) has been eliminated from <20 countries. More than 500,000 new cases of *B. melitensis* infection are reported each year.

Transmission

Ingestion of unpasteurized dairy products, especially soft white goats' cheeses, and raw meat. Exposure to infected animal tissue/secretions is an occupational hazard for farmers and abattoir workers.

Clinical

After an incubation period of 1 week to several months, every system can be involved and so the range of symptoms is enormous. Commonly there is acute or insidious persistent fever with chills, arthralgias, septic arthritis, back ache, spinal tenderness signifying osteomyelitis, granulomatous hepatitis, meningoencephalitis, endocarditis, and epididymo-orchitis and other genitourinary infections.

Diagnosis

At the base hospital or after return home in the case of long incubation periods, blood, marrow, and other cultures (prolonged, using special media) and serology (IgG agglutinins difficult to interpret) may prove diagnostic. Laboratory workers are at high risk of transmission, ensure you have informed the lab that brucellosis is a potential diagnosis so they can instigate adequate safety precautions.

Treatment

Doxycycline (oral 100 mg twice a day) and rifampicin (oral 600–900 mg/day) for 6 weeks, or doxycycline for 6 weeks and gentamicin (5 mg/kg IV) for 7–10 days, or streptomycin (0.5–1.0 g/day IM) for 21 days are the most effective regimens.

Prevention

Avoid unpasteurized milk and milk products, especially cheeses and undercooked meat products in parts of the world where brucellosis is prevalent, such as Africa, the Middle East, and Latin America.

Diphtheria

Diphtheria (*Corynebacterium diphtheriae*) usually infects the upper respiratory tract or skin (p. 503) and its toxin can affect the heart, nerves and kidneys. Although largely eliminated by childhood vaccination, diphtheria still occurs in developing countries and has increased in the former Soviet Union.

Transmission

From human to human by aerosol or contact with respiratory tract secretions.

Clinical

After an incubation period of 2–5 days there is inflammation of mucosae usually of the fauces, nasal cavity, trachea, larynx or bronchi, development of the classic greyish-yellow pseudomembrane covering tonsils, pharynx and larynx, local lymphadenopathy, and swelling of the neck ('bull neck'). Diphtheria can cause skin ulcers apparently indistinguishable from simple bacterial ulcers, but they have an area of anaesthesia round them which can be detected by testing pinprick sensation (→ Skin, p. 312).

Treatment

High-dose benzylpenicillin (12 g each day in six divided doses) or erythromycin will eliminate the infection but antitoxin is needed for severe toxic effects, and emergency tracheostomy or needle cricothyroidotomy (→ p. 207–208) may be needed to relieve airway obstruction. Suspected diphtheria warrants immediate evacuation.

Prevention

(See → p. 28.) Childhood immunization in combination with tetanus and pertussis is routine in most countries. For boosting immunity in adult travellers, adsorbed diphtheria (low dose) and tetanus vaccine (formol toxoids) is recommended for adults and adolescents.

Leptospirosis

Leptospirosis is a zoonotic infection by *Leptospira icterohaemorrhagiae* and related strains or serovars, affecting rats, dogs, pigs, sheep, cattle, other mammals including humans, and reptiles and amphibians throughout most parts of the world. Increasing numbers of cases are being detected in South Asia. Leptospirosis is an occupational disease of farmers and sewer workers. Those involved in freshwater sports (canoeing, sailing, water skiing) and exposure to watery, flooded environments are also at risk. During the 10-day Eco-Challenge-Sabah 2000 multisport endurance race, 26% of 304 athletes caught leptospirosis. Andy Holmes, a British Olympic gold medal oarsman, died of leptospirosis in 2010.

Transmission

Infection is acquired when broken skin or intact mucosae are in contact with fresh water contaminated by infected mammals' urine.

Clinical

The incubation period is 2–26 (mean 10) days. Most infections are subclinical or mild but in ~10% severe features, including jaundice, hepatorenal failure, pulmonary haemorrhage, and shock may develop. Symptoms include fever, rigors, headache, myalgia, backache, painful tender calves, meningism, and GI and pulmonary haemorrhages. Jaundice and subconjunctival haemorrhages are common signs.

Treatment

Early treatment with oral doxycycline (100 mg twice daily for 1 week) or parenteral ceftriaxone are the treatments of choice.

Prevention

Avoid contact with fresh water likely to be contaminated by rats and other mammals especially if you have skin abrasions. Doxycycline in the dose taken for malaria prophylaxis (100 mg each day) or 200 mg once each week is protective. Post-exposure prophylaxis after immersion in a river or lake might be appropriate in some circumstances.

Lyme disease

Lyme disease, named after Lyme, in Connecticut, US, is the most common vector-borne disease in North America, where there are ~20,000 new cases reported each year. About 1000 new cases per year are diagnosed in the UK. It is an infection of northern boreal forests common in northern Europe, north-eastern, mid-Atlantic, and north-central US states in people aged 5–14 years and 45–54 years. In N. America it may be accompanied by other tick-borne infections—babesiosis and ehrlichiosis. Lyme disease also occurs throughout forested Europe where it may be accompanied by TBE virus in central and eastern Europe. It is caused by *Borrelia burgdorferi sensu stricto* in North America and by *B. burgdorferi sensu lato* (*B. burgdorferi, B. garinii,* and *B. afzelii*) in Europe. Lyme disease has not been found in tropical countries or in Australia.

Transmission

From mice, deer, and other mammals to humans is by bites of hard (*Ixodes*) ticks.

Clinical

After an incubation of 7–10 days, a red macule/papule and later an expanding red ring (erythema migrans) usually appears around the tick bite site (➔ Colour plate 11) and may be associated with local lymphadenopathy, fever, chills, headache, myalgia, arthralgia, and meningism. The classic erythema migrans does not always appear. Neuroborreliosis, most commonly unilateral facial nerve palsy and radiculopathy are the commoner secondary manifestations in European Lyme, while arthritis is more common in North America. Carditis with heart block, and other rashes may occur.

Diagnosis

Confirmed by serology at the base hospital.

Treatment

Early treatment with oral doxycycline 100 mg twice daily for 14–21 days is curative. Treat erythema migrans empirically. About 15% of patients show a mild exacerbation of symptoms (Jarisch–Herxheimer reaction) within 2 h of starting treatment.

Prevention

Anti-tick measures (➔ Skin, p. 308–309) are important. Chemoprophylaxis before tick attachment is not justified and afterwards only within strict criteria.

Websites

℘ http://www.cdc.gov/lyme/
℘ https://www.gov.uk/government/collections/lyme-disease-guidance-data-and-analysis

Melioidosis

Melioidosis, a dangerous infection caused by soil-dwelling *Burkholder pseudomallei*, is increasingly recognized in South-East Asia, Norther Australia, and the tropical Americas, and as an imported travellers' diseas Infection is usually through exposure of skin lesions to wet fields and flood rarely by ingestion of infected fresh water and inhalation. Severe case are usually immunosuppressed by diabetes mellitus, chronic renal failur urinary lithiasis, alcoholic cirrhosis, malignancy, or corticosteroid or other immunosuppressant treatment. Infection may be latent for many decades (e.g. in US veterans of the Vietnam war).

Clinical features

Local infections and abscesses may involve cutaneous/subcutaneous tissues, lungs, parotids, lymph nodes, bones, joints, liver, spleen, genital tract, and brain. A septicaemic illness is the commonest presentation, often associated with a primary pneumonia but chronic fever and weight loss also occur. Case fatality varies from >40% in South-East Asia to 14% in Australia.

Diagnosis

Can be confirmed only where there are good bacteriological facilities. The organism may be cultured and detected by PCR.

Treatment

Involves drainage of collections of pus and prolonged antimicrobial therapy, first with parenteral ceftazidime or a carbapenem (for at least 14 days), then with oral trimethoprim–sulfamethoxazole for 12–20 weeks.

Prevention

Vulnerable people should avoid exposure to wet or inundated areas in endemic areas, especially if they have open wounds.

Meningitis

Bacterial (pyogenic) meningitis is an acute infection involving the meninges and CSF. Common causes in younger people are the meningococcus (*Neisseria meningitidis*), pneumococcus (*Streptococcus pneumoniae*), and *Haemophilus influenzae* type b (Hib) although all they are increasingly controlled by routine childhood vaccination. Meningococcal meningitis is common across the sub-Sahelian zone of Africa, extending from Senegal to the Sudan ('meningitis belt'; ➲ Fig. 2.1, p. 32), where there are annual cold season epidemics of group A or C disease. Outbreaks may also occur where there are gatherings of people from all over the world, such as in Mecca for the Hajj (check ℘ http://www.promedmail.org for news of current epidemics).

Other causes of acute meningitis include viruses (e.g. herpes simplex, enteroviruses, mumps, etc.); causes of more insidious meningitis/encephalitis are tuberculosis, fungi (e.g. *Cryptococcus*), free-living amoebae (*Naegleria, Acanthamoeba*, and *Balamuthia*) and even worms (e.g. *Angiostrongylus*).

Transmission

By aerosol from infected carriers or cases.

Symptoms

Fever.
Headache.
Photophobia.
Nausea.
Vomiting.
Diarrhoea.
Myalgia.

Meningococcal meningitis

A non-blanching petechial/purpuric rash is characteristic. It is initially macular, often starts on the forearms or shins, and may be visible on the conjunctivae. It spreads over the trunk and face and may become vasculitic with geometrical areas of skin necrosis. Stiff neck (meningism) is the diagnostic sign of meningitis. Ability to flex the neck so that the chin touches the chest or shake the head from side to side virtually excludes meningism. Impairment of consciousness and seizures (children) are ominous developments. Very rapid evolution to classic meningococcal sepsis (profuse rash, shock, bleeding, peripheral gangrene, multiple system failure) occurs in a minority of cases. Meningococcal sepsis can also occur in the absence of meningitis.

Pneumococcal meningitis

There may be an obvious source of infection (e.g. pneumonia, otitis media).

Diagnosis

Unless the diagnosis can be rapidly confirmed by lumbar puncture and CSF examination (unlikely in most expeditions), suspicion of bacterial meningitis warrants immediate, parenteral, preferably IV, antibiotic treatment, and urgent evacuation to the base hospital.

Treatment

Ceftriaxone or cefotaxime (2 g IV or IM 12-hourly) are the antibiotics of choice, covering all causes of bacterial meningitis except *Listeria monocytogenes* (special risk in pregnant women and some immunosuppressed patients; add ampicillin). Benzylpenicillin 2.4 g IV or IM 4-hourly is effective for meningococcal infection. If parenteral treatment is impossible amoxicillin 2 g 4-hourly, or chloramphenicol 100 mg/kg each day in four divided doses can be given by mouth. Adjuvant corticosteroids (dexamethasone 10 mg IV four times daily) should be started pre-antibiotics, in anyone suspected of having pneumococcal meningitis. Steroid should be continued for 4 days if pneumococcal is confirmed, otherwise it should be stopped if an alternative cause is identified.

Prevention

(See ➲ p. 29–32.) Hib vaccine (since 1992), meningococcal group C vaccine (since 1999), and conjugated pneumococcal vaccine since 2006 have been routinely offered to children in Britain. Travel to the African meningitis belt (➲ Fig. 2.1, p. 32) or other areas of current epidemic meningococcal meningitis, justifies group A,C,W135,Y vaccine ('ACWY Vax'). A recombinant protein multicomponent meningococcal group B vaccine is now available. Contacts are treated with ciprofloxacin (500 mg single dose) or rifampicin (600 mg twice daily for 2 days).

Plague

Plague is a bacterial infection carried by rodents and transmitted to human by the bite of an infected rat flea. There is usually gross lymphadenopath at the site of the flea bite (this is the so-called bubo that gives the disease its name of bubonic plague). The infected person may die from a sepsis syndrome. The bacteria may spread to the lungs to give a pneumonia and the bacteria then become transmissible via the airborne route (pneumonic plague). About 2700 cases and 200 deaths from plague are reported each year (case fatality 7%), mainly from Madagascar and other African countries, and southern Asia, but a few are from the western US (Fig. 15.4). Warning of an impending epidemic is a die-off of rats, mice, marmots, etc.

Prevention

If your expedition is going to a notorious plague area (see 'Website') and an epidemic is in progress, consider going elsewhere or taking preventive measures such as avoiding rodents and their parasites, and taking chemoprophylaxis (doxycycline, ciprofloxacin, or co-trimoxazole). No vaccines are currently available.

Website

🔗 http://www.cdc.gov/plague/

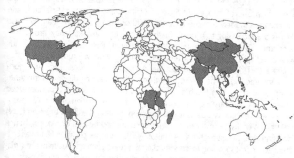

Fig. 15.4 Countries reporting plague cases to the WHO 2013–2018.

Q fever

Q fever is a disease caused by the bacteria *Coxiella burnetii*. These bacteria naturally infect some animals, such as goats, sheep, and cattle. *C. burnetii* bacteria are found in the birth products (i.e. placenta, amniotic fluid), urine, faeces, and milk of infected animals. People can get infected by breathing in dust that has been contaminated by infected animal faeces, urine, and birth products and by consuming dairy products. Some people are asymptomatic; those who become unwell usually develop flu-like symptoms including fever, chills, fatigue, and muscle pain. Complicating organ involvement can occur, such as endocarditis.

Diagnosis

Confirmed by serology or PCR at a base hospital.

Treatment

Doxycycline (100 mg PO twice daily) for 14 days is indicated for acute infection. If organ involvement is confirmed, doxycycline and hydroxychloroquine are recommended for at least 18 months.

Prevention

There is no vaccine. Careful hygiene after animal contact and avoiding unpasteurized dairy products will reduce the risk.

Website
https://www.cdc.gov/qfever/healthcare-providers

Tetanus

Tetanus remains endemic in developing countries and still carries a high case fatality. All patients with contaminated wounds should have their tetanus vaccination history reviewed. A tetanus toxoid booster may be indicated (→ Immunizations, p. 28).

Tuberculosis

TB is the world's most prevalent bacterial infection, infecting 2 billion people, one-third of the world's population. The incidence is 8.8 million new cases of active disease and 1.1 million deaths each year, 23% of which are in India and 17% in China. Throughout most of Africa, Eastern Europe, Asia, and Latin America the incidence exceeds 50/100,000 of the population/year. All these figures are increasing as a result of the human immunodeficiency virus (HIV) pandemic. The causative organism, *Mycobacterium tuberculosis*, shares the genus with other species of mycobacteria, environmental or non-tuberculous mycobacteria (NTM) that are not usually pathogenic to humans. They are more commonly found in the environment, sometimes causing disease in immune-compromised patients (such as *M. avium* complex in HIV-immunosuppressed patients) but only rarely causing problems in the immunocompetent. All mycobacteria have the characteristic staining property that the Ziehl Neelsen (ZN) stain taken up by their cell walls is not decolourized by acid or alcohol, hence 'acid and alcohol-fast bacteria' (AAFB or AFB). Many people are infected as children, sometimes leading to serious clinical disease such as disseminated ('miliary') TB. In most cases, infection is controlled by a normal immune response and held dormant as latent TB infection—this may be reactivated at any time to produce clinical TB disease. It is more likely to occur in someone who becomes immune suppressed due to cancer, HIV infection or immune suppressive drugs such as steroids and the new biologic agents such as infliximab.

Transmission

Transmission is by aerosol created by coughing and, to a far less extent, by ingestion of *M. bovis*-infected (unpasteurized) milk.

Clinical

Typically, if the immune response is inadequate, infection involves the lungs (apical cavitating pneumonia), mediastinal nodes, or pleura during the period up to 2 years after exposure or much later from reactivation of latent infection. Pericardium, lymph nodes (e.g. scrofula of the cervical nodes), kidneys, genital tract, bones, joints, gut or peritoneum, spleen, brain or meninges (tuberculous meningitis), or any other organ may be affected. Fulminant miliary or disseminated TB is most common in children and immunocompromised patients. More commonly, TB develops insidiously. No symptom is diagnostic, but a chronic productive cough lasting for weeks and associated with malaise, weakness, wasting, anorexia, and the classical fever and night sweats are typical presentations of pulmonary TB, the commonest form of the infection.

Diagnosis (at a base hospital)

Confirmed by staining or culturing *Mycobacterium* in sputum or else where or detecting characteristic histopathology in biopsies. Mantoux ski testing has been largely superseded for diagnosis by a blood test. An IGRA (Interferon Gamma Release Assay) blood test can detect active and latent TB and distinguish these from immunity due to BCG vaccination.

Treatment

Quadruple therapy with isoniazid, rifampicin, pyrazinamide, and ethambutol or streptomycin is usually effective, but drug resistance is emerging. Multidrug resistant (MDR-TB) and extensively drug-resistant (XDR-TB) infections have been reported. Adjuvant steroids have been shown to have beneficial to outcomes in TB meningitis.

Prevention

(See ⮕ Immunizations, p. 28.) Intradermal BCG vaccination (⮕ Colour plate 9) provides variable but potentially valuable protection against TB (especially miliary TB and tuberculous meningitis in children) and leprosy. Those born in hyperendemic countries should have been given BCG at birth (look for the scar). BCG vaccination of Mantoux/interferon-gamma negative expedition members is recommended if the destination is in a hyperendemic area and if the programme involves mixing with local people in crowded high-risk environments such as hostels, prisons, refugee camps, hospitals, or clinics. HIV-immunocompromised people should consider taking prophylactic isoniazid (300 mg each day with pyridoxine 50 mg/kg each day) or isoniazid with rifampicin. However, there are potentially serious drug interactions with antiretrovirals and so expert advice should be sought.

Website

℘ http://guidance.nice.org.uk/CG117

Leprosy

Mycobacterium leprae causes leprosy, a skin disease of historic and global importance which is unlikely to infect short-term travellers. It has, however, affected expatriates who have lived for long periods in socially deprived conditions (e.g. missionaries in Papua New Guinea). It affects the skin and peripheral nerves. Diagnosis is confirmed by skin biopsy and demonstration of acid-fast bacilli at specialist centres. Treatment is with dapsone, clofazimine, and rifampicin.

Atypical mycobacteria

These *Mycobacterium* spp. usually cause chronic skin and soft tissue infection. Transmission is by direct inoculation or inhalation. They may need to be considered in chronic non-healing wounds in travellers on return from the expedition and require specialist diagnosis and treatment in a referral centre in the home country.
They include:
- *M. marinum* (⮕ p. 314–315): soft tissue granulomas spreading up the limb lymphatic drainage in fish handlers and tropical fish enthusiasts.
- *M. chelonae* and *M. fortuitum*: similar presentation to *M. marinum* but derived from soil inoculation.
- *M. avium/intracellulare*: causes painless mycobacterial lymphadenitis usually of the cervical or submental glands in children, *or* disseminated disease with fever in HIV/AIDS patients.
- *M. ulcerans*: causes Buruli or Daintree ulcer, an infection of subcutaneous fat leading to expanding ulcers.

Typhoid and paratyphoid (enteric fevers)

Infections by *Salmonella typhi* and *S. aratyphi* A, B, and C are still common in the Indian subcontinent, Vietnam, and Indonesia (100–1000 cases/100,000 population/year). Worldwide, there are an estimated 15–30 million cases and 500,000 deaths each year. Although they are caused by salmonellae, these conditions differ radically from other *Salmonella* infections, being pure human pathogens with no zoonotic reservoir and causing primarily a bacteraemia rather than a luminal GI infection.

Transmission

By faecal–oral spread from water and food infected by human carriers (up to 1% of the population in some communities).

Clinical

After an incubation period of 3–60 (usually 7–14) days, the illness starts insidiously with fever, headache, malaise, abdominal discomfort, some bowel disturbance (often constipation but sometimes diarrhoea), cough, sore throat, and epistaxis. Signs include a slow pulse rate in relation to the fever, hepatosplenomegaly, a blanching macular rash on the abdomen ('rose spots'), rhonchi in the chest, and abdominal tenderness (especially right iliac fossa). Untreated patients may develop severe complications in the second to fourth weeks of illness: perforation, intestinal haemorrhage, shock, and coma.

Diagnosis

By blood, stool, urine, or bone marrow culture.

Treatment

Because of increasing antibiotic resistance, oral azithromycin for non-severe cases (10–20 mg/kg/day for 7 days) is recommended. More severe cases will require parenteral ceftriaxone (50–60 mg/kg/day for 7–14 days) or oral cefixime (20 mg/kg/day for 7–14 days).

Prevention

Strict food and water hygiene (→ Chapter 3) are crucial. Effective injectable and oral vaccines, covering typhoid but not paratyphoid, are available and strongly recommended for all expeditions to developing countries (→ Immunizations, p. 28).

Typhus

Rickettsial bacteria cause a large variety of arthropod-borne acute febrile diseases in most parts of the world, usually with a distinctive rash. Louse-borne epidemic typhus (*Rickettsia prowazeckii*) remains an epidemic threat in poorer countries, mite-borne scrub typhus (*Orientia tsutsugamushi*) is prevalent throughout South-East Asia (Fig. 15.5), tick-borne Rocky Mountain spotted fever (RMSF) (*R. rickettsii*) is one of the most dreaded infections in North America, and tick-borne African tick fever (*R. africae*) is commonly acquired by safari travellers in Southern Africa.

Transmission

By tick or mite saliva during their blood meal, by louse or flea faeces inoculated through skin or mucosae by scratching.

Clinical

After an incubation period of 4–14 (average 7) days, fever, chills, headache photophobia, nausea, vomiting, abdominal pain, and cough may develop

This is followed 3–5 days later by a generalized maculopapular and eventually petechial rash (→ Colour plate 12). A papule appears at the site of the infected bite in spotted fevers such as African tick fever, RMSF and Mediterranean boutonneuse fever, and in scrub typhus (→ Colour plate 12). This evolves into a black-scabbed eschar with lymphangitis and local lymphadenopathy (→ Colour plate 13). Severe multisystem complications may ensue.

Diagnosis

Confirmation is serological and by PCR.

Treatment

Early treatment with oral doxycycline 200 mg once a day for 7 days, azithromycin 1 g stat then 500 mg for 2 days, or chloramphenicol 2 g in four divided doses each day for 2–3 days is appropriate for clinically suspected rickettsial infections. The therapeutic response is often dramatic and diagnostic.

Prevention

Vaccines are not generally available. Doxycycline in the dose taken for malaria prophylaxis (100 mg each day) or 200 mg once each week is protective. Scrub typhus is suppressed rather than eradicated and so it may appear after cessation of chemoprophylaxis. Prevention of tick, louse, flea, and mite infestation is crucial (→ p. 308–309).

Website

℗ http://www.cdc.gov/ncidod/dvrd/rmsf/index.htm

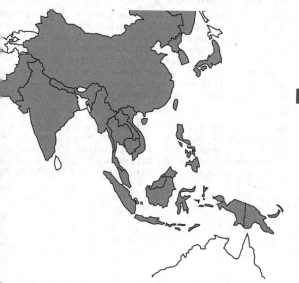

Fig. 15.5 Distribution of scrub typhus in South-East Asia.

Malaria

Malaria occurs throughout the tropics: north to Kyrgyzstan, south to north-eastern South Africa, west to Mexico, and east to Vanuatu in the western Pacific, an area inhabited by >40% of the world's population (Fig. 15.6).

Malaria caused an estimated 241 million cases of fever in 2020, 75% in Africa, 25% in South-East Asia. It killed an estimated 627,000 people, the majority young children and pregnant women in sub-Saharan Africa.

Human malaria parasites

- *Plasmodium falciparum* causes life-threatening falciparum malaria, also called 'malignant tertian malaria'.
- *P. vivax* causes vivax malaria or 'benign tertian malaria', although it can cause severe disease.
- *P. ovale* causes ovale malaria, also 'benign tertian malaria'.
- *P. malariae* causes malariae malaria or 'quartan malaria'.
- *P. knowlesi* causes life-threatening knowlesi malaria, transmitted from monkeys in South-East Asia, especially Borneo.

Transmission

Female *Anopheles* mosquitoes bite between dusk and dawn, transmitting malaria while they suck human blood. Transmission transplacentally (congenital malaria), via blood transfusion, marrow and organ transplant, needlestick, and nosocomially through contaminated injections is also reported.

Imported travellers' malaria

In 2018, 1683 cases (six deaths) of imported malaria were reported in the UK, most of which were caused by *P. falciparum*; 85% of cases were in people travelling to visit friends and relations. Over the past 10 years, an average of six deaths have been reported each year, mostly in people who had not taken prophylaxis. Most of the deaths could have been prevented if travellers had been better educated about mosquito protection and correct chemoprophylaxis and if they had sought prompt medical attention when they fell ill during the first few weeks or months after returning home.

Incubation

The minimum interval between an infective mosquito bite and the first symptom (incubation period) is about 7 days, but most travellers with falciparum malaria become ill within a month of returning home; exceptionally, there may be a delay of more than a year with other forms of malaria. More than 1% of vivax infections present more than a year after leaving the tropics.

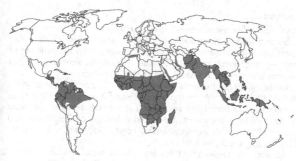

Fig. 15.6 Distribution map for malaria. An interactive map providing details of the current distribution of different malarial types can be found at: 🖰 https://malariaatlas.org/explorer/#/

Symptoms

- Acute severe fluctuating fever with rigors.
- Severe headache.
- Pain in muscles and back.
- Nausea.
- Diarrhoea.
- Loss of appetite.
- Postural hypotension.
- Prostration.
- *Absence* of sore throat, rash, lymphadenopathy.

Classic periodicity of fever is uncommon but the fever often recurs at the same time every day.

Signs

- There may be none and the patient may be afebrile.
- Petechiae, tender enlarged liver and spleen, pale conjunctivae, and jaundice are worth looking for.
- Falciparum malaria in non-immunes (those who have not acquired temporary immunity to malaria through repeated infections) can be a rapidly evolving and potentially life-threatening disease (exceptionally, first symptom to death in 24 h). Worrying features are severe prostration, impaired consciousness (cerebral malaria), seizures, profound anaemia, deep jaundice, hypoglycaemia, shock, renal failure, spontaneous systemic bleeding (suggesting DIC), and respiratory distress.

Diagnosis

(See ℘ http://www.malaria-reference.co.uk/)

Suspect malaria in anyone who develops acute fever >7 days after entering, or within a few months of leaving, a malarious area whether or not they have taken prophylaxis. Consider unusual risks of infection, such as 'runway', 'airport', 'needlestick', and transfusion malarias.

Classic microscopy: this remains the best way of confirming the diagnosis but will be impracticable for most expeditions. Thick and thin blood films, preferably made from finger prick blood at the bedside rather than from blood stored in anticoagulant, are stained with Field's or Giemsa stain and examined (oil immersion, high power). If negative, repeat daily for 72 h before rejecting the diagnosis of malaria.

Rapid malaria antigen tests: these are a convenient alternative to microscopy for expeditions but some training is essential. The tests are quick, sensitive, and species-specific.

The BinaxNOW® malaria test (℘ https://www.alere.com/en/home/products-services/infectious/malaria.html) is available in the UK and approved by the US FDA.

Differential diagnosis

At the base hospital, malaria must be distinguished from other tropical fevers (typhoid, typhus, relapsing fevers, leptospirosis, dengue, and other viral haemorrhagic fevers), less exotic infections such as glandular fever (EBV), pyogenic bacterial infections, meningitis, viral hepatitis, viral encephalitis, HIV seroconversion illness, and heatstroke.

Treatment

Suspected malaria warrants immediate evacuation.

See UK malaria treatment guidelines: ℘
http://www.journalofinfection.com/article/S0163-4453(16)00047-5/pdf and

WHO malaria treatment guidelines: ℘
http://apps.who.int/iris/bitstream/10665/162441/1/9789241549127_eng.pdf

Falciparum malaria

- Wherever *P. falciparum* infection may have been acquired, assume that it is chloroquine resistant.
- For adults who can swallow tablets and keep them down:
  - Artemether-with-lumefantrine (Riamet®, Coartem®, or co-artemether): adult and children >12 years and >35 kg in weight dose four tablets at 0, 24, 36, 48, and 60 h *or*
  - Proguanil hydrochloride-with-atovaquone (Malarone®): adult dose four tablets (children 11–20 kg, one tablet; 21–30 kg, two tablets; 31–40 kg, three tablets) daily for 3 days (best avoided if Malarone® has been used for prophylaxis) *or*
  - Quinine sulphate: adult dose 600 mg (children 10 mg/kg) 8-hourly for 5–7 days followed by either doxycycline 200 mg for 7 days or (pregnant women or children) clindamycin 450 mg three times daily (children 20–40 mg/kg in three divided doses) for 5 days.

- During the first trimester, pregnant women should be treated with quinine + clindamycin, but in the second and third trimesters, artemisinin combination treatment (ACT), e.g. artemether-with-lumefantrine, is considered safe.

Severe falciparum malaria

For adults who are vomiting and unable to swallow and retain tablets or who have severe prostration, impaired consciousness, jaundice, profound anaemia, hypoglycaemia, renal failure, spontaneous systemic bleeding/DIC, black urine, or respiratory distress:

- Sodium artesunate is the drug of choice despite emerging resistance in South-East Asia (http://www.cdc.gov/malaria/diagnosis_treatment/artesunate.html): loading dose 2.4 mg/kg by IV injection followed by 1.2 mg/kg by IV injection daily for a minimum of 3 days, followed by oral antimalarial, e.g. artemether-with-lumefantrine.
- Artemether: loading dose 3.2 mg/kg by IM injection followed by 1.6 mg/kg by IM injection for a minimum of 3 days followed by oral antimalarial (e.g. artemether-with-lumefantrine).
- Quinine dihydrochloride; loading dose 20 mg/kg by IV infusion over 4 h (or IM), then, after 8 h, maintenance dose 10 mg/kg by IV infusion over 4 h (or IM) 8-hourly until able to swallow tablets. Complete the course with quinine sulfate followed by either doxycycline 200 mg for 7 days (*not* for children or pregnant women) or clindamycin 450 mg three times daily (children 20–40 mg/kg in three divided doses) for 5 days. *Quinine may cause hypoglycaemia!*

For severe malaria in areas with established artemisinin resistance (South-East Asia) give parenteral artesunate and parenteral quinine together in full doses.

Consideration will need to be given pre-deployment as to how real the risk of malaria is at the expedition location and what empiric treatment agents will be carried and used.

'Benign' malarias

For adults, chloroquine (BASE) 600 mg (usually four tablets) (children 10 mg BASE/kg) followed by 300 mg after 6–8 h (children 5 mg BASE/kg) followed by 300 mg daily for 2 days (children 5 mg BASE/kg) (total dose ~25 mg BASE/kg body weight). Eradicate liver cycle with primaquine (⊕ p. 520) (beware of G6PD-deficiency!). In New Guinea and adjacent areas of Indonesia (e.g. Lombok), *P. vivax* has become resistant to chloroquine. A double dose of chloroquine or the standard dose of mefloquine, followed by a 4-week course of primaquine, can be used to treat such resistant infections.

Severe *P. vivax* and *P. knowlesi* malaria is increasingly reported. It should be treated as for *P. falciparum*. In many cases malaria speciation will not be available. In these situations, treat as for *P. falciparum*.

Prevention of malaria

Assessing the risk

Within malarious countries, the areas of malaria transmission may be patchy, depending on environmental factors such as temperature, altitude, vegetation, and season. There is no malaria transmission in some African capital cities that are at a comparatively high altitude, such as Addis Ababa and Nairobi, and in other areas malaria transmission occurs only during a brief rainy season. Seek reliable local advice about malaria transmission at the places and times when the expedition will be there. Even within a transmission area, the risk of being bitten by an infected mosquito can vary from less than once per year to more than once per night. The risk of catching malaria during a 2-week visit without any protection has been estimated at about 0.2% in Kenya and 1% in West Africa.

People who are especially vulnerable to malaria, including pregnant women (Box 15.3), should seriously reconsider whether they really need to enter a malarious area.

> **Box 15.3 Principles of personal protection against malaria**
> - Awareness of risk: vulnerable individuals, such as pregnant women, infants, splenectomized or otherwise immunocompromised people, should avoid entering a malarious area
> - Anti-mosquito measures: kill, exclude, repel, and avoid mosquitoes
> - Sensible clothing: long sleeves and long trousers between dusk and dawn
> - DEET-containing insect repellent applied to exposed skin
> - Insecticide (pyrethroid)-impregnated mosquito bed net or screened (air-conditioned) accommodation sprayed with insecticide each evening
> - Vaporizing insecticide in the sleeping quarters (burning mosquito coil, electrical, knock-down insecticide)
> - Chemoprophylaxis: Malarone®, doxycycline, or mefloquine or other drugs, depending on the particular geographical area (➲ p. 517–520). (*Remember that there have been NO deaths in UK travellers who have complied with an appropriate chemoprophylaxis regimen*)
> - Standby treatment: co-artemether, quinine, or Malarone®
> - In case of feverish illness within a few months of return: see a doctor and mention malaria specifically!
> - Avoid all alternative/homeopathic remedies for prevention or treatment of malaria (🔗 https://www.gov.uk/government/publicati ons/malaria-homeopathic-remedies)

Anti-mosquito measures
- *Sleeping quarters:* malaria-transmitting mosquitoes bite in or near human dwellings during the hours of darkness and so the risk of infection can be reduced by insect-proofing sleeping quarters or by sleeping under a mosquito net. Individual, lightweight, self-supporting mosquito nets are available. Protection against mosquitoes and other biting invertebrates (sandflies, lice, fleas, bed bugs, ticks) is greatly enhanced by sleeping under insecticide-treated nets (ITNs). The net is soaked in a pyrethroid insecticide such as 10% permethrin (75 mL or 200–500 mg per m² of material every 6 months). Even better, long-lasting insecticidal nets (LLINs) are factory-treated to retain their activity for at least 20 washes and 3 years of use. Screens and curtains can also be impregnated with insecticide. In addition, bedrooms should be sprayed in the evening with a knock-down aerosol insecticide (e.g. Etofenprox®, Malathion®,

Deltamethrin®) to kill any mosquitoes that may have entered the room during the day. Mosquitoes may also be killed or repelled by vaporizing synthetic pyrethroids (D-allethrin, S-bioallethrin, transfluthrin) on an electrical vaporizing mat (such as No Bite® and Buzz Off®) where electricity is available, or over a methylated spirit burner. Burning cones or coils of mosquito-repellent 'incense' may also be effective.

- *Protective clothing:* to avoid bites by any flying insect, high-necked, light-coloured, long-sleeved shirts, and long trousers afford better protection than vests and shorts. To avoid malaria-transmitting mosquito bites, this sensible clothing should be worn, particularly after dark, even on the beach. Cotton clothes and ankle bands can be impregnated with DEET and other materials can be impregnated with permethrin insecticide.
- *Repellents:* exposed areas of skin should be rubbed or sprayed with repellents containing DEET or p-methane-diol ('Mosiguard Natural'). Insecticide-containing soaps and suntan oil are available.

Antimalarial chemoprophylaxis: two strategies

Two different strategies have been proposed for antimalarial chemoprophylaxis. In areas of high incidence (>10 cases of malaria per 1000 of the local population per year) such as West Africa, the risk of infection outweighs the risk of side effects of taking antimalarial drugs and so chemoprophylaxis is justified. However, in areas of low incidence (<10 cases of malaria per 1000 of the local population per year), such as Central America and Southeast Asia, the risk of taking antimalarial drugs outweighs the risk of infection and so reliance is placed on full anti-mosquito measures and carrying a course of standby emergency treatment (SBET) to be taken if the traveller develops symptoms suggestive of malaria while out of reach of medical care (Table 15.1).

- *Compliance:* the failure of travellers to take their antimalarial tablets regularly, and in particular to continue taking them for long enough after leaving the malarious area (4 weeks for all but Malarone® which need only be taken for 7 days), also reduces the effectiveness of chemoprophylaxis. During bouts of vomiting and diarrhoea (traveller's diarrhoea), these drugs may not be adequately absorbed.
- *Choice of drug:* risk of contracting malaria should be balanced against the relative efficacy and risk of side effects of a particular prophylactic drug.

> No antimalarial drug offers absolute protection. Much depends on compliance. Travellers who become feverish and ill, especially in the early months after their return should consult a doctor and mention the possibility of malaria. If there is any doubt, referral to an infectious/tropical disease unit for exclusion of malaria is an urgent necessity. Antimalarial prophylactic drugs should be stopped until the diagnosis is confirmed or rejected.

Chemoprophylactic drugs and combinations

Atovaquone–proguanil (Malarone®)

This is a safe, effective, and most convenient prophylaxis but it is an expensive drug. Malarone® acts on liver stage parasites and so needs be taken for only 7 days after leaving the malarious region. The dose is one tablet each day for adults. It is not approved in pregnancy but could be used if there is no alternative in the second and third trimester. A register of accidental use in the first trimester has found no evidence of birth defects.

Doxycycline

This tetracycline antibiotic has proved useful for prophylaxis in areas where mefloquine resistance is prevalent, such as the Thai–Cambodian border region. It gives some protection against other travellers' diseases such as typhus, leptospirosis, and some types of travellers' diarrhoea. One 100 mg tablet should be taken every day. Side effects include oesophagitis, photosensitive rashes, skin irritation, diarrhoea, and oral/oesophageal or vaginal thrush. It should be taken while standing up on a full stomach with plenty of fluid to reduce the risk of it becoming stuck in the oesophagus and causing irritation/ulceration. It is best avoided in pregnant women and is contraindicated in children <12 years.

Mefloquine

Mefloquine is effective against some multiresistant *P. falciparum* strains but has some unpleasant side effects: nausea, stomach ache, and diarrhoea in 10–15% of people who take it; insomnia and nightmares; giddiness and ataxia (unsteadiness and incoordination) in some; and a rare 'acute brain syndrome' (psychosis and even seizures).

Contraindications include: a history of previous adverse reactions to this drug, hypersensitivity to quinine, depression, any type of neuropsychiatric disease, and epilepsy. Airline pilots, scuba divers, those who have suffered a traumatic brain injury, and those whose work demands manual dexterity should choose another drug unless they have already proved tolerant of mefloquine.

Adult dose is 250 mg once a week.

Start weekly mefloquine 4 weeks before leaving for the malarious area in case side effects demand a change in treatment. If side effects are going to emerge, it is usually on the third or fourth dose of mefloquine. All antimalarial drugs that kill parasites in the bloodstream must be continued for 4 weeks after return so that late-emerging parasites (hepatic merozoites), protected as long as they remain in the liver, are eliminated when they enter the circulation.

Proguanil and chloroquine

Proguanil—adult dose two tablets (each of 100 mg) every day—and chloroquine—two tablets (each of 150 mg BASE) once a week—is no longer recommended for Africa, the Amazon region, South-East Asia, Assam, and Oceania but remains effective prophylaxis elsewhere. It is safe in pregnancy and (in a lower dose) in children. The only side effects are rare mouth ulcers, mild indigestion, and hair loss. The combination is available in the UK as Paludrine®/Avloclor®.

Chloroquine taken for up to 5–6 years continuously in the dose recommended for prophylaxis against malaria does not cause damage to the eyes, but those who have taken it for >6 years continuously (total cumulative dose approaching 100 g) should have their vision checked.

Table 15.1 Choice of prophylactic strategy in different geographical areas: chemoprophylaxis or standby emergency treatment

Country	Strategy	Drug
Central America + Hispaniola	SBET	Chloroquine
South America: Brazil— Rondônia, Roraima, Acre; Guyana, Suriname, French Guiana—interior	Chemoprophylaxis	Malarone®, mefloquine, or doxycycline
South America: other malarious areas	SBET	Riamet® or Malarone®
Africa (including Madagascar): malarious areas	Chemoprophylaxis	Malarone®, mefloquine, or doxycycline
Middle East: malarious areas	SBET	Riamet® or Malarone®
Central India, Assam, SE Bangladesh*	Chemoprophylaxis	Chloroquine-proguanil/ Malarone®, mefloquine, or doxycycline*
Some parts of Burma, Laos, Cambodia, Vietnam*	Chemoprophylaxis	Malarone® or doxycycline
Rest of Indian subcontinent and Southeast Asia + China: malarious areas*	SBET	Riamet® or Malarone®
Lombok, Eastern Indonesia, New Guinea, Solomon Islands	Chemoprophylaxis	Malarone®, mefloquine, or doxycycline
Vanuatu	SBET	Riamet® or Malarone®

*For more details see: https://assets.publishing.service.gov.uk/government/uploads/system/uploads/attachment_data/file/833506/ACMP_Guidelines.pdf

Pregnant women

Pregnant women should avoid entering a malarious area because of the risks to them and their fetus. If exposure is unavoidable, full anti-mosquito precautions and chemoprophylaxis are essential. The hazards of getting malaria, particularly *P. falciparum* malaria, during pregnancy exceed the small but finite hazard of adverse effects to the baby of the antimalarial drugs. Proguanil and chloroquine are safe. Mefloquine may be an acceptable alternative where there is a high risk of infection and this combination is ineffective. Doxycycline and Malarone® should be used only if there is no alternative.

Standby emergency treatment

SBET is appropriate for two categories of travellers:
1. Those visiting areas of low malaria risk (Table 15.1) who are not taking antimalarial chemoprophylaxis.
2. Those visiting remote areas with a high risk of malaria who are taking appropriate chemoprophylaxis (in case of infection breaking through their prophylaxis).

Both groups should carry a course of standby treatment to be taken if they develop a malaria-like fever but do not have ready access to hospitals and diagnostic laboratories. This must not delay their seeking medical treatment at the base hospital as soon as possible. Appropriate drugs for standby treatment are:

- Artemether-with-lumefantrine (Riamet®, Coartem®, or co-artemether): adult dose four tablets at 0, 24, 36, 48, and 60 h or
- Quinine sulfate: adult dose 600 mg 8-hourly for 5–7 days followed by either doxycycline 200 mg for 7 days or clindamycin 450 mg three times daily for 5 days or
- Proguanil hydrochloride-with-atovaquone (Malarone®) four tablets daily for 3 days (unless in category 2 this drug is being taken for prophylaxis).

Prevention of the 'benign' malarias (P. vivax, ovale, and malariae)

Weekly chloroquine or mefloquine prevent *P. vivax*, *ovale*, and *malariae* malarias. However, *P. vivax* and *P. ovale* can establish themselves in the liver despite chloroquine prophylaxis and may re-emerge to cause relapsing infections months or years later. Primaquine, adult dose 15 mg a day for 2 weeks, eradicates latent liver infection (hypnozoites) and should be given to travellers who have spent more than a few months in areas where these species are endemic (beware of G6PD deficiency!). In parts of Indonesia, particularly Irian Jaya, and in Papua New Guinea, Thailand, the Philippines, and the Solomon Islands, Chesson-type strains of primaquine-resistant *P. vivax* require a 4-week course of primaquine.

Useful websites and other information

♪ http://travelhealthpro.org.uk/factsheet/52/malaria
♪ http://www.who.int/malaria/publications/atoz/9789241549127/en
♪ https://www.gov.uk/government/collections/malaria-guidance-data-and-analysis

Advice on prophylaxis

♪ https://www.gov.uk/guidance/mrl-reference-diagnostic-and-advisory-services#advisory-service

Emergency advice for malaria treatment

- Hospital for Tropical Diseases, London, UK:
  - Emergency Admission: Tel: +44 (0)20 7387 9300 and ask for the Duty Doctor.
  - Tel: +44 (0)20 34567890 and ask for Duty Tropical Diseases Doctor.

Other protozoal infections

Leishmaniasis

Leishmania can cause a spectrum of skin, mucosal membrane, and visceral infections in humans and animals in the Mediterranean, Middle East, Africa, Asia, and in North, Central, and South America (Fig. 15.7). An estimated 1.5–2 million cases of cutaneous leishmaniasis and 500,000 cases of visceral leishmaniasis (kala-azar) occur each year.

Transmission

Leishmania are transmitted from infected humans or animals by the bite of tiny sandflies (Phlebotomus, Lutzomyia).

Clinical

- Cutaneous leishmaniasis: days to months after the infected sandfly bite, a nodule appears that grows, crusts, and ulcerates over weeks to months. The classic 'oriental sore' is 1–5 cm in diameter, painless with raised edges and granulating apple jelly base, and small satellite lesions on an exposed area (➡ Colour plate 14). Lesions may slowly heal or persist, recur, and spread.
- Mucocutaneous leishmaniasis: infection with some Latin American Leishmania presents with a cutaneous ulcer but (sometimes years) later destructive lesions develop in the nasopharyngeal mucosa.
- Visceral leishmaniasis (kala-azar): there is fever, massive splenomegaly, hepatomegaly, wasting, hypersplenism, and secondary bacterial infection. Post-kala-azar dermal leishmaniasis may develop, after apparent recovery. HIV-immunosuppressed patients are especially vulnerable.

Diagnosis

Scrapings from the nodular edge of the sore are stained with Giemsa and examined microscopically. Mucosal lesions are biopsied. Scrapings and biopsies can be tested by PCR. Kala-azar can be confirmed serologically (direct agglutination test or rK39 dipstick test) (➚ http://bmj.com/cgi/doi/10.1136/bmj.38917.503056.7C) and in hospital, intracellular amastigotes can be seen in splenic or bone marrow aspirate, liver or lymph node biopsy or buffy coat.

Treatment for cutaneous leishmaniasis

Small sores can be excised, larger ones can be injected with sodium stibogluconate twice weekly for 2–3 weeks or the lesions can be left to heal. Oral fluconazole 200 mg/day for 6 weeks is proving effective for cutaneous Old World leishmaniasis caused by L. major and L. tropica. For infections acquired in Latin America; unless L. brasiliensis, L. panamensis, and L. guyanensis, which carry the risk of mucosal involvement, can be excluded; prolonged courses of IV treatment with drugs such as sodium stibogluconate, pentamidine, paromomycin (L. aethiopica), ketoconazole or fluconazole (L. major, L. mexicana) are needed. For kala-azar, oral miltefosine or prolonged courses of IV treatment with drugs such as sodium stibogluconate or amphotericin B are needed. None of these treatments are likely to be urgent and expert advice should be sought after return.

Prevention

Avoid bites by nocturnally active sandflies tiny enough to penetrate ordinary mosquito nets but deterred by pyrethroid-impregnated bed and face nets, wear sensibly ample clothing, and apply DEET-containing repellent to skin, cotton clothing, and ankle bands.

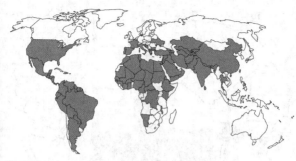

Fig. 15.7 Leishmaniasis distribution worldwide.

African trypanosomiasis (sleeping sickness)

An estimated 40,000 new cases of sleeping sickness occur each year in a number of smallish areas scattered throughout West, Central, East, and southern Africa (Fig. 15.8). There is currently a resurgence of the disease in Angola, Central African Republic, Uganda, Nigeria, and adjacent countries following the breakdown of control measures. A few foreign travellers, especially to the game parks of eastern and southern Africa, have been infected.

Transmission

Tsetse flies (*Glossina*) transmit the trypanosomes causing Gambian sleeping sickness (*Trypanosoma brucei gambiense*) between humans and those causing Rhodesian sleeping sickness (*T. b. rhodesiense*) between humans and animal reservoir hosts (game, antelopes, etc.).

Clinical

A small ulcer with a scab ('chancre') may appear at the site of the infected tsetse fly bite and, within the next few days, intermittent fever begins, associated with headache, loss of appetite, and enlargement of lymph glands, especially in the posterior triangle of the neck. Eventually, there is invasion of the CNS, and patients become apathetic, sleepy, and eventually comatose.

Diagnosis

By finding motile trypanosomes in lymph node aspirates, blood, or CSF and by serology.

Treatment

Pentamidine or suramin are used before CNS invasion. Drugs used after CNS invasion (detected by CSF examination), melarsoprol, eflornithine, and nifurtimox are toxic. Fexinidazole is a new oral drug for the treatment of *T. b. gambiense*.

Prevention

Chemoprophylaxis is not feasible. Avoid tsetse fly bites by wearing sensible clothing (light-coloured, not blue) and applying repellents.

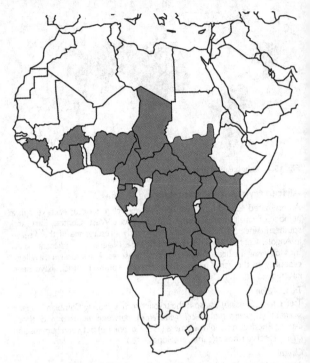

Fig. 15.8 Distribution of African trypanosomiasis.

American trypanosomiasis (Chagas' disease)

In Latin America, there are 300,000 new cases of *Trypanosoma cruzi* infection each year and there are 7–8 million chronically infected people, especially in Brazil, Bolivia, and the countries further south. The Southern Cone control programme reduced transmission by >65%, from an estimated 700,000 new cases per year in 1983, to <200,000 cases per year in 2000.

Transmission

Transmission from a variety of peri-domestic opossums and other mammals is usually by inoculation of faeces of blood-sucking triatomine bugs (➔ Insect bites, p. 292) and not by their bites. Rarely, transmission by drinking juices made from berries of açaí or bacaba palms or cane sugar 'garapa' in which infected bugs have been accidentally ground up, by blood transfusion and other parenteral routes, transplacentally, and via breast milk has been documented.

Clinical

Bugs frequent traditional mud and thatch huts (up to 10,000 per hut). They drop onto the faces of sleeping humans where they feed, defecate, and infect. Waking with a swollen painful eye (Romaña's sign) indicates conjunctival infection. A chancre (chagoma) appears at the site of skin infection. A febrile systemic illness may follow and, eventually, debilitating chronic dilatation may affect the heart, oesophagus, bowel, ureters, and other organs after invasion, multiplication in macrophages, and destruction of autonomic innervation. Cardiomyopathy is a major cause of death.

Diagnosis

Can be confirmed in the acute phase by finding the trypanosomes in blood smears, by isolating them in clean bugs fed on the patient's blood, ('xenodiagnosis') or by serology.

Treatment

Early benznidazole ('Rochagan' Roche) 5–7 mg/kg each day in two divided doses for 60 days is essential in an attempt to limit invasion of tissues.

Prevention

In endemic areas, avoid sleeping quarters conducive to bug infestation, or apply repellents to exposed surfaces and mattresses and sleep under a pyrethroid-impregnated net (➔ p. 516). Avoid uncooked palm or cane sugar juices that have been left unprotected.

Filarial worms

Onchocerciasis (river blindness)

In parts of East, West, Central, and southern Africa, Yemen, and north-eastern South America (Fig. 15.9), pernicious little black flies (e.g. *Simulium damnosum*) transmit this infection from human to human in the vicinity of fast-flowing rivers, streams, and waterfalls.

Clinical

The adult filarial worms live in subcutaneous nodules, especially around the waist. They produce enormous numbers of microfilariae which cause irritation and changes in the pigmentation and texture of the skin and damage the eyes, eventually causing river blindness. Foreign travellers have contracted onchocerciasis after only brief stops in the transmission zone. They may present a year later with a localized or generalized itchy red macular/maculopapular rash.

Diagnosis

Eosinophilia is usual. Microscopic examination of skin snips taken from affected areas reveals wriggling microfilariae. ELISA and PCR are sensitive and specific.

Treatment

Ivermectin (dose 150 micrograms/kg) followed by 6 weeks of doxycycline 200 mg once daily, then a further stat dose of ivermectin is effective treatment. However, this may cause damaging exacerbation of lesions in the eye and skin, and initiation of therapy should therefore be supervised in a hospital.

Prevention

Wear light-coloured clothing (long sleeves and long trousers) and apply DEET-containing repellents to exposed areas of skin. Avoid unnecessary stops and camping near *Simulium*-infested waters.

Elephantiasis (lymphatic filariasis)

Throughout vast areas of tropical America, Africa, Asia, and the western Pacific, mosquitoes (*Culex* and *Anopheles* spp.) transmit filarial infections that cause fever and chronic inflammation with obstruction of the lymphatic system, producing grotesque lymphoedema of the limbs and scrotum and other complications such as chyluria, lymphuria, and pulmonary eosinophilia (Fig. 15.10). Mosquito vectors can be controlled by insecticides, etc. and excluded by using mosquito nets; population-based chemoprophylaxis with diethylcarbamazine has proved effective. If your expedition is going to an endemic area, find out more from the websites given below.

Websites

℘ http://www.who.int/mediacentre/factsheets/fs102/en/
℘ https://www.cdc.gov/parasites/lymphaticfilariasis/
℘ https://www.gaelf.org

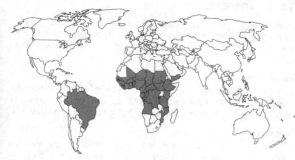

Fig. 15.9 World distribution of onchocerciasis.

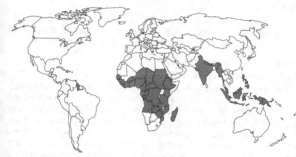

Fig. 15.10 World distribution of lymphatic filariasis.

Worm infections

Passing a wriggling worm-like object in the stools, or even worse vomiting one up, is a singularly unpleasant experience. Intestinal worm infections are enormously prevalent in developing countries where they cause much debility.

Transmission

Worms can be transmitted by ingestion of their eggs or cysts in food (e.g. *Ascaris*, tape worms, liver flukes), by human contact (e.g. pin worms), or percutaneously by filariform larval worms (hook worms and *Strongyloides*).

Diagnosis

Identify the worm that has been passed. Suspect infection if someone has anorexia, malaise, and weight loss, and looks anaemic. Confirmation is by identifying specific helminth eggs in the stool. There may be significant blood eosinophilia.

Prevention

Ensure that all food, especially meat, fish, and green vegetables and salads, is thoroughly cooked, that people wear proper shoes, especially in areas contaminated by human faeces, and that latrines are properly constructed.

Round worms (nematodes)

'Round worm' (Ascaris lumbricoides)

(12–35 mm long, 2–6 mm thick, pale brown with white longitudinal lines.) Looks like an earth worm. It may be found in the stool, emerging from the anus, or even the nose or mouth. Infection is acquired by ingesting eggs in uncooked food, especially green vegetables and salads fertilized with human faeces. There are usually no symptoms except for mild cough or asthma when larvae are migrating through the lungs. Rarely, a worm may block the appendix, bile duct, or pancreatic duct, causing acute inflammation. A mass of worms may obstruct the intestine.

Hook worm (Ancylostoma, Necator)

(7–13 mm long, 0.3–0.6 mm thick, white, grey, reddish brown.) Infection is usually acquired when larvae that have hatched from human stools on the ground penetrate the skin of a bare foot and travel via lymphatics and the lungs into the gut where they attach to the jejunal mucosa. Symptoms (tiredness, anaemia, oedema) result from chronic blood loss. Infection with dog and cat hookworms causes 'cutaneous larva migrans' (➲ Colour plate 2).

Strongyloidiasis (Strongyloides stercoralis)

(2.5 mm long.) Larvae in moist soil penetrate exposed skin and disseminate in the bloodstream, eventually reaching the small bowel. A skin eruption 'larva currens' may be the only evidence of infection. Cough, tracheitis, wheeze, and gut symptoms may develop and, in immunosuppressed people, hyperinfection may cause potentially fatal diarrhoea, Gram-negative septicaemia, pneumonia, and meningitis.

Whip worm (Trichuris)

(30–50 mm long, greyish-white or pink.) Whip worm infection is acquired by ingesting eggs. Massive infections cause anaemia, colitis with blood and mucus in the stools, and sometimes appendicitis and rectal prolapse. Visible worms may be passed.

Pin worms (Enterobius vermicularis)

(2.5–13 mm long, white.) Lay their eggs around the anal verge, causing intense nocturnal pruritus ani, scratching and excoriation of perianal skin, and insomnia. Eggs contaminate the microenvironment and are spread among the family by ingestion or inhalation. The host is reinfected by licking contaminated fingers. Diagnosis is confirmed by microscopic detection of eggs stuck to strips of sellotape applied to the anal margin on waking.

Treatment

All these round worm infections can be treated with albendazole 400 mg single dose or mebendazole 100 mg twice each day (first line for whip worm) for 3 days. However, those with hookworm infection may need haematinics for iron deficiency, and treatment of pin worm infection should include the whole household and must be repeated after 1 week.

Flukes

Schistosomiasis (bilharzia)

This trematode infection occurs in Africa, the Middle East, eastern South America, China, and South-East Asia (Fig. 15.11). Infection is acquired through contact with fresh water from lakes and sluggish rivers, usually by bathing or washing with water taken from these sources. Infected humans contaminate the lake by defecating or urinating into it and infect, in turn, the intermediate snail hosts. Snails release tiny cercariae into the water which burrow through the skin of bathers.

Clinical

The earliest symptom of possible infection is 'swimmer's itch', experienced soon, sometimes minutes, after contact with infected water. Some people develop an acute feverish illness associated with an urticarial rash and blood eosinophilia a few weeks after infection ('Katayama fever'). Later symptoms include passing cloudy or frankly blood-stained urine or dysentery and, rarely, ascending paralysis and loss of sensation in the lower limbs. Travellers usually get worried about bilharzia when they get back from their trip and remember bathing in forbidden lakes or hear that schistosomiasis has been diagnosed in another member of the party.

Diagnosis

Search for characteristic ova in stool, urine (midday, centrifuged, end-stream sample is optimal) or rectal biopsy, or by serology.

Treatment

One to two doses of praziquantel 40 mg/kg orally.

Prevention

Avoid bathing in brackish fresh water sources in endemic areas. Local advice may be misleading. Lake Malawi, officially declared free of bilharzia, has been the source of many imported cases of bilharzia in the UK over the last few years.

Screening of returned travellers

Although routine screening is not indicated, groups of people travelling with and presumed to have shared the same exposure as a confirmed case deserve to be tested, as do those who were at particularly high risk. Ova can be detected as soon as 3–4 weeks after exposure. If asymptomatic travellers are screened, wait 3 months after exposure before doing serology. Many travellers who have swum in Lake Malawi have purchased praziquantel locally to take immediately. However, their purchase may not contain any active praziquantel, and taking it immediately post-exposure (swim) is far too early in the life cycle for it to be effective.

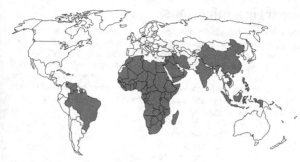

Fig. 15.11 Geographic distribution of schistosomiasis.

Liver flukes

Liver fluke *Fasciola hepatica* (20–30 × 8–13 mm) and intestinal fluke *Fasciolopsis buski* (20–75 × 8–20 mm) infections result from ingestion of metacercariae attached to water cress, water chestnuts, and other freshwater plants. Liver fluke (*Clonorchis*, *Opisthorchis*) (7–25 × 3–5 mm) infections acquired by eating freshwater fish are very common in South-East Asia and China. Anorexia, RUQ abdominal pain, tenderness and hepatomegaly, and episodes of cholangitis are typical of liver fluke infection. Nausea, anorexia, abdominal discomfort, and lienteric diarrhoea (passing undigested food) are typical of heavy *F. buski* infections.

Treatment

Praziquantel 25 mg/kg three times daily after meals for 2 days is effective for all flukes except *F. hepatica*, which should be treated with triclabendazole 2 doses 10 mg/kg, 12 h apart.

Tape worms (cestodes)

Beef (*Taenia sagginata*) (4–12 m long, 5–7 mm thick whitish, semi-transparent) or pork (*T. solium*) (3–8 m long, 5–7 mm thick, yellowish) tape worms are acquired by eating inadequately cooked meat containing viable cysticerci (e.g. 'measly' pork). Passing a long tape worm through the anus or seeing the elongating and contracting whitish reproductive segments (proglottids) (18–30 × 5–7 mm) in the stool or vomitus are the commonest symptoms, but nausea, abdominal pain relieved by eating, pruritus ani, and weight loss are common. Neurocysticercosis, a complication of *T. solium* infection, presents with seizures. This results from swallowing faecally contaminated food containing *T. solium* eggs. The larval tapeworms settle in tissue like muscle and brain and form cysts. It is the pressure and scarring of the cysts in the brain that can cause seizures.

Treatment

Niclosamide 2 g as a single morning dose or praziquantel 10–20 mg/kg as a single dose after breakfast is effective for gut tapeworms. It is important to exclude brain lesions before treatment with praziquantel. Treating neurocysticercosis is more complex, and expert advice should be sought.

Emerging infections

Over the past decade, a number of entirely new pathogens have emerged as important causes of (sometimes epidemic) human disease; some known pathogens have mutated into drug-resistant strains and others have re-emerged. Members of expeditions to remote areas might, like 'sentinel animals', be exposed to some of these known emerging and unknown re-clusive pathogens enzootic in wild animals. They should be aware of current epidemics to assess risk and plan prevention.

℘ http://www.cdc.gov/mmwr/
℘ http://www.promedmail.org/
℘ http://www.who.int/wer/en/
℘ http://wwwnc.cdc.gov/eid/
℘ https://travelhealthpro.org.uk/outbreaks

Coronavirus disease 2019 (COVID-19)

This infection emerged in Wuhan, China, in December 2019 and has resulted in a global pandemic. As of September 2022, there have been >612 million cases with 6.5 million deaths affecting all continents. The virus appears very transmissible but less pathogenic than SARS or MERS-CoV. It is thought to have been derived from bats via wild pangolins sold in the market in Wuhan.

Transmission
Airborne droplets and close human-to-human contact.

Clinical
After an incubation period of 1–14 days, fever (>38°C), myalgia, lethargy, malaise, chills, non-productive cough, sore throat, and loss of taste/smell may develop, although the magnitude of symptoms is very variable. There may be progression to severe respiratory distress, while hypercoagulability syndromes can produce multisystem effects including renal failure and stroke. Mortality is highest in the elderly, those with pre-existing cardio-respiratory morbidity and the obese. Significant morbidity may follow severe infection, so-called long COVID.

Diagnosis
PCR of nasopharyngeal secretions and serology.

Treatment
Supportive treatment may include non-invasive respiratory support or ventilation. Dexamethasone reduces mortality in seriously ill patients. Remdesivir, molnupiravir, and other antiviral agents are used in the treatment of patients.

Prevention
The use of face masks and social distancing help to reduce the spread of illness. Vaccination reduces the risk of serious illness and death. In February 2022 four vaccines were available in the UK—Moderna, Oxford/AstraZeneca, Pfizer/BioNTech, and Janssen.

Emerging bacteria

New antibiotic-resistant strains of bacteria are constantly emerging (℘ http://www.cdc.gov/drugresistance/).

Drug-resistant strains are increasingly important globally causing infections which may not respond to conventional antibiotics.

Emerging antibiotic-resistant strains. Some examples are:

- Penicillin-resistant pneumococci which cause pneumonia or meningitis. These are usually sensitive to ceftriaxone.
- Meticillin (MRSA) and vancomycin-resistant *Staphylococcus aureus*, which may be community acquired, and Panton–Valentine leucocidin (PVL)-positive strains of *S. aureus*. The majority of strains of *S. aureus* causing skin and soft tissue infection in the US and several other countries are resistant to flucloxacillin which is the mainstay of staphylococcal treatment. Strains that produce the toxin PVL may cause more severe systemic and recurrent infection. Group A streptococci (GAS), *Streptococcus pyogenes*, although not antibiotic resistant, can cause very severe septic shock by toxin-mediated immune modulation. The focus is usually soft tissue, although it can be the throat or genital tract. The recognition and management of impending sepsis is crucial. In the absence of a hospital, fluid resuscitation and oral linezolid (600 mg 12-hourly), expensive and probably difficult to acquire, may be an effective holding measure for severe MRSA and invasive GAS.
- Extended spectrum beta-lactamase (ESBL)-producing *Escherichia coli*, carbapenemase-producing *Klebsiella pneumoniae* (with New Delhi Metallo-beta-lactamase-1 (NDM-1)), and other Gram-negative organisms have become highly resistant to many if not all antibiotics. These multiresistant organisms pose a major global health hazard. They cause the same infections as sensitive Gram-negative organisms (i.e. urinary, biliary, and intra-abdominal sepsis), but fail to respond to conventional antibiotics. In many countries, such organisms have entered the food chain through water and food and are selected out as the predominant bowel organisms by antibiotic treatment. They are usually carried harmlessly but should be considered when infections fail to respond to treatment. Microbiology investigations may be essential to establish sensitivity.
- *Stenotrophomonas maltophilia* and other environmental pseudomonads may become important in critically ill patients, particularly those with intravascular lines, ventilation, and who have also received broad-spectrum antibiotics. These organisms are also multiresistant, although cotrimoxazole is the treatment of choice for *Stenotrophomonas*.
- Vancomycin- and teicoplanin-resistant *Enterococcus faecium* are important in certain hospital units. Linezolid is active against these organisms.
- Multiresistant gonococci, fluoroquinolone-resistant typhoid bacilli (*Salmonella typhi*), and tetracycline-resistant scrub typhus (*Orientiatsutsgamushi*) all require expert management.
- *Acinetobacter baumannii* is an intrinsically multiresistant bacterium associated with some recent blast victims from Afghanistan and Iraq. It has caused some nosocomial outbreaks.
- *Rhodococcus equi* can cause severe lung disease in HIV-immunocompromised people, and *Arcanobacterium haemolyticum* causes bacterial pharyngitis. Both are diphtheria-like bacteria.
- Emerging rickettsia-like organisms include *Ehrlichia chaffeensis* which causes human monocytic ehrlichiosis, *Anaplasma phagocytophilum*

(human granulocytic anaplasmosis), and *Ehrlichia ewingii* (human granulocytic ehrlichiosis) are rare pathogens. Diagnosis is available by PCR at the Rare and Imported Pathogens laboratory, Public Health England.

Other emerging pathogens

Cyclosporiasis

Since 1996, the coccidian protozoan, *Cyclospora cayetanesis*, has been increasingly recognized as a cause of giardiasis/cryptosporidiosis-like GI symptoms in travellers. There have been some epidemics related to imported berries, herbs, and salads.

Balamuthia mandrillaris

A free-living amoeba of tropical fresh water environments that can cause devastating cutaneous, nasal, and intracerebral disease.

Microsporidiosis

Many species of protozoan microsporidia (e.g. *Encephalitozoon* spp.) are now recognized as causes of keratoconjunctivitis and GI, biliary, urinary, and respiratory tract, and muscle infections in severely immunocompromised people.

Sexually transmitted infections

Definition

Any disease transmitted by sexual contact.

Epidemiology

Sexually transmitted infections (STIs), although mostly curable, are often asymptomatic, are easily transmissible, can cause serious complications, and can affect anybody.

Incidence

The exact data for infections worldwide are unknown, although the WHO estimated 376 million new cases of curable STIs globally in 2016, with the largest numbers in South/South-East Asia, sub-Saharan Africa, Latin America, and the Caribbean.

Causes

Of the eight main infections transmitted sexually, four are curable: bacterial STIs *Chlamydia trachomatis*, *Neisseria gonorrhoeae*, and syphilis (*Treponema pallidum*), and *Trichomonas vaginalis* (a parasitic flagellate protozoan). The remaining four are incurable though preventable and treatable viral STIs: HIV, herpes simplex virus (HSV), human papillomavirus (HPV or warts), and HBV. Hepatitis types A and C can also be transmitted sexually.

Risk factors

Any unprotected sexual contact, including skin-to-skin contact (for HSV and HPV), and fluid-to-fluid contact.

Prevention

Must be considered prior to travel:
- Hepatitis A and B vaccination (➔ Immunizations, p. 28).
- Practise safe sex.
- Avoid sexual contact with higher-risk groups (e.g. sex workers).
- Barrier contraception/condoms—take them with you. Condoms purchased abroad may not conform to British safety standards and may break.
- Protected oral sex: some infections (e.g. chlamydia and gonorrhoea) can also be carried in the throat and can be transmitted this way. Hepatitis A can be transmitted through oral–anal routes. Use flavoured condoms and dental dams (squares of latex for oral–vaginal/oral–anal contact).

Treatment

For up-to-date STI treatment guidelines see the website of the British Association for Sexual Health and HIV (BASHH): ℘ https://bashh.org/guidelines

Sexual assault
See ➔ p. 182.

Urethral discharge

Definition
Pus/fluid coming from the urethral orifice in the glans penis.

Causes
Most common causes are chlamydia, gonorrhoea, and non-specific urethritis (NSU). HSV can also cause urethral discharge but would usually be accompanied by painful genital sores/blisters.

Organisms

Chlamydia
- Caused by bacterium *Chlamydia trachomatis*.
- Transmitted via oral/vaginal/anal contact, or direct inoculation of infected secretions from one mucous membrane to another.
- About 50% of men are asymptomatic.
- Typically clear/white urethral discharge ± dysuria.

Gonorrhoea
- Caused by bacterium *Neisseria gonorrhoeae*.
- Transmitted via oral/vaginal/anal contact, or direct inoculation of infected secretions from one mucous membrane to another.
- About 10% of men are asymptomatic.
- Typically yellow/green urethral discharge ± dysuria.

Non-specific urethritis (NSU)
(Assuming *Chlamydia* and gonorrhoea are not the cause.)
- Up to 30% have no bacterial pathogen.
- Possible causes are *Trichomonas vaginalis* (1–17%), *Mycoplasma genitalium* (20%), urinary tract infection, *Candida*, foreign bodies, chemical irritation (e.g. soaps, washing powders).
- Typically clear/white discharge may only be present on urethral massage ± dysuria.

Investigations
These depend on the equipment available. Ideally, a Gram-stained urethral smear to confirm diagnosis of gonorrhoea and NSU, leucocyte esterase dipstick for NSU on first-catch urine, nucleic acid amplification test (NAAT) test on a first-catch urine for chlamydia and gonorrhoea, and culture on urethral swab for gonorrhoea.

Management
- Avoid sexual contact to prevent further transmission.
- Ensure partner(s) are informed and treated prophylactically.
- Ideally, test the patient as soon as possible to avoid STI complications.
- Consider treating if investigations are not possible and there is uncomplicated infection (no testicular pain, no eye symptoms).
- If patient is treated, recommend full STI screen when they return home.

Treatment

BASHH guidelines suggest:

- Chlamydia: doxycycline 100 mg twice daily for 1 week (beware photosensitivity) *or* azithromycin 1 g stat *or* erythromycin 500 mg four times a day for 7 days (less efficacious than doxycycline and more likely to cause side effects).
- Gonorrhoea: ceftriaxone 500 mg IM (or other third-generation cephalosporin) *plus* treatment for chlamydia is current global recommendation. Other regimens include cefixime 400 mg PO stat *or* ciprofloxacin 500 mg PO stat *plus* treatment for chlamydia *but* high resistance worldwide.
- NSU: treat as for chlamydia.
- If treating blind, consider drug regimen that could treat chlamydia and gonorrhoea plus UTI such as ofloxacin 200 mg twice daily for 1 week.

Complications

- Epididymo-orchitis—inflammation of one or both testes (presentation usually with unilateral testicular pain).
- Sexually acquired reactive arthritis (SARA)—immune response in the joints to a bacterial STI, causing pain ± swelling and stiffness at one or more joints.
- Conjunctivitis.
- (Uncommon) gonococcal metastatic septicaemic arthritis and skin lesions.

Vaginal discharge

Definition

Fluid coming from the vagina. A 'normal' vaginal discharge is usually clear/milky, does not smell, may change during a woman's cycle, and keeps the vagina healthy. Changes in vaginal discharge that may indicate a problem are:

- Increase in quantity.
- Change in colour or smell.
- Irritation, itchiness, soreness, or burning.

Causes and symptoms

See Table 15.2.

Investigations

Microscopy of Gram-stained vaginal smears may allow diagnosis of gonorrhoea, candidal *infection*, and bacterial vaginosis. Direct observation by a wet smear for *Trichomonas*. Ideally more complicated lab tests are employed if they are available, e.g. NAAT for chlamydia and gonorrhoea.

Management

- Avoid sexual contact to prevent further transmission.
- Ensure partner(s) are informed and treated prophylactically.
- Ideally, test the patient as soon as possible to avoid STI complications.
- Suggest testing rather than treating blind if possible.
- Consider treating blind if confident of diagnosis (e.g. patient has had same previously) and suitable medication available.
- If patient treated, suggest full STI screen when they return home.

Table 15.2 Vaginal discharge causes and symptoms

Infection	Typical symptoms
Chlamydia	70% asymptomatic
	Purulent vaginal discharge, dysuria, intermenstrual/postcoital bleeding, low abdominal pain
Gonorrhoea	50% asymptomatic
	Increased/change in discharge (especially colour and smell), low abdominal pain
Trichomonas vaginalis	10–50% asymptomatic
	Change in vaginal discharge (varying thickness, sometimes frothy, often yellow/green), vulval irritation, dysuria, offensive odour
Bacterial vaginosis	Thin/watery, white/grey, homogeneous, offensive, fishy-smelling discharge. Not STI
Candidiasis (thrush)	Thick, white, curdy 'cottage cheese' discharge, vulval itching, soreness, and erythema. Vulval fissures, external dysuria. Not STI

Treatment

BASHH guidelines suggest:
- Chlamydia and gonorrhoea: see ➲ Urethral discharge, p. 537.
- *Trichomonas*: metronidazole 2 g orally stat.
- Bacterial vaginosis: only treat if symptomatic—metronidazole 400 mg twice daily for 5 days.
- Avoid soaps/shower gels/scented products to genital area.
- Candida: clotrimazole pessary (varying dosages), clotrimazole cream or fluconazole 150 mg stat capsule. Avoid soaps/shower gels/scented products to genital area, avoid tight-fitting clothes. Oral treatments and cream are preferable on expedition.

Complications

Untreated chlamydia/gonorrhoea can lead to:
- Pelvic inflammatory disease (➲ p. 417)—upper genital tract inflammation, causes low abdominal pain, pyrexia, systemic illness.
- Possible infertility owing to scarring/blocking of fallopian tubes.
- SARA—immune response in the joints due to a bacterial STI, causing pain ± swelling and stiffness at one or more joints.
- Conjunctivitis.
- (Uncommon) gonococcal metastatic septicaemic arthritis and skin lesions.

Genital sores and ulcers

Open wounds of skin or mucous membrane in genital area. If lesion originates from sexual contact, causative organisms are likely to be syphilis or genital herpes (Table 15.3).

Syphilis

Caused by bacterium *Treponema pallidum*, it is currently increasing in Western countries.

There are three stages:
- Early (primary, secondary, and early latent <2 years).
- Late (late latent >2 years).
- Tertiary (with neurological and cardiovascular involvement).

Syphilis is transmitted via oral/vaginal/anal contact, blood-to-blood contact, or mother-to-baby contact (vertical transmission).

The incubation period is 9–90 days for primary symptoms.

Genital herpes

- Caused by HSV type 1 or 2.
- Transmitted via skin-to-skin contact (oral/vaginal/anal).
- Incubation period is typically 2–10 days but can be years.

Investigations/diagnosis

For experienced medical practitioners, visual diagnosis is possible. Dark ground microscopy from lesions in early syphilis can confirm infection, otherwise serological test for *Treponema pallidum* is performed. Early false-negatives are possible, so repeat if there is high clinical suspicion. HSV viral culture from swab from genital lesions is ideal.

Management

- Avoid sexual contact to prevent further transmission.
- Test patient as soon as possible to avoid complications if STI present.
- Suspected syphilis needs infection confirmation, specialized medical attention, and supervised treatment.
- Consider self-treating herpes if the patient gives a history of HSV, and there appears to be uncomplicated infection (no urinary retention).
- Avoid sharing towels/flannels as there is a very slight risk of transmission.

Treatment

BASHH guidelines suggest:
- *Early syphilis:* benzathine benzylpenicillin 2.4 MU IM *or* (if penicillin allergy) doxycycline 100 mg PO twice daily for 14 days. Treatment differs in pregnancy, if neurological/ophthalmic involvement in early syphilis and in late latent syphilis.
- *Herpes:* treatment needs to be started within 5 days of the first symptoms. Aciclovir 200 mg five times per day for 5 days *or* famciclovir 250 mg three times per day for 5 days *or* valaciclovir 500 mg twice per day for 5 days *and* saline bathing, topical anaesthetic agents, and analgesia.

Table 15.3 Genital sores and ulcers

Infection	Typical symptoms
Syphilis	Primary: single, painless, indurated ulcer (chancre) with a clean base discharging clear serum. Regional lymphadenopathy
	Secondary: multisystemic involvement, generalized polymorphic rash, often affecting palms and soles
Genital herpes	Painful blisters/sores and ulceration of genital/perianal area. May be accompanied by burning, tingling, itching, dysuria, and urethral/vaginal discharge. Systemic symptoms of fever are common in primary infection. Chronic condition, symptoms can recur

Complications
- Syphilis—reactions to treatment (Jarisch–Herxheimer/anaphylaxis).
- Herpes—urinary retention, secondary bacterial infection.

Differential diagnoses
- Behçet's disease (chronic immune condition). Symptoms of mouth ulcers ± genital ulcers, skin lesions, eye and joint inflammation.
- Chancroid (caused by bacteria *Haemophilus ducreyi*, mainly found in developing countries).
- Trauma—possible cause if patient recalls specific incident.

Genital lumps and other sexually transmitted infections
See Table 15.4.

Table 15.4 Genital lumps and other sexually transmitted infections: causes and symptoms

Infection	Typical symptoms
Genital warts	Small, pink/white lumps, sometimes 'cauliflower-shaped', itchy, usually painless. Visually same as warts elsewhere
Molluscum contagiosum	Small, round, 'spots', often have white head or small dimple in centre
Folliculitis	Infected hair follicle causing painful pus-filled swellings in genital area, erythema; may have yellow head

Genital warts

- Caused by HPV.
- Transmitted through sexual contact (including skin-to-skin contact).
- Treated with cryotherapy, podophyllotoxin 'paint' or imiquimod.
- Psychological distress is the main difficulty; treatment can wait until repatriation as complications are unlikely.

Molluscum contagiosum

- Caused by species of molluscipoxvirus.
- Transmitted through sexual contact (including skin-to-skin contact).
- Avoid sharing towels/flannels/clothing.
- Treatment (if required) with cryotherapy.

Folliculitis

- Infected hair follicle—often bacterial cause.
- Common in areas that rub (e.g. buttocks and groin).
- May burst by itself; keep area clean, saline bathing.
- Treat with antibiotics if no improvement.

Human immunodeficiency virus

Definition

HIV is a retrovirus that suppresses the body's immune response and is responsible for acquired immunodeficiency syndrome (AIDS), a collection of specific opportunistic infections.

Incidence

HIV disproportionately affects sex workers, men who have sex with men, and people who inject drugs. There were an estimated 37.9 million living with HIV at the end of 2018, 21% unknowingly, with 1.7 million new infections that year. The areas with the highest prevalence of HIV are sub-Saharan Africa, South-East Asia, Russia, the Caribbean, and South America. See: ℘ http://aidsinfo.unaids.org

Transmission

HIV is present in blood (including menstrual blood), semen, and vaginal fluids. Transmission can occur if infected fluids pass between people. There are three main routes of transmission:

- Unprotected sexual contact (including oral sex).
- Blood-to-blood contact.
- Mother-to-baby transmission.

Risk factors

- Unprotected sexual contact.
- Injecting drug use/sharing injecting equipment.
- Needlestick injuries/contaminated sharps.
- Contaminated blood products.
- Mucous membrane exposure (e.g. splash of blood/semen/vaginal fluid into the eye).

HIV prevention

- Safe sex—condom use for all sexual activity (➲ STI prevention, p. 536).
- Avoid sexual contact with higher-risk groups (e.g. sex workers, high-incidence countries).

- Ensure safe injecting equipment/sharps.
- Pre-exposure prophylaxis is a drug taken by HIV-negative people before and after sex to reduce the chance of HIV infection. It is available in the UK from sexual health clinics.

Post-exposure prophylaxis

This is an emergency measure and should be considered where there is felt to have been a significant risk of HIV exposure. This comprises a 4-week course of antiretroviral (anti-HIV) medication, started up to 72 h (but ideally ASAP) after possible exposure to attempt to abort HIV infection. It is not guaranteed to prevent infection and may have side effects. It was previously used for healthcare workers following needlestick injuries from HIV-positive patients but is now also considered after sexual exposure.

The currently recommended first-line regimen is Truvada® and Raltegravir® for 28 days (for latest updates refer to ℅ http://www.bashh. org.uk). Treatment is very expensive (~£1000 for 28 days), so 'starter packs' of 3–5 days could be taken on expedition with immediate repatriation to continue treatment. If the expedition does not have PEPSE, some countries may have the recommended drugs available to buy—seek advice in the local area.

Common side effects of PEPSE are diarrhoea, nausea, and vomiting, so antiemetics (domperidone 10–20 mg three times a day when required) and antidiarrhoeals (loperamide 4 mg stat followed by 2 mg after each loose motion to maximum of 12 mg in 24 h) may be needed.

Risk–benefit analysis should be undertaken and decisions made in each case. Consider whether the person might already be infected with HIV and their ability to adhere to (vital) and tolerate the drug regimen, especially in remote areas (Table 15.5).

The same regimen could be considered if an expedition member was heavily contaminated with blood or body fluids, e.g. when delivering first aid to a member of the local population in an area of high HIV prevalence.

Table 15.5 Risk of HIV transmission following an unprotected sexual exposure from a known HIV positive individual, not on treatment

Type of exposure	Estimated median (range) risk of HIV transmission per exposure
Receptive anal intercourse	1.11% (0.042–3.0%)
Insertive anal intercourse	0.06% (0.06–0.065%)
Receptive vaginal intercourse	0.1% (0.004–0.32%)
Insertive vaginal int ercourse	0.082% (0–0.004%)
Receptive oral sex (fellatio)	0.02% (0–0.004%)
Insertive oral sex (receiving fellatio)	0%

℅ http://www.bashh.org/documents/4076.pdf

Chapter 16

Expedition mental health

Chapter editor
James Moore

Contributors
Jon Dallimore
Karen Forbes
Debbie Hawker
James Moore
Marc Shaw
Michael Jones (1st edition)
Ian Palmer (1st edition)

Introduction

Expeditions by definition involve travel, usually into remote areas, and include activities unlikely to form part of a normal working week. Any change from the normal pattern of life can be stressful, and participants must adapt to a multitude of novel experiences, enjoyable and otherwise. Most fit, healthy, and well-prepared individuals should adapt readily to the physical and psychological effects of stress, but occasionally travellers encounter circumstances that can result in long-term mental health sequelae.

Small groups may consist of companions who are previously acquainted in other settings, and an informal process of selection may have occurred. Those in larger groups may have had little or no contact with other participants prior to the journey, especially if the group has been organized as a charity trek, adventure race, or commercial expedition. The lack of familiarity before the expedition may particularly put participants more at psychological risk. In addition, the longer the expedition, the more stressful or arduous the activity, and the poorer the preparation, the greater the likelihood that psychological problems will surface.

Stressors in the wilderness

The physical demands of the expedition

The physical demands of the expedition are likely to cause a lowered reserve for dealing with other stressors, including making new relationships within the group.

If participants have joined their first expedition, they may be unprepared for the intensity of contact involved in sharing tents or cramped sleeping accommodation. Experienced members may be intolerant of the difficulties experienced by those unused to, e.g. close quarter living, jungle-style sanitation, the reduced opportunity for keeping clean, and the absence of home comforts. In polar extremes, 24 h daylight or darkness are well-recognized causes of stress, leading to illnesses such as 'seasonal affective disorder' (SAD)—a problem documented by early explorers. If possible, plan a team-building exercise before the expedition that introduces some of these stressors to observe how people may adapt to the physical demands of the expedition.

Cultural adjustment

During an expedition, contact with indigenous peoples may be limited or very intense. The opportunity for developing understanding of different cultural values may be limited by language barriers unless fluently bilingual interpreters are present.

Factors which may reduce cultural transitional stress include:
- Previous exposure to that culture and knowledge of local languages.
- Understanding cultural adaptation and local values and customs.
- A flexible, resourceful temperament, and the ability to tolerate ambiguity with a good sense of humour.
- An understanding of the physical geography and history of the region to be travelled.

All these factors should be borne in mind when screening potential expedition team members.

Pre-existing problems

Increasing numbers of individuals with a prior medical history of mental health problems are undertaking expeditions, and this can result in problems during the expedition and possibly a need for repatriation. Problems are most likely if members have a pre-existing psychological morbidity that was either not declared, or considered unimportant, during the selection process (➲ Team selection, p. 548, and ➲ Psychiatric illness, p. 550–554).

Considerations before departure

Assessing vulnerability

Some form of psychological health screening of potential expedition members is highly desirable and becomes increasingly important for longer expeditions. An acute psychosis, although rare, may cripple the progress of an expedition until repatriation can be organized. In addition, losing a member of the team because of illness may affect the overall skills of the group.

No screening process will ever distinguish perfectly between those who will thrive on an expedition and those who will develop problems; however, the risks of serious adverse events can be reduced with some simple measures. Information should be sought from several sources, for example:

Application forms

These should be constructed carefully so that all questions have to be answered (➲ Pre-existing medical problems, p. 48). GPs completing medical forms should be informed that any prior psychological history is fundamentally important, and that non-disclosure could be detrimental to the safety of both the applicant, and the rest of the team. Non-disclosure may invalidate medical insurance. However, it is also important to stress that disclosure of mental health issues is primarily to enable individuals to prepare for the rigours of expedition life and not necessarily to prevent them from participating.

Work references

Work references are particularly important because they are provided by people in regular contact with the candidate who see them when they are not trying to create a specific impression.

Interviews

Interviews should be at the core of any selection process. Panel members must include those involved in the expedition, individuals who have previous experience in the field in similar situations, and are aware of small group dynamics and their influence on morale and psychology of the group. The interview can include:
- *Employment history:* relationships at work and the reasons for job changes should be explored. Candidates who give up easily may not be the best team members for a physically and psychologically demanding expedition.
- *Personal and family mental health history:* the assessor should ask about any consultations with the GP for any form of emotional ill health and any previous referrals for psychiatric help or counselling, as well as any untreated episodes.
- *Substance abuse:* any abuse of alcohol or drugs should be noted. Insight into any past difficulties, and healthy strategies for dealing with any future problems would balance concerns about previous substance abuse.
- *Adaptability and resilience to deal with stressful events:* it can be helpful to ask the candidate to describe how they have been affected by stress in the past. What sort of things do they find stressful? What are their

vulnerability points and their coping mechanisms? How adaptable are they to change?
• *Personal relationships:* individuals have many different motivations for embarking on an expedition. Recent relationship failures are often cited as motivation for adventure. For all this, however, although individuals may feel mentally stable, their coping mechanisms for the rigours of an expedition may be weakened.

Unsuitability due to mental health

Each expedition will be different, and the ability to help those with complex psychological needs will depend on the location, purpose, duration, staffing levels, and medical competence of the team.
• *Serious mental illness:* includes schizophrenia, bipolar disorder, hypomania, severe depression, or anxiety. People with schizophrenia are more prone to psychotic breakdown when their environment is altered; bipolar and manic disorders often require potent medication for control, and failure to take medication may lead to relapse. Those on lithium need access to laboratory monitoring and are at risk of lithium toxicity in the event of dehydration. Expeditions tend to be stressful, and are not suitable for most people with serious mental illness.
• *Untreated psychological disorder:* any current psychological disorders should have been treated and followed by a symptom-free period where the individual has been able to cope with other stressful situations.
• *Anxiety, depression, or panic attacks:* repeated episodes of anxiety and depression will raise concern.
• *Recent loss:* following recent bereavement, divorce, or broken relationship, it is wise to delay before potentially stressful trips.
• *Eating disorders* (⊕ p. 552–553): previous anorexia nervosa or bulimia nervosa must have been controlled for a year or two such that the applicant has healthy eating routines, does not engage in self-induced vomiting or laxative abuse, and is maintaining a satisfactory BMI.
• *Deliberate self-harm and previous suicide attempts:* a recent psychiatrist's report is advised and may be required to ensure that the individual is safe to travel to a remote area, has resolved any outstanding issues, can manage their distress in other ways, and will not be a risk to themselves.
• *Drug or alcohol abuse:* a period of abstinence or recovery of 1 year is suggested following a rehabilitation programme, coupled with a contractual agreement not to misuse substances while on expedition.

Pre-expedition preparation

As with any other pre-existing medical condition, individuals with a history of mental illness should have coping mechanisms and appropriate treatment planned prior to departure. In some instances, it might be prudent to create a contract between the individual, the team leader, and a medical professional detailing:
• What is considered acceptable behaviour while on expedition.
• What individuals should do if they feel they are struggling to cope.
• The consequences of crossing any pre-determined boundaries.
• A repatriation plan.

For example, for a person with an eating disorder:
- Agree a pre-arranged acceptable calorie intake.
- Agree that if unable to maintain the pre-arranged food input, the individual will discuss this issue with a named individual.
- Agree treatment strategies and a plan of action, e.g. communication with relative/counsellor via satellite phone, dietary changes, or change in level of activity.
- Agree that failure to respond to pre-agreed strategies will result in curtailing of expedition activities, followed by repatriation.

All parties involved should sign this agreement. It will also be necessary to review insurance policies and ensure individuals have appropriate repatriation cover.

Expedition leaders or medical officers have a responsibility to receive some mental health first-aid training. See ➔ p. 45.

Stresses on an expedition

Human resilience increases when basic needs are attended to: varied food and sufficient water, shelter, rest, and time for recreation. Poor living conditions and excessive tiredness result in poor decision-making. Common causes of stress include relationship problems, poor leadership, lack of control, poor understanding of roles, and a lack of support. Such stressors should be explored before departure to try to match expectations to organization. Appropriate pressure leads to excitement and improves performance; although excessive and unrelenting pressure can cause team members to feel overwhelmed and exhausted. Strategies that can boost resilience include:
- Ensuring basic needs are met as far as possible.
- Reviewing expectations—are they realistic?
- Clarifying areas of uncertainty.
- Talking things through. A formal structure should be in place for information to be shared and complaints to be aired early.
- Taking time out where possible—including for leaders.

Mental health conditions

Psychopathology in people working overseas, even after rigorous selection, is common, and those engaged in expeditions and other prolonged visits into wilderness locations are at risk.

Anxiety disorders

Anxiety may be generalized or focused on particular concerns such as snakebite or flying. Features are as for panic disorder (see later paragraph).

Anxiety about health is normal when travelling internationally, but can be a problem if it becomes extreme or remains, despite reassurance. It may be made worse on expeditions which are isolated from competent medical help.

Aviophobia (fear of flying) is experienced by up to 2.5-5% of air passengers. Behavioural therapy, and in particular systematic desensitization, is a very effective treatment, and medication such as beta-blockers or one-off doses of benzodiazepines can complement physical technique.

and cognitive strategies to overcome the fear. There are several UK-based courses such as:

ℹ www.virtualjetcentre.co.uk/fear-of-flying/

ℹ www.gatwickairport.com/booktrip/Travel-advice/fear-of-flying/

Panic disorder is the presence of recurrent panic attacks; a discrete period of intense fear or discomfort, involving at least four of the following symptoms:

Palpitations.

Sweating.

Shaking.

Shortness of breath or feeling of choking.

Chest pain.

Nausea/abdominal symptoms.

Dizziness.

Feelings of unreality or being detached from oneself.

Fear of losing control or going crazy.

Fear of dying or 'impending doom'.

Numbness or tingling sensations.

Chills or hot flushes.

Management of anxiety or panic consists of calm reassurance and, in the case of rapid breathing, breathing in and out of a paper bag or cupped hands. The 5–4–3–2–1 'grounding technique' encourages individuals to name five things they can see, four things they can feel, three things they can hear, two things they can smell, and one thing they can taste.

If symptoms persist, an expert opinion should be sought. Anxiolytic drugs or/and psychological therapies may be advised.

Depression

It is important to distinguish clinical depression from the low mood which all people experience from time to time. Homesickness, concerns about how one may cope, environmental stressors, and fatigue may all produce similar symptoms during an expedition. Depression may follow a clear trigger such as bereavement but it may have no obvious precipitant. Characteristic features of clinical depression include:

Low mood (particularly in the morning).

Lack of motivation and low energy levels.

Poor sleep, particularly early morning wakening.

Persistent weepiness.

Preoccupation with worries or feelings of guilt.

Excessive alcohol consumption.

Possible suicidal thoughts. Those with active plans for suicide are at high risk. Asking about suicidal plans does not increase the risk of the person harming themselves.

Management of depressed people is likely to require expert help in the form of psychological therapy and/or medication, particularly if there are suicidal features. Repatriation may be required.

Psychosis and acute confusional states

Psychoses are severe mental illnesses and are rare, but they can develop while travelling and may be provoked by medication such as mefloquine

(Lariam®) or illicit drugs such as marihuana, amphetamines, and cocaine. However, it is important to remember that physical illness may be the cause for abnormal behaviour: see ⊃ Delirium/confusion, p. 270–271.
- Protozoal tropical infections—cerebral malaria, African trypanosomiasis (sleeping sickness), and amoebic dysentery.
- Bacterial infections—typhoid and meningitis.
- Other causes—hypoglycaemia, head injury, viral encephalitis, hypoxia.

Features of psychosis/acute confusion include:
- Bizarre behaviour.
- Paranoia.
- Disinhibition.
- Hallucinations, delusions.
- Thought disorder.
- Pressure of speech.
- Disorientation in time, place, or person.
- Lack of insight.

In practice, it may be difficult to distinguish between physical and psychiatric illness. Absence of fever, lack of orientation in time and place, and auditory hallucinations tend to point towards a psychiatric problem. Visual hallucinations tend to indicate physical illness.

A psychotic or confused patient may not cooperate with treatment or safety procedures. Approaches to increase engagement include:
- Maintaining a calm environment.
- Repeated gentle persuasion.
- Explaining what is happening.
- Acknowledging that the situation may be frightening for them.
- Treating them as normally as possible.
- Avoiding physical restraint unless vital for their own safety.

Someone with an acute psychotic illness should be evacuated for expert assessment and treatment, usually with a psychotropic medication. Consider sedation with olanzapine 5–10 mg PO (available in orodispersible form). Haloperidol 0.5–3 mg two to three times daily is an alternative and can be used in delirium; it may need to be given with an anticholinergic such benzhexol or procyclidine. Mental health laws and access to support will differ between countries, or may be absent.

Eating disorders

Approximately 2% of adult females and occasionally males have been diagnosed with an eating disorder. The main eating disorders are:
- *Anorexia nervosa*: a conscious reduction in calorific input alongside preoccupation with eating, shape, or weight. Symptoms include severe weight loss, dizziness, abdominal pain, growth of soft, fine hair (lanugo) all over the body, amenorrhoea, perfectionist behaviour, excessive exercising, or covert micro-exercising.
- *Bulimia nervosa*: individuals become caught in a cycle of over-eating large quantities of food, then purposefully vomit, omit food, or take laxatives as a method of 'purging'. Symptoms may include abdominal pains, mood changes, irregular periods, puffy cheeks, sore throat, halitosis, and kidney and bowel problems.

- *Binge eating disorder (BED):* individuals consume large amounts of food in relatively short periods of time. Unlike patients with bulimia nervosa they do not purge.
- *Eating disorders not otherwise specified:* individuals who display partial signs and symptoms of the previous three eating disorders.

Eating disorders are complex. It is unlikely that issues causing these illnesses will be resolved on expedition. It is not unusual for the care of an individual suffering from an eating disorder to become stressful, particularly around meal times, as they seek increasingly more covert ways of reducing their calorific intake. Mealtime behaviour for someone with an eating disorder such as anorexia nervosa might include:

- Delaying eating.
- Dissecting or tearing food into tiny pieces.
- Playing with or hiding food.
- Offering food to other members of the team.
- Covert micro-exercising which may be confused with agitation.

Strategies for managing mealtimes may include:

- Acknowledging the eating difficulty but reinforcing the need to start/ continue eating.
- Firm but supportive prompting.
- Ensuring others around the table act as role models.
- Maintaining contact after mealtimes, allowing food to digest, preventing opportunities for purging and an opportunity to offer support feedback, while recognizing the need for potential repatriation.

It is important to avoid the emotional game of dietary chess, where success or failure rides on an individual's ability to hide food or make someone complete a meal. Firm but supportive care, where clarity of boundaries and consequent repercussions must be paramount.

Neurodiversity

Increasing numbers of adolescents embark on youth expeditions. Some of these have disabilities such as attention deficit hyperactivity disorder (ADHD) or autism spectrum conditions that will require careful considera-tion and planning to enable a safe trip.

- *ADHD:* a term used to describe hyperactive children and adolescents who have difficulty concentrating. Symptoms include appearing constantly distracted, an inability to sit still, and poor social skills. Problems such as autism, conduct disorders, and neurological conditions are found to coexist in children with ADHD.
  Autism spectrum conditions: characteristics include difficulties with communication, social interaction, behaving flexibly or having repetitive patterns of behaviour Asperger's syndrome is a common autism spectrum condition, associated with high-functioning individuals.

Preparation is the key to providing effective adjustments and support for people with neurodiverse conditions, but relies on individuals disclosing sensitive and often stigmatized conditions prior to departure. As with some psychological conditions, contracts detailing acceptable behaviour, bound-ries, and repercussions are important. Some ADHD medicines may have customs restrictions and should be carried with the appropriate documentation. While away, management strategies should include:

- Encouragement, positive support, and plenty of praise.
- Consistency, fairness, and appropriate discipline.
- Breaking tasks into smaller, simpler components.
- Providing simple instructions for tasks or responsibilities.
- Individuals with neurodiverse conditions are often misunderstood, feel stigmatized and become marginalized. These issues become a barrier to effective communication and support. Fostering an atmosphere of mutual respect will maximize effective management.
- See ℗ www.adhdfoundation.org.uk and ℗ www.autism.org.uk for useful information and further reading about these conditions.

Nocturnal enuresis

About 1–2% of adolescents over the age of 15 suffer from bed-wetting. Although the causes can be physiological, the effects are psychological, affecting self-esteem and confidence. While on an expedition, individuals may attempt to control the volume of urine created by drinking less which in adverse environments can lead to potentially hazardous dehydration.

Desmopressin (1-deamino-8-D-arginine vasopressin or DDAVP) is a potent antidiuretic used in the management of nocturnal enuresis, causing increased water reabsorption in the renal tubules. If taken too often (something a nervous or embarrassed expedition member might do), or taken alongside the increased fluids often required in hot and humid climates, it can result in a dangerous risk of hyponatraemia (⮕ p. 806).

Hyponatraemia may also be induced with the concomitant use of NSAIDs.

Psychological reactions to traumatic events

(See also ⤷ Death on an expedition, p. 184, and ⤷ Sexual assault, p. 182.)

Most expeditions will be completed with only minor untoward events. However, anyone taking a group into the field, particularly those responsible for young people, must be aware of how to care for the group's psychological welfare should illness, accident, or, at worst, death occur. These events might occur within the group while on expedition, but it is also possible that leaders might be responsible for informing an expeditioner of events that have occurred at home. Possible traumatic events include:

- Death on the expedition.
- Grave illness or injury.
- A member of the team going missing.
- A hostage situation.
- Death or serious illness of a relative or close friend at home.

In some situations, the whole group will have witnessed what has happened. In others, the leader may have to inform a member or members of the group about a traumatic event or its repercussions. See ⤷ Box 16.1, p. 560, for some guidance on how to do this. Further details are available at: ℘ https://dartcenter.org/sites/default/files/breaking_bad_news_0.pdf

When a traumatic event occurs, leaders should assume that some people may be stunned and bewildered, or react with incapacitating anxiety or anger. The leader, and/or medic, needs to identify quickly how people are reacting and use them appropriately. Those reacting effectively may be needed to help in rescue efforts or to ensure the safety of the others. It is important to note, all team members will respond to traumatic events in their own way, and this may be incongruent with their role or position. For example, a team leader may become incapacitated or incapable of leading. The leadership reaction to negative expedition outcomes should be included in pre-departure discussions, along with a range of planned responses.

What should the leader and medic do?

In the event of a disaster, the leader must ensure rapidly that they and the rest of the team are safe; the rest of the team cannot be put at risk and the victim may already be lost or dead. The leader, rescuers, other group members, family and friends, and expedition organizers may all experience different psychological reactions. The psychological care of the victim and the rest of the group are the leader and medic's responsibility, as well as maintaining their own well-being. They should provide accurate information in a timely fashion to the victim and all others involved.

Care of the victim

While an ill or injured group member is awaiting evacuation, their physical comfort, security, and dignity must be maintained, e.g. ensuring they are covered and have privacy. If the person is conscious, they should be kept informed about what is happening. They may be very distressed or bewildered. It is important to be patient and honest, to allow them time to talk and to accept what may be muddled and rapidly changing thoughts and emotions, and reassure them these are normal.

If the victim is unconscious, their right to privacy and dignity must still be respected. It should also be assumed they can hear; they should have company, be kept informed, and be spared pessimistic conversations happening around them.

Psychological first aid

Psychological first aid should be offered to the rest of the group. This includes:

- Ensuring safety (including from unhelpful rumours or media).
- Practical help (e.g. food and shelter).
- Providing information.
- Offering comfort and reassurance; helping people calm down.
- Agreeing how people outside the group should receive information. Relatives/friends of everyone involved ought to receive information in an appropriately supportive manner, not through uncontrolled use of social media.
- Facilitating contact with family members.
- Listening, but not pressuring people to talk.
- An important aim is to reduce arousal levels as this will reduce the risk of PTSD developing (⊃ p. 558–561). A free manual on psychological first aid is available at: ℘ https://www.who.int/mental_health/publi cations/guide_field_workers/en/

Care of the group

Having ensured the initial safety of the group, the leader is responsible for ensuring their needs for food, water, and shelter are met, and then for providing a supportive environment. In a small, functional group this may be relatively simple and possible on a one-to-one basis.

In a larger group, particularly if fault or blame might be apportioned around the cause of the traumatic event, the task will be more difficult and the leader might choose to arrange a debriefing meeting 24 h or longer after the event, after the practicalities of medical care, evacuation, and informing relatives have been completed. The primary aim of this meeting would be to facilitate a supportive emotional environment and get a functional team home. In most instances, it is inappropriate to attempt to establish causality of an event, or attribute blame, immediately after it has occurred. Many facts surrounding critical incidents only become visible after proper investigation and without the added complications of acute emotional attachment.

An operational debriefing concentrates on evaluating procedures and dealing with practical matters. The team may also agree on the next steps (e.g. whether to continue the expedition or return home).

A critical incident debriefing provides an opportunity for the group to talk about the facts of what has happened, and their thoughts and feelings. The process must be non-judgemental. Common responses to trauma are normalized, and people are taught that these usually disappear naturally with time. Information is provided about helpful coping mechanisms. Group support is encouraged, future plans are discussed, and people are told how to obtain further help if it is needed. Critical incident debriefing should not take place too soon (within 24 h of a traumatic event), and sufficient time should be allocated for the process (at least 2 h). It can occur remotely (e.g. over the internet).

Debriefing should be facilitated by an individual with sufficient skills or experience as, done incorrectly, it can cause short- or long-term distress.

Reactions to traumatic events or bad news

Group members witnessing or being involved in a traumatic event and an expeditioner given bad news from home may react in similar ways.

To be bereaved is to be deprived of someone or something of value. We may grieve for a person, but we may also grieve for other losses, such as friendship, hope, or our perceptions of safety and immortality. People who are grieving may have feelings of numbness, sadness, anxiety, anger, guilt, or yearning; they may experience physical sensations of a 'flight or fright' reaction, with dry mouth, hollow stomach, breathlessness, or tachycardia; they may be confused, bewildered, disbelieving, and disorientated. In close relationships they may even have auditory or visual hallucinations of the person who has died. Their behaviour may be altered, with crying, restlessness, loss of appetite, sleep disturbance, and absent-mindedness, which could compromise the individual's safety on an expedition.

Bereavement and loss are a normal part of life. The vast majority of people who are bereaved of someone close to them, or who experience a traumatic event, recover with time and the support of family and friends. In the aftermath of such an event, individuals should be reassured that the jumble of emotions, sensations, thoughts, and behaviours they are experiencing are normal and does not mean there is something wrong with them or they are 'going mad'. Expeditioners who are so distressed by grief they might compromise their own or the group's safety might have to be evacuated, but there may be good arguments for keeping a supportive group together. Evacuation may also be necessary to facilitate attendance at a funeral, which is an important part of the grieving process.

It is important to stress that difficulty with grieving or PTSD may occur even with good leadership, because of the person's pre-existing personality or mental health, or because of the nature of the event. The leader's job is to provide a supportive environment so that recovery is encouraged, where possible, and to get the team home safely.

Post-traumatic stress disorder

Symptoms of PTSD may develop after experiencing 'a stressful event of an exceptionally threatening or catastrophic nature'. Sufferers involuntarily re-experience the event or aspects of it and these 're-experiencing symptoms' may feel very real, frightening, and distressing. Victims often have recurrent flashbacks or nightmares and may avoid triggers reminding them of the event, or return continuously to why it happened or how it could have been avoided. They may have emotional numbing or be in a constant state of alertness, being fearful, irritable, easily startled, and having difficulties with concentration and sleeping. Such symptoms are normal up to 6 weeks after an incident. Persistent problems indicate the need for psychiatric or psychological input.

Who develops post-traumatic stress disorder?

The chances of developing PTSD are higher in women than in men and differ according to the traumatic event. The risk of developing PTSD is highest after rape (about 20% in women), other sexual attack, being threatened with a weapon, and kidnapped or taken hostage. About 10% of people seeing accidents, death or injury, and natural disasters will go on to develop PTSD.

Psychological reactions to a crisis or tragedy

When the tragedy becomes known to the expedition, team members may go through a variety of reactions: grief, guilt, acceptance, and then resolution:

* 'This can't have happened.'
* 'I don't believe it.'
* 'This is ridiculous—he was only here in this camp an hour ago.'
* 'Tell me that again!'

Psychological debriefing is the generic term for immediate interventions following trauma (usually within 3 days) that seek to relieve stress with the intent of mitigating or preventing long-term pathology. In the first days after the death of a colleague, expeditioners are advised to:

* Talk about the dead colleague, talk about the death, talk about their positive and negative feelings for their colleague. Talk about the nightmares and any other symptoms that may result, and acknowledge that these reactions are normal after such an event and usually get better by themselves, with time.
* In the first 8 weeks expeditioners should not try to push flashbacks, intrusive images, or nightmares away. These are all ways the psyche is trying to work through and make sense of an abnormal situation.
* Advice should be given *not* to drink or indulge in recreational drugs 'more than normal', as both impede the brain's processing of the trauma.
* All within the group need to remind themselves that they are not going crazy (a common feeling). The phrase 'reacting normally to an abnormal situation' can be helpful.
* Avoidance of discussion of the incident is one predictor of PTSD. The whole group may slowly confront the situations that they are trying to avoid. In the early stages after the incident this involves talking about the event and about the dead colleague by name. Such discussion may include the need or desire either to continue with the journey or to return home, and may predispose to feelings of selfishness (that turn into guilt), selflessness, remorse, blame, and whether there is willpower to go on. Collectively the expedition survivors might talk in terms of:

* 'We were shocked.'
* 'We thought we'd have to quit.'
* 'We decided to continue to honour our fallen friend.'
* 'This is what he/she would have wanted us to do.'

Symptoms of PTSD may develop several weeks (or longer) after the event, and team members affected should then seek help through their GP or healthcare professional. NICE guidance[1] suggests the principles of care of people with PTSD are peer support, maintaining safe environments, and involving and supporting families and carers. Some people will need to go on to individual or group trauma-focused cognitive behavioural therapy.

- An expedition plan should include a coordinated psychosocial response to possible disasters. If they occur, the leader's responsibility is to ensure everyone's safety, that basic needs are met, and people are supported to go over the events and express emotions without being judged, and are offered comfort and reassurance. The leader should advise group members who are struggling to seek help on their return home.

Box 16.1 Breaking bad news: the 'SPIKES' acronym

S—Setting up the interview

- Prepare yourself.
- Have as much information as possible.
- Think about the questions the person will ask.
- Ensure privacy, avoid interruptions.
- Involve significant others.
- Sit down.
- Make eye contact.

P—assess Perception

- What do they already know?
- What do they think has happened?

I—obtain the person's Invitation

- Gain permission to give more information, e.g. 'Can I tell you what happened this afternoon?' or 'I need to tell you what happened this afternoon' or 'Can I tell you what happened to [name].'

K—give Knowledge and information

- Give a warning: 'I'm afraid I have some bad news for you about [name].'
- Avoid blurting it all out—give information in small chunks.
- Avoid excessive bluntness, but be honest, clear, and avoid euphemisms.
- Check for understanding periodically.
- Respect the level of knowledge the person wants, e.g. some will just want to know the person is injured or has died while some will want to know how and why.

E—address Emotions with empathic responses

- Observe for emotional responses.
- Identify the emotion and the reason for it to yourself.

---

1 ℞ https://www.nice.org.uk/guidance/ng116

- Empathize: e.g. 'I can see you are really upset.' 'This must be very difficult for you.' 'I'm so sorry this has happened.'
- Avoid 'I know how you feel': you don't.
- Give time and respect silence.
- Use touch if appropriate.

S—Strategy and Summary

- Summarize what has been said.
- Agree what should happen next for expedition members, e.g. does the person wish to stay on the expedition, or do they want to go home, or who would they like to 'buddy' them?

Adapted from a protocol for breaking bad news to patients with cancer: Baile WF, et al. SPIKES—a six-step protocol for delivering bad news. *Oncologist.* 2000;5:302–311.

Serious psychological threats

The most extreme psychological threats of an expedition relate to death, serious accident or illness, RTC, mugging/assault/carjacking, or kidnapping/hostage-taking.

Unfortunately, kidnapping and hostage-taking remain prevalent in many areas of the world. They probably represent the most extreme and sustained form of psychological (and sometimes physical) abuse.

It is important to be aware of any such risks in the locations to be explored (https://www.gov.uk/foreign-travel-advice). Clear contingency plans are advisable. A reputable 'survival in hostile region' course may help in learning how to avoid becoming captured. The course should include training in how to cope if kidnapping does occur (see following section).

Surviving kidnapping

All kidnappings are undertaken for gain, usually after careful surveillance. Captors are criminal and/or political; while of perceived value, captives of criminals are relatively safe. The fate of political hostages is less certain. Kidnappers' previous behaviour is the best predictor of outcome. Kidnapping is not personal; most victims are a pawn in another's game. The aim of those kidnapped is to survive.

Kidnapping may be conceptualized in three phases:

- Capture.
- Incarceration.
- Release.

Capture

Kidnappers obtain compliance through extreme violence, dominance, and uncertainty. Capture and release are the most dangerous times of kidnapping. If escape is unlikely, heroics should be avoided. Weapons should not be used, unless the captive is skilled in their use. Sensory deprivation may be used to isolate the captive and is disorientating, by design. After the initial shock of abduction, there may be a short-lived euphoria at having survived, followed by a pattern of enforced sensory deprivation, threat, abuse, and hardships.

On abduction:

- Be calm, composed, patient, polite, and cooperative.
- Obey all orders.
- Keep quiet unless spoken to.
- Move slowly and deliberately—ask first.
- Listen closely to what is going on.
- Keep clothes and belongings if possible.
- Rest/sleep/eat/drink whenever possible/offered.
- Inform captors of any medical requirements.

Incarceration

Immediately establish a routine that focuses on maintaining physical and mental hygiene, health, and fitness. Physical health requires eating the food and drink offered. Physical fitness improves resistance to infection, raises mood, and may allow for a successful escape attempt. Mental fitness requires awareness of uncontrollable (external) and controllable (internal) self-induced) stressors. A positive frame of mind is important. Release is the most likely outcome; someone will be working for release of hostages.

A primitive existence will develop, centred upon bodily functions, sleeping, and eating in an atmosphere of intimidation and ruthlessness. Self-questioning and blame are destructive to self-esteem and self-worth, and lead to inertia, depression, and despair. Emotional lability is common. Any pre-existing psychological or psychiatric predispositions may be triggered. Physical activity is the best counter to this.

Compassion is required for those who are not coping well. Captors' attempts to 'split' the group will severely worsen the situation for all captives. Maintaining clear lines of communication and interest in each other's welfare is protective. The intimacy engendered by enforced proximity and shared adversity may lead to deep personal attachments/antipathies. A group leader should be appointed if taken as a group.

Captors vary in their abilities to mistreat their charges. Dehumanization promotes maltreatment. Trying to understand captors and developing rapport by active listening and drawing attention to your human needs (e.g. hunger, thirst, and bodily functions) may be beneficial.

To prevent dehumanization:
- Remain calm and courteous.
- Develop rapport and negotiate (with care) for basic needs.
- Act to maintain self-respect and dignity.
- Avoid whining, begging, or arguing.
- Prepare for a long captivity.
- Seek information on captors, time, place, and deadlines.
- Look for humour in all things and help each other.

Keep the mind active: chess, writing/reciting poems, plots of plays, films, novels.
- Focus on previous good experiences.
- What to do if/when.
- Monitor body language.
- Do not believe all given information.
- Maintain religious or spiritual beliefs—without irritating others.

Release

Maintain belief in rescue and be patient. Peaceful resolution is the default option, as violent conclusion may involve killings. Deadlines are dangerous for all parties. Any escalation of violence by kidnappers will increase the likelihood of an armed solution. Thus always assume there are plans for a forceful solution. Think ahead; obtain as much information as possible about deadlines. Armed forces are most likely to enter through windows or doors, thus stay away from portals, locate a safe place, and wait.

On hearing gunfire or explosion:
- Go to ground.
- Keep your hands visible at all times.
- Make *no* attempt to help.
- Make *no* sudden movements.
- Follow all instructions immediately.
- Rescuers will assume you are a kidnapper—expect extremely firm handling.
- Never exchange clothing with captors.

There is a natural euphoria on release. This may be tempered if locally employed individuals remain behind or were killed. Relationships formed during captivity may influence the healing process. Problems present before capture will remain unresolved. Depending on the event, consideration should be given to the competing physical, psychological, and social variables, and the variety of interested parties involved, such as family, friends, colleagues, employers, pressure groups, politicians, doctors, and media.[2]

Resource

See 🕭 https://www.hostageinternational.org for further information, including guidelines to help families cope, and advice on handling the media.

2 Palmer I. What to do if you are taken hostage. *BMJ Career Focus*. 2004;329:157–158.

Recreational drugs and alcohol

Worldwide, levels of drug abuse are rising, with evidence suggesting illegal drug use in up to one-third of some groups of travellers. Drug use on expeditions is rare, although do not assume that expedition members are immune to inquisitive behaviour, especially if the expedition finds itself located among bushes of wild plants such as marihuana.

The consequences of drug misuse on expedition are considerable, ranging from life-threatening illness to life-threatening judicial sentencing. In addition, the consequences might not be confined to the individuals participating, but also to other expedition members not partaking in drug use. Have clearly explained policies on drug use and the consequences thereof and make them known before the expedition.

When managing drug abuse on expedition, consider the implications of involving local authorities, especially the police. Advice should be sought carefully and involve the expedition leadership team. However, decisions such as these should not prevent the patient from receiving life-saving hospital treatment.

General approach

The average expedition medical kit is unlikely to contain the appropriate medicines for managing an individual who is under the influence of drugs.

Immediate management

- Rapid assessment of the patient (ABCDE (➜ p. 236–237); measure P, BP, RR, conscious level, temperature, glucose level.
- Resuscitation where appropriate.
- Medical and nursing care, including:

Rule out organic, psychiatric, and medicinal reactions as cause of signs and symptoms of drug misuse (see following section).

Removal and safe storage or destruction of drugs.

Consider further expedition participation and repatriation of individual.

Considerations

- Drugs are not always taken alone—always consider alcohol.
- The patient's condition might change abruptly: continue to monitor.

Basic drug categories and field management

Stimulants

Examples: amphetamines, cocaine, khat, betel nut, crystal meth.

Effects: euphoria, increased confidence, anxiety, mood swings, reduced appetite, rapid pulse, sexual arousal, dehydration.

Field management: treat high body temperature with cooling and fanning. Give fluids if there is dehydration. Consider small doses of benzodiazepines for agitation.

Dissociatives

Examples: nitrous oxide, ketamine, methoxetamine (MXE).

Effects: panic, hallucinations, euphoria, disconnected/numb.

Field management: reassurance and close observation.

Empathogens

Examples: mephedrone, MDMA, PMA.

Effects: sweating, anxiety, depression, mood swings, sexual arousal, connected, understanding, sense of belonging.

Field management: supportive treatment only.

Psychedelics

Examples: ayahuasca, LSD, NBOMes, psilocybin ('magic mushrooms').

Effects: hallucinations, poor coordination, increased body temperature, disorganized thoughts and distorted perceptions, anxiety, euphoria, paranoia, panic.

Field management: observation and supportive treatment as needed.

Opioids

Examples: codeine, fentanyl, heroin, methadone, naltrexone, oxycodone.

Effects: euphoria, relaxation, pain relief drowsiness, impaired concentration, reduced sex drive, sweating, constipation.

Field management: airway and respiratory support. If RR <10 breaths/min: naloxone at a dose of 0.8 mg IV repeated every 2–3 min until RR ≥10 breaths/min.

Cannabinoids

Examples: cannabis and butane hash oil.

Effects: anxiety, dry mouth, paranoia, poor motivation, loss of memory, bloodshot eyes, feeling of relaxation/calm.

Field management: reassurance and monitoring. Supportive measures.

Hallucinogenics

Examples: phencyclidine, LSD, 'magic mushrooms'.

Field management: mainly supportive—quiet reassurance, calm, and quiet environment. In severe agitation, consider benzodiazepines.

Depressants

Examples: alcohol (see also next section), benzodiazepines, GHB, Kava.

Effects: nausea/vomiting, euphoria, confidence, mood swings, coma.

Field management: airway and respiratory support. Observation until effects have worn off.

For detailed information about drugs of abuse see Australian Alcohol and Drug Foundation: ℘ https://adf.org.au/drug-facts/#wheel

Alcohol

Alcohol misuse is a leading cause of preventable death/illness either via excessive ingestion or as a co-factor in accidents. Be aware that alcohol is illegal in some countries with strict penalties for possession. Excessive alcohol consumption may also be culturally unacceptable in some areas.

- Alcohol is a problem when an individual's consumption has a recurrent adverse effect on day-to-day activities including those of others. Even small amounts of alcohol can adversely affect perception, reaction time, and decision-making. Traditional/homemade alcohol may be of unpredictable potency and purity posing additional risks.
- Policies on alcohol should be made clear at the outset of the expedition including what code of conduct is expected of participants.
- Individuals with alcohol dependence are unlikely to have declared this during a detailed medical screening process. Sudden alcohol withdrawal symptoms are a real possibility on expeditions where access to alcohol is limited or not possible.

Management of alcohol withdrawal
- Consider offering a benzodiazepine.
- If this is unavailable and the patient is becoming increasingly agitated, one could consider providing small quantities of an alcoholic drink to prevent acute withdrawal symptoms.
- Chlordiazepoxide can be used for the treatment of delirium tremens.
- Beware of the risk of acute alcohol withdrawal seizures.
- Further information is available at ℘ www.drinkaware.co.uk

After the expedition

For the majority, expeditions are positive experiences that enhance self-esteem and self-awareness. Expeditions will change all those involved, particularly individual participants. It takes time for the 'system' to readjust to the returnee and vice versa. Readjustment requires acceptance, adjustment, and accommodation and is something that is very often not prepared for, particularly in relation to expeditions requiring months or years of preparation.

For many, a period of 'reverse culture shock' is normal and this may include a period of mourning. Reconnection with enjoyable activities at home and contact with other expedition members is helpful. Accept that change is irrevocable and inevitable but not necessarily negative.

- Most expeditions pass without disaster, but with minor disagreements/personality clashes.
- After the initial excitement of returning, it is common to miss the camaraderie of the expedition; a feeling of anti-climax is an inevitable consequence of a successful trip.
- Far more attention is given to the process of team building at the beginning of an expedition than to team separation at the end ... neither should be ignored!

Practical steps:
- Circulating a list of contact details, or an organized reunion a few months after coming home, as well as getting expeditioners to contribute to an expedition report.
- Untreated, symptoms can persist for years leading to significant disability/distress. Get expert help!

Severe physical or mental problems persisting >3 months or those interfering with day-to-day function merit the following:
- It is vital that physical causes are thoroughly excluded with a detailed medical history and physical examination and appropriate investigations. Once this process is complete, other factors which may be generating symptoms can be explored.
- Where appropriate, referral to a GP and/or counsellor with experience of mental health problems associated with travel and/or traumatic illness and injury.

Resources

A web-based guide to the management of stress disorders can be found at: ℅ http://www.ncbi.nlm.nih.gov/books/NBK159725/

The Expedition Psychology Project: ℅ http://wp.lancs.ac.uk/expeditionpsychology/

Chapter 17

Risks from animals

Author
David A. Warrell

Acknowledgements for advice on attacks by large animals
Jim Bond
Robert Conway
John Davies
Lloyd Figgins
Simon Fox
Beth Healey
Lucy Whitton

Animals that can cause severe trauma

Animals, wild and domesticated, especially large ones, should always be treated with great respect and not approached unnecessarily. Popular TV wildlife programmes have tended to diminish our perception of the risk posed to travellers by giant pachyderms and apex predators. Tigers, lions, leopards, and other big cats, hyenas, domestic dogs, jackals, wolves, bears, elephants, rhinos, hippopotamuses, buffaloes, bison, wild and domestic cattle, moose, elk, other large deer and antelopes, domestic and wild pigs, rams, tapirs, chimpanzees, baboons, ostriches, cassowaries, and even ferrets have killed people.

Learn about the likely hazards by asking the local residents. Be vigilant at all times. Beware of wandering alone and unprotected, especially between dusk and dawn when most attacks by large mammals occur. Travel in groups, do not stray from vehicles, and do not take dogs with you—they attract large predators. A competent look-out armed with a large-calibre rifle (0.375 or more) is essential if you are working in the open where big game animals roam. However, firearms can become a danger and a liability unless they are in the hands of an experienced warden, ranger, or hunter.

Black and brown bears

All bears, even giant pandas, are potentially dangerous carnivores. Mothers with cubs are responsible for 80% of attacks on people. In North America, backpackers and campers in national parks are victims of daytime or evening attacks. From 2010 to 2019, black bears (*Ursus americanus*) were responsible for about ten deaths, brown bears (*U. arctos*), including grizzlies and Kodiak bears, for 18 deaths, and polar bears for two deaths. Brown bears also kill and injure people in Romania, Scandinavia, and other parts of Europe. Asian sloth bears (*Melursus ursinus*) killed 48 people and injured 687 in Madya Pradesh, India (1989–1994).

Prevention

In bear country, hikers should travel in groups, making plenty of noise so that bears are not taken by surprise. Never go too close (e.g. to photograph them), especially when there are cubs about and keep away from carrion and garbage tips that attract scavenging bears. Warning signs that the bear is irritated include standing up, hissing or growling, yawning, and head swinging. If a bear approaches or charges you, avoid eye contact and do not attempt to hide, run away, or climb a tree. When it is within a distance of 10 m, it may be repelled by discharging a pepper spray (10% capsicum oleoresin) towards its eyes. If this fails and the attacker is a grizzly bear, roll into a ball, interlocking your hands behind your neck, protecting your face with your elbows, and your back with your backpack. Stay in this position for long enough to ensure that the bear has gone away. If the attacker is a black bear, growl, shout, and fight back with any available weapon. Do not store food in camp but hang it in a tree >100 m away, 4 m from the ground and >1.25 m away from the tree trunk.

Polar bear

Polar bears (*U. maritimus*) are the most predatory, aggressive, and dangerous of all bears, killing six people in Canada (1965–1985), and attacking

50 people in Svalbard (Spitzbergen, Norway) (1973–1986) (➜ Wildlife in cold regions, p. 643). In 2011, an English expeditioner was killed by a starving polar bear while camping near Von Post glacier in Svalbard. In Arctic regions, keep a look out for these increasingly hungry animals. Travel in groups, carry a firearm (minimum calibre 0.308 with expandable lead core bullets or 12-bore shot gun) and flares, and know how to use them. If you see a bear, make a lot of noise, keep as far away as possible, and remain up-wind so that it senses your presence and will not be startled by your sudden appearance. If the bear approaches, fire a flare or warning shot, but at 25 m shoot to kill if it continues to advance, aiming at the chest or shoulder. Protect camps with bear fences with trip wires, take it in turn to be on bear watch and use guard dogs. At close quarters, use pepper spray, hit the bear on its nose or shoot it.

Websites

🔊 http://kho.unis.no/doc/Polar_bears_Svalbard.pdf
🔊 https://www.pc.gc.ca/en/pn-np/mtn/ours-bears/securite-safety/ours-humains-bears-people

Big cats

Attacks by lions, tigers, leopards, American mountain lions (cougar, puma), jaguars, and other large felines are increasing in many areas. Big cats usually attack humans from behind, seizing the head or throat and shaking the victim to break the cervical spine or biting at the base of the skull. Severe scratches are inflicted.

Lion

In Kenya and Tanzania there were historical epidemics of fatal attacks by man-eaters. Between 1990 and 2005, 563 human deaths and 308 injuries were reported in south-east Tanzania. Lions are attracted to farms by marauding bush-pigs but end up killing farmers sleeping in shelters in their fields.

Mountain lion (puma, cougar)

In North America, there are an average of 5.6 mountain lion attacks and 0.8 deaths each year.

Tiger

India is famous for its man-eaters. In the Sundarbans (India–Bangladesh border), tigers kill up to 100 people every year during daylight attacks.

Leopard

In India and Pakistan, individual man-eating leopards have claimed hundreds of lives. As human population and farmlands expand, leopards increasingly coexist, even in suburban areas, and the incidence of attacks is rising. Leopards usually attack at night and may enter dwellings.

Prevention

Big cats are best observed from a vehicle, hide, or from the back of an elephant. Females with cubs and solitary males are the most aggressive. Firearm protection is necessary for walking safaris in dangerous areas. Long-term camps should be protected by high fencing and campfires. In the

Sundarbans, wearing face-like masks on the back of the head reduced tiger attacks on villagers and in Botswana, cows were protected from lions by having eyes painted on their rumps. If you are attacked, fight for your life, using any available weapon and making as much noise as possible.

Cattle, camels, and horses

Domesticated and wild beasts of burden can lethally kick, bite, crush, and bolt! Treat them with great respect and stand well clear of the head or tail ends unless you are an expert. Between March 2000 and March 2020, 98 people were killed by cattle in the UK. Of those, 22 were members of the public, with the rest being either farmers or farm workers.

Dogs and wolves

Bites by domestic and feral dogs are common worldwide. More than 200,000 patients bitten by dogs attend hospital in England and Wales each year. In the US, each year, dogs bite 4.5 million people: 885,000 require medical attention (reconstructive surgery in 31,000) and 12 are killed. Children are especially vulnerable. Walkers and joggers in both urban and rural areas frequently encounter aggressive dogs guarding their owners' properties and strays.

Unless they are rabid, wolves usually keep away from humans and rarely attack, but there have been fatalities, especially in children, in Europe (Estonia, Poland, Spain, Russia, Belarus), Iran, India, and North America.

Prevention

Avoid dogs' territories as far as possible and do not disturb bitches with puppies or dogs that are eating or sleeping. Carry a heavy stick or club and fill your pockets with stones. If attacked, avoid eye contact and do not run away, but shout, protect yourself with your backpack, and fight back with sticks and stones.

Websites

℞ https://www.avma.org/resources-tools/pet-owners/dog-bite-prevention

℞ https://www.cdc.gov/mmwr/preview/mmwrhtml/mm5226a1.htm

Elephants

Elephants (maximum height 4 m, weight 7000 kg) are the largest land animals and are highly dangerous. Each year, they kill about 300 people in India and 50 in Sri Lanka and Kenya. Humans may be grasped by the trunk, thrown high in the air, trampled, and then gored. A high proportion of attacks prove fatal. Elephants attack because they are guarding calves or territory, are sick, injured, frightened, or, in the case of bulls, are in 'musth', episodes of increased testosterone production indicated by black oily discharge from temporal glands (between the eye and ear), urinary incontinence, priapism, green algal staining of the penis, and extreme aggression. Early warning signs of irritation before a charge are trumpeting, raised head and trunk, spread ears, swaying body, and lashing tail. 'Mock' charges and attacking charges, with lowered head and curled trunk, may be indistinguishable.

Prevention

Always treat elephants with extreme respect and caution even if they are working or performing animals. Walking safaris in elephant country are dangerous. Experienced rangers with firearms of appropriate calibre are essential. If you sight elephants, travel downwind of them, avoiding, in particular, cows with calves, and solitary bulls. If charged by an elephant, it is futile to run or try to climb a tree. The only hope is to face the animal, shout, and wave your arms. Vehicles may not provide adequate protection.

Hippopotamuses

These massive (maximum height 1.65 m, weight 4500 kg) and irritable African herbivores wallow on the beds or banks of rivers and lakes by day, remaining submerged for periods of up to 6 min. They come ashore to graze at night. Especially in Kenya, Tanzania, Niger, and Botswana, they are notorious for capsizing canoes and drowning their occupants (usually fishermen), for trampling people underfoot and, in water or on land, inflicting terrible bite wounds with their 50 cm-long canines. However, they kill fewer people than elephants, lions, or crocodiles.

Prevention

Avoid swimming, diving, and canoeing in hippo-infested waters. Look out for ripples suggesting a submerged animal and, when it emerges, for warning yawn and grunting. If you are in a boat, escape into deeper water. On land, never block a grazing hippo's trail or its retreat to the water and beware of cows with calves. You cannot outrun a hippo. If charged, hide behind or climb a tree.

Hyenas

Campers resting by day or sleeping in the open at night in Africa have been seized by the head and severely mauled by hyenas causing horrific head and facial injuries. Attacks and deaths are reported from Malawi, Mozambique, Ethiopia, Kenya, and elsewhere.

Pigs and peccaries

Wild, domesticated, and feral pigs are armed with sharp tusks and can attack swiftly and unexpectedly, especially in Melanesia. Penetrating abdominal injuries with prolapse and strangulation of the intestine, pneumothorax, open fractures, laceration of tendons, and artery and nerve injuries have been described.

Prevention

For protection against these lethal animals in Papua New Guinea, an expert's considered advice was 'Carry two spears'.

Crocodiles and alligators

Between 1928 and 2009, 567 encounters with alligators (*Alligator mississippiensis*) (maximum length 4.6 m, weight 453 kg) were reported in the US, 139 provoked by handling, and 24 fatalities. Florida is worst affected. The black caiman (*Melanosuchus niger*) (maximum length 6 m, weight 400 kg) is the most dangerous crocodilian of the Amazon region. Nile crocodiles (*Crocodylus niloticus*) (6.1 m, 900 kg) kill about 1000 people each year in Africa. A famous American infectious diseases physician was seized by a crocodile from a canoe on the Limpopo River, Botswana, in March 2006, and an experienced South African tour guide was taken from a kayak on the Lukuga River, DR Congo, in December 2010. In northern Australia, 27 deaths from 60 attacks by the salt water crocodile (C. porosus) (7 m, 2000 kg) have been reported since 1876. This species is responsible for many attacks and killings in the Purari-Kikori delta region in the Gulf of Papua New Guinea. Mass killings by crocodiles have been described in the Nile at the time of Alexander the Great, in the Second World War (Japanese army off Ramree Island, Burma), and recently after flooding in Ethiopia. Many victims are killed outright and eaten, their bodies never recovered. Victims reaching hospital usually survive but most will require debridement, amputations, and skin grafting; 40% are left with permanent deformities. Fatalities are increasing in Ethiopia, Tanzania, Malawi, and Papua New Guinea. *Pseudomonas*, *Enterococcus*, *Aeromonas*, *Clostridium*, *Serratia*, *Citrobacter*, *Bacteroides*, *Burkholderia*, and *Vibrio*, including *V. vulnificus*, have been implicated in crocodile/alligator bite infections (◯ Marine wound infections, p. 314–315).

Prevention

Take advice from local people. Walkers should keep well away from the water's edge. Avoid footpaths by lakes, rivers, and waterfalls. Do not pitch camp too close to water, do not attract crocs by throwing in waste food and keep children and dogs under control. Never bathe between dusk and dawn. Canoeing is hazardous in croc-infested waters. Do not trail extremities in the water. If attacked on land, run. If attacked in the water, fight back hitting the animal on the nose and eyes with any available weapon.

Sharks

Between 1958 and 2018, 2785 shark attacks were reported with 439 deaths (averages of 46 attacks and seven deaths each year). Most attacks are in Florida, Australia, and South Africa. Surfers and wind surfers are most at risk, followed by swimmers, snorkelers, divers, and waders. Great white (*Carcharodon carcharias*) (length 6 m females, 4 m males, weight 2250 kg), tiger (*Galeocerdo cuvier*) (5.5 m, 900 kg), and bull (*Carcharhinus leucas*) (3.5 m, 360 kg) sharks are the most dangerous, but >70 species that grow longer than about 2 m are potentially lethal. Sharks can inflict truly appalling wounds, resulting in devastating blood loss from severed arteries, causing shock, and the risk of drowning. Common targets are buttocks, thighs, or shoulders. The rough placoid scales can cause abrasions.

Prevention

Avoid bathing in shark-infested waters, between sand bars and the deep ocean, where dead fish have been thrown into the water, where many sea birds are feeding, and where there is sewage effluent. Reduce risk by bathing in groups, close to the shore, only in daylight, and not if you are injured or menstruating. Do not wear jewellery or brightly coloured or patterned clothing. Spear fishermen should not carry their catch. Avoid looking like a seal, a major prey species of dangerous sharks, when you are lying on a surf board. Neither splash excessively nor swim with pet dogs. If attacked by a shark, fight back, hitting it on the nose and clawing at its eyes and gills. Get out of the water as soon as possible. Surface swimmers and surfers are usually targeted rather than divers. Scuba divers who encounter sharks can avoid attacks by descending to the ocean floor, hiding beneath rocks or reefs, and staying in groups. Various chemical and electrical field repellents, chain mail protective suits, and 'bang sticks' (firearms) have been developed but none is of proven benefit.

Website

🔗 http://www.flmnh.ufl.edu/fish/sharks/isaf/2012summary.html

Other fish

Most fish can inflict a painful and damaging bite if handled carelessly on a line or in a net, with a high risk of infection (⊖ Marine wound infections, p. 314–315). Barracudas, marlin, sailfish, titan trigger fish, and rays can be aggressive. In the great river systems of South America, piranhas are capable, at the very least, of biting a chunk out of a foot or hand trailed over the side of the boat. Tiny catfish (Portuguese 'candirú', Spanish 'canero'), their tropism for the gills of the large fish that they parasitize confused by the smell of urine, may, like aquatic leeches, penetrate the urethra, vagina, or anus of bathers, especially women who are menstruating. At Hospital Santa Rosa, Puerto Maldonado, Peru, some half a dozen cases are seen at the local hospital every year. Indo-Pacific marine gar fish or needle fish (*Tylosurus*) can leap out the water at night, attracted by a light, and fatally impale the fisherman.

Prevention

Prevention of all these unusual hazards is to take local advice and to take sensible precautions (e.g. don't bathe in the nude!).

Treatment of trauma caused by animals

First aid of severe injuries

- Secure the victim out of danger and out of the water.
- Control bleeding by direct pressure or tourniquet.
- Close perforating injuries with pressure dressings.
- Start IV fluid volume repletion.
- Evacuate to the base hospital.
- Assume that all injuries are infected. Clean wounds urgently and thoroughly with soap and water and apply iodine and alcohol solutions. For multiple/severe dog- and cat-bite wounds and bites of face and hands, start prophylactic co-amoxiclav, doxycycline, or erythromycin. For other bites, use penicillin, an aminoglycoside (e.g. gentamicin for 48 h) and metronidazole; for marine wounds see ➒ p. 314–315.
- Cover risk of tetanus and rabies.

Emergency treatment at the base hospital

- Replace blood loss.
- Attend to local mechanical complications such as fractures, tension pneumothorax, damage to large blood vessels, perforation of the bowel, and lacerations of other abdominal viscera.
- Debride or amputate dead tissue, removing animals' teeth, etc.
- Irrigate with saline and betadine and drain.
- Delay primary suturing for 48–72 h, except for head and neck wounds which should be sutured immediately.

Further reading

Packer C, Ikanda D, Kissui B, et al. Lion attacks on humans in Tanzania. *Nature*. 2005;436: 927–928 https://doi.org/10.1038/436927a

Packer C, Swanson A, Ikanda D, et al. Fear of darkness, the full moon and the nocturnal ecology of African lions. *Plos One*. 2011;6(7):e22285. https://doi.org/10.1371/journal.pone.0022285

Woodroffe R, Thirgood S, Rabinowitz A (eds). *People and Wildlife: Conflict or Coexistence* Cambridge: Cambridge University Press; 2005.

Venomous land animals

Travellers' fears about venomous animals are usually exaggerated. Although most parts of the world, especially the tropical regions, are inhabited by animals with potentially lethal venoms, it is the local people (agricultural workers, hunters, and their children) rather than travellers who suffer. However, venomous bites and stings have caused a few fatalities in travellers, explorers, and researchers. Risk is reduced by sensible behaviour, protective clothing, and training in prevention and treatment.

Before embarking on an adventurous journey, find out about the local venomous fauna of your wilderness destination. If it is infested with dangerous animals or if the purpose of your expedition involves high exposure (e.g. zoological or botanical surveys in a rain forest), proceed as follows:

- Decide whether to take your own supply of antivenom (antivenin, antivenene or anti-snakebite serum or anti-snake-venom); this is justified only if the expedition is at high risk of venomous bites and stings, the area is more than a few hours' evacuation time from medical care, and your party includes someone capable of injecting the antivenom IV and dealing with the anaphylactic reaction that it may provoke.
- Check the availability of antivenom at the nearest (base) hospital.
- Identify a national centre for antivenom production, supply, and treatment (see ➋ p. 605, for addresses and websites of foreign manufacturers). Antivenoms for bites by foreign snakes cannot be ordered in UK.
- Acquire the necessary knowledge about preventing and treating envenoming. Educate the expedition members at an early stage about prevention and first aid, and rehearse skills, treatment, and evacuation of bite/sting victims.

Snakebite

Snakebite is an important cause of death in agricultural communities in some parts of West Africa, Burma, the Indian subcontinent, New Guinea, and among indigenous Amerindians of the Amazonian region. In India alone, there were an average of 58,000 snakebite deaths each year. Most parts of the world are inhabited by venomous snakes (Fig. 17.1). The medically important groups are elapids, vipers, pit vipers, back-fanged (colubrid) snakes and burrowing asps (Figs. 17.2–17.4).

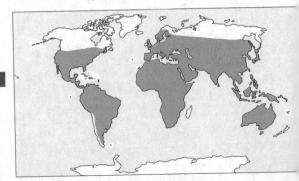

Fig. 17.1 Map of venomous land snake distribution.

Europe
- Vipers only, e.g. adder *Vipera berus*, long-nosed viper *Vipera ammodytes*.

Africa and the Middle East
- Elapids (Fig. 17.2), e.g. cobras and spitting cobras (*Naja*), mambas (*Dendroaspis*).
- Vipers (Fig. 17.3), e.g. saw-scaled vipers (*Echis*), puff adders (*Bitis*), desert horned-vipers (*Cerastes*).
- Colubrids (Fig. 17.4), e.g. boomslang (*Dispholidus*), twig snake (*Thelotornis*).
- Burrowing asps (*Atractaspis*) (Fig. 17.4).

Asia
- Elapids, e.g. cobras (*Naja*) and kraits (*Bungarus*).
- Vipers, e.g. Russell's vipers (*Daboia*), saw-scaled vipers (*Echis*).

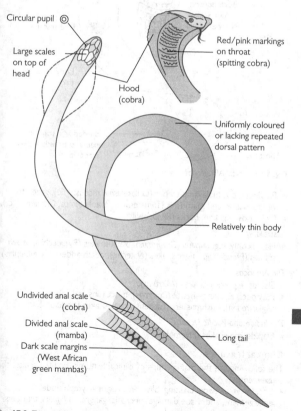

Circular pupil

Large scales on top of head

Hood (cobra)

Red/pink markings on throat (spitting cobra)

Uniformly coloured or lacking repeated dorsal pattern

Relatively thin body

Undivided anal scale (cobra)

Divided anal scale (mamba)

Dark scale margins (West African green mambas)

Long tail

Fig. 17.2 Typical African elapid snake.

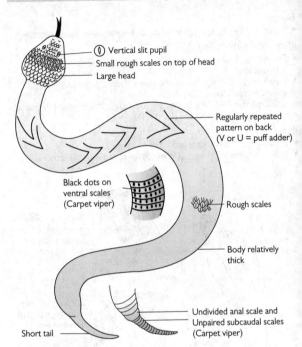

Fig. 17.3 Typical African viper.

- Pit vipers, e.g. Malayan pit viper (*Calloselasma rhodostoma*), green tree vipers, habus, and mamushis (*Trimeresurus, Protobothrops, Gloydius*, etc.).
- Colubrids, e.g. keel-backs (*Rhabdophis*).

Australasia
- Elapids only, e.g. taipans (*Oxyuranus*), black snakes (*Pseudechis*), brown snakes (*Pseudonaja*), tiger snakes (*Notechis*), death adders (*Acanthophis*)

The Americas
- Elapids, e.g. coral snakes (*Micrurus*).
- Pit vipers, e.g. lance-heads (*Bothrops*), moccasins and cantils (*Agkistrodon*), bushmasters (*Lachesis*), rattlesnakes (*Crotalus, Sistrurus*).

The Indian and Pacific Oceans
- Elapids, sea snakes (*Hydrophis*).

Clinical features

The following are the main groups of clinical features *[and the snakes th* *cause them]*:
- Local pain, swelling, bruising, blistering, regional lymph node enlargement, and tissue damage (necrosis/gangrene) *[vipers, pit vipers, burrowing asps, some cobras]*.

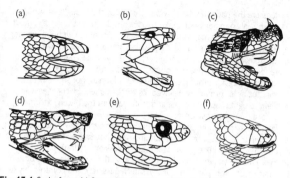

Fig. 17.4 Snake fangs. (a) Sea snake. (b) Cobra. (c) Viper. (d) Pit viper. (e) Back-fanged snake (boomslang). (f) Burrowing asp.

- Incoagulable blood (20 min whole blood clotting test—see ⊃ p. 586), persistent bleeding from bite wound, and spontaneous systemic bleeding (from gums, nose, skin, gut, genitourinary tract) *[vipers, pit vipers, Oceanian (Australia and New Guinea) elapids, colubrids]*.
- Shock (hypotension) *[vipers, pit vipers, burrowing asps]*.
- Descending paralysis progressing from ptosis and external ophthalmoplegia to bulbar and respiratory muscle paralysis *[elapids, a few vipers and pit vipers]*.
- Generalized skeletal muscle breakdown (rhabdomyolysis) (generalized myalgia, muscle tenderness, and myoglobinuria-black/'cola-coloured' urine positive for blood on stix testing) *[sea snakes and a few other elapids, vipers, pit vipers]*.
- Acute kidney injury (oliguria/anuria, ECG changes of hyperkalaemia) *[sea snakes, a few other elapids, a few vipers (especially Russell's vipers), pit vipers and colubrids]*.

Treatment of snakebite

First-aid treatment of snakebite must be applied immediately by the victim or other people who are on the spot.

First-aid treatment of snakebite
- Reassure the bitten person.
- Do not interfere with the bite site in any way.
- Immobilize the victim, especially their bitten limb, using pressure pad immobilization (PPI) or pressure bandage immobilization (PBI) (see following section).
- Arrange urgent evacuation to medical care.
- Treat pain.
- *Do not* attempt to catch or kill the snake (smartphone pictures are useful).
- Avoid all traditional, herbal and 'quack' remedies.

- *Reassure* the patient, who may be terrified by the thought of sudden death: only a minority of snake species are dangerous; even the most notorious species may, on 10–80% of occasions, bite without injecting enough venom to be harmful ('dry bites'); the risk and rapidity of death from snakebite have been greatly exaggerated—lethal doses of venom usually take hours (cobras, mambas, sea-snakes) or days (vipers, rattlesnakes, and other pit vipers) to kill a human, not seconds or minutes as is commonly believed; *correct treatment is very effective.*
- *Remove* tight rings, bracelets, and clothing from the bitten extremity before it becomes swollen.
- *Immobilize* the whole patient, especially their bitten limb, with a splint or sling to delay spread of venom from the bite site. PPI or PBI are effective but training is necessary (see following section).
- *Evacuate* the victim to medical care (e.g. to the expedition doctor, clinic or base hospital), as quickly, safely, passively, and comfortably as possible: vehicle, motorbike, bicycle, boat, or stretcher are suitable. Ideally, the patient should lie in the recovery position (➜ p. 248–249) to minimize the risk of aspirating vomit (a common early symptom of systemic envenoming) and should keep as still as possible to avoid exercising any part of the body, especially their bitten limb (muscle contraction pumps venom through veins and lymphatics). Don't waste time before starting the journey; get going!
- Give analgesia as snakebite can be very painful: paracetamol or codeine are suitable but avoid aspirin or non-steroidal anti-inflammatory agents as they increase the risk of bleeding.
- Do not attempt to catch or kill the snake: but if it has been killed already, take it along as useful clinical evidence. Never handle a dead snake with bare hands; even a severed head may strike! Smartphone images of head, back, and belly, are useful.
- Do not use traditional methods: incisions, suction, tourniquets, electric shock, ice packs, instillation of potassium permanganate crystals, herbs, black/snake stone, etc. are useless and potentially harmful.

Pressure pad immobilization and pressure bandage immobilization

These first-aid treatments are important for elapid bites that can cause rapidly evolving paralysis and some viper bites that can cause early life threatening shock. However, in the field, snake identification is usually uncertain. Immediate application of PPI or PBI is therefore recommended for all cases of snakebite except where such dangerous snakes can be confidently ruled out (e.g. Europe and north of latitude 43°). Pressure can be released later if an elapid bite can be confidently excluded. The aim is to empty and compress lymphatics and veins draining the bite site (in the case of PPI) or the bitten limb (in the case of PBI), to delay systemic spread of venom toxins into the systemic circulation where they may cause early death. This can be achieved with an external pressure of 50–70 mmHg (roughly equivalent to the firm binding of a sprained ankle).

- *PPI*: a firm pad ~8 × 8 × 3 cm thick, made for example by folding a bandage or piece of cloth, or using foam rubber, is applied directly over the bite site, using a broad non-elastic circumferential bandage around the bitten limb (Fig. 17.5a).

- *PBI:* the whole bitten limb is bound, using several robust elastic
  bandages (10 cm wide, 4.5 m long)[1] and incorporating a splint (e.g.
  SAM® splint), starting around the fingers or toes and finishing at the
  armpit or groin (Fig. 17.5b). Don't bind too loosely! If it is too tight,
  it will obstruct arterial blood flow, like a tourniquet, the limb will
  become ischaemic, cyanosed, and very painful, and peripheral pulses
  at the wrist or ankle will be impalpable.

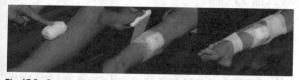

Fig. 17.5a Pressure pad immobilization. Application of pressure pad directly over
the bite wound, bound in place, and the bitten limb immobilized with a splint.

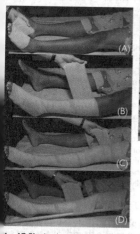 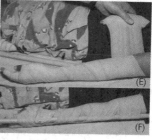

Fig. 17.5b Applying pressure immobilization bandages. A–C: firm binding of
the bitten limb with wide elasticated bandages, starting beyond the bite site, and
extending up to the groin; D: incorporating a splint; E–F: same for upper limb with
elbow extended. Images courtesy of Dr David Williams.

Mölnlycke Setopress® PEC high compression bandage Type 3c, 10 cm × 3.5 m, applied at
>40 mmHg using visual pressure guide, is recommended. https://www.molnlycke.com/products-
solutions/setopress/

Indications for antivenom treatment

Any of the following:

- Spontaneous systemic bleeding (➔ Clinical features, p. 582–583).
- Incoagulable blood: failure of the patient's blood to clot solid when placed in a new, clean, dry, glass vessel and left undisturbed for 20 min *or* persistent bleeding (>30 min) from the fang punctures or other wounds, including venepuncture sites.
- Shock: low or falling BP or cardiac arrhythmia.
- Paralysis (➔ p. 583).
- Black/dark red-brown/'cola-coloured' urine (indicating rhabdomyolysis or massive haemolysis or impending acute kidney injury: declining urine output, increasing serum creatinine/blood urea).
- Local swelling: involving more than half the bitten limb *or* swelling after bites on the fingers and toes *or* swelling after bites by snakes whose bites have a high risk of causing necrosis.
- Mild local swelling alone is not an indication for antivenom. Never give antivenom unless you have adrenaline (epinephrine) available to treat early anaphylactic reactions to the antivenom, and are able to recognize the features of anaphylaxis (see following 'Administration of antivenom' section and ➔ p. 56, 256–257).

Choice of appropriate antivenom

Before giving antivenom make sure that its range of specificity includes the snake likely to have bitten your patient.

Most antivenoms are polyvalent and are able to neutralize venoms of the medically important venomous species of the region for which it is intended. For example, in India, all antivenoms cover the 'big four' venomous species: spectacled cobra, common krait, Russell's viper, and saw scaled viper; in Latin America, some antivenoms cover the local lanceheads, rattlesnakes, and bushmaster (*Lachesis*). Monovalent antivenoms can be used if only one dangerous species occurs in the area (e.g. adder *V. beru* in UK, Netherlands, Belgium, Luxemburg, Poland and Scandinavia), if the snake has been reliably identified, or if a diagnostic clinical syndrome of envenoming appears. For example, in the savanna region of northern third of Africa, incoagulable blood is virtually diagnostic of saw-scaled/carpet viper (*Echis*) bite.

Administration of antivenom

- Give prophylactic adrenaline/epinephrine, adult dose 0.25 mg of 0.1% SC before starting antivenom to reduce the risk of a severe reactions.
- For optimal effect, administer antivenom by slow IV injection (2 mL/min) or IV infusion diluted in 250–500 mL isotonic fluid over 30–60 min
- Initial dose depends on the type of antivenom, species of snake, and severity of symptoms: commonly four to five 10 mL ampoules. Exactly the same dose is given to children and adults.
- Watch the patient closely for at least 2 h after starting antivenom for signs of anaphylaxis: restlessness, fever, itching, urticarial rash, angioedema (swelling of lips, gums, tongue, and throat), vomiting, breathlessness and wheezing, tachycardia, and fall in BP.

- Treat anaphylaxis immediately with adrenaline/epinephrine, adult dose 0.5 mL of 1 in 1000 solution IM (lateral thigh); this can be repeated after 10 min if it is not effective. Asthmatic reactions require additional inhaled bronchodilator.
- Repeat initial dose after 6 h if the blood remains incoagulable when retested, or after a few hours if bleeding, shock, or paralysis are undiminished.

Only in an extreme emergency should untrained people administer antivenom; e.g. when the victim is many hours away from medical care, develops severe envenoming, and is deteriorating (Fig. 17.6). Only in this unusual situation, give antivenom by multiple deep IM injections into the thighs (not the buttocks). Massage injection sites to increase absorption and apply firm pressure bandages to control bleeding.

Treatment of complications
- *Hypovolaemic shock:* massive external bleeding or leakage of blood and tissue fluid into a swollen limb may leave the patient with an inadequate circulating volume so that the BP falls (check for postural drop of >20 mmHg in systolic BP from lying to sitting up). Transfusion with plasma expanders such as 0.9% saline or Hartmann's solution may be needed.
- *Respiratory failure:* from respiratory obstruction from bulbar paralysis, prolapsed tongue, or inhaled vomitus; or respiratory muscle paralysis; must be treated by re-establishing an airway; giving oxygen by any available means; and by assisting ventilation, mouth-to-mouth or by bag-valve mask, endotracheal tube, laryngeal mask airway, or i-gel™, whatever is available and effective in the circumstances.
- *Acute kidney injury:* some patients become anuric or oliguric soon after bites by Russell's vipers, some pit vipers, Oceanian elapids, and sea snakes. They must be managed conservatively until they reach the base hospital. Correct hypovolaemia by giving IV fluid until the jugular venous pulse becomes visible when the patient is propped up at 45°, then restrict fluids and give paracetamol 1g 6-hourly (adult dose) to protect the kidneys.
- *Wound infection* may be introduced by the snake's fangs or by ill-advised tampering at the bite site producing delayed local inflammation (difficult to distinguish from envenoming) or an obvious abscess which should be aspirated. A tetanus toxoid booster is appropriate immediately after the bite. In cases of obviously infected or necrotic wounds, treat with antibiotics such as metronidazole, co-amoxiclav, or chloramphenicol.
- *Surgical complications:* at the base hospital, necrotic tissue should be debrided and the skin defect covered with split skin grafts. Fasciotomy to relieve suspected compartment syndrome (e.g. anterior tibial compartment) is almost never indicated and should be considered only after normal haemostasis has been restored with adequate antivenom treatment and persistently raised intracompartmental pressure confirmed by direct measurement (e.g. using a Stryker pressure monitor).

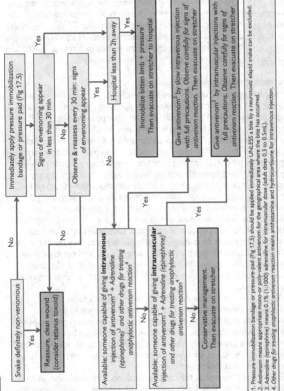

Immediately apply pressure immobilization bandage or pressure pad (Fig 17.5)

Snake definitely non-venomous → No

Yes → Reassure, clean wound (consider tetanus toxoid)

No → Signs of envenoming appear in less than 30 min

No → Observe & reassess every 30 min: signs of envenoming appear

Yes → Hospital less than 2h away

Yes → Immobilize bitten limb + pressure[1] Then evacuate to hospital

No →

Available: someone capable of giving **intravenous** injection of antivenom[2] + Adrenaline (epinephrine)[3] and other drugs for treating anaphylactic antivenom reaction[4]

Yes → Give antivenom[2] by slow intravenous injection with full precautions. *Observe carefully for signs of antivenom reaction.* Then evacuate on stretcher

No →

Available: someone capable of giving **intramuscular** injection of antivenom[2] + Adrenaline (epinephrine)[3] and other drugs for treating anaphylactic antivenom reaction[4]

Yes → Give antivenom[2] by intramuscular injections with full precautions. *Observe carefully for signs of antivenom reaction.* Then evacuate on stretcher

No → Conservative management. Then evacuate on stretcher

1. Pressure-immobilization bandage or pressure-pad (Fig 17.5) should be applied immediately UNLESS a bite by a neurotoxic elapid snake can be excluded.
2. Antivenom means appropriate mono- or poly-valent antivenom for the geographical area where the bite has occurred.
3. Adrenaline (epinephrine) means 0.1% (1:1000) adrenaline for intramuscular dose (adult dose 0.3 to 0.5mL).
4. Other drugs for treating anaphylactic antivenom reaction means antihistamine and hydrocortisone for intravenous injection.

Fig. 17.6 Algorithm to guide use of antivenom in remote wilderness situations.

Paralysis caused by Asian cobras and Australasian death adders may respond to anticholinesterases such as neostigmine, or physostigmine. Atropine 0.6 mg is given IV followed by 0.02 mg/kg neostigmine bromide/methylsulfate by IM injection (adult doses). If there is an improvement in muscle power within the next 20–30 min, treatment can be continued with SC neostigmine methylsulfate, 0.5–2.5 mg every 1–3 h up to 10 mg/24 h maximum (adult dose).

Spitting cobra-induced eye injuries

Spitting cobras occur in Africa and parts of South-East Asia. They can spray venom defensively for a metre or more towards the glinting eyes of a perceived aggressor. Venom falling on the conjunctivae causes agonizing chemical conjunctivitis with profuse tearing, leucorrhoea, and blepharospasm. Corneal ulceration, infection, and permanent blindness may result.

Emergency treatment

Irrigate the eye(s) immediately with large volumes of any available bland fluid, ideally water under the tap (but milk or even urine is better than nothing: 'Please urinate into my eye'!). Single (only!) instillation of LA (e.g. tetracaine) or 1% adrenaline (epinephrine) eye drops with oral paracetamol relieves pain. Exclude corneal abrasions by fluorescein staining or slit lamp examination and apply prophylactic topical antibiotic (e.g. tetracycline, chloramphenicol). Prevent posterior synechiae, ciliary spasm, and discomfort with topical cycloplegics (e.g. 2% atropine). Give topical antihistamine for allergic keratoconjunctivitis. Topical or IV antivenom and topical corticosteroids are contraindicated.

Prevention of snakebites

Do

- Avoid all snakes and snake charmers.
- Open and shake out sleeping bags and clothing before use.
- Tap boots before wearing to dislodge any unwanted inhabitants.
- Check ground before sitting at the base of trees.
- Wear boots, socks, and long trousers when walking in undergrowth or deep sand.
- Wear boots and use a torch and a prodding stick when walking off or on a track at night, especially after heavy rain and also when relieving yourself at night (many snakes are most active in the dark).
- Be cautious and wear gloves when collecting firewood.
- Remember that banks and streams are common snake haunts.
- Travel with a local guide who is much more likely to see camouflaged snakes.
- Sleep off the ground (hammock or camp bed), or use a sewn-in ground sheet and mosquito-proof tent, or sleep under a mosquito net that is well tucked-in under your sleeping bag or mat. This will protect against night-prowling kraits (Asia) or spitting cobras and burrowing asps (Africa) which often bite people while they are asleep on the ground.

Do not

- Put hands blindly down inside rucksacks—empty out contents.
- Put hands or poke sticks into burrows or holes.

- Put hands up onto branches or ledges that can't be seen.
- Swim in rivers matted with vegetation in which snakes may be hiding or in muddy estuaries favoured by sea snakes.
- Straddle logs—better to step up onto them then over.
- Disturb, corner, provoke, or attack snakes. Never handle them, even if they are said to be harmless or appear to be dead (some snakes sham death!).
- Move, if you do corner a snake by mistake. Snakes strike only at moving objects so keep absolutely still until it has slithered away although this demands almost inhuman *sangfroid*!

Lizard bite (parts of Middle and Central America only)

Gila monster (*Heloderma suspectum*) (up to 55 cm long) of south-western USA and adjacent Mexico and the Mexican beaded lizard or escorpión (*H. horridum*) (up to 80 cm) of western Mexico south to Guatemala are the only dangerously venomous lizards. However, some monitors (*Varanidae*) (notably the Komodo dragon (*Varanus komodoensis*)) and other lizards have now been shown perhaps to secrete mildly venomous saliva but are far more likely to cause harm by physical trauma. Helodermids' venom glands and grooved fangs are in their lower jaws. They only bite people who attack/handle them, hanging on like bulldogs, making it very difficult to disengage and increasing the exposure to envenoming. Lever its jaws apart with a screw driver, put it under the tap, place its four feet on the ground or introduce some alcohol into its mouth.

There is immediate severe local pain, spreading tender swelling, erythema and regional lymphadenopathy, weakness, dizziness, tachycardia, hypotension, syncope, angioedema, sweating, rigors, tinnitus, nausea, and vomiting. No fatal cases are confirmed.

Treatment

Antivenom is not available. A powerful analgesic may be required. Hypotension should be treated with plasma expanders and perhaps adrenaline or noradrenaline depending upon response.

Arthropods

Bee, wasp, hornet, yellow jacket, and ant sting hypersensitivity (Hymenoptera)

Stings by these insects are a common nuisance in many countries. Bees (*Apidae*) and wasp-like insects including yellow jackets and hornets (*Vespidae*), occur worldwide. Fire ants (*Solenopsis*) inhabit the Americas and jumper ants (*Myrmecia*) are found in Australia (especially Tasmania). Stings by all these hymenoptera can cause rapidly developing, potentially-lethal, systemic anaphylaxis in ~2–4% of the population who have become sensitized to their venoms by a previous sting. Other people may develop delayed, massive and persistent local swelling and inflammation which is unpleasant but not life-threatening.

Clinical

Symptoms of anaphylaxis can evolve in seconds. They include urticaria, angioedema, shock, unconsciousness, bronchoconstriction, GI symptoms (nausea, vomiting, diarrhoea), double incontinence, and, in women, uterine contractions. Venom-specific IgE is detected by radioallergosorbent test (RAST) or prick skin/patch testing, confirming hypersensitivity (➲ Treatment of anaphylaxis, p. 56, 256–257).

Prevention

People who have had anaphylaxis must carry self-injectable adrenaline (e.g. EpiPen®, Emerade®, Jext®) with them at all times, but most have little idea how to use it in an emergency (Fig. 17.7). The technique should be practised with an EpiPen®Trainer. Allergic subjects should wear an identifying tag (e.g. MedicAlert™ or MediTag™) to indicate their problem (e.g. 'allergic to wasp stings—give adrenaline') in case they are found incoherent or unconscious.

Desensitization: those with a history of systemic anaphylaxis to a sting and who are RAST or skin test-positive for the appropriate venom can be effectively desensitized before the expedition. Control of the hypersensitivity takes about 8 weeks, while cure takes 3–5 years.

1. Pull off the grey safety cap, as shown in diagram (a).
2. Hold the auto-injection as shown in diagram (b) and place the black tip on your thigh, at right angles to your leg. Always apply to the thigh.
3. Press hard into your thigh until the auto-injection mechanism works and hold the device in place for 10 seconds. The EpiPen® unit can then be removed. Massage the injection site for 10 seconds

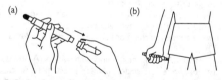

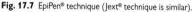

Fig. 17.7 EpiPen® technique (Jext® technique is similar).

Mass attacks

In tropical countries, rock climbers and other travellers have been attacked by large swarms of aggressive bees, resulting in fatal falls. In Zimbabwe, a man survived 2000 bee stings despite terrible symptoms of massive histamine release. Some accidents could have been prevented by seeking local advice. Thundery weather is known to upset bees but a perceived threat to their nest is the commonest provocation.

In the face of an attack, run away very fast, ideally into undergrowth, or immerse yourself under water. For climbers, a fall is the greatest danger. First, secure yourself, then use anorak, rucksack, or tent for protection. South Asia has aggressive giant honey bees 3 cm long and in South America there have been many deaths from mass attacks by furious swarms of

Africanized ('killer') honey bees. Multiple stings can cause haemolysis, rhabdomyolysis, bronchospasm, pneumonitis, and acute kidney injury. No antivenom is commercially available.

Blister beetles ('Spanish fly', 'Nairobi eye', rove beetles)

These beetles exude vesicating fluid containing cantharidin or paederin when inadvertently touched or trapped (e.g. in antecubital fossa when elbow is flexed), causing erythema, itching, and formation of large, painless, thin-walled blisters. 'Spanish fly' (*Cantharis vesicatoria*, family Meloidae) is iridescent green. 'Nairobi eye' and similar blistering conditions in Australia and South East Asia are caused by paederin-containing secretions of rove beetles (*Paederus*, family Staphylinidae; Fig. 17.8). Toxin from crushed beetles or blister fluid is easily spread to other sites such as the eye by fingers. Treatment is palliative.

Moth and caterpillar sting ('lepidopterism', 'erucism')

These insects, in particular brightly coloured, hairy caterpillars, such as the sycamore tussock moth (*Halysidota harrisii*), can cause local pain, inflammation, nettle rash, blistering, and arthritis on contact. In northern South America, stings by giant silkworm moth caterpillars (*Lonomia obliqua* and *L. achelous*) (➔ Colour plate 15), can result in incoagulable blood, acute kidney injury, and fatal systemic bleeding. A Canadian tourist, stung in Peru, died after returning home to Canada. Treatment is non-specific (antihistamines, corticosteroids, analgesics) except in the case of *Lonomia*, for which an effective specific antivenom is manufactured in Brazil.

Spider bite

The most dangerous genera of spiders are:
- *Latrodectus*—black/brown widow spiders (Americas, southern Europe, Southern Africa, Australia, New Caledonia; Fig. 17.9).
- *Phoneutria*—wandering, armed or banana spiders (Latin America; Fig. 17.10).
- *Atrax* and *Hadronyche*—(Sydney) funnel web spiders (Australia).
- *Loxosceles*—brown recluse spiders (Americas, southern Africa, and Mediterranean).

Many completely innocent (hobo, wolf, white-tailed, sac) spiders have been vilified as causes of 'necrotic arachnidism', attributable to other ulcerative conditions.

Clinical

Bites usually happen when the victim brushes against a spider that has crept into curtains, clothes, or bedding. *Latrodectus*, *Phoneutria*, and *Atrax* are neurotoxic, causing local puncture marks and surrounding erythema, severe pain spreading from the bite site, cramping abdominal or chest pains simulating an acute abdomen or MI, muscle spasms, weakness, profuse sweating, salivation, goose flesh, fever, nausea, vomiting, priapism, anxiety, feelings of doom and alterations in pulse rate and BP. Local pain, sweating, and gooseflesh at the site of bite are useful signs. Some genera of Old World tarantulas (Theraphosidae) can cause severe muscle spasms. *Loxosceles* venom is necrotic, causing evolution, over a few hours at the site of bite, of pain

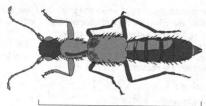

Fig. 17.8 Nairobi eye beetle.

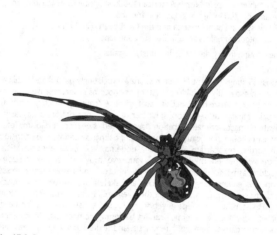

Fig. 17.9 Brown widow spider *Latrodectus geometricus*.

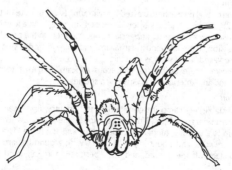

Fig. 17.10 Brazilian wandering spider *Phoneutria*.

and a circumscribed lesion ('red-white-and-blue sign') and scarlatiniform rash (➔ Colour plate 16). Rarely, there are systemic effects: fever, haemoglobinuria, coagulopathy, and acute kidney injury.

Deaths are unusual except among children. Antivenoms are manufactured in countries such as South Africa, Australia, Mexico, and Brazil, where severe spider bites are common.

Scorpion sting

The most dangerous scorpions are:

- *Leiurus quinquestriatus*, *Androctonus* spp., *Hemiscorpius lepturus*, and *Buthus* spp. in North Africa and the Middle East.
- *Parabuthus* spp. in South and North-East Africa.
- *Centruroides* spp. in North America (15000 stings by *C. exilicauda* per year reported in Arizona, US) and Mexico.
- *Tityus* spp. in Latin America and the Caribbean (Fig. 17.11).
- *Hottentotta tamulus* in the Indian subcontinent.

All are found in dry desert or hot dusty terrains.

Clinical

Almost all stings (except *H. lepturus*) are excruciatingly painful and fatalities do occur, especially in children. Systemic symptoms reflect release of autonomic neurotransmitters, initially acetylcholine (causing vomiting, abdominal pain, pancreatic secretion, sphincter of Oddi constriction, bradycardia, salivation, nasolacrimal secretion, generalized sweating, priapism, etc.) then catecholamines (causing piloerection, palmar sweating, hypertension, tachycardia, myocarditis, pulmonary oedema, and ECG abnormalities). *Centruroides* envenoming causes erratic eye movements, fasciculations, muscle spasms simulating tonic–clonic seizures, and respiratory distress. *Parabuthus* envenoming causes ptosis and skeletal and respiratory muscle paralysis; some species can squirt their venom. *Hemiscorpius lepturus* (Iran, Iraq, Pakistan, and Yemen) envenoming causes a distinctive syndrome of painless sting, local erythema, bruising, blistering and necrosis, bleeding tendency, myocardial damage, haemolysis, and acute kidney injury with high case fatality.

Treatment

The severe local pain is best treated by infiltrating LA at the site of the sting (e.g. 1–2% lidocaine), ideally by digital block if the sting is on a finger or toe. Otherwise, powerful opiate analgesia may be required. In the base hospital, hypertension, acute left ventricular failure, and pulmonary oedema may respond to vasodilators such as prazosin.

Antivenoms are available for dangerous African/Middle Eastern, South African, Indian, American, and Australian species.

Prevention

When establishing camp in scorpion-infested country, first clear the area of rocks, undergrowth, and debris to expose the scorpions. By night, a UV lamp is a useful adjunct as it makes scorpions fluoresce. They hide in cracks, crevices, and under rubbish. Don't walk around in bare feet, be sure to sleep off the ground, and use a permethrin-impregnated bed net.

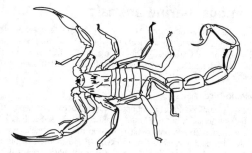

Fig. 17.11 Brazilian scorpion *Tityus serrulatus*.

Always shake out your boots and shoes before putting them on (see also ➋ Prevention of snakebite, p. 589–590).

Other venomous invertebrates

Centipede stings, inflicted by their pincer-like forcipules just behind the jaws, are very painful and can cause local swelling, redness, lymphangitis, blistering and necrosis. Stings by the most dangerous genus, *Scolopendra*, up to 35 cm long (➋ Colour plate 17), sometimes cause vomiting, sweating, headache, hypotension, and fever, with very rare reports of fatalities in the Philippines, Thailand, and Rodrugues Islands (RGS Shoals Capricorn Programme Western Indian Ocean 1998–2001). Hypersensitization may lead to anaphylaxis.

Millipedes can squirt highly irritant defensive secretions, causing blistering and staining of skin and mucosae. No specific treatment is available.

Giant freshwater water bugs (beetles) (Belostomidae) can inflict painful bites.

Tick species in North America (e.g. *Dermacentor* spp.), eastern Australia (*Ixodes holocyclus*), and Europe can inject a neurotoxin while sucking blood. If one of your team develops an ascending flaccid paralysis while in these countries, search hairy areas and the external auditory meatus, and detach any ticks as soon as possible using the correct technique (➋ p. 308–309). Paralytic symptoms should then subside.

Venomous marine animals

Although venomous bites and stings can occur in temperate waters, the risk is much greater in tropical seas (Indo-Pacific, Red Sea, Eastern Mediterranean, and Caribbean). Often, the animal is not seen or identified, but the circumstances and symptoms may be helpful in establishing the likely cause (➡ Fig. 17.17, p. 602).

Sea-snakebite

Sea-snakes occur in colossal numbers in warmer oceans, estuaries, rivers, and a few inland lakes, but not in the Atlantic or the Red Sea (Fig. 17.12). They are encountered mainly by fishermen in the Indo-Pacific region but bite only if handled (e.g. while being picked out of hand nets or off fishing lines). Heads and tails may be difficult to distinguish. Bites are usually pain-less leaving small puncture marks, often multiple and containing broken-off teeth. The principal symptoms of envenoming are progressive myalgia and muscle tenderness with trismus, passing dark (cola-coloured) urine (myoglobinuria), ptosis, descending paralysis threatening respiratory failure, and acute kidney injury. Rhabdomyolysis can be so severe that potassium released from damaged muscles causes cardiac arrest. Hyperkalaemia may be controlled with IV calcium chloride, sodium bicarbonate, or insulin and glucose. Treatment is the same as for other snakebites (➡ p. 583–587). Wet suits are protective against the bites of all but the longest-fanged and most aggressive of sea snakes.

Fish sting

More than 1200 species of fresh water and especially marine fish are ven-omous, but only about 200 species can cause dangerous stings. They inhabit both tropical and temperate waters. Important species include: stingrays, mantas, catfish, weevers, toadfish, stargazers, stone lifters, scorpion fish, stone fish (*Synanceja verrucosa* is the most deadly), sharks, and dogfish. Their venomous spines are in the gills, fins, or tail. Beautiful lion, zebra, tiger, turkey, or red fire fish (*Pterois*, *Dendrochirus*; Fig. 17.13) are popular aquarium pets. Stingrays are common in the oceans and in rivers of South America and Equatorial Africa. If trodden upon, they lash their tails, impaling the ankle with a venomous spine (Fig. 17.14).

Stings occur when fish are:

- Handled by fishermen or tropical aquarium keepers.
- Trodden on or touched by bathers and waders on beaches or by people fording rivers in the Amazon region, especially in the dry season.
- Irritated by swimmers and scuba divers around coral reefs.

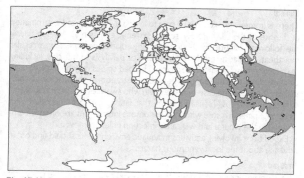

Fig. 17.12 Distribution of sea snakes.

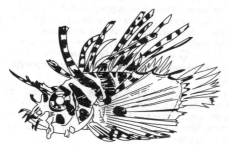

Fig. 17.13 Lion fish *Dendrochirus*.

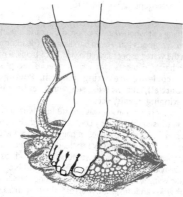

Fig. 17.14 Stinging action of stingray.

Clinical

There is immediate excruciating pain followed by swelling and inflammation at the site of the sting. Rarely, severe systemic effects may develop during the following minutes or hours: vomiting, diarrhoea, sweating, irregular heartbeat, cardiac arrest, fall in BP, spasm or paralysis of muscles, including respiratory muscles, and fits. Stingrays' barbed spines may be large enough to cause fatal trauma (pneumothorax, penetration of thoracic or abdominal organs), as in the case of Steve Irwin who swam over a large ribbon-tail stingray (*Taeniurops/Taeniura meyeni*) that fatally punctured his heart with its spine. Spines invested with their venomous integument are often left embedded in the wound and will cause infection unless removed.

Expeditions involving activities in aquatic environments should find out in advance about the local venomous hazards.

First aid

The agonizing local pain is dramatically relieved by immersing the stung part in hot but not scalding water. Test the temperature with your own elbow. If you have a thermometer, check that the temperature does not exceed 45°C. Hotter water will cause a full thickness scald. Ad hoc methods of local heating have been described: a lighted cigarette, cigar or lighter advanced to within inches of the wound, or a damp towel wrapped round a hot engine block. Alternatively, 1% lidocaine or some other LA can be injected, ideally as a digital block (➔ p. 627–628). The venomous spines of stingrays and catfish are often barbed but must be removed as soon as possible.

Antivenom

Seqirus (formerly CSL) Australia produces an antivenom for stonefish (genus *Synanceja*) that covers stings by some other scorpion fish. Exceptionally, a stung patient might need mouth-to-mouth respiration and chest compressions. Atropine (0.6 mg IV for adults) should be given if there is hypotension attributed to bradycardia.

Infection

Both venomous and non-venomous fish wounds can become infected with unusual marine pathogens (➔ p. 314–315).

Prevention

Employ a shuffling gait when wading or prod the sand ahead of you with a stick to disturb venomous fish. Avoid handling fish (dead or alive) and keep clear of fish in the water, especially in the vicinity of tropical reefs. Footwear, the thicker the better, protects against most species except stingrays.

Cnidarian (coelenterate) sting: jellyfish, Portuguese man o' war ('blue bottle'), sea nettle, sea wasp, cubomedusoids, sea anemones, stinging corals, etc.

The tentacles of these marine animals are studded with millions of stinging capsules (nematocysts) triggered by contact to fire their venomous stinging hairs into the skin. This produces lines of painful blisters and inflammation in distinctive patterns. Hypersensitivity may lead to recurrent urticarial rashes over many months. The venom of some species, such as the notorious box jellyfish (*Chironex fleckeri* and *Chiropsalmus* spp.) of Northern Australian and Indo-Pacific waters, has caused >70 deaths since 1883. Severe systemic effects can result in cardiorespiratory arrest within minutes of the stings.

'Irukandji' syndrome is caused by *Carukia barnesi* and other tiny transparent cubomedusoids. There is severe musculoskeletal pain, anxiety, trembling, headache, piloerection, sweating, tachycardia, hypertension, and pulmonary oedema starting within about 30 min of the sting and persisting for hours.

Other medically important jellyfish include Portuguese men o' war (*Physalia*) which are worldwide in distribution, and have caused a few fatalities and local gangrene caused by arterial spasm (➲ Colour plate 18); *Stomalophis nomurai* of the north-west Pacific, China, and Japan which can cause fatal pulmonary oedema; the sea nettle (*Chrysaora quinquecirrha*) which is very widely distributed but is most common in Chesapeake Bay, on the east coast of the US, and the mauve stinger (*Pelagia noctileuca*), which can swarm in enormous numbers causing stinging epidemics in the Adriatic and other parts of the Mediterranean.

Coral cuts are common injuries inflicted by coelenterates in tropical waters. Painful superficial grazes and cuts result when tender areas of the body are inadvertently brushed against coral outcrops. Mechanical injury from the spiky calcified crust is combined with envenoming and the risk of a marine bacterial infection (➲ p. 314–315).

Sea bathers' eruption or 'pica-pica': hypersensitization to nematocysts of tiny (16 × 13–20 mm) larvae of sea anemones and thimble jellyfish, such as *Linuche unguiculata* and *Edwardsiella lineata* causes intense itching of areas of skin covered by swimming costumes. This develops while swimming in tropical or sub-tropical waters, or, more often, after leaving the water and showering. Persisting itchy maculopapular rashes erupt, sometimes with malaise, headache, mild fever, GI symptoms, and pain passing urine.

Treatment

- Remove the victim from the water to prevent drowning and resuscitate if collapsed, cyanosed and pulseless.
- Prevent further discharge of nematocysts by washing or shaving off adherent tentacles using sea water:
  - *Do not use* commercial vinegar or acetic acid solution and pressure immobilization, formerly recommended for *Chironex* spp. and other cubozoans; and *do not use* alcoholic solutions, such as methylated spirits and suntan lotion, formerly used for *Chrysaora quinquecirrha* and *Physalia physalis* stings. They may provoke nematocyst discharge.
- Relieve agonizing pain:
  - Hot water treatment (as for fish stings; ➲ p. 596–598) has proved more effective than ice.
  - Lidocaine hydrochloride spray is the most promising topical analgesic and prevents nematocyst discharge of *Chiropsalmus quadrumanus*, *Chrysaora quinquecirrha*, and *Physalia physalis* nematocysts.

Treat severe envenoming:
- CPR on the beach has saved lives.
- Antivenom for box jellyfish, 'Sea wasp' (*C. fleckeri*), is manufactured in Australia. Ideally, give IV, but it has been given on the beach by surf lifesavers by IM injection.

Coral cuts: should be cleaned and debrided as far as possible, irrigated, cleaned with antiseptic, and dressed. Infection should be treated promptly (➲ p. 314–315).

- Sea bathers' eruption: remove swimming costume and rinse body with sea water. Machine wash costume. Apply 1% hydrocortisone lotion to rash. For systemic symptoms try oral antihistamine or prednisolone.

Sea urchin and starfish injuries (echinoderms)

The sharp venomous spines and grapples of some sea urchins may become deeply embedded in the skin, usually of the sole of the foot when the animal has been trodden upon. Wounds may be stained blue-black. Soften the skin with 2% w/w salicylic acid ointment and then pare down the epidermis to a depth at which the spines can be removed with forceps. If the spines are visible, try to remove them immediately. If not, they are absorbed over several days provided they are broken into small pieces in the skin. If they penetrate a joint or cause infection, surgical removal is necessary.

Molluscs: octopus bite and cone shell sting

The blue-ringed octopuses of the Indo-Australasian region rarely exceed 20 cm in diameter but have caused fatal envenoming after unnoticed, painless bites (Fig. 17.15). Cone shells (Fig. 17.16) are beautiful collectors' items but they can envenom by harpooning and implanting a venom-charged arrowhead. Stings may be unnoticed, causing spreading numbness and paralysis. Beware of picking up these attractive animals bare-handed. Their stings can be fatal. No antivenom is available. Treatment of mollusc bites and stings is purely supportive, based on the knowledge that their venoms (tetrodotoxin in the case of the blue-ringed octopus) are ion-channel agonists/antagonists that may cause paraesthesiae, paralysis, and cardiac arrest.

Annelids: bristle worm bites and stings

Most species of these polychaete annelid marine worms (e.g. lugworms, sandworms) are <10 cm long but one species grows to 3 m. Their paddle-like parapodia are armed with sharp setae that can become embedded causing pain and irritation while bites can also be painful. Some species may inject toxins by stinging and biting.

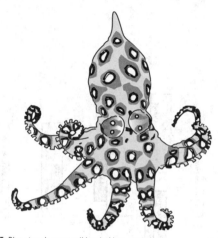

Fig. 17.15 Blue-ringed octopus (*Hapalochlaena maculosa*).

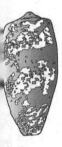

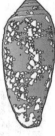
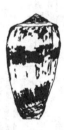

Conus geographus   *Conus textile*   *Conus aulicus*   *Conus striatus*

Conus tessulatus   *Conus abbas*   *Conus tulipus*   *Conus lividus*

Fig. 17.16 Cone shells.

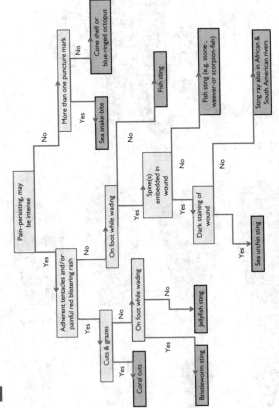

Fig. 17.17 Diagnosis of envenoming of unknown cause in a tropical sea.

Poisonous fish and shellfish

Everywhere, but especially in the tropics, the flesh of many species of fish, shellfish, and other marine animals is dangerously poisonous, always or seasonally, to humans and other animals.

Ciguatera poisoning

Symptoms develop 1–6 h after eating warm-water shore or reef fish (groupers, snappers, parrot fish, mackerel, moray eels, barracudas, and jacks). There may be 500,000 cases each year and, in some Pacific Islands, up to 1% of the population is affected each year, with a case fatality of 0.1%. GI symptoms resolve within a few hours, but paraesthesia and myalgia may persist for a week or even months.

Tetrodotoxin poisoning

Scaleless porcupine, file, trigger, puffer, and sunfish (order: Tetraodontiformes) become poisonous at certain seasons. Puffer fish ('fugu') is popular in Japan. Neurotoxic symptoms develop 10–45 min after eating the fish and death from respiratory paralysis may follow 2–6 h later. There may be no GI symptoms. Skin changes include erythema, petechiae, blistering, and desquamation. 'Zombification' in Haitian 'ju-ju' has been attributed to the use of this toxin. Tetrodotoxin, ultimately derived from bacteria, accumulates in parrotfish (*Scaridae*), Californian newts (*Taricha*), toads (*Atelopus*), blue-ringed octopuses ($\bigodot$ p. 601–602), starfish, eggs of horseshoe crabs (*Limulidae*), certain species of angelfish, polyclad flatworm, *Chaetognatha* (arrow worm), nemertean (ribbonworm), and xanthid crab.

Scombroid poisoning (histamine-like syndrome)

Bacterial contamination and decomposition of dark-red-fleshed fish (tuna, mackerel, bonito, skipjack), and canned sardines and pilchards generates histamine. *An early warning is immediate tingling or smarting of the lips and tongue at the first mouthful with a peppery flavour!* A few minutes to a few hours later, there is flushing, burning, sweating, urticaria, pruritus, headache, abdominal colic, nausea, vomiting, diarrhoea, bronchial asthma, giddiness, hypotension, and collapse.

Paralytic shellfish poisoning

Bivalve molluscs (mussels, clams, oysters, cockles, and scallops) become toxic when there is a 'red tide' of algal blooms. Many fish, sea birds, and mammals perish. Within 30 min of ingestion, paralysis begins and may progress to fatal respiratory paralysis within 12 h in 8% of cases. Milder GI and neurotoxic symptoms (neurotoxic shellfish poisoning) without paralysis may occur.

Treatment

- In all cases, give repeated doses of activated charcoal which is of unproven benefit but is unlikely to do harm.
- In acute ciguatera poisoning, mannitol (1.0 g/kg or 500 mL of 20% solution in adults given IV over 45 min) may reduce the risk of neurotoxicity.
- Scombroid poisoning responds to antihistamines and bronchodilators.
- Severe cases of paralytic poisoning require assisted ventilation.

- Victims of tetrodotoxin poisoning have recovered despite fulfilling the criteria for brain death.

Prevention

Note! Marine poisons are not destroyed by cooking or boiling.

Do

- Take local advice about what it is safe to eat.

Don't eat

- Seafood if there is an obvious 'die off' of marine life (rows of dead fish and sea birds on the shore).
- Shellfish if there is a 'red tide'.
- Very large reef fish (ciguatera poisoning) and any parts of any fish other than muscle (i.e. no skin, viscera, gonads, roe, etc.).
- Notorious poisonous species such as Moray eels (ciguatera), parrotfish (saxitoxin and others), large sharks (ciguatera, carchatoxin, trimethylamine), marine and fresh water puffer fish (tetrodotoxin/ saxitoxin) and, especially, horseshoe crabs' eggs, a delicacy in Thailand (*Carcinoscorpius rotundicauda*—Thai 'mengda' and *Tachypleus gigas*— Thai 'mengda chaan').
- Livers of any carnivorous polar mammal (polar bear, seals, cetaceans, huskies, etc.) because of the risk of fatal vitamin A toxicity.

Advice on venomous bites and stings

United Kingdom

TOXBASE® Administered by National Poisons Information Service (Edinburgh) website (registered users): ℘ http://www.toxbase.org 24/7 poisons information in the UK: Tel.: 0344 892 0111; email: mail@ toxbase.org

United States

American Association of Poison Control Centers 24/7 help line: Tel. 1-800-222-1222.
Miami-Dade Fire Rescue Anti-Venin Bank: Tel. 1-305-468-5900.

Useful websites

Snakebite in South and South-East Asia

℘ https://www.who.int/snakebites/resources/9789290225300/en/

Snakebite in Africa

℘ https://www.who.int/snakebites/resources/9789290231684/en/
℘   http://www.sun.ac.za/english/faculty/healthsciences/Clinical%20P harmacology/Poison%20Information%20Centre/Pages/default.aspx

Envenoming worldwide

℘ http://www.toxinology.com/
℘ http://www.vapaguide.info/

Antivenoms: general

℘ https://www.who.int/bloodproducts/snake_antivenoms/snakeantiven omguide/en/
℘ http://www.antivenoms.toxinfo.med.tum.de/

Australian antivenoms
🔎 http://www.toxinology.com/generic_static_files/cslavh_antivenom.html

South African antivenoms
🔎 http://www.savp.co.za/

Marine: Australia
🔎 http://www.anaesthesia.med.usyd.edu.au/resources/venom/marine_enven.html

Plants and fungi

Author
David A. Warrell

Dangers of living off the land

The abundance of appetizing, fragrant, and diverse fruits, tubers, leaves, and fungi offered by the wilderness environment may tempt the expeditioner to 'live off the land'. This ideal is enthusiastically encouraged in some military survival exercises and by certain heroic TV personalities! However, without expert guidance such attempts may prove lethal. In Europe, especially in France, Scandinavia, and Russia, enthusiastic amateur mushroom hunters seek novel gustatory experiences, but every year thousands are poisoned and hundreds die. Toxic plants and fungi are easily confused with edible ones and it is salutary that even expert botanists and mycologists are occasionally poisoned. You should not be reassured by seeing wild animals and birds feeding with apparent impunity. They have adapted to avoid poisoning in many clever and evolutionary ways. For example, Zanzibar's red colobus monkeys (*Piliocolobus kirkii*) eat charcoal to prevent poisoning by phenolic compounds in the Indian almond (*Terminalia catappa*) and mango (*Mangifera indica*) leaves that are their staple diet. Sometimes poisoning results from rash experimentation in quest of psychedelic experiences, using fungal psilocybin or tropane-containing plants. In South India and Sri Lanka, toxic plants are commonly employed as a means of self-harm (e.g. yellow oleander—*Cascabela thevetia* and Kerala suicide nut—*Cerbera manghas* or *C. odollam*). Herbal remedies may contain toxic ingredients, some staple crops (e.g. cassava) may be poisonous if inadequately cooked, and starvation may drive people to eat dangerous plants (e.g. grass peas).

Since recognizing danger is the secret of survival, an essential adjunct to this chapter is a profusely illustrated guide, CD-ROM (e.g. ℘ http://www.kew.org/data/poisplts.html), or website covering the poisonous (and edible) plants and fungi of the expedition's location.

Prevention of plant and fungal poisoning

Do

- Educate expedition members about the local toxic flora.
- Rely on your own food supplies.
- Confine collection of food from the environment to what you can identify with certainty as being safely edible or what is confidently recommended by local indigenous people.
- *Remember!* Cooking does not destroy fungal toxins!

Don't

- Experiment.
- Eat 'forbidden fruits': those resembling familiar cultivated fruits may be highly poisonous. To a non-expert, the death cap toadstool looks very like an edible mushroom (➲ p. 612).
- Eat wild fungi and certainly none with white gills (➲ p. 612).
- Accept invitations to inhale, 'snort', or ingest the local psychedelic brew: a splitting headache, nausea, vomiting, and terrifying hallucinations are more likely than any pleasurable trance or 'out-of-body' experience.

Irritant effects of plants on skin

Contact dermatitis is by far the commonest risk posed by plants. Examples include stinging nettles, euphorbias, and 'dumb cane' (*Dieffenbachia*).

Allergic dermatitis may be caused by a large variety of plants, notably poison ivy (*Toxicodendron (Rhus) radicans*) whose leaves have a trifoliate pattern ('leaves of three, leave them be'), (Pacific) poison oak (*Toxicodendron diversilobum*), primula (*Primula obconica*), and citrous fruits. Some plant saps are photosensitizing, resulting in erythema, papules, vesicles, bullae, and persistent hyperpigmentation confined to exposed areas.

Treatment

Treatment is based on immediate decontamination by washing with water, followed by symptomatic use of systemic antihistamines and topical corticosteroids.

Prevention

To avoid further contact, try to identify the cause. Since photosensitization is a common sequel, try to reduce solar exposure. In general, avoid unnecessary contact of bare skin with plants, especially those that have stinging hairs or are exuding latex or sap. If your expedition is botanical, learn to recognize some of the most notoriously irritant plants in advance and wear gloves when necessary.

Effects of eating poisonous plants

When to suspect plant poisoning
Within minutes to hours (exceptionally 24 h) after ingesting any part of a wild fruit, plant, or fungus (mushroom or toadstool):
• Nausea, vomiting, abdominal colic, and/or diarrhoea.
• Confusion, hallucinations, or convulsions.
• Atropinic, nicotinic, or muscarinic symptoms.
• Cardiac arrhythmias.
• Flushing in response to alcohol ingestion.
• Oliguria/anuria.

Effects on gut

Many of the plants that cause contact dermatitis also irritate the gut. Cuckoo pint/arum lily, dumb cane, and many other plants have an irritant sap containing oxalate crystals. Ingestion causes immediate soreness, reddening, and blistering of buccal mucosa, salivation, and dysphagia. Most poisonous plants cause rapidly evolving nausea, abdominal cramps, vomiting, and diarrhoea (e.g. laburnum, anemone, hellebore, horse chestnut, ivy, privet, pokeweed, and snowberry). Some even more toxic plants cause severe GI symptoms after a delay of several hours up to 2 days (e.g. autumn crocus (*Colchicum autumnale*), glory lily (*Gloriosa superba*), jequirity bean (*Abrus precatorius*), and castor oil bean (*Ricinus communis*)).
  See ➔ Colour plate 19.

Effects on cardiovascular system

Bradycardia, heart block, other arrhythmias, ECG changes ('digoxin effect'), and GI irritation are caused by foxglove (*Digitalis purpurea*), white/pink oleander (*Nerium oleander*), yellow oleander (*Cascabela thevetia* also known as *Thevetia peruviana*), monkshood (*Aconitum napellus*), yew (*Taxus baccata*), and death camas (*Zigadenus*).

Effects on nervous system

• Hallucinogenic: e.g. cannabis (*Cannabis sativa*), khat (*Catha edulis*), morning glory (*Ipomoea*), and peyote (*Lophophora williamsii*).
• Convulsant: e.g. cowbane (*Cicuta virosa*), ackee (*Blighia sapida*), and nux vomica (*Strychnos nux-vomica*). Cowbane poisoning causes gastroenteritis, increased secretions, and long-lasting intense episodes of generalized tonic–clonic convulsions, resulting in severe metabolic acidosis and multiple organ failure. Consumption of unripe ackee fruit is responsible for 'Jamaican vomiting sickness' associated with hypoglycaemia and fatal encephalopathy.
• Atropine-like: e.g. deadly nightshade (*Atropa belladonna*), angel's trumpet (*Brugmansia suaveolens*) (➔ Colour plate 20), and thorn apple or Jimson weed (US) (*Datura stramonium*) and related species such as devil's trumpet (*D. metel*). Clinical effects are 'red as a beet, dry as a bone' (flushed, hot, red, dry face), tachycardia, and dilated pupils (mydriasis) and, in serious poisoning, arrhythmias, urinary retention, psychosis, convulsions, coma, and fatal respiratory failure. Some of these plants are hallucinogenic and therefore desirable to some people.

- Nicotine-like: e.g. spotted hemlock (*Conium maculatum*) (➲ Colour plate 21), responsible for killing Socrates and Hamlet's father, first stimulates and then paralyses autonomic ganglia, and can cause convulsions and respiratory arrest.

Effects on liver

Pyrrolizidine alkaloid-containing plants such as comfrey (*Symphytum officinale*) can cause hepatic veno-occlusive disease, which has occurred mainly in Jamaica, India, and Afghanistan. Nausea, abdominal pain and distension, hepatomegaly, and sometimes fever and vomiting develop a few days after ingestion.

Effects on kidneys

Oxalate-rich plants such as rhubarb (*Rheum rhabarbarum*), dock, and sorrel (*Rumex*), and plants containing other nephrotoxins may damage the kidneys. Rhubarb stems contain much less oxalate than the leaves and are safe to eat if cooked.

Poisonous food plants

Staple food plants in many tropical countries can be poisonous if inadequately soaked, dried, fermented, or cooked:
- Cassava (*Manihot esculenta*), sweet potato, yam, some fruit kernels, pips, and cherry laurel (*Prunus laurocerasus*) can cause acute or chronic cyanide poisoning if inadequately boiled.
  - Especially in Africa, tropical ataxic neuropathy and spastic paraparesis ('konzo') are attributed to cassava poisoning.
- Lathyrism is an epidemic paralytic disease (e.g. in the Denbia depression of Ethiopia) caused by oxalyldiaminopropionic acid in grass peas (*Lathyrus sativus*).
- Favism occurs in some Mediterranean and Middle Eastern countries. Those with congenital G6PD deficiency may develop intravascular haemolysis after eating broad (fava) beans (*Vicia faba*).

Fungal poisoning

Fungal poisoning is usually sporadic and accidental but occasionally may be homicidal, suicidal, or epidemic. In Europe (especially France, Scandinavia, and Russia), where there are many enthusiastic collectors and connoisseurs of wild mushrooms, poisoning is more common than elsewhere in the world. Between 2010 and 2017, 10,600 people were poisoned by mushrooms in France with 22 reported deaths.

The toxicity of fungi varies with location and season, from year to year, and with individual susceptibility.

The deathcap, the world's deadliest mushroom or toadstool, looks superficially like an edible mushroom (*Agaricus*) but it has white gills (radiating linear structures under the mushroom's cap) and a sac or volva at its base, whereas the edible mushroom has dark brown or black gills and no volva at the base of its stem (Fig. 18.1).

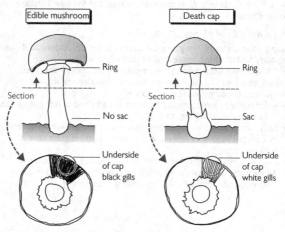

Fig. 18.1 Distinguishing edible mushrooms from death cap.

Poisoning with early symptoms (within a few hours)

- *GI symptoms:* vomiting, diarrhoea, and abdominal pain are usually transient but sometimes more intense, resulting in fluid and electrolyte disturbances. They may be caused by many species of common fungi, including honey agaric (*Armillaria mellea*) and *Boletus luridus*.
- *Cholinergic effects (muscarinic poisoning):* abdominal pain and diarrhoea, sweating, lacrimation, salivation, miosis, bronchorrhoea, and sometimes bronchospasm, bradycardia, and hypotension may develop 5–120 min after ingesting *Inocybe* and *Clitocybe* mushroom species.

- *Confusion (ibotenic poisoning)*: nausea, vomiting, confusion, disorientation, anxiety, euphoria, hallucinations, visual disturbances, ataxia, muscle cramps, and coma may develop 20–120 min after ingestion of panther cap (*Amanita pantherina*), fly agaric (*Amanita muscaria*), and *Amanita strobiliformis*.
- *Hallucinations (psilocybin poisoning)*: LSD-like, mainly visual hallucinations are induced by eating 'magic mushrooms' (*Psilocybe, Conocybe, Gymnopilus, Panaeolina, Panaeolus, Pluteus*, and *Stropharia* spp.). Within 30 min, there is mydriasis, tachycardia, euphoria, confusion, dizziness, and vomiting.
- *Antabuse-like reactions (coprine poisoning)*: eating ink cap (*Coprinus atramentarius*) or club foot (*Clitocybe clavipes*) may produce a reaction similar to that induced by disulfiram. If alcohol is drunk within 72 h of eating the fungi, there is flushing of the skin, metallic taste, sweating, mydriasis, nausea, vomiting, anxiety, confusion, dyspnoea, severe headache, tachycardia, chest pain, and hypotension.

Poisoning with delayed symptoms (6 h to several days)

- *Gastroenteritis with hepatotoxicity and nephrotoxicity (amatoxin poisoning)*: may result from eating the deathcap (*Amanita phalloides*; Fig. 18.1), destroying angel (*Amanita virosa*), fool's mushroom (*Amanita verna*), *Conocybe filaris*, and some *Galerina* and *Lepiota* spp. Abdominal pain and vomiting, but in particularly severe cases, watery or bloody diarrhoea, starts 6–24 h (usually 12 h) after ingestion, leading to dehydration. After a period of apparent recovery, lasting up to 72 h, fatal hepatorenal failure may supervene.
- *Gastroenteritis with neurological symptoms (gyromitrin poisoning)*: there is gastroenteritis with a feeling of bloating, severe headache, vertigo, pyrexia, sweating, diplopia, nystagmus, ataxia, cramps, delirium, and sometimes coma, lethargy, hypoglycaemia, hepatic damage, haemolysis, and renal damage starting 2–24 h after ingesting false morel (*Gyromitra esculenta*) or inhaling fumes while it is being cooked.
- *Renal damage (orellanine poisoning)*: may develop 2–17 days after eating *Cortinarius* spp. There is fatigue, intense thirst, headache, chills, paraesthesiae, tinnitus, and abdominal, lumbar, and flank pain. After a transient polyuric phase, oliguria and anuria may ensue.
- *Ergotism ('St Anthony's fire')*: results from eating cereal crops whose seed heads are infected with the hard, purplish-black fruiting bodies of *Claviceps purpurea*. Symptoms include vasoconstriction, leading to peripheral gangrene and muscular tremors, convulsions, and hallucinations.

Treating plant and fungal ingestion

First aid

- Gastric lavage is potentially dangerous and is discouraged because of the risks of aspiration and trauma to pharynx and oesophagus.
- Give the patient a glass of milk to drink provided they are fully conscious and not vomiting.
- Give oral activated charcoal 50 g immediately, followed by 25 g every 2 h for at least 48 h (this is not evidence based but is very unlikely to be harmful).

At the base hospital

Severe cases will require supportive treatments for organ failure such as mechanical ventilation and renal dialysis, with therapy for hypovolaemia, acid–base disturbances, hypoglycaemia, cardiac arrhythmias, and convulsions.

- For *cholinergic (muscarinic) symptoms*—atropine (adult 0.6–1.8 mg IV).
- For *central and peripheral anticholinergic (atropine-like) effects*—physostigmine (adult 1–2 mg IV) to control hallucinations, delirium, and psychotic behaviour.
- For *confusion or hallucinations*—tranquillizers such as diazepam (adults 5–10 mg).
- For *psychotic behaviour*—chlorpromazine or haloperidol may be required.

Specific antidotes

- For poisoning by yellow oleander, other *Apocynaceae*, and any plant containing cardiac glycosides: digoxin-specific antibodies (ovine Fab fragments such as Digibind® or DigiFab®).
- For severe autumn crocus (*Colchicum autumnale*) poisoning: colchicine-specific Fab antibodies.
- For amatoxic fungal poisoning: infuse silibinin (silybin, silymarin) 5 mg/kg IV over 1 h, followed by 20 mg/kg/24 h (available in Germany but not in the UK or US) or large doses (300,000–1,000,000 U/kg/day by continuous IV infusion) of benzylpenicillin. Acetylcysteine might reduce liver damage. In severe cases, liver transplantation is life-saving.
- For gyromitrin fungal poisoning: pyridoxine 25 mg/kg over 30 min, glucose IV, and promote diuresis.

Reference

Poisonous Plants and Fungi in Britain and Ireland. ISBN 1 900347 92 X. Interactive CD-ROM from Publications Sales, Royal Botanic Gardens, Kew, Richmond, Surrey TW9 3AE, UK. ℘ http://www.kew.org/data/poisplts.html

Advice about plant and fungal poisoning

United Kingdom

TOXBASE® administered by National Poisons Information Service (Edinburgh) website (registered users): ℘ http://www.toxbase.org
24/7 poisons information in the UK: Tel. 0344 892 0111; email: mail@toxbase.org
Plants and fungi identification: telephone advice service for urgent poisoning case enquiries—Kew Gardens: Tel. +44 (0)020 8332 5000.

United States

American Association of Poison Control Centers:
℘ https://aapcc.org/24/7 help line: Tel. 1-800-222-1222.

Chapter 19

Analgesia and anaesthesia in remote locations

Chapter editor
Chris Johnson

Contributors
Rose Buckley
Rachael Craven
Chris Johnson
Joe Silsby (1st edition)

Reviewers
Edi Albert
Spike Briggs
Harvey Pynn

NB: this chapter has been extensively revised since the previous edition of this handbook. Many painkilling and anaesthetic drugs are misused as recreational substances, and legislation controlling their transport and prescription has been tightened internationally. The penalties for inadvertently failing to comply with local laws on the importation or prescription of drugs can be very severe.

Anaesthetic techniques, both local and general, require expertise and experience. They should be attempted only by appropriately trained personnel except, possibly, in circumstances where life or limb are threatened (e.g. urgently freeing a trapped casualty or dealing with a fracture dislocation of a limb that has obstructed the blood supply).

Introduction to analgesia and anaesthesia

'Analgesia' (from the Greek) means without pain, while 'anaesthesia' means 'without feeling'. Pain is defined as 'an unpleasant sensory and emotional experience associated with actual or potential tissue damage or described in terms of such damage'. Mild pain may simply be unpleasant, but severe pain can incapacitate. Relatively trivial injuries such as blisters can make movement difficult while severe toothache prevents sleep and destroys morale. When the cause of a pain is uncertain or indicates a serious underlying condition, it becomes associated with anxiety and fear. The pains associated with serious injury or conditions such as renal colic can be overwhelming and reduce the strongest individual to dependence upon others. Painful conditions are often self-limiting and simple analgesics will enable the traveller to continue, but if the cause of the problem is unknown or the pain is very severe, evacuation will have to be considered to establish the cause and to provide ongoing care.

Pain is personal. Something that one individual may regard as trivial can overwhelm another. Pain relief must therefore be tailored to the needs of an individual. Common painful problems that may be encountered on an expedition include:

- Headache—tension headache, migraine, hangover, altitude.
- Blisters.
- Bites and stings—bees, wasps, scorpions, larger animals.
- Burns and scalds.
- Period pains.
- Wounds and haematomas.
- Sprains and fractures.
- Dental ailments (➔ Chapter 11).

This chapter discusses different ways to relieve pain and discomfort in the field, primarily through the use of painkilling medications together with local anaesthesia (LA) and regional anaesthesia. Good medical and nursing care which include splinting, wound management, pressure relief, hydration, and psychological support have important roles in relieving distress.

LA or regional anaesthesia (➔ p. 625–631) may also be required for the treatment of wounds and minor surgical complaints.

There are very rare but important circumstances such as entrapment or serious trauma which demand urgent treatment to save life or limb. Most expeditions will never encounter such problems or will be able to call upon the help of local services to assist. However polar expeditions, ships' crews and scientific teams may spend prolonged periods in isolation, where accidents and acute surgical conditions can develop and medics on such trips may require anaesthetic skills.

LA and regional anaesthetics do not affect a person's conscious level but strong painkilling drugs and other forms of sedative (including alcohol) may cause drowsiness or sleep. A 'sedated' person will, however, always be rousable by vocal or tactile stimulation.

Anaesthetic drugs deliberately render a person unrousable so that surgical procedures can be undertaken. Anaesthesia is always potentially hazardous as the patient can no longer look after their own airway and other physiological parameters may be affected.

Treating pain

The 'analgesic ladder'.

Current techniques of pain relief depend upon the use of increasingly potent treatments, used singly or in combination until the patient is comfortable. A low dose of several different drugs is preferable to a higher dose of just one. See Table 19.1.

Painkilling drugs may be given:

- *Topically*—as skin rubs.
- *Transcutaneously*—some opiate drugs such as buprenorphine and fentanyl are available as skin patches and have been used by field expeditions. They are legally controlled drugs. LA skin patches (5% lidocaine) can also help relieve pain.
- *Inhaled*—volatile painkilling agents such as methoxyflurane.
- *Orally*—as liquids (for children), tablets, caplets, or capsules.
- *Rectally*—as suppositories; particularly useful if a patient is vomiting, for instance with a renal or abdominal colic.
- *IV*—if there is secure venous access.
- *IM.*
- *LA blocks* can be used to relieve localized pain.

Different medical conditions require different methods of pain relief and taking a selection of formulations in the medical kit may be beneficial.

Table 19.1 The analgesic ladder

Mild pain	Physical measures (see below)
	Paracetamol
Moderate pain	Physical measures
	Paracetamol *plus*
	NSAIDs:
	• Ibuprofen
	• Diclofenac
	• Naproxen
	Note contraindications to use of NSAIDs
If moderate pain uncontrolled	Combine paracetamol and ibuprofen and consider codeine
Severe pain	Physical measures
	Paracetamol *plus*
	Ibuprofen *or* codeine
	Tramadol (if available)
	Morphine (if available)
	Methoxyflurane (Penthrox®)
	Ketamine
	If appropriate (e.g. fracture) consider LA block
Children and small (<50 kg) adults require lower doses	

Physical measures can significantly reduce pain and discomfort. These can include:

- Reduction and splinting of fractures.
- Rest, ice, compression, and elevation (RICE) of sprains.
- Appropriate dressing of blisters, scalds, and grazes.
- Heat pads or cold compresses for some pains and bruises.
- Appropriate positioning, padding, and use of slings to minimize strain on injured areas.
- Gargles for throat and mouth washes for dental pain.
- A *simple painkiller*, such as paracetamol (acetaminophen), will be safe for most people.
- A *NSAID* such as ibuprofen, naproxen, or diclofenac can be given orally, rectally, or as a skin rub. About 15% of the population cannot take NSAIDs—see ➋ p. 621.
- *Codeine* is a drug that works very well in some people, but leaves others feeling light-headed and dreadful.
- *Tramadol* is a powerful painkiller which is reasonably safe to use as it rarely causes respiratory depression. It can be taken by mouth or injected but can make some people feel sick, dizzy, or disoriented so initial supervision is required to see if these side effects develop.
- *Opiates*, of which morphine is the most common, are powerful painkillers but frequently produce sedation, dizziness, and nausea. Individual tolerance to these drugs varies and the drug dosage should be titrated to provide effective pain relief but minimize sedation and respiratory depression.

Codeine, tramadol, and opiates are all popular recreational drugs controlled by legislation that varies between countries. Medications sold over the counter in one locality may be prohibited elsewhere. Expeditions planning to travel to very remote locations may need to take powerful painkillers, in which case you must be aware of the appropriate licensing and storage procedures for each country you visit, including those you transit. If in doubt, do not take them.

- *Inhalational drugs:* at low concentrations, the volatile anaesthetic drug methoxyflurane (Penthrox®) (➋ p. 623–624) is an effective painkiller and its use should be considered if a casualty needs to be released from entrapment or transported in difficult circumstances.
- *LAs:* local infiltration and nerve blockade (➋ p. 625–631) with a suitable drug such as lidocaine, levobupivacaine, or ropivacaine can reduce the pain of fractures and very painful bites/stings. 5% lidocaine topical skin patches can reduce the pain of fractured ribs.
- *IV/IM ketamine:* for those with appropriate skills and experience ketamine (➋ p. 622, 636–637) may be appropriate either as an anaesthetic or, in lower doses, as a painkiller to assist in the release of a trapped casualty or to enable initial manipulation of severe injuries prior to evacuation.
- *Anxiety and stress* make pain worse both psychologically and because muscles tense around the affected part of the body. Try to calm the patient and enable them to relax. If available, very small doses of

anxiolytic drugs (e.g. diazepam, midazolam) can help particularly during the reduction of a fracture but must be used with extreme caution if the patient has received potent painkillers, as respiratory depression or deep sedation may result. As with powerful painkillers, possession of these drugs is now controlled by legislation and we do not recommend that mobile expeditions carry them.

- Any patient who has been given significant amounts of pain relief must be appropriately supervised and monitored (➔ p. 254–255).
- *Alcohol* can have very unpredictable effects when combined with painkillers and should be avoided. Respiratory depression is a serious, potentially life-threatening side effect of opiate drugs.
- *Naloxone* (➔ p. 622) reverses the effects of opiate drugs and can save lives.
- *Nausea and vomiting*. Severe pain or the sight of an injury can make people feel sick. Nausea is also an unpleasant side effect of some painkilling drugs and is also common with colic pains. Antiemetic drugs such as prochlorperazine or cyclizine may help.

Pharmacology of painkillers and associated drugs

Table 19.1 and the following list contain only a small range of basic drugs but used in combination these will be adequate for most situations. A wide range of long-acting oral and transcutaneous painkillers are now manufactured, and if your expedition medical kit contains these, read about their benefits and drawbacks. If painkilling preparations are purchased from a local pharmacist, read the small print carefully to determine what they contain; often it will simply be an expensive combination of the types of drugs listed in Table 19.1.

Topical painkillers

Topical painkillers include preparations of NSAIDs and LAs. Drug concentrations vary and some formulations include other constituents such as menthol that act as 'counter-irritants'.

- *Lidocaine 5%*: useful for jellyfish stings and can aid in removal of splinters.
- *Bonjela®* (cetalkonium chloride + choline salicylate): used to treat mouth ulcers, cold sores, and sore spots in the mouth. 1.5 cm gel rubbed into mouth up to 3-hourly.
- *NSAIDs*: many companies produce topical formulations of NSAID drugs for treatment of arthritic, muscular and back pain. Be aware of varying strengths, and contraindications to use of these drugs (➔ p. 621).

Paracetamol (acetaminophen in North America)

- Available as tablets, caplets, capsules, suppositories, and IV infusion.
- Dose 1 g 4–6-hourly. Maximum dose 4 g per day.
- IV paracetamol 1 g in 100 mL (15 mg/kg 6-hourly for patients <50 kg) infused over at least 15 min is an excellent painkiller for patients with established IV access.
- Allergy is rare.
- Familiarity should not breed contempt—paracetamol is a cheap and remarkably effective painkiller.
- Never exceed recommended dose—fatal liver damage can result.
- Avoid in people with existing liver disease such as alcoholics.

NSAIDs

- Available as tablets/capsules, suppositories, skin rubs, or IV/IM preparations.
- Commonest NSAIDs are:
  - *Ibuprofen* 400 mg four times daily, although the dose can be increased to a maximum of 2400 mg per day for short periods. Available topically, as liquid or tablets.
  - *Diclofenac* 50 mg orally three times daily (also effective as suppositories up to 150 mg/day). Parenteral preparations also available.
  - *Naproxen* 500 mg initially then 250 mg every 6–8 h. Maximum dose after first day: 1.25 g/daily.
- Parenteral preparations of diclofenac need to be diluted and given in a flowing IV infusion. Avoid IM route unless no alternative available as drug can cause sterile abscesses.
- NSAIDs should not be used in patients with:
  - Allergy to this group of drugs.
  - Kidney disease.
  - Some asthmatics.
  - Heart disease.
  - Bleeding tendency or taking anticoagulants.
  - Peptic (stomach) symptoms.
- When given orally, NSAIDs are best taken with or soon after food, and swallowed with plenty of fluids.
- The combination of dehydration with NSAIDs can cause renal damage. This is a particular risk in endurance athletes, especially in hot climates, who may take painkillers prior to or immediately after exercise when they may be significantly dehydrated. Paracetamol is a better choice under these circumstances.

Codeine

Low-dose codeine or dihydrocodeine is commonly mixed with paracetamol or an NSAID to improve effectiveness and these combination tablets are sold by pharmacies in the UK.

Higher-dose codeine: 30–60 mg tablets up to 240 mg per day.
- Avoid if allergic, should not be given to children <12 years.
- Do not combine with alcohol or benzodiazepine drugs.
- Should be avoided by those with sleep apnoea syndrome.
- Codeine is illegal in some countries, check online if you plan to include codeine-containing compounds in your medical kit.
- Individuals metabolize codeine differently; some people find it an effective painkiller while it makes others feel awful.
- Side effects include drowsiness, confusion, giddiness, nausea, vomiting, and confusion.

Tramadol

Tramadol 50–100 mg 4–6-hourly as capsules or by injection is an effective painkiller with a relatively safe side effect profile, although some people will experience nausea or other GI symptoms. It has become a drug of abuse and its use is now legally restricted in many countries, so it can no longer be recommended as a routine component of expedition medical kits.

Opiates

Opiate painkillers originated from the opium poppy and common derivatives include morphine and heroin. They have been used as effective painkillers for millennia. A wide range of opiate painkillers, natural and synthetic, have been developed, several of which are now manufactured and sold illegally. As a result, most countries have introduced strict controls over their possession and use, and this handbook can no longer recommend that such drugs should be routinely carried by expedition medics. However, there will be circumstances, for instance at remote scientific bases, at sea, or in very remote areas, when casualty evacuation will be difficult and where an adequate supply of the strongest painkillers is appropriate, provided that all licensing and dispensing controls are adhered to. Street purchases of opiate painkillers contain unpredictable quantities of various drugs and can be lethal.

Morphine
- Morphine can be given orally (as tablets or a fluid), IV or IM 10 mg 2–4-hourly. Higher dosage may be appropriate in carefully monitored patients.
- Allergy is very rare.
- May be combined with paracetamol and NSAIDs but not with codeine.
- Can cause respiratory depression, drowsiness, giddiness, nausea, vomiting, and confusion.
- Constipation develops if used repeatedly.
- Anyone given a strong opiate requires appropriate nursing and careful monitoring (➔ p. 254–255).

Ketamine
Ketamine (➔ p. 632, 636–637) is an effective analgesic for acute pain, although there is no general agreement on the optimum dose or method of administration. Usually given IV or IM it may also be administered orally, nasally, SC, or rectally. Subanaesthetic dosages are not well defined but IV rates of 0.5 mg/kg given over 30 min to 1 h have been recommended.[1]

Opiate antidote
Naloxone is a specific antagonist to the effects of opiate drugs and is a very effective treatment if someone takes or is administered excessive amounts of an opiate. Dose is 400 micrograms IV or IM repeated regularly (every 2 min) until effective. Up to 4 mg may be required in severely poisoned patients. Its duration of effectiveness is shorter than that of many of the drugs it antagonizes, so the patient should be very closely monitored and repeat doses given if necessary. Naloxone can result in the sudden arousal of someone, possibly in pain, and they may then become restless and distressed.

Antiemetics
Nausea and vomiting are relatively common side effects of both trauma and the analgesic drugs used to treat the pain. Commonly available drugs include:
- *Prochlorperazine* 12.5 mg IM 6-hourly or 20 mg tablet initially then 10 mg after 2 h PO.

1 ⌕ https://www.ncbi.nlm.nih.gov/pmc/articles/PMC5609085/

• *Cyclizine* 50 mg three times daily orally, IM or IV.
Other possible drugs are listed in the travel sickness section (➲ p. 750–751).

Inhalational drugs

Penthrox®

Methoxyflurane is an obsolete anaesthetic agent used nowadays at a lower vapour concentration to provide analgesia for moderate to severe pain using a Penthrox® inhaler (Fig. 19.1). Each Penthrox® unit contains 3 mL of pure methoxyflurane.

• Methoxyflurane has a characteristic fruity smell.
• Pain is relieved after six to ten inhalations.
• Patients can assess their own level of pain and titrate the amount they inhale.
• A 3 mL bottle of Penthrox®, used continuously, will last about 25–30 min. Used intermittently it will last longer and patients should be advised to inhale the lowest possible dose to achieve pain relief.
• The safety limit for the drug is unknown but the manufacturer recommends an upper limit of 6 mL/day or 15 mL/week. Excessive use could result in kidney failure.
• Penthrox® is not licensed for use by anyone <18 years.
• The drug is contraindicated in anyone who has:
  • A family history of malignant hyperpyrexia.
  • Hypersensitivity to any of the fluorinated anaesthetic drugs including any form of liver failure resulting from an anaesthetic.
  • Clinically significant renal failure.
  • Altered level of consciousness as a result of head injury, drugs, or alcohol.
  • Cardiovascular or respiratory instability.

Website

🔗 https://www.medicines.org.uk/emc/product/1939/smpc

1. Ensure the Activated Carbon (AC) Chamber is inserted into the dilutor hole on the top of the PENTHROX Inhaler.

2. Remove the cap of the bottle by hand. Alternatively, use the base of the PENTHROX Inhaler to loosen the cap with a ½ turn. Separate the Inhaler from the bottle and remove the cap by hand.

3. Tilt the PENTHROX Inhaler to a 45° angle and pour the total contents of one PENTHROX bottle into the base of the Inhaler whilst rotating.

4. Place wrist loop over patient's wrist. Patient inhales and exhales PENTHROX through the mouthpiece to obtain analgesia. First few breaths should be gentle and then breathe normally through Inhaler.

5. Patient exhales into the PENTHROX Inhaler. The exhaled vapour passes through the AC Chamber to adsorb any exhaled methoxyflurane.

6. If stronger analgesia is required, patient can cover dilutor hole on the AC chamber with finger during use.

7. If further pain relief is required, after the first bottle has been used use a second bottle if available. Alternatively use a second bottle from a new combination pack. Use in the same way as the first bottle in step 2 and 3. No need to remove the AC Chamber. Put used bottle into the plastic bag provided.

8. Patient should be instructed to inhale intermittently to achieve adequate analgesia. Continuous inhalation will reduce duration of use. Minimum dose to achieve analgesia should be administered.

9. Replace cap onto PENTHROX bottle. Place used PENTHROX Inhaler and used bottle in sealed plastic bag and dispose of responsibly.

Fig. 19.1 How to use a Penthrox® inhaler.

Local anaesthesia

LA can be used in several different ways:

- By infiltration into and around an affected area, e.g. wound infiltration prior to exploration or suturing.
- By numbing the nerves supplying a specific area, e.g. the nerves supplying a specific digit following a scorpion sting.
- By regional blockade of an area such as the forearm or hip following a fracture.
- Useful blocks include:
  - Digital blocks of fingers and toes (➲ p. 627–628).
  - Ankle blocks for foot injuries.
  - Fascia iliaca blocks for hip and leg injuries (➲ p. 630–631).

Emergency department physicians and anaesthetists will be most familiar with using ultrasound to define the nerves that require LA blockade. However, in the absence of ultrasound equipment most common blocks can be positioned reasonably accurately using anatomical landmarks. Short-bevelled LA needles make it easier to identify the relevant tissue layers and skilled practitioners may wish to include a few such needles in their medical kit. If a short-bevelled LA needle is unavailable the tip of a conventional hypodermic needle can be blunted by tapping it a few times against the sterile exterior of its sheath.

LAs can be a very effective adjunct to other forms of pain relief and are commonly used in the emergency department and to relieve postoperative pain.

LA may result in both a numb limb and weakness of the affected area. A numb arm should always be protected by padding and a sling, while patients should not attempt to walk on a numbed leg.

If a LA block is used to relieve severe pain, for which a patient has already received a high dose of painkilling drugs, the sudden reduction in pain levels may lead to the patient falling asleep, potentially with a degree of respiratory depression. Regular observations are essential.

Local anaesthetic drugs

Lidocaine and prilocaine have a rapid onset and short duration of action, while levobupivacaine and ropivacaine last longer and are better suited for long-duration pain relief.[2]

Lidocaine

Most widely available LA. Short acting.

- Dose: 3 mg/kg plain lidocaine to a maximum of 300 mg; or 7 mg/kg with adrenaline (epinephrine) 1:200,000 up to maximum of 500 mg.

Prilocaine

Good if large volumes will be required and is fairly safe but relatively short acting.

- Dose: 6 mg/kg plain or 9 mg/kg with adrenaline (epinephrine) to a maximum of 400 mg.

🔖 https://www.frca.co.uk/article.aspx?articleid=100816

Levobupivacaine

Levobupivacaine is the S-enantiomer of bupivacaine and acts for longer, with an improved side effect profile compared with bupivacaine.
- Available as either 0.25% or 0.5% solutions.
- Dose: 2 mg/kg without adrenaline or 2.5 mg/kg with adrenaline, to maximum of 150 mg.
- Avoid intra-articular injection as it is toxic to cartilage.

Ropivacaine

A less cardiotoxic alternative to bupivacaine, it is probably a better drug to use, when available.
- Various concentrations available for different indications.
- Dose: up to 200 mg or 10–20 mg/h as a continuous infusion.

To calculate a drug dose
- Drugs in solution are quoted as percentage concentrations.
- 1% means 1 g of drug has been dissolved in 100 mL of solvent. So: 1% solution = 10 mg/mL; 0.25% solution = 2.5 mg/mL.
- If your casualty weighs 70 kg and you are using lidocaine the maximum safe dose for lidocaine is 3 mg/kg, which for this patient is 3 × 70 = 210 mg.
- Therefore, the maximum volume of lidocaine you can infiltrate is: 210/10 = 21 mL of the 1% solution or 210/20 = 10.5 mL of the 2%.

Symptoms and signs of local anaesthetic overdose

See Table 19.2.

Table 19.2 Symptoms and signs of LA overdose

Mild	Moderate	Severe
Perioral tingling	Restlessness	Fits
Tinnitus	Slurred speech	Coma
Metallic taste	Nystagmus	Hypotension
Blurred vision	Tremor	Dysrhythmias
		Cardiac arrest

Treatment of local anaesthetic overdose

- Stop injection.
- Resuscitate using ABC approach.
- Diazepam 10 mg IV or other benzodiazepine for fits.

Local infiltration anaesthesia

When to use it

Minor surface surgery such as:
- Wound suturing.
- Small superficial abscesses—although LAs are less effective in the presence of infection.
- Digital blocks.
- Dental work (➔ Chapter 11).
- Pain relief—following some animal bites and stings.
- Topically on the surface of the eye or other mucous membranes (tetracaine—➔ p. 347, 589, 668).

Advantages
- Safe.
- Easy to learn.
- Minimal equipment required.
- Additional monitoring unnecessary.

Disadvantages
- Not appropriate for large or multiple areas if maximum safe dose will be exceeded.
- LA toxicity, while rare, is a challenge to treat in remote situations.
- Not always effective, especially if affected area is inflamed or infected.
- Inadvertent intravascular injection may cause systemic toxicity even without using the 'maximum' dose.

Local infiltration techniques

First calculate the maximum safe dose for your casualty (➔ p. 626).

If you think a large volume may be required, consider using a LA solution containing adrenaline (epinephrine) 1:200,000 unless it is an area supplied by end arteries such as fingers, toes, penis, or tip of ear.

Wound infiltration
- Wearing sterile gloves, clean the skin with antiseptic solution.
- Draw up calculated volume of LA into syringe.
- Using a 23 or 25 G needle, inject SC along both sides of the wound. Aspirate prior to injection to avoid intravascular injection.

Alternatively, inject in a diamond shape around the wound or abscess with a single entry point at either side of the area to be anaesthetized.

Digital nerve block
See also ➔ Fig. 14.6, p. 628.
- Used for surgery distal to the base of the proximal phalanx of fingers or toes.
- Never use adrenaline (epinephrine)-containing solutions.
- If available, choose a 25 mm 25 G needle.
- Infiltrate LA on either side of the base of the proximal phalanx, in a vertical plane from the dorsal surface until the needle almost reaches the palmar surface (Fig. 19.2). Inject 2–3 mL of 1% lidocaine or prilocaine, or the same dose of 0.25% bupivacaine on each side of the digit, then add a small additional dose over the dorsum of the digit.

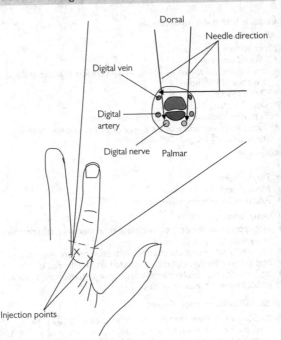

Fig. 19.2 Digital nerve block.

Haematoma block

- Used to reduce fractures of the distal radius and ulna or occasionally also distal tibia and fibula.
- Not suitable for use on open fractures.
- Wear sterile gloves and clean the skin with antiseptic solution.
- Palpate the fracture line and introduce the needle into the fracture site aspirating as you go to identify fresh blood from the fracture haematoma (Fig. 19.3).
- Once in the haematoma, inject 6–8 mL of 2% lidocaine (for a 70 kg adult), plus a further 2–3 mL in ulna styloid area.
- Onset of anaesthesia takes about 10 min.

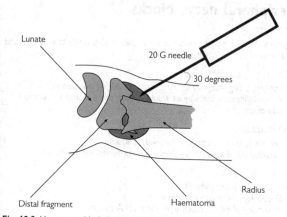

Lunate

20 G needle

30 degrees

Radius

Distal fragment

Haematoma

Fig. 19.3 Haematoma block showing injection into haematoma at fracture site.

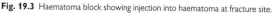

Peripheral nerve blocks

What they are

Injection of LA around a nerve or nerve plexus to provide anaesthesia and analgesia in its area of distribution.

When to use them

- Longer-lasting analgesia for limb fractures during evacuation.
- When infiltration techniques would require more than the maximum safe dose.

Advantages

- Longer-lasting anaesthesia than with infiltration.
- Larger area of anaesthesia than can be provided with infiltration.

Disadvantages

- Technically more difficult.
- Possibility of damage to a nerve.
- Possibility of intravascular injection and LA toxicity.

Fascia iliaca block

(See Fig. 19.4.) This block has been identified as a block suitable for non-specialist practitioners since its injection point, when performed correctly, is away from both nerves and major blood vessels, and is therefore relatively safe.[3]

- *Indication:* analgesia for femoral shaft and neck of femur fractures, anterior thigh, and above-knee amputation.
- *Equipment:* single-bevel LA needle (if available), 1–2 mL 1% lidocaine for skin infiltration, 50 mL syringe, and chosen LA.
- *Method:*
  - Calculate maximum safe dose of LA (see ❷ To calculate a drug dose, p. 626), this is a volume-dependent block so you need to choose a percentage that will allow you to inject a large volume, e.g. 30 mL 0.25% levobupivacaine.
  - Ensure you have IV access.
  - Identify your landmarks: a line connecting the anterior superior iliac spine and the pubic tubercle divided into thirds. Mark the injection point 1 cm caudal to the junction of the lateral and middle third (Fig. 19.4).
  - Clean the skin with antiseptic.
  - Infiltrate skin at injection point with 1% lidocaine.
  - Using a LA single-bevel needle pierce the skin at the injection point at right angles to the skin.
  - Advance the needle cranially at an angle of 60° until you have felt two 'pops' of fascia lata and fascia iliaca.
  - Aspirate before injecting and every 5 mL during injection to ensure no intravascular placement.

---

3 https://rcem.ac.uk/wp-content/uploads/2021/10/Fascia_Iliaca_Block_in_the_Emergency_Department_Revised_July_2020_v2.pdf

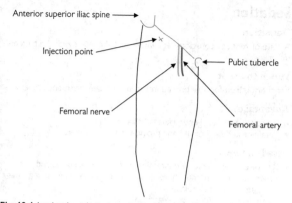

Anterior superior iliac spine

Injection point

Femoral nerve

Pubic tubercle

Femoral artery

Fig. 19.4 Landmarks and injection point for fascia iliaca block.

Axillary nerve block

This block is technically more demanding than the fascia iliaca block, and since the injection point is by a major nerve plexus and large blood vessels it has a higher risk of both nerve damage and intravascular injection. However, in experienced hands it is an excellent block to use in the field for both anaesthesia and analgesia of the upper limb.

Sedation

Definition

A state of reduced consciousness where verbal contact with the patient is maintained.

When to use it

For short, uncomfortable procedures to provide anxiolysis and amnesia.

Advantages

- May avoid need for general anaesthesia.
- Ketamine and methoxyflurane provide analgesia as well.

Disadvantages

- Risk of cardiorespiratory depression with benzodiazepines and ketamine, therefore must have resuscitation equipment including a bag/valve/mask system available.
- Benzodiazepines have no analgesic effects.
- Caution if using opiates with sedatives as easier to oversedate.

Techniques

Ideally the same level of monitoring and oxygen as for general anaesthesia.

Benzodiazepines

- Midazolam 0.07–0.1 mg/kg IV or diazepam 0.05–0.1 mg/kg IV.
- Titrate to response, give 1–2 mg doses and allow at least 3 min between each dose for effect.
- Anxiolysis and amnesia but no analgesia.
- Flumazenil 0.1–1 mg can be used to reverse the effects of benzodiazepines.
- Be aware of restrictions on transport and use of this class of drugs (➔ p. 42).

Ketamine

- Dose 0.3–0.8 mg/kg IV or 2–4 mg IM.
- Titrate to effect using a divided dose.
- Allow 5–10 min for IM effect.
- Provides anxiolysis, amnesia, and analgesia.

Methoxyflurane (Penthrox®/green whistle)
See ➔ p. 623–624.

Introduction to field anaesthesia

Know your limits

All anaesthetics are potentially hazardous; an anaesthetic given by inexperienced hands can cause more harm than good. When selecting a technique consider:

- The risks and benefits to the patient—both of operating and of doing nothing.
- The physiological state of the patient. If they have lost blood or are dehydrated due to illness, pre-anaesthetic resuscitation is vital.
- The drugs and equipment available.
- The effects and side effects of the chosen anaesthetic technique.
- What help is available; simultaneously trying to operate and look after a patient is very difficult.
- The capabilities of the anaesthetic administrator and of the surgeon.
- LA or regional anaesthesia is usually safer than general anaesthesia.
- Airway management requires considerable expertise—ventilating using a bag and mask can be technically difficult, and unskilled attempts may result in inadequate ventilation or distention of the stomach.
- Mal-placement of a tracheal tube or laryngeal mask airway will obstruct breathing and can kill. Airway adjuncts should be used only after appropriate training and knowledge of how to identify correct placement.
- The side effects of potent drugs and complications of anaesthesia or surgery can be difficult or even impossible to deal with in remote locations.

When to give an anaesthetic

Avoid anaesthesia if possible

Some conditions usually treated by surgery are more safely dealt with in the field by IV fluid resuscitation, analgesia, and antibiotics. Examples include acute surgical conditions such as suspected appendicitis, where conservative management should normally allow sufficient time for evacuation of the patient (➔ Acute appendicitis, p. 412–413).

Life- or limb-saving situations

Sedation or anaesthesia may be essential to save life or limb before evacuation. Examples include:

- Upper or lower limb fracture-dislocation with occlusion of the blood supply requiring immediate reduction to restore the blood supply and save the limb before evacuation.
- Entrapment of a casualty by rockfall requiring amputation or vigorous manipulation of a limb for extraction.

Treatment to prevent complications

Other situations may not require evacuation but do need treatment to prevent further complications. Examples include removal of foreign bodies from tissues, incision of abscesses, and cleansing and suturing of superficial lacerations and wounds. Often LA techniques provide a safe and effective way of anaesthetizing for these procedures.

> Use general anaesthesia in the field only as a last resort when there is no other option.

Ketamine anaesthesia

Ketamine is widely used in field and developing world anaesthesia. Its ease of administration should not tempt the inexperienced to use it except in desperate circumstances.

When to use it

- For general anaesthesia, if LA and regional anaesthetic techniques are not possible.

Advantages

- Sole agent required for induction and maintenance of anaesthesia.
- Increases sympathetic tone so BP well maintained even in shocked patients.
- Respiration is not depressed (especially useful at altitude).
- Airway is normally well maintained.
- Strong analgesic.
- Doses can be given as IV boluses, IV infusions, or IM.
- Can be used in low 'sedative-analgesic' doses for reduction of fractures, splint application, small abscess drainage, and burns dressings.

Disadvantages

- Drug ampoules dispensed in a variety of strengths, check carefully.
- Anaesthetized patients often have involuntary movements; their eyes may remain disconcertingly open.
- Salivation increases. Consider atropine (0.6 mg IV) at induction.
- Aspiration and respiratory arrest are still possible, so full resuscitation equipment must be available.
- Some patients get unpleasant hallucinations following ketamine anaesthesia.

Monitoring

Continuous clinical assessment, together with BP and pulse oximetry, represent the minimum acceptable level of monitoring. ECG and capnography are highly desirable but may not be available in critical situations.

Technique

- Obtain IV access.
- Apply monitoring, and oxygen if available.
- Check and have available resuscitation equipment including airway and bag/valve/mask assembly.

Induction

- IV dose for anaesthesia: 1–2 mg/kg. Onset 1–2 min, lasts 10–15 min.
- IM dose for anaesthesia: 8–10 mg/kg IM. Onset 5 min, duration 20–30 min.

It is safer to give a smaller dose and titrate to effect than to give the full dose straight off. You can always give more but you can't take it out!

Maintenance

- Give intermittent bolus 0.5–1 mg/kg IV every 15–20 min.

Or

- Continuous infusion for longer cases:
  - Add 500 mg of ketamine to a 500 mL bag of crystalloid fluid (= 1 mg/mL), run at 2–4 mg/kg/h.
  - Stop infusion 30 min before expected end of procedure.

To set up an infusion

- Most drip sets are 20 drops per mL (but check packaging).
- If you use an infusion concentration of 1 mg ketamine/mL then a rate of:
  - (Patient's weight in kg) drops/min = 4 mg/kg/h.
  - That is, if the patient weighs 70 kg, then 70 drops/min equates to ~4 mg/kg/h.
- In the absence of more sophisticated equipment, set drops/min rate by timing against watch, and then ask an assistant to regularly check that the rate does not vary.

Emergence

- 'Emergence phenomenon' can be unpleasant.
- Try to permit patient to wake naturally in a quiet and calm environment.
- Consider IV benzodiazepine, such as diazepam or midazolam 0.1 mg/kg with induction.

Further reading

Craven RM, Edgcombe H, Gupta B (eds). *Oxford Specialist Handbook of Global Anaesthesia.* Oxford: Oxford University Press; 2020.

Mahoney PF, Jeyanathan J, Wood P, et al. (eds). *Anaesthesia Handbook.* Geneva: International Committee of the Red Cross; 2017.

Warman P, Conn D, Nicholls B, et al. (eds). *Oxford Specialist Handbook of Regional Anaesthesia, Stimulation and Ultrasound Techniques.* Oxford: Oxford University Press; 2014.

Chapter 20

Cold climates

Chapter editor
Chris Imray

Contributors
Ian Davis
Chris Johnson
Clive Johnson
Barry Roberts
Howard Oakley (1st and 2nd editions)

The polar environment

Wilderness medicine in a cold or polar environment involves all the challenges of remote medicine but with additional climatic stresses that impact on all aspects of living, travelling, and surviving. In addition to being cold and windy, these regions are often extremely remote and may include dramatic high-altitude mountains, ice fields, and glaciers—hostile yet beautiful environments under imminent threat from global warming.

Weather

The characteristic feature of cold climates is that the temperature remains below freezing for lengthy periods of the year, resulting in accumulations of snow and ice. Polar environments surround both poles and extend to lower latitudes during winter, similar conditions are found at high altitude anywhere on earth. The predominance of snow and ice in a polar landscape disguises the fact that many of these areas have very little precipitation; Antarctica is one of the driest places on earth, but winds move the snow around, regularly generating blizzard conditions. Sub-arctic continental environments such as the Yukon, Alaska, and Siberia have bitterly cold winters, but their summers can be mild or even hot, with a rich diversity of wildlife, flowers, insects, and even a significant risk of huge forest fires.

The dominant factors in polar and cold climates are air temperature, wind speed, and sunlight. Around freezing point, high humidity (freezing fog) can make conditions feel bitterly cold, but humidity falls at lower temperatures and ceases to be a significant influence.

The windchill index combines temperature and windspeed to estimate the hazards to humans of the environment. In practice, it is easier to use online calculators[1] or one of the numerous downloadable weather apps to judge the hazard of the environment. For those without communication links, Fig. 20.1 and Fig. 20.2 provide equivalent information.

Prevailing meteorological conditions may be modified by local circumstances; for instance, wind speed and therefore windchill are reduced by contour features, trees, and clothing, but increased by skiing or travelling on a skidoo. Temperatures may be lower in sheltered valleys but travel that is safe in the valley can become dangerous when crossing an exposed and windy pass. Bright sunshine raises the apparent temperature considerably. Careless behaviour can lead to frostbite in conditions that should pose a low physical risk. (See Table 20.1.)

---

1 ℘ http://www.onlineconversion.com/windchill.htm

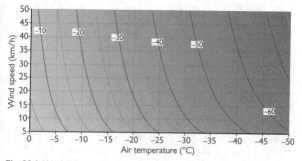

Fig. 20.1 Wind chill index. Reproduced with the permission of the Minister of Public Works and Government Services Canada, 2007.

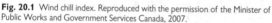

The following are approximate values

Temperature (°C) Wind (km/h)	−15	−20	−25	−30	−35	−40	−45	−50
10	*	*	22	15	10	8	7	2
20	*	30	14	10	5	4	3	2
30	*	18	11	8	5	2	2	1
40	42	14	9	5	5	2	2	1
50	27	12	8	5	2	2	2	1
60	22	10	7	5	2	2	2	1
70	18	9	5	4	2	2	2	1
80	16	8	5	4	2	2	2	1

*Frostbite unlikely.
The wind speed, in km/h, is at the standard anemometer height of 10 m (as reported in weather observations).

Frostbite possible in 2 min or less	2
Frostbite possible in 3–5 min	5
Frostbite possible in 6–10 min	10

Fig. 20.2 Wind chill—minutes to frostbite. Reproduced with the permission of the Minister of Public Works and Government Services Canada, 2007.

Table 20.1 Polar environment risks

Environmental	Medical
Low temperature	Hypothermia
High winds	Frostnip
Whiteout	Frostbite
Avalanche	Sunburn
Crevasse	Snow blindness
Shifting sea ice	Trench foot
Wildlife (especially bears)	Polar thigh
Thin lake, stream, or marsh ice	Contaminated water
Transport (ski and skidoo)	Dehydration
Insects in summer season	Malnutrition
	Slips and falls
	Recreational hazards

Risk assessment

(See also **Avalanches, p. 678–683.)

Novice travellers in cold environments may encounter many hazards—most of them unfamiliar:

- Visitors to snowy areas want to enjoy the recreational opportunities, but the environment is not always accorded the respect it demands. Icy areas around living accommodation are a common place for injuries—spread grit or ash to improve grip.
- Skiing, snowboarding, and sledging are hazardous, and an expedition with scientific goals and limited medical backup must minimize the risk that team members injure themselves during travel to project areas or in their leisure time.
- Rocks may be frost-fractured and unstable, while ice climbing is a high-risk pastime.
- Steep snow slopes can avalanche and glaciers are often crevassed.
- Gullies in hills and mountains may be filled with soft deep snow, possibly with a stream running underneath.
- Falling through lake or river ice is very dangerous and is particularly likely to occur during the spring thaw.
- Tracked vehicles have small turning circles and unprotected machinery. Noise and limited visibility prevent their drivers from being fully aware of their surrounding—skiers and pedestrians must stay well away. Skidoos range from slow load-haulers to racing vehicles; keep your legs and arms inboard, follow trail rules, and beware of wire fences.
- Cold weather and alcohol don't mix. Drunkenness leads to injuries and the risk of hypothermia and/or frostbite.
- Many circumpolar peoples have low alcohol tolerance and should not be encouraged to drink alcohol, particularly when they are in the field.[2]

2 Savchenko M, Bokhan N, Plotnikov E. Analysis of alcohol dependence in indigenous peoples in Northern Siberia. *Arch Psychiatry Psychother*. 2015;3:14–20. https://doi.org/10.12740/APP/58735

Wildlife in cold regions

(See also ➲ Chapter 17.)

Animal life at the two poles differs considerably.

South polar regions

In the south, hazards are rare away from the coast. Animals should be observed from a sensible distance and well back from the sea ice edge. Research scientists are at greater risk.

Killer whales and *leopard seals* are potential threats in or on the water and ice edge.

Fur seals bite intruders in their colonies, while *bull elephant seals* will aggressively guard their territory.

At both poles, *birds*, particularly *terns*, will attack intruders on nesting sites by flying at their heads; an umbrella or walking pole may prevent collisions.

Northern polar regions

In northern areas, *bears*, *wolves*, *elk*, and *moose* pose substantial threats. By far the commonest problem occurs on roads at night. *Moose* use roads as convenient thoroughfares and as salt licks, as a result they are frequently hit by cars, sadly often with fatal results to both animal and humans. In Newfoundland there are about 700 moose/vehicle collisions each year, and *elk* create serious problems for Scandinavian drivers. Away from roads, these large animals can also be a threat. Avoid approaching male moose during the autumn rutting season, and do not stray between a mother and her calf. At other times, the animals are generally placid and can be safely observed from a distance.

Bears are a danger. In North American tourist areas, national park rangers monitor bear activity and offer advice about travel, closing campsites and trails if aggressive bears have been reported. Advice on dealing with a bear encounter is widely available.[3]

Most *bears* prefer to keep away from humans and will move on if parties make noisy progress through the wilderness. *Brown and grizzly bears* usually hibernate in winter and are the greatest threat if early autumn snow forces them down from the mountains into tourist areas. Do not leave food where it is accessible to bears. They become accustomed to this easy source of food, threaten humans, and then have to be culled or transported to very remote areas. Travellers on back-country trails should carry pepper sprays.

Polar bears are a very serious danger, particularly in areas such as northern Canada and Svalbard (Spitzbergen). Campsites can be protected by a perimeter alarm system of rape attack alarms, ropes, bells, or empty cans; sledge dog teams can be spanned around the periphery, it may be essential to carry firearms, and clearly appropriate training is crucial (➲ Polar bear, p. 572–573). The risk of polar bear attack is reduced if visitors stay in cabins instead of tents, use trip wires that detonate explosives, use guard dogs, and deploy someone on polar bear watch who is armed.

During the summer, huge numbers of *biting insects* breed in the ponds and marshes of low Arctic regions; clothing with ankle and wrist elastics, and midge hoods will make life bearable.

3 🔗 https://bearsafety.com

Travel in cold climates

Improvements in transport, navigation, equipment, and communications have made access to remote polar areas much easier. Using a combination of fixed and rotary winged aircraft and coastal craft, logistic companies can supply and support polar expeditions, but travel remains costly and weather restricted, sometimes making casualty evacuation very difficult.

Once at the destination, travel may involve traditional technologies such as by walking, snowshoes, dog sleds, or skis, or more modern solutions such skidoos, superjeeps, ski cats, or kite skis. Environmental hazards such as crevasses and avalanches, and meteorological variations such as diurnal temperature change or whiteout may affect route timing and choice. Deep and drifting snow may disguise the shape of the land making it difficult to interpret maps. Navigation may utilize maps and a compass but be aware that, close to the Poles, magnetic deviation from the grid north of maps may be considerable and changes each year. Satellite navigation and digital maps greatly enhance a traveller's ability to navigate in difficult weather and terrain, but only so long as the device's batteries last.

Whiteout

Whiteout is a meteorological condition where there is a complete lack of contrast. Visibility may be excellent but with no differentiation between an overcast sky and snow, or everything may be masked by fog and the visibility poor. With no visual points of reference, it is easy to walk or ski over a cornice or crevasse, travel in circles, or even fall over while standing still. Though sometimes necessary, travel in whiteout is undesirable and may be very hazardous. Whenever practical, stay on well-marked routes or consider bivouacking until conditions improve.

Search and rescue

Avalanche transceivers are essential in mountainous areas and familiarity with their expeditious use is vital if buried victims are to have a chance of being extricated alive. See ➔ Chapter 21.

Mobile phone coverage extends to fairly remote areas of Scandinavia and Iceland. Satellite phones are valuable though expensive when beyond the range of terrestrial equipment and essential if you have arranged a 24 h 'doctor on call' emergency service. In 2021, only the Iridium system guarantees polar coverage. Checking the adequacy of coverage of any system prior to departure is essential. Short-wave radio communications can be disrupted by auroral activity. Satellite beacons (emergency position-indicating beacons (EPIRBs)) are useful particularly if a satellite phone fails due to loss, damage, or drained batteries. but require sophisticated SAR services in the area. The SPOT device is a small simple and cheap (~£150) one-way tracking and messaging service, while the Garmin inReach® uses the Iridium satellite network to both send and receive text messages (~£400). (See also ➔ Avalanche transceivers p. 680–681.)

Environmental impact of humans

Polar and cold environments are threatened by global warming, their habitats fragile and vulnerable to the increasing numbers of visitors. The concept of sustainable ecotourism needs to be championed. Visits to Antarctica are governed by the environmental protocol of the Antarctic Treaty and most commercial tour operators belong to the International Association of Antarctic Tour Operators (IAATO). Protocols limit the numbers of people allowed to visit the most sensitive areas, such as the McMurdo Sound Dry Valleys, and historic huts. Arctic areas have no similar recognized protection but all visitors to these precious areas need to be aware of the impact of their visit and try to minimize its effects (➲ Assessing an expedition's environmental footprint, p. 126–127).

Humans in polar areas

Humans have little ability to acclimatize to cold environments. The only proven physiological response to chronic cold exposure is the Lewis 'hunting response'. Fit, experienced workers who regularly expose their hands to temperatures below +5°C can develop a cyclical vasodilatation of the skin vessels that enables them to maintain higher mean hand temperatures than new arrivals in a cold environment. At a time when hunting and fishing required hand agility at low temperatures, this mechanism had survival benefit. However, most modern polar travellers will not regularly expose their hands to such low temperatures, and those who do, run the risk of suffering recurrent minor cold injury instead of acclimatizing. Indigenous peoples in circumpolar areas have a short, stocky build, suggesting that an endomorphic body shape has survival benefits in very cold climates. People who enjoy bathing in cold water habituate to sudden cold water exposure, reducing their cold shock response (→ p. 652).

Travellers in cold, dry climates encounter few problems if the temperature is above −10°C. As temperatures fall further:
- The need to humidify dry air causes the nose to drip—facial and anorak hood encrustation with icicles develops.
- Lips become dry and cracked—a good moisturizing sunscreen is essential. During prolonged arctic journeys travellers can have serious problems with lip ulceration and bleeding. Suitable lip salves may help but should be oil rather than water based.
- Bright sunlight can cause snow blindness (→ p. 668–669), but sunglasses or goggles can be difficult to use in very cold conditions as condensation from forehead or eyes freezes on their surface. Two-layer goggles are more resistant to fogging.
- Category 4 lenses let through <8% of light and are suitable for activities like skiing, mountain climbing, high-altitude hiking, and desert trekking. Spare eye protection should be carried.
- Strong sunlight and UV light reflecting off a bright reflective snow or ice surface greatly increases the risk of sunburn on any exposed skin. Protect skin with high SPF creams, including the undersides of chin, ears, and nose.
- Strenuous exercise in very low temperatures, below −40°C, can result in chest pain, possibly caused by very cold air reaching the bronchi. Asthma is commoner among cross country skiers than in the general population.

Chronic conditions that may be exacerbated by cold dry air include:
- Cold-induced asthma.
- Peripheral circulatory problems, including Raynaud's syndrome and chilblains, and the presence of cold agglutinins in the blood.
- Angina.

Children in cold weather

Children can safely be taken into cold climates but must be dressed properly and closely supervised as they can lose body heat rapidly. Early signs of chilling include grumpiness and a reluctance to move. Young children should not be carried in backpacks in the cold; the parent may slip and fall while the youngster's legs can become constricted by the base of the pack resulting in poor circulation and cold injury to the legs. Ski pulks—sledges for towing youngsters in the snow—are popular in Scandinavia; legislation bans their use if the air temperature is below −10°C. Parents or guides should regularly check to ensure that their charges' hands and feet have not become numb. An exercising adult may be unaware of how cold the resting youngster has become.[4]

Accommodation, heat, light, and fuel

Polar expeditions will usually choose a permanent building as a base camp for their work. When the camp involves several buildings, doorways should be linked by hand-lines, as it is easy to become disorientated in darkness or a blizzard. This particularly applies to latrines sited some distance from the base. Fire is a serious threat in areas where water is not available to extinguish flames. Store fuel away from the main base building, there should also be an emergency dump of clothing and food in case of a serious conflagration.

For prolonged polar travel, MSR stoves (with appropriate spare parts) using liquid fuel (white 'gas' aka naptha) is the preferred choice. If using gas in extreme cold and at high altitude, for cooking gas cylinders should be warmed (body warmth or sunlight) before use. Consider keeping the cylinder in the sleeping bag at night. When in use, raise the cylinder off the cold ground using a thin insulating board. Consider the mix of fuels being used. Pure propane has a boiling point of −42°C but requires a heavy steel canister to safely contain it. Butane has a boiling point of −1°C but does not vaporize well when the temperature drops well below freezing. In cold weather, an appropriate cold weather blend is the best solution and usually a mix of 80–85% iso-butane and 15–20% propane is optimal (e.g. MSR IsoPro® fuel, Snow Peak GigaPower® fuel, or Jetboil JetPower® fuel).

Snow holes are warmer than tents in extreme conditions, but more laborious to construct. Tents and snow holes must be positioned away from avalanche runs and trails; both should be well marked so that vehicles and skiers do not accidentally cross them, and they can be re-located in poor weather.

When camping on glaciated terrain, camps need to be carefully assessed by a roped climber using an avalanche probe to rule out hidden crevasses and mark the safe perimeter using bamboo canes or 'wands'. Only then should the team unrope and, once unroped, they should remain inside the designated safe area at all times.[5]

Carbon monoxide poisoning

Carbon monoxide (CO) poisoning and dangerously low oxygen levels are both serious risks in closed areas if cooking stoves are used. If a candle flame burns low or goes out, oxygen levels are dangerously low. CO from cooking stoves is odourless and causes insidious poisoning. Headache and nausea usually precede unconsciousness, but the cause may not be apparent to fatigued travellers, or at altitude where such symptoms are common. Tents designed for extreme conditions are very windproof, particularly if they

4 ℘ https://www.norwegianamerican.com/rudolph-dont-sulk-pull-santas-pulk/

5 Imray C, Tipton M, Dhillon S, et al. Surviving in a crevasse. *Lancet*. 2013;381(9881):1903–1904. https://doi.org/10.1016/S0140-6736(13)61161-7

become partially buried in drifting snow; ventilators may block with conden-sation and must be checked regularly. Cooking with the tent door partially open in all but the most extreme weather is strongly recommended. Deaths have occurred. Supplementary oxygen should be given to a survivor and the victim evacuated.

Water

Fresh water can usually be obtained by melting snow and is safe to drink unless it comes from an area frequented by animals or birds. Clear and sep-arate designation of the latrine area and water source has to be established from the outset. Using a small volume of water at the base of a pan of snow greatly increases the speed at which the snow (mainly air) will melt and also reduces the risk of incomplete fuel combustion and CO production. Large amounts of fuel[6] are needed to melt snow, particularly at very low temper-atures, so whenever practical, dig or drill through overlying snow to obtain stream water running below. The upper layers of sea ice usually contain little salt and are potable. In the Northern hemisphere, deer and beaver may live close to apparently pristine melt streams and can contaminate the water with *Giardia*. Glacier outwash streams contain fine, highly abrasive rock dust in suspension; this is a powerful laxative. If in doubt, filter water and then boil or sterilize it (➜ Water purification, p. 108–114).

Because polar air is very dry, sweat evaporates quickly and fluid losses may be underestimated. Dehydration is a risk during the first days of an expedition; even if people do not feel thirsty, they should drink sufficiently to ensure that they pass dilute, pale urine. A combination of malaise, head-ache, and raised body temperature is common when groups first arrive in the cold; this may be a mild form of heat exhaustion. Bathing in cold climates is a masochistic pastime. On shorter expeditions and when facil-ities permit, people and clothes should be washed whenever possible to prevent fungal skin infections and boils. In the field, 'wet wipes' can provide a practical way of maintaining hygiene. However, without washing, the Inuit and members of prolonged field expeditions develop a natural balance with their body oils and the risk of infection reduces. To avoid offence, it is wise to shower shortly after returning to heated accommodation!

Food

Around base camp, or travelling using motorized transport, energy re-quirements will be similar to those of an outdoor worker in the UK (3000 kcal/12,000 kJ per day), but man-hauling sledges and cross-country skiing are extremely energetic pastimes requiring two to three times this energy intake and eating enough is challenging. Typically, a 5–10 min rest every hour to snack and rehydrate is the only way of adequately fuelling during a strenuous climb. A greater proportion of the diet is likely to be made up of fatty foods, and a wide selection of high-calorie snacks and foods should be available. In the past, polar expeditions have lived off the land, but nowadays most Arctic species are protected and licences required be-fore they are hunted. The internal organs of some polar animals contain toxic amounts of vitamin A and should never be eaten. When travelling in areas where big mammals hunt, you should ensure that food is stored

6 At least double the fuel requirements for your stove if temperature is −40°C.

appropriately. Airtight containers in rucksacks and animal-proof food dumps reduce the risk of unwanted visitors.

Sanitation

Polar environments are extremely fragile ecosystems in which organic matter degrades very slowly. Removing waste is your gift to future generations. In Antarctica, expeditions are required to ship out all their waste, including faeces and sanitary materials. National Parks in North America, Canada, and Greenland also have specific requirements about waste disposal, which is a 'pack in—pack out' policy.

Supplies

Cold will affect many items, including batteries, contact lens fluids, and drugs. Aqueous drugs freeze, crystallize, and may degrade in the cold, so powdered preparations and plastic containers should be selected whenever possible. Critical items can be kept warm by body heat or heat packs used to maintain temperature.

Detailed advanced planning is required to accurately predict food and fuel consumption. Contingency plans and adequate reserves are essential. Stoves are lifesavers in the hostile polar environment and spare parts or a spare stove are essential. The optimal choice of fuel will depend upon a number of factors including the numbers travelling, the destination, the duration, and the ease of re-supply.

Preparations for a polar trip

- Dental check-up, as problems may be exacerbated by the cold.
- If you take regular medication, make sure you take enough to last the entire trip plus extra in case of delays. Inform other team members, so they are aware of the dose and where the medication is kept.
- If you wear spectacles, take a spare pair and have prescription sun glasses made. Make sure ski goggles are the type that fit easily over glasses.
- Make sure that boots fit well and are 'broken-in' before starting out. Physical and mental endurance are essential on multi-day trips. Middle-aged participants in 'adventure' holidays that involve long distances skiing, snow-shoeing, or pulling sledges must have trained and prepared properly.
- Consider rabies vaccination if the disease is endemic among local sledge dogs.
- Comprehensive insurance is essential; it remains difficult, dangerous, and very expensive to evacuate casualties from remote polar areas.
- Tents, skis, and other equipment must be appropriate to the area visited and capable of surviving extreme conditions.

Just having the appropriate equipment is not enough. Familiarity with when and how to use it is often overlooked and is just as important. Inexperienced polar travellers are a potential hazard to both themselves and their companions.

Clothing

Careful consideration needs to be given to the range and choice of clothing taken to cold and polar regions. Active individuals will typically use a flexible layering system, with a wicking non-absorbable base-layer (e.g. merino wool) building up through a series of insulating layers to an outer wind/waterproof shell. Those riding on sledges or skidoos may prefer a heavily insulated overgarment, though these can restrict movement. The final choice will vary between individuals and will reflect the ambient temperature, the wind chill, the altitude, their susceptibility to cold, and the activity undertaken. Synthetic and natural fibres and fabrics have different advantages and disadvantages; these need to be understood if the benefits are to be fully utilized.

Clothing should be adequate to prevent body cooling, but excessive clothing results in a build-up of body heat and sweating, which is undesirable as perspiration condenses in clothes, reducing their insulation. Although modern breathable synthetic fabrics function adequately in cold dry climates, some experts prefer cotton 'Ventile®' shell garments. After prolonged use without washing, woollen base layers such as merino are less malodorous than synthetics. Energetic cross-country skiers often wear thin garments, but must carry windproofs in case conditions change; the groin area can become painfully cold and requires effective thermal protection, e.g. using thermal windproof underpants. If such 'wind-pants' are not worn, the penis is alarmingly vulnerable to frostbite. At any rest or meal break, conserve heat by putting on a belay jacket or zipping up anorak vents, and by putting on scarf, hats, and gloves.

Mittens are superior to gloves at retaining peripheral heat in very cold climates and should be used with wrist or child loops. Chemical hand warmers are useful when hands or feet become uncomfortably cold and are a great morale booster for children in the snow but should be used with caution if peripheries have become numb, as there is the risk of thermal heat injury. Loose fitting, well-insulated footwear, with gaiters to prevent snow getting onto socks, are desirable. Battery-powered heated insoles are available if feet are to be exposed to the cold for lengthy periods at low exercise levels; for instance, when travelling by skidoo, or making scientific observations. However, the practicality of using any electrical or chemical technique over sustained periods is unrealistic. Whenever possible, boots should be warmed and dried; over a period of days, they accumulate moisture and can freeze if taken off in a tent overnight.

Eyes

Eyes must be protected from UV glare by appropriate sunglasses or goggles (see ➲ Snow blindness (photokeratitis), p. 668–669). For those with visual defects, contact lenses, prescription sunglasses, or spectacles with photochromic lenses all work reasonably well. Wearing ordinary spectacles under goggles is cumbersome. Anyone whose vision is so poor that they always need to wear glasses or contact lenses must plan to avoid the difficulties that would arise from loss or breakage: as a minimum, a spare pair of spectacles should be taken. Below −20°C, glasses invariably mist over, and contact lenses may be preferable. However, contact lenses can adhere or even freeze to the eye. Forced or clumsy removal can then result in corneal abrasion, requiring topical treatment with antibiotics and LA (➲ Contact lenses, p. 347).

Metal spectacle frames can become very cold and cause cold injury if in direct contact with the skin; opticians sell silicone sheaths that cover the side arms. Plastic-framed glasses or snow goggles are preferable but become brittle at low temperatures. Carry spare filters for goggles as these too can crack after prolonged exposure to the cold.

Infectious diseases in polar areas

In the past, imported infectious diseases such as diphtheria, measles, and TB tragically decimated circumpolar indigenous populations, but infectious diseases are nowadays uncommon in polar areas. Some sledge dogs carry rabies, and inoculation is advisable if the expedition is visiting an endemic area. STIs have a worldwide distribution. After prolonged residence in a cold climate—e.g. over-wintering on a polar base—travellers will be particularly susceptible to URTIs.

An increasing number of visitors are being airlifted onto the Antarctic plateau (2500 m+) to compete in races or personal challenges. The combination of cold and altitude with pre-existing URTIs has resulted in several incidents where previously fit individuals have developed severe pulmonary symptoms, possibly from a combination of infection and altitude sickness.

Cold shock

Sudden immersion in very cold water, such as falling through ice, or slipping off a riverbank can result in the victim experiencing a cold shock, which is the probable cause of death in many drownings.

Effects include:
- The immediate shock of the cold water leads to sudden and uncontrollable hyperventilation which, if the victims head is below the surface, may result in drowning.
- Immersion in very cold water can lead to heart arrhythmias, which in turn can precipitate cardiovascular collapse.
- Peripheral vasoconstriction from the cold can suddenly elevate BP, again leading to cardiac problems in the unfit.

Habituation to cold water reduces the effects of these responses, and many people enjoy bathing in very cold water. Novices tempted by a 'polar plunge' should, however, be cautious initially and try to ensure both that assistance is available if they encounter problems swimming and that their face remains above the surface when they initially enter the water.

Hypothermia

Accidental hypothermia is defined as an unintentional drop in core temperature to 35°C or below. The Wilderness Medical Society (WMS) updated its clinical guidelines for the management of accidental hypothermia in 2019.[7]

Hypothermia is a drop in the victim's core body temperature to an extent that their ability to function normally is impaired. Normal core temperature is 36–37°C. Temperatures <35°C cause progressive symptoms similar to drunkenness and described as the 'umbles': the victim fumbles, grumbles, mumbles, stumbles and then tumbles. They may shiver uncontrollably, but do not always do so and—rejecting help—may vehemently deny that anything is wrong. Untreated, they will eventually become comatose and die (Table 20.2). Individuals vary widely in their tolerance to cold, with no consistent correlation between core temperature and symptoms.

In the field, diagnosis can be difficult, but consider hypothermia if anyone is behaving strangely or making poor progress on a cold day. Anyone whose torso feels 'as cold as marble' should be treated as a cold casualty.

Once in a warm location, diagnosis can be confirmed by measuring body temperature using a low reading rectal thermometer, preferably a calibrated electronic device with the sensor inserted to 15 cm beyond the anal sphincter. Conventional oral thermometers do not measure low body temperatures, and infrared tympanic membrane thermometers can be inaccurate by several degrees, particularly when the ear has been exposed to cold winds, heat, or water. In severe hypothermia, once the airway has been protected, an oesophageal temperature probe will provide the most accurate readings of core temperature.

Prevention

Hypothermia is uncommon in a properly clothed fit person, but develops if someone is exhausted, injured, lost, short of food or water, or if their clothing is inadequate or wet, especially in windy conditions. Typically, it develops insidiously over several hours but death (usually from 'cold shock' or drowning when disabled by hypothermia) can occur within minutes if someone is immersed in cold water.

If you suspect one member of a group is hypothermic then, unless there is an obvious reason such as inadequate clothing or water immersion, it is likely that the whole party is at risk, particularly if there will be additional delays as a result of treating the casualty.

7 Dow J, Giesbrecht GG, Danzl DL, et al. Wilderness Medical Society clinical practice guidelines for the out-of-hospital evaluation and treatment of accidental hypothermia: 2019 update. *Wilderness Environ Med.* 2019;30(4S):S47–S69. https://doi.org/10.1016/j.wem.2019.10.002

Table 20.2 Stages of hypothermia (WMS)

Individuals' responses to hypothermia will vary		
Stage	Core temperature (°C)	Symptoms
Cold stressed not hypothermic	>35	May complain of cold and shiver but remains active and coordinated
Mild hypothermia	35–32	Complains of cold, shivering, poor fine motor coordination
Moderate hypothermia	32–28	Violent shivering, stumbling, confusion. May appear alert until finally collapses
Severe hypothermia	<28	Shivering stops, reduced level of consciousness progressing to stupor, paradoxical behaviours such as burrowing and undressing, bradycardia and tachyarrhythmias, reduced respiration, cold diuresis, organ failures, and death. If in cold water, drowning is probable
Profound hypothermia	<24	Victim unconscious. The chance of survival drops significantly because of the risk of cardiac ventricular fibrillation or asystole.

Following consensus discussions, this classification is recommended by the WMS, but varies from the 'Swiss' hypothermia classification and that recommended by the American Heart Association.

Field management

The clinical signs guiding hypothermia treatment are:
• Level of consciousness.
• Alertness.
• Shivering intensity.
• Physical performance.
• Cardiovascular stability including BP and heart rhythm.

These signs are easier to assess in the field than attempting to measure core body temperature. WMS have produced a 'Cold Card'. The front side of this card (Fig. 20.3) indicates the field management recommended, dependent upon the characteristics that the patient is showing.

The aim of treatment is to restore the body heat of the victim, but the needs of everyone else in the group must also be considered:
• Seek shelter—building, tent, snow hole, survival bag, or group shelter.
• Remove damp outer clothing. Wrap casualty in additional dry insulation such as a sleeping bag or extra down jacket. If this is impossible, place inside a heavy plastic bag and seal around the neck to eliminate evaporative heat loss. A foil wrap close to the skin may be beneficial but is unsuitable without additional insulation.
• Lie down and insulate from the ground using, for instance, ropes, sleeping mats or rucksacks.

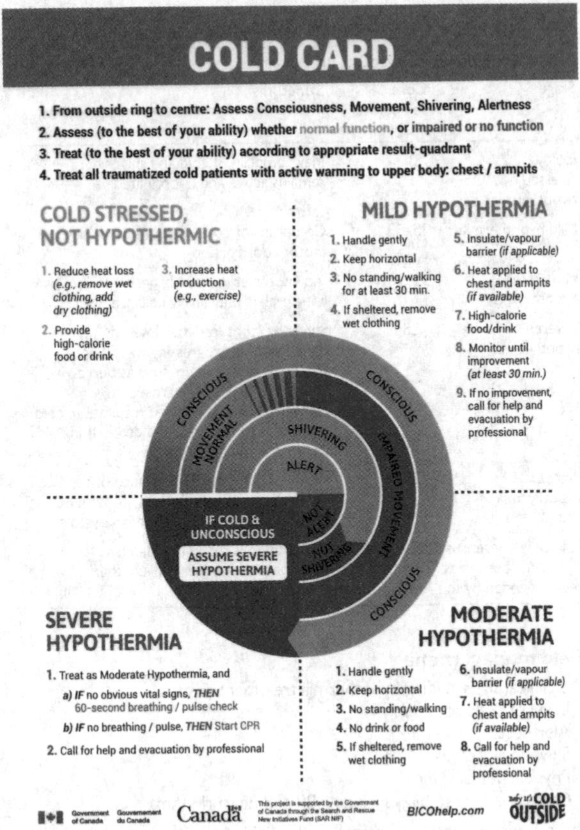

COLD CARD

1. From outside ring to centre: Assess Consciousness, Movement, Shivering, Alertness
2. Assess (to the best of your ability) whether normal function, or impaired or no function
3. Treat (to the best of your ability) according to appropriate result-quadrant
4. Treat all traumatized cold patients with active warming to upper body: chest / armpits

COLD STRESSED, NOT HYPOTHERMIC

1. Reduce heat loss (e.g. remove wet clothing, add dry clothing)
2. Provide high-calorie food or drink
3. Increase heat production (e.g. exercise)

MILD HYPOTHERMIA

1. Handle gently
2. Keep horizontal
3. No standing/walking for at least 30 min.
4. If sheltered, remove wet clothing
5. Insulate/vapour barrier (if applicable)
6. Heat applied to chest and armpits (if available)
7. High-calorie food/drink
8. Monitor until improvement (at least 30 min.)
9. If no improvement, call for help and evacuation by professional

IF COLD & UNCONSCIOUS
ASSUME SEVERE HYPOTHERMIA

SEVERE HYPOTHERMIA

1. Treat as Moderate Hypothermia, and
   a) *IF* no obvious vital signs, *THEN* 60-second breathing / pulse check
   b) *IF* no breathing / pulse, *THEN* Start CPR
2. Call for help and evacuation by professional

MODERATE HYPOTHERMIA

1. Handle gently
2. Keep horizontal
3. No standing/walking
4. No drink or food
5. If sheltered, remove wet clothing
6. Insulate/vapour barrier (if applicable)
7. Heat applied to chest and armpits (if available)
8. Call for help and evacuation by professional

Government of Canada Gouvernement du Canada Canada This project is supported by the Government of Canada through the Search and Rescue New Initiatives Fund (SAR NIF) BICOhelp.com Baby it's COLD OUTSIDE

Fig. 20.3 WMS/Canadian Cold Card.

- If conscious:
  - Restore body heat by providing warm drinks, warming the air with a stove, and sharing the body heat of unaffected rescuers.
  - Large chemical heat pads are recommended if available but ensure that they do not cause burns. Keep checking the skin.
  - Do not give alcohol.
  - Ensure casualty rests and is kept under close supervision until fully recovered.

- If unconscious or body temperature very low (<32°C):
  - Ensure breathing does not obstruct, try to prevent further heat loss, arrange urgent evacuation if feasible.
  - Rewarm using any method that can be improvised.
  - Support circulation with warmed IV fluids if available.

It may be very difficult to tell whether a hypothermic casualty is dead or alive. Breathing will be slow and shallow, while the pulse may be slow, and palpable only in the neck and groin. If unsure, assume that the casualty is alive. In an isolated base camp, the best that can be done is to keep the victim as warm as possible, ensure that their breathing does not obstruct and, if possible, infuse some IV fluids at (40–42°C) to maintain hydration and raise temperature. The patient needs to be turned regularly to ensure that they are not lying in one position for a prolonged period.

Advanced life support for hypothermia

Advanced life support measures are summarized in the nomogram (Fig. 20.4). Measures such as intubation or the insertion of a supraglottic airway can precipitate intractable ventricular fibrillation but may sometimes be a necessary risk. Similarly, starting external cardiac massage may tip the unstable hypothermic heart into ventricular fibrillation. Once started, cardiac massage should be maintained until the patient has been rewarmed or delivered to a hospital. Intermittent CPR can be used if necessary—5 min on, 5 min off.

If you do start CPR in the field, it is clearly difficult to give evidence-based advice on how long to continue. Following immersion in very cold water, there have been cases of full recovery following several hours of chest compressions. The most effective form of rewarming from severe hypothermia is extracorporeal circulatory rewarming, but this will require rapid evacuation to a tertiary care hospital. Declaring a victim dead is more confidently done if they are warm, but the difficulty here lies in warming up someone in the wilderness enough to be able to do this.

Sequelae

Recovery from mild hypothermia is usually uneventful, although the victim may feel exhausted for hours or a few days. Although rare, fulminating acute pancreatitis can cause rapid deterioration during or after rewarming.

Severe hypothermia, especially if the patient has been unconscious for some time, requires careful monitoring in hospital. Extracorporeal warming with warm air (e.g. Bair Hugger™) is important, while cardiopulmonary bypass is recommended to rewarm a profoundly hypothermic casualty. Arrhythmias, muscle damage, and kidney failure can develop. Maintaining the patient at 33°C for 48 h before fully rewarming may reduce complications.

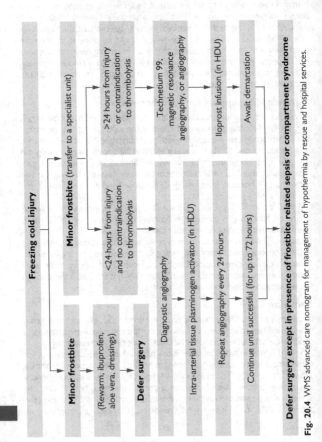

Freezing cold injury

Minor frostbite

(Rewarm, ibuprofen, aloe vera, dressings)

Defer surgery

Minor frostbite (transfer to a specialist unit)

<24 hours from injury and no contraindication to thrombolysis

>24 hours from injury or contraindication to thrombolysis

Technetium 99, magnetic resonance angiography, or angiography

Iloprost infusion (in HDU)

Await demarcation

Diagnostic angiography

Intra-arterial tissue plasminogen activator (in HDU)

Repeat angiography every 24 hours

Continue until successful (for up to 72 hours)

Defer surgery except in presence of frostbite related sepsis or compartment syndrome

Fig. 20.4 WMS advanced care nomogram for management of hypothermia by rescue and hospital services.

Freezing cold injuries

See Fig. 20.5.

Frostnip

Frostnip is a superficial reversible freezing of the skin surface, which resolves completely within 30 min of starting to rewarm the frozen part. In the field, it looks as though pale wax has been dropped on the skin. Typically affecting parts of the body that are exposed to prevailing cold and wind, such as chin, cheeks, and earlobes, frostnip is rare if the environmental temperature is above −10°C, but common in conditions below −25°C. Strong winds, either natural, or generated by travel (running, skiing, or skidooing), increase the risk. Some experienced cold-weather travellers believe they can feel the onset of frostnip as a sudden burning 'ping' sensation. Once established, the lesions are numb and painless.

Pathophysiology

There is vasoconstriction of the cutaneous blood vessels endothelial cell damage and freezing of the outermost layers of the skin. Deeper tissues are unaffected.

Prevention

Proactive behaviour by assessing the weather conditions and taking appropriate steps is key to avoiding most cold injuries. Novice visitors to very cold climates must be constantly aware of the dangers of the environment.

- Use a system of 'buddy' pairs if travelling in adverse conditions, with the buddies checking each other regularly for cold injuries.
- Protective clothing (multiple loose layers are ideal).
- Avoid clothing that constricts blood flow to any part of the body.
- Stay dry and avoid prolonged cold exposure.
- Try to protect your face from high winds using a facemask or the hood of an anorak.
- Use shelter as much as possible to reduce force of wind.
- Wear a windproof, insulated hat that covers the ears.
- Wear gloves to protect your fingers, and in extreme cold, appropriately attached insulated mitts with child loops.
- Wear appropriately insulated boots, socks should not cramp feet.
- Maintain adequate nutrition and hydration.
- Avoid alcohol and smoking.
- Consider supplemental oxygen.
- Chemical and/or electrical hand and foot warmers for short severe exposure (such as a summit bid).
- Metal in contact with the skin (e.g. metal-framed spectacles, earrings, or other facial piercings) increases risk of local cold injury.

For men, the protective value of beards is a hotly debated topic. In some Scandinavian countries, ointments are sold that are claimed to reduce the risk of cold injury. Evidence suggests that these are ineffective and some may actually increase the risk of injury.

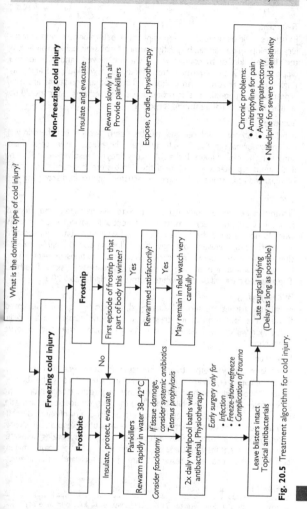

Fig. 20.5 Treatment algorithm for cold injury.

Treatment

Frostnip should be treated as soon as possible, before permanent tissue injury develops. The skin can be gently warmed by blowing exhaled air across the affected skin, or by contact with a warm ungloved hand. Do not rub nipped areas. Once rewarmed, the affected area will look red and may tingle or burn. Frostnip is an indication that weather conditions are hazardous and that additional skin protection is required or shelter should be sought. No additional treatment is required.

Sequelae

Initially the area will look red and may be slightly swollen, but the skin will return to normal rapidly. Once frostnipped, the affected areas of skin are susceptible to repeat injury. If the cold injury does not resolve within 30 min, if a zone is repeatedly injured, or if the skin blisters, the condition should be regarded as frostbite, the casualty evacuated, and treated accordingly.

Frostbite

Frostbite is freezing of body tissues, with extensive damage to the affected areas. This type of injury is most likely to occur in novices in polar areas who do not care for themselves properly. Serious frostbite injury is rare in experienced travellers, but develops following serious injury, immersion in cold water, or when extreme weather conditions prevent travel. Dehydration and high altitude substantially increase the risk of frostbite. The affected part will be cold, white, numb, and rigid (Table 20.3).

Pathophysiology

Frostbitten tissues are seriously damaged, cell structures being disrupted through the formation of ice crystals and osmotic damage to the cells. Circulation will cease in the affected area with muscles frozen and no nerve conduction.

Prevention

Consider carefully whether travel is necessary in severe weather conditions, dress appropriately, drink sufficient fluids, and pair off using the 'buddy' system. Avoid tight clothing and boots that may restrict circulation. Tape gloves to clothing (or use 'child loops') so that they cannot be lost in a gale, and carry spare hat, gloves, and socks. Do not ignore painfully cold hands and feet; try to rewarm affected parts as soon as possible and seek shelter urgently. Never immerse hands or feet in seawater near freezing: seawater typically freezes at temperatures below the freezing point of tissues, making severe frostbite a common result. Beware of cold fuels and gas canisters.

Table 20.3 Features of frostbite

Early features (➔ Colour plate 22)	Late features (➔ Colour plate 23)
Affected part feels cold and possibly painful	White and waxy skin with distinct demarcation from uninjured tissues
Continued freezing produces paraesthesia and/or numbness	Woody, insensate tissues
Areas of blanching blending into areas of apparently uninjured skin	Progression to bruising and blister formation (usually upon thawing)

Predisposing factors

- *General:* unusually cold weather, prolonged exposure to cold, inadequate clothing, inadequate use of appropriate clothing, homelessness, psychiatric illness, dehydration, old age, ethnicity, high altitude.
- *Systemic disease:* peripheral vascular disease, diabetes mellitus, Raynaud's disease, sepsis, previous cold injury.
- *Pharmaceutical:* beta blockers, sedatives, neuroleptics, smoking.
- *Trauma:* any immobilizing injury but especially head and spinal injuries, and proximal limb trauma compromising distal circulation.
- *Intoxication:* alcohol and illicit drug use.

Field management

Frostbite injuries are serious and the casualty will usually need to be evacuated. Although undesirable, a victim can continue to travel with a frozen limb, but, once the affected area has been thawed, they will be incapacitated. Try to protect the numb area from further damage until shelter is reached.

Initial base management

- Once shelter and safety are reached, the limb can be thawed.
- Give the victim painkillers—the rewarming process can be very painful.
- Place the affected part in warm at ~40°C. Ensure that the water never becomes hot enough to cause additional thermal damage. Stir the water constantly to ensure good heat transfer.
- Once warmed, protect the damaged areas from pressure and do not allow them to re-freeze.
- Cover raw areas with sterile dressings and change regularly.
- Wherever possible leave blisters intact, although some experts suggest aspirating with a sterile needle.
- Consider treatment with a simple antibiotic such as flucloxacillin if an infection might be developing.
- Ibuprofen provides both pain relief and has an anti-prostaglandin effect which may improve healing.

Severe frostbite

The only reason for delaying rapid rewarming is if an arm or leg is very badly frozen. In such cases, the cellular structure of the deep tissues can be seriously damaged and the patient requires urgent transfer to hospital. As the tissues thaw, they swell, and pressures in the deep fascial compartments may exceed arterial pressure, leading to complete ischaemia of the limb. Fasciotomy prior to rewarming can prevent this disaster but requires full investigation prior to surgery (Fig. 20.5). (See also → Crush injuries, p. 295, 837–838.)

Thrombolysis and/or iloprost

In individuals who have sustained a severe frostbite injury and where they can be evacuated to a major vascular or plastics unit within 72 h of the injury (this may be possible, e.g. in Alaska, the European Alps, or Scotland), it may be possible to reduce final tissue loss by the use of intra-arterial recombinant tissue plasminogen activator (rt-PA) and/or iloprost.[8] IV iloprost should be considered first-line therapy for severe frostbite <72 h after injury. Contraindications to thrombolysis (associated major trauma, recent stroke, GI bleed, etc.) need to be ruled out.

Iloprost is a prostacyclin analogue with vasodilatory properties that mimic the effects of a sympathectomy. It may also affect platelet aggregation and therefore decrease microvascular occlusion. Intravenous iloprost remains off license in USA,

Cauchy et al.[9] published a randomized controlled trial comparing iloprost and iloprost/rt-PA arms. The amputation rates were 0% and 3.1%, respectively. The administration of iloprost is via an IV infusion. The administration and dose regimens are available online.[8] The infusion is continued for 6 h/day for 5–8 days. The advantages of iloprost compared to rt-PA are that it does not require radiological intervention during administration and can be managed on a general or vascular ward. Iloprost can be used when there is a history of trauma or when the exposure occurred over 24 h ago, unlike rt-PA where trauma is a contraindication and efficacy is reduced beyond 24 h.

Sequelae

In the early phase after rewarming, the affected area will look red, blistered, and severely swollen. Raw areas leak copious amounts of serous fluid. Later, peripheral parts of affected limbs will turn black and mummify. Systemic antibiotics and tetanus prophylaxis should be given to anyone who has significant amounts of dead or dying tissue.

The mainstay of continuing treatment is the whirlpool bath into which affected parts are placed for 30 min twice daily. An appropriate antibacterial should be added to the water. Exposure in a warm environment and early mobilization should be encouraged; smoking should be forbidden.

In temperate climates, where frostbite is very rare, vascular surgeons are familiar only with dry gangrene caused by vascular insufficiency. Such patients have deep-seated, often painful, gangrene, and require amputations. Frostbite injuries can look very similar but the damage is usually more superficial and, unless infection develops, surgical interventions should be avoided until a natural demarcation line becomes obvious between dead and healthy tissue. Better scanning techniques and anti-prostaglandin drugs are improving the outlook for patients with serious frostbite injuries.[10,11,12]

8 Handford C, Buxton P, Russell K, et al. Frostbite: a practical approach to hospital management. *Extrem Physiol Med.* 2014;3:7. https://doi.org/10.1186/2046-7648-3-7

9 Cauchy E, Benoit Cheguillaume B, et al. A controlled trial of a prostacyclin and rt-PA in the treatment of severe frostbite. *N Engl J Med.* 2011;364(2):189–190 https://doi.org/10.1056/NEJMc 1000538

10 Hallam MJ, Cubison T, Dheansa B, et al. Managing frostbite. *BMJ.* 2010;341:c5864. https://doi.org/10.1136/bmj.c5864

11 Wilderness Medical Society. *Practice Guidelines for the Prevention and Treatment of Frostbite.* http://www.wemjournal.org/article/S1080-6032%2811%2900077-9/fulltext

12 Russell KW, Imray CH, McIntosh SE, et al. Kite skier's toe: an unusual case of frostbite. *Wilderness Environ Med.* 2013;24(2):136–140. https://doi.org/10.1016/j.wem.2012.11.013

Internet and satellite phones frostbite advice

A virtual opinion or more specialized advice can be sought from anywhere in the world using a combination of digital images and satellite phones.[13]

Non-freezing cold injury

Non-freezing cold injury is a protean condition that occurs in cold, wet conditions ('trench foot'), shipwreck survivors ('immersion foot'), wet jungle ('paddy foot'), even those with dependent and immobile legs ('shelter limb'). Common to these is a period of relative ischaemia in the feet or hands, during which there is impairment or loss of sensation, followed by hyperaemia when they are rewarmed, often accompanied by persistent and severe pain. Predisposing factors are similar to those of frostbite, but tissues do not freeze. Cold exposure is longer in duration, typically 24–72 hours or days, although non-freezing cold injury can occur in <6 h. Individuals of African ethnicity are particularly susceptible to developing the condition.

Pathophysiology

Although less understood than frostbite, current evidence suggests that cold and ischaemia damage nerves and the vascular endothelium in local tissues. Rewarming then results in further damage from free radicals and inflammation.

Prevention

High standards of foot care are essential, with frequent regular replacement of wet socks with dry ones and wiggling of toes to try to maintain local blood flow. Even assiduous care can only postpone the onset of injury, so periodic removal from cold, wet conditions is also necessary. Footwear that relies on eliminating evaporative heat loss ('vapour barrier') or surrounding the feet with impermeable materials leads to accumulation of sweat next to the skin, resulting in non-freezing cold injury. Foot care routines and drying are even more important when rubberized or impermeable boots are worn.

Management

Cases that present before rewarming must be allowed to rewarm slowly, and thus non-freezing cold injury must be distinguished from frostbite which should be rapidly rewarmed. Sometimes the only clue is that socks remained wet and did not freeze. Many cases present after rewarming, with florid redness, swelling, and pain. As this is neuropathic in origin, conventional approaches to pain management are unsuccessful, but early administration of amitriptyline in a single 10–25 mg dose a couple of hours before sleep normally brings relief. Dosage can be increased to 100 mg or greater if necessary, but patients must be cautioned about drowsiness, and must not drive, operate machinery, etc. Other similar drugs such as gabapentin or pregabalin can be considered. Severe cases may develop blistering sloughing of skin, and gangrene, which should be managed as for severe frostbite once slow rewarming has completed.

Sequelae

Long-term sequelae are more common following non-freezing cold injury and include chronic pain and sensitization to the cold. Specialist advice important, and interference with sympathetic innervation, even brief trial blocks, must be avoided, as it worsens the prognosis.

Chilblains

An example of non-freezing cold injury which is uncomfortable but causes little or no impairment of function. As with other injuries of this type it is caused by repeated exposure of bare skin to wet, windy, cold conditions. It commonly affects the hands, toes, cheeks, even knees of inadequately clothed adventurers.

The chilblain area is characterized by red, warm, tender, swollen and itchy skin. Drying and cracking of the skin may occur.

Treatment consists of warm protective clothing and simple painkillers such as ibuprofen or paracetamol. Hydrating creams such as Balmosa® may also help.

Snow blindness (photokeratitis)

Snow blindness is sunburn of the corneal and conjunctival epithelium covering the front of the eye. Like sunburn, there is a delay between exposure and development of symptoms, usually some 6–12 h. The eye becomes red, swollen, gritty, and very painful. In serious cases victims are incapacitated, as spasm of the eyelids means that they are unable to open their eyes and they develop a severe headache.

Pathophysiology

UV light is a component of sunlight. Because light is reflected off snow, levels of UV radiation in polar areas can be several times greater than in temperate or tropical areas; additionally, in spring, thinning of the ozone layer allows increased amounts of these wavelengths to penetrate the atmosphere. The radiation causes an inflammatory response, with oedema and multiple dry areas over the superficial cornea. The whole surface epithelium of the eye may come away, a process associated with considerable lacrimation. Healing then occurs and subsequent long-term problems are very rare. The retina of the eye is unaffected.

Prevention

UV rays can penetrate cloud so good-quality sunglasses (category 4) should be used in both clear and brightly overcast conditions. Both the front and the side of the eye should be shielded, either by suitable side flaps or by wrap-around spectacles. Should proper sunglasses have been lost, damaged, or rendered useless by recurrent condensation, an effective emergency solution is to recreate Eskimo eye protection by cutting two thin eye slits in a piece of wood, paper, plastic, or fabric, use elastic or string to hold it to the head and use this as a shield for the eyes (Fig. 20.6).

Treatment in the field

- Ensure that the patient has no history of foreign bodies entering the eye. Contact lenses should be removed if still in place.
- Rest in a darkened room or tent.
- Give simple painkillers, such as paracetamol 1 g 4-hourly or ibuprofen 400 mg 8-hourly to relieve pain and headache. In severe cases, a more powerful painkiller such as codeine may also be needed.
- Flushing the eye with clean water or saline solutions may relieve discomfort.
- Eye drops that relax ciliary muscle spasm of the pupil (e.g. tropicamide 0.5%) can help in moderate to severe cases, but should not be used if the patient suffers from glaucoma.
- If available, one dose of LA eye drops such as tetracaine 0.5% (amethocaine) relieves the initial discomfort, but repeated doses of LA drugs are no longer recommended as they may delay healing and increase risk of accidental abrasion.

- Chloramphenicol eye ointment 1% three to four times daily is soothing and may prevent infection, although there is some evidence that the regular use of eye ointments may actually slow the healing process.
- The eyes can be double-padded (➲ Fig. 10.8, p. 352) to provide relief from photophobia and blinking.

Sequelae

Most cases of snow blindness will recover within 72 h. Seek help and follow up if:
- Infection develops.
- There is evidence of visual loss persisting after eye drops have been discontinued.

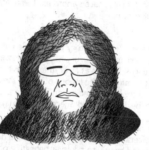

Fig. 20.6 Traditional polar sunshades.

Skin problems

Solar energy is intense in polar areas with strong reflections off the snow, and the radiation intensity may exceed that in equatorial regions. High latitude (owing to thinning of the ozone layer) and altitude increase the risk of sunburn, and a high factor (SPF 50+) sun cream should be applied liberally. Sunburn is particularly uncomfortable when rays reflected upwards off the snow burn the eyelids and underside of the chin and nostrils.

When persistently exposed to the cold, lips are particularly vulnerable to severe and painful chapping. They may crack and bleed. It is not certain whether this injury is due to sunburn, cold injury caused by the persistent evaporation of moisture from their surface, or the activation of herpetic cold sores. There is no guaranteed protection, but regular application of a moisturizing sunblock may reduce symptoms. The benefits of antiviral cold sore creams are unknown.

Polar thigh

Polar thigh is a thermal/inflammatory process seen in long-distance polar skiers. The exact mechanism of injury has yet to be determined but tends to affect the mid thighs. It starts as an erythematous rash, often urticarial in appearance. Most commonly the lesions occur on the anterior and medial aspects of the mid-thigh. A combination of friction, cold, and prolonged exercise seem to be features and anecdotally it may be more common in women.

- Focal infection develops leading to cellulitis and sometimes tissue necrosis with ulceration. It can be very painful and debilitating.
- It can be prevented by using a silk layer beneath wool base layers and wearing a down skirt over your ski trousers.
- Treat the itchy red lesions with topical steroid cream at an early stage and take antibiotics if local infection develops. Serious cases may need evacuation.

Problems of prolonged polar travel

These often occur during exploration, and more recently as a result of the rise in polar racing and challenge trips where individuals or groups are exposed to long periods on the ice.

Health

- Respiratory problems are common—cold, dry air.
- Feet—blisters.
- Hands and lips—cracking of skin.
- Psychological factors and team dynamics:
  - Depression.
  - Poor self-care.
  - Team breakdown.
  - Inability to feel positive.
  - Snow blindness.

Technical issues

- Losing tent, tent fire.
- Fuelling injury, stoves not lighting.
- Poor navigation.
- Not knowing how to repair kit.
- Running out of food or fuel.
- Communication failures.
- Inability to charge batteries.
- Unpredictability of weather.
- Inability to evacuate unless medical emergency and well insured.
- Nutrition and scurvy.

Male/female differences in ultra-endurance polar travel

Sustained polar ski travel has always been very challenging. Nutritional issues were a major problem and contributed to the ultimate demise of Robert Falcon Scott in 1912. The Stroud/Fiennes Antarctic crossing was notable for many reasons including the enormous metabolic tariff and associated weight loss.

There has been increasing interest in sustained polar travel over 61–67 days. Potential differences in male/female performance in ultra-endurance polar travel have been studied through the RGS Global Polar and Altitude Metabolic Research Registry.[14] Mean calorie intake in the men was 6461 kcal/day and women was 4939 kcal/day, $p = 0.004$. No difference was found in any of the normalized (corrected for weight) energetics measures studies between men and women.

Resource

For Antarctic news and information, see: ℜ http://www.bas.ac.uk

14 Hattersley J, Wilson AJ, Gifford R, et al. A comparison of the metabolic effects of sustained strenuous activity in polar environments on men and women. *Sci Rep.* 2020;10(1):13912 https://doi.org/10.1038/s41598-020-70296-4.

Mountains and high altitude

Chapter editor
Chris Imray

Contributors
Jon Dallimore
Barry Roberts
Jeremy Windsor
Charles Clarke (1st edition)
Christopher Moxon (1st edition)
Annabel H. Nickol (1st and 2nd edition)
Andrew J. Pollard (1st and 2nd edition)
George W. Rodway (1st and 2nd edition)

The high-altitude environment

Physical characteristics

High altitude is defined as any altitude >2500 m and is found on all the world's continents. See Table 21.1. While the world's highest peaks are only accessible to well-equipped mountaineers, substantial areas of the American Rockies, the Andes, and the Tibetan plateau are accessible by road. About 140 million people permanently reside above 2500 m, while similar numbers travel to altitude for work or recreation each year. These numbers are rising dramatically. Visitors to Kilimanjaro National Park have nearly doubled in the years between 2003 and 2012. Between 1993 and 2018, the annual number of trekkers and mountaineers visiting Nepal increased from 69,619 to 187,692 (170%). A similar increase has been seen above 6000 m: in the 40 years between 1950 and 1990, 19,810 climbers attempted the highest peaks in Nepal compared to 30,141 between 1990 and 2006.

Mountains do not have to be high to be dangerous—between 2013 and 2020 there have been 15–20 fatalities each year in the Scottish Highlands. Anyone venturing onto the hills should have adequate knowledge of their environment and appropriate equipment to manage any difficulties they encounter.

Table 21.1 Altitude and associated physiological changes

Zone	Height (m)	Arterial saturation	Physiological changes
Intermediate	1500–2500	>90%	Altitude sicknesses rare. Physiological changes detectable
High	2500–3500	>85–90%	High-altitude illnesses are common with rapid ascent
Very high	3500–5800	>80%	Altitude sickness common. Hypoxaemia occurs during exercise. Highest permanent habitation is 5800 m
Extreme	>5800	<75%	Marked hypoxaemia at rest. Progressive deterioration occurs despite acclimatization
'Death zone'	>8000	~55%	Prolonged acclimatization is essential (>6 weeks). Most climbers require supplementary oxygen for safe ascent. Time spent above this altitude is very limited

Weather

Weather conditions can be extreme in the mountainous and high-altitude regions of the world. High winds and severe cold may be encountered, though intense heat and strong UV can also be problematic (→ Solar skin damage, p. 284–285).

Travel and navigation in the mountains

The terrain will dictate the safest and most expeditious means of travel, both to and from base camp as well as on the mountain. High-altitude terrain often requires ropes for safe passage and crevasses, ice falls, or avalanches may be encountered. Crampons, snow shoes, or skis can aid progress while in snowy areas supplies may be brought in using sledges or pulks. GPS and satellite mapping can aid navigation, but must not be relied upon in steep terrain; often a map, compass, and direct vision are the only realistic ways of navigating through difficult mountainous terrain.

Risk assessment

Comprehensive risk assessment is vital for safe travel within these challenging environments and should reflect both the objectives of the expedition together with the skill base and experience of the individuals concerned.

Environmental impact of humans

Mountain environments are particularly susceptible to the effects of global warming; glacial retreat is now visible in most mountain regions. The delicate ecosystems can be adversely affected by the increased numbers visiting these regions with demands of tourism resulting in deforestation to provide fuel (e.g. in Nepal), and pressure on water supplies (e.g. the Atacama desert). The impact on local communities can vary: tourism can bring money and improved standards of living, but traditional lifestyles may be irrevocably disrupted. Expeditions must plan to minimize their impact on the environment and this may, for instance, include the need to remove all human and other waste (e.g. Alaska, Antarctica).

Animal, bird, and insect life

While very few predatory animals live at high altitude and particularly above the snow line, precautions against aggressive animals including domestic animals, and diseases with insect vectors (→ Chapter 17) need to be taken when travelling to and from high-altitude areas.

Risks of mountaineering

Specific risks in the mountains include:
- Avalanche (→ Avalanches, p. 678–683).
- Ice or rock fall.
- Adverse weather.
- Reduced atmospheric pressure and oxygen availability.
- Steep and slippery surfaces.
- Navigation.
- Equipment failure.
- Human factors.
- Difficulties accessing food, fuel, water, shelter, and medical help.

Climbing and mountaineering have always been high-risk activities associated with significant death and injury rates, especially when expeditions ascend above 7000 m. Dedicated and experienced climbers accept these risks, but increasingly adventure travellers are buying guided ascents of the great peaks, which may expose them to hazards beyond their skill and understanding.

Mortality rates vary according to a number of factors including the altitude, the technical challenges encountered, and the ability of individuals to acclimatize. They range from 0.031% on Mount Rainier, 0.308% on Denali, to 1.3% on Everest. The death rate on Everest via standard routes is higher for climbers than for Sherpas (2.7% vs 0.4%).[1]

Factors influencing risk in the mountains

- *Choice of area, mountain, and route:* popular, non-technical peaks are likely to be considerably safer than new technical routes in remote areas. A survey of New Zealand mountain climbers in 83 expeditions to unclimbed technical objectives found a mortality rate of 4.3%.
- *Activity:* downhill skiing in resorts is safer than off-piste skiing. Deaths from technical mountaineering in New Zealand are more than 1000 times more common than during treks in Nepal.
- *Access to definitive treatment:* life-threatening injuries at altitude require urgent treatment. Helicopters can rarely rescue stranded mountaineers above 6000 m and require good visibility. At lower altitudes weather conditions may delay evacuation for several days and victims may need to be carried long distances or managed on the mountain.
- *Resources, experience, and expertise of the party:* without a comprehensive medical kit and the expertise to use it, lives can be quickly lost. To prevent life-threatening injuries and illness inexperienced members need close supervision from their guides. The recent trend for commercial organizations to market very challenging objectives as 'adventure holidays' or 'charity treks' to the general public places inexperienced travellers at risk and demands excellent risk management, which is not always apparent.
- *Search and rescue (SAR):* the terrain, remoteness, likely weather, available communications, and local SAR resources all need to be factored when planning an expedition to mountainous regions. Facilities vary enormously between, for instance, the European Alps and the Antarctic Plateau.

Causes of death in the mountains

- *Trauma:* traumatic injuries resulting from falls and collisions are the commonest cause of death in the mountain environment.
- *Cold injury and hypothermia:* since ambient temperature falls by ~5.5°C for every 1000 m of height gain, hypothermia and cold injury increase significantly with gains in altitude and can quickly complicate injuries and illnesses.
- *Sudden cardiac death:* the commonest cause of non-traumatic deaths in the mountain environment. Accounts for 52% of deaths during downhill skiing and 30% of mountain hiking fatalities.

1 Firth PG, Zheng H, Windsor JS, et al. Mortality on Mount Everest, 1921–2006: descriptive study. *BMJ.* 2008;337:a2654. https://doi.org/10.1136/bmj.a2654

- In keeping with other deaths that occur during physical activity, extensive coronary artery disease is usually found at postmortem.
- *High-altitude illness:* covered extensively in subsequent sections on high-altitude headache (acute mountain sickness (AMS)), high-altitude pulmonary oedema (HAPE), and high-altitude cerebral oedema (HACE). However, it should be noted that some adventure holiday organizations and charity treks are encouraging people to climb mountains faster than is desirable: this is a particular problem with Kilimanjaro and some Andean mountains where access treks are short.

Avalanches

An avalanche is a sliding mass of snow, which may contain rocks, ice, or other debris. Avalanches are released by either an increase in stress (fresh snow or weight of a climber, skier, or snowmobile) or a decrease in strength of the snow pack caused by the heat of the sun and water percolation. In Europe and North America, ~150 people die annually in avalanches[2]; estimates suggest that 90% of victims have triggered the avalanche themselves. Death rates in the high mountain ranges are unknown.

In high mountains snow can fall at any time of year, and wilderness travellers will have to evaluate the risks of terrain and snow pack for themselves. Knowledge of avalanche assessment, prudent group management strategies, and the skills and equipment to effect the rescue of avalanche victims are prerequisites to back-country mountainous snow travel both in summer and winter.

Avalanche deaths result from:
- Burial and suffocation: 65% of deaths.
- Collision with obstacles: 25% of deaths.
- Hypothermia and shock: 10% of deaths.

Overall, only 50% of victims fully buried by an avalanche survive; shallow burial and rapid retrieval significantly improve survival rates.

At up to 15 min buried, survival rates are 90%, but by 35 min the chance of survival is reduced to 30% (Fig. 21.1). Burial depth is related to survivability (Fig. 21.2). These data emphasize the importance of groups being trained in SAR techniques as the 'golden 15–30 minutes' are likely to have passed before the arrival of any external SAR team.

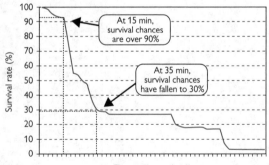

Fig. 21.1 Full burial survival rates.

2 http://www.avalanche.ca/cac/library/avalanche-accidents

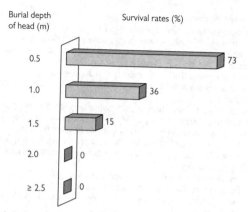

Fig. 21.2 Survival rates by burial depth.

Travel in avalanche-prone areas
- Plan your route to follow safe terrain.
- Are you starting early enough and moving fast enough to avoid sun-exposed slopes later in the day?
- Avoid terrain traps where deep burial is more likely.
- Avoid areas where there is clear evidence of past avalanche activity—including uprooted vegetation, rocks, soil, and snow and ice debris.
- Beware gaps in the vegetation (past avalanche paths?).

Crossing high-risk terrain
- Ensure that avalanche transceivers are set to send.
- Remove ski pole straps, undo all buckles (ski safety straps, rucksack).
- Zip up clothes, put on hat and gloves, cover mouth with a scarf.
- Move gently, one at a time, on a predetermined 'safe' line.
- Don't stop or regroup until you reach an 'island of safety': a ridge, rock outcrop, hill top, forest, or other area out of all potential avalanche paths.
- Use signals to indicate when it is safe for the next person to cross.

Search and rescue
If caught in an avalanche:
- Shout to attract attention.
- Jettison poles, rucksacks, and skis—they will drag you down.
- Try to get to the edge of the avalanche and out of its path.
- Fight to stay on the surface using a swimming motion, particularly just before the avalanche settles.
- Cover your mouth as the avalanche settles and fight to create an air pocket around your face.

Avalanche transceivers
- All modern transceivers operate on a frequency of 457 kHz.
- The transceiver must be worn on the body under clothing, so it cannot be ripped off in an avalanche. It should *not* be in a rucksack or pocket.
- Turn it on, put it on, and leave it on all day.
- Test transceivers daily—this ensures they are turned on.
- Transceivers are in SEND mode unless switched to RECEIVE mode to conduct a search.
- Use lithium batteries which operate normally in very low temperatures. As lithium batteries discharge, they do not lose power but they suddenly go flat without any warning, so carry spare batteries.
- Each type of transceiver has specific performance advantages, but all of them require training, education, and practise for maximum proficiency in search situations.
- Transceiver models differ in four significant ways:
  - The range at which they first detect a signal.
  - How distance and direction to the victim is displayed—audible signals, lights, or digital number displays.
  - How the unit deals with more than one buried victim—a multiple burial scenario.
  - Some models incorporate the 'on button' into the harness strap so it is impossible to wear the device without turning it on. Other models can be worn in the 'off' mode and require the user to activate a switch, which introduces scope for human error.

For these reasons it is important for groups to practise transceiver searching together to appreciate the differences between transceiver models and the search patterns recommended by the manufacturer.

Probe
For detailed searching—or searching for a victim with no transceiver—a proper avalanche probe is necessary. A probe is a thin, sectional aluminium pole, like a tent pole, which assembles into a 2–3 m length that can penetrate even dense snow. You cannot probe effectively with ski poles or ice axes.

Shovel
Effective digging requires a proper shovel since skis, hands, trekking poles, ice axes, and skis are slow and ineffective. Strong (metal preferable), light, collapsible shovels are essential.

Other technologies

With 65% of deaths occurring as a result of suffocation and burial shortly after the avalanche, new approaches have been developed:

* The RECCO® system. Some outdoor clothing, boots, helmets, and other equipment is equipped with a RECCO® reflector which 'enables rapid directional pinpointing of a victim's precise location using harmonic radar'. The two-part system consists of a RECCO® detector used by professional rescue groups and RECCO® reflectors. The RECCO® system is not intended for self-rescue and is not an alternative to transceiver use in the back-country.
* *Snorkel:* the Avalung® provides the user with the potential to breathe fresh air directly from the snowpack, rather like a snorkel. In addition, by diverting exhaled air away from the fresh air intake zone it is said to reduce the risk of rebreathing carbon dioxide and so suffocation.
* *Airbags:* another technique (a number of models are available including Airbag Safety Systems, Mammut, and Back Country Access) uses a deployable air bag system stored in a rucksack. Once in an avalanche the climber or skier pulls an activation handle that rapidly inflates from a re-usable gas cartridge a large (~200 L) air bag, so reducing the risk of burial and creating an air pocket. Initial reports were very encouraging, and although more recent research is not quite so impressive, airbags do reduce absolute mortality if used appropriately.

If a party member is caught in an avalanche

* Stop, think, and assess further risk to rescuers before going to help.
* Watch the victim carefully to estimate where they are buried.
* Look for clues as to the path they were swept down—clothing and equipment on the surface—note the last spot seen.
* Count survivors so you know how many victims you are searching for. Multiple burials complicate the transceiver search.
* Make a visual search for any sign of the victim sticking clear of the snow before starting a more complex transceiver search.
* Start a transceiver search; turn rescuers' transceivers to receive.
* Probe search once you have narrowed down the transceiver search.
* Dig the victim out from downhill side.
* Turn the victim's transceiver off in case of multiple burials.
* Administer medical attention.
* Once all victims have been rescued, switch *all* transceivers back to send.

Extrication priorities

(See Fig. 21.3.) Rapid extraction of victim is crucial, greatly increasing survival (Fig. 21.2) and regular practice is essential.

* Burial <60 min: extricate as fast as possible. Clear the airway. If the victim is in a critical condition, suspect acute asphyxia or mechanical trauma. Treat accordingly.
* Burial >60 min: assume hypothermia and extricate as gently as possible. Check carefully for an air pocket around the victim's face and for a clear airway; both are paramount to a favourable outcome.
* Following a complete burial (head and trunk), the victim should be monitored for 24 h to observe for pulmonary complications (aspiration and pulmonary oedema) in a hospital with intensive care facilities.

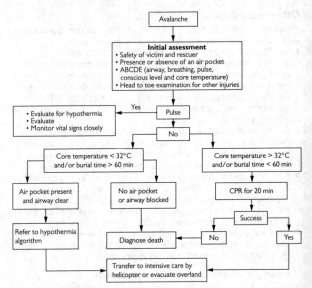

Fig. 21.3 Management of avalanche casualties.

Avoiding avalanches

Terrain factors

High risk:
- Slope angles between 30° and 45°.
- Smooth ground surface (grass, scree, or ice).
- Lee side, high near the ridge line.
- Aspect:
  - Wind direction—lee slopes or in gullies on cross-loaded slopes.
  - Solar radiation—sun after recent snowfall.
  - Shade—cold temperatures inhibit snow pack stability and prolong the dangers.
- Terrain traps:
  - V-shaped gullies reaching to ridges, or stream beds.
  - Slopes that end in cliffs.

Lower risks are associated with:
- Slope angle <30°—with no steeper slopes above.
- Densely forested areas.
- Ridges.
- Tops of knolls and small hills offering 'islands' of safety.
- Wide valleys, away from the run-out zone from surrounding slopes.

Prevailing weather conditions

The following factors *reduce* the stability of the snow pack:
- Rapid accumulation of recent, fresh snow.

- Temperature—rapidly warmer temperatures close to 0°C after snow fall. Or persistently low temperatures (−5°C to −10°C).
- Intense solar radiation.
- High winds (>50 km/h).

The following factors *increase* the stability of the snow pack:
- Warm temperatures encourage rounding of snow grains.
- Warm/cold cycles.

Observation of snow landscapes

Danger signs to look for:
- Any obvious avalanche activity (debris, crown lines, avalanche paths).
- Obvious snow slabs that break off beneath your feet.
- 'Sun balls' rolling down the slope.
- Evidence of wind redistribution—scoured ridges and slopes, snow drifts, deep pockets of snow in hollows and gullies.
- Unmistakable 'whoomf' or cracking sounds underfoot, evidence of the snow pack settling, slabs, or poorly bonded layers.

'If you don't know, don't go'.

Human factors

Expert knowledge of snow pack evolution and high-risk terrain is worthless if human factors override 'snow science' and objective decision-making.
- Decision-making—have clear, prudent decisions been made or does the group blindly carry on in the face of new information? Groups tend to lend more weight to information that supports their assumptions and pay less attention to information that challenges those assumptions.
- Leadership—who is coordinating decision-making and making unpopular proposals to change the route or plan in light of new information?
- Group size—larger groups equate to a greater load on susceptible snow slopes, are generally less manageable, and more prone to a 'go with the flow' mentality.

Skill level:
- Do members of the group have the necessary technical skills to alter their route and move on terrain that takes them out of avalanche danger?
- Fitness level—is the group strong enough to turn back to safety or choose a safer route even if it is more physically demanding (longer, uphill)?
- Discipline—will everyone follow safe travel procedures?

Conclusion

Assessing the snow, developing a sense of which route to take, and generally getting a feel for the level of risk in a snowy mountain environment is not a science and is hard to learn from a book. Even one day spent in the mountains with a knowledgeable friend or mountain guide practising the techniques outlined and applying the 'science' will substantially raise your understanding of the hazards associated with snow travel and make you a safer, more respectful mountain traveller. Make sure that everyone in the party is properly equipped and trained to respond effectively in an avalanche emergency. There is no point in being the only 'expert' if you are the one buried in an avalanche.

Preparing to travel to altitude

Preparations

- Physical and mental endurance are essential on multi-day trips. Preparation is vital—especially for middle aged individuals who may have limited physical fitness.
- Anecdotally, some experienced high-altitude mountaineers have deliberately gained weight in order to offset later losses; however, this should not be due to lack of exercise!
- Make sure that all clothing and equipment fits well. It is vital that boots must be 'broken in' before starting out.
- Appropriate insurance is essential; it remains difficult, dangerous, and very expensive to evacuate casualties from remote mountain areas.

Having appropriate equipment is not enough; familiarity with when and how to use it is just as important. The affluent but inexperienced mountaineer is a potential danger to both themselves and their companions.

Clothing

Clothing for travel to high altitude needs to be appropriate for the conditions expected and there is much overlap in the clothing advice for travel to cold (⊙ Clothing, p. 650–651). The relative advantages (insulation below freezing) and disadvantages (poor insulation when wet, weight, and cost) of natural fibres such as down over manmade fibres need to be fully understood.

Medical kits for altitude

A medical kit appropriate for remote mountain travel (⊙ Chapter 28) needs additional drugs to treat AMS, HAPE, and HACE. These include acetazolamide, dexamethasone, and nifedipine. Consider emergency medical oxygen if travelling above 6000 m particularly if travelling across a plateau such as in Tibet, as descent is impractical. A portable hyperbaric chamber is a practical alternative. It is worth considering giving each mountaineer climbing above 6000 m their own mini-medical kit with drugs for HACE and HAPE. These need to be easily accessible and close to the body in order to prevent freezing.

Pre-departure medical preparations

- Medical checks should identify commonly undertreated medical conditions such as acid reflux, asthma, and minor dermatological conditions. These can often deteriorate in the mountain environment.
- Dental checks are necessary as changes in diet, ambient temperature, and pressure can worsen pre-existing dental problems.
- Prior to ascent, training should be given on how to give injections.
- Those who wear spectacles should take a spare pair and have prescription sunglasses made. Make sure ski goggles are of a type that fit easily over glasses, if necessary.
- Many GPs can advise on the risks of travelling to altitude with common medical conditions.
- Those with diabetes mellitus can travel to altitude provided they are stable, have a good understanding of their condition and can manage appropriately in the remote environment.

- In collaboration with the GP and hospital specialist, a clear management plan must be put in place for anyone heading to altitude with significant disease. This should include steps to optimize the condition before departure and a step-by-step plan to follow in the event of an exacerbation.
- Any individual on regular medication needs an adequate supply of drugs, stored appropriately to minimize the effects of heat and cold, readily available in a day sack, with a backup supply in their main kit bag, and a reserve supply stored with the expedition medic.

Website

Further information can be found at: ℘ www.theuiaa.org/mountaineering/people-with-pre-existing-conditions-going-to-the-mountains

Humans at altitude

While high-altitude illnesses tend to dominate consideration of the risks of high altitude, more mundane problems can cause hazard and accidents. These include:

- Exhaustion and dehydration.
- Hypothermia and local cold injury.
- UV keratitis (snow blindness).
- Poor visibility: whiteout or problems with masks and spectacles.
- Communication difficulties in poor weather.
- Unstable, steep, and slippery terrain.
- Onset of darkness before descent complete.
- Poor decision-making.

Campcraft

High mountain environments are similar to polar regions (➡ Chapter 20). Tents, skis, and other equipment must be appropriate to the area visited and capable of surviving extreme conditions. Clean and plentiful fresh water supplies (or clean snow) and appropriate and separate siting of latrines are important.

Cooking and eating equipment

Lightweight liquid gas stoves are essential to the success of any expedition, together with a plentiful supply of fuel especially if fresh water is to be obtained from melting snow. Check what is available locally, e.g. white gas (liquid) fuel tends to be the norm in Alaska. At high altitude, propane fuels burn at a lower temperature than butane and a 20/80 propane/butane mix is the best compromise in most situations (➡ p. 647). Failure of a stove can be a disaster and each stove set must include spares, cleaning tools, windshield, stove stand, and matches in a waterproof container. The equipment should be designed for high-altitude use and will need to be thoroughly tested before departure. At high altitude, all team members should carry a minimum of a cooking pot, lightweight plastic bowl (keeps food warmer than metal), and a metal spoon (doesn't break easily), together with a small scrubber and sterilizing 'wipes' for cleaning.

Sanitation

This is covered in detail in ➡ Humans in polar areas, p. 646.

Nutrition at altitude

In mountaineering, as in war, it seldom pays to defer a meal if an opportunity for eating offers; at the best the next opportunity may be long in coming, at the worst it may never come again.

(H. Tilman 1938)

A 5–20% decrease in body weight is typical after time spent at high/extreme altitude. Although fat reserves tend to be metabolized first during an expedition, loss of significant amounts of muscle protein also occurs, leading to a dramatic effect upon performance. Weight loss at altitude is due to:

- A rise in basal metabolic rate of 10–30%.
- An increase in energy expenditure (5000 kcal/day).
- Symptoms of AMS (lethargy, nausea, vomiting, and anorexia).

- Limited availability of food, water, and fuel.
- Possible changes in the absorption of fat, carbohydrate, and protein.
- Alteration in bowel flora and GI infection causing diarrhoea, abdominal pain, and anorexia.

As in all other environments, meticulous attention to kitchen and culinary hygiene as well as personal hygiene will reduce the incidence of GI upsets.

Any expedition venturing above 3500 m will need a period of acclimatization to ensure appetite and physical performance are optimized. Little, however, is gained from spending long periods of time above 5000–6000 m. At these altitudes the appetite falters, cooking is difficult and weight loss soon becomes apparent.

Where possible, the responsibility of choosing menus and purchasing food should be given to an experienced member of the team. Ideally, local cooks and kitchen staff should be employed. If this is impossible, the quartermaster should be responsible for providing:

- A wide variety of safely prepared meals, snacks, and 'packed lunches', together with an abundant supply of clean, cold water.
- A warm, well-lit mess tent large enough to accommodate the entire expedition comfortably.
- Adequate cooking utensils and crockery, together with appropriate cooking and storage facilities.

Hydration

Climbers need to drink 3–4 L of fluids each day. Dehydration develops quickly at high altitude; a water deficit of as little as 2% has been shown to reduce performance. Water at high altitude is often obtained from melting snow, which should be gathered from fresh, uncontaminated sources and added slowly to warm water. Melting large bowls of snow is inefficient and tends to lead to the formation of condensation on the outside of pans, which can extinguish the stove's flame.

Diet

In recent years, carbohydrate-rich diets have been widely used on high-altitude expeditions. Theoretically, these not only raise the respiratory exchange ratio (R) and improve the partial pressure of oxygen in the alveoli, but they also reflect the preference tissues have for glucose over free fatty acids at altitude. This results in:

- An increased work tolerance and capacity to produce anaerobic energy.
- Improved mental acuity.
- An increased tolerance to altitude and reduction in symptoms of AMS.

A combination of simple and complex carbohydrates should be used to provide a sustained source of energy.

Snacks

During expeditions, small snacks eaten every 2–4 h provide invaluable sources of energy. A good mixture of carbohydrates can be found in power gels, muesli bars, nuts, dried fruit, flapjacks, and biscuits. In addition, modest quantities of simple carbohydrate 'treats', such as boiled sweets and chocolate bars, provide a useful boost to morale.

Meals

Noodles, potatoes, rice, pasta, polenta, and couscous provide ideal sources of carbohydrate. These can be combined with small amounts of meat, fish, eggs, pulses, and vegetables, and flavoured with chillies, garlic, pepper, pickles, powdered cheese, butter, or olive oil. Breakfasts are essential for both rehydration and calorie consumption and should include cereals (porridge or muesli) and breads (chapattis, rotis, etc.) supplemented with spreads (chocolate, peanut butter, etc.) or preserves. At high altitude, foods should be pre-prepared and should only need the addition of hot water (noodles, 'instant' potato). It is vital to sample foods first before taking them to high camps. This provides information on preparation (cooking time, amount of water required) and, most importantly, palatability.

Supplements

In general, additional vitamins and minerals are not necessary during high-altitude expeditions. However, those with iron or folate deficiencies may benefit from supplements, as red cell production is an essential feature of acclimatization.

Sleep at altitude

(See also ➲ Chapter 21.)

At high altitude, cold, harsh living conditions and psychological stress can disrupt rest and sleep. Hypoxia directly disturbs sleep by causing a cyclical variation of respiration, known as 'periodic breathing'.

Pathophysiology of sleep disordered breathing at altitude

Peripheral chemoreceptors in the brain and blood vessels identify hypoxia and trigger an increase in the rate and depth of breathing. However, this lowers the partial pressure of carbon dioxide in the body below the apnoeic threshold. During sleep, this leads to a pause in breathing (apnoea) to allow the partial pressure of carbon dioxide to rise. As this increases, hypoxia becomes more pronounced and ventilation increases. This often coincides with awakening or lightening of sleep. If the duration of sleep is not extended, fatigue is likely to quickly develop.

Prevalence

Periodic breathing and central apnoeas are nearly universal in native low-landers at high altitude. This is in contrast to Sherpa natives who as long-standing high-altitude dwellers experience a blunting of their hypoxic ventilatory response. With increasing altitudes, the proportion of the night spent in periodic breathing increases.

Implications

Poor sleep, together with hypoxaemia, is likely to impair judgement, reduce vigilance, and compromise safety at extreme altitude. Sleep disturbance at altitude is a feature of HAPE and HACE and group members should be able to recognize and take rapid action if someone develops either of these conditions.

Treatment of periodic breathing

Periodic breathing and nocturnal hypoxaemia diminish with acclimatization. Graduated, slow ascent, allows time for acclimatization and will improve sleep quality. When severe, descent should be considered.

- Increased sleep duration may compensate in part for reduced sleep quality. This is often impractical during climbing expeditions!
- At extreme altitudes, oxygen supplementation during sleep improves sleep quality.
- Acetazolamide significantly reduces periodic breathing at altitude. It also helps prevent and treat altitude-related illness (➲ Drugs in altitude illness, p. 701–702).

High-altitude physiology

Hypoxia and reduced atmospheric pressure

While the percentage of oxygen remains constant at all altitudes, the barometric pressure and partial pressure of inspired oxygen falls with ascent (Table 21.2 and Fig. 21.4). Above 2500 m this has an impact upon the carriage of oxygen in the blood (arterial oxygen saturation) and the movement of gas into the cells. At an altitude of 5000 m the barometric pressure and partial pressure of oxygen fall by half. Only through a series of physiological processes, collectively known as acclimatization, is survival possible. Two of the best-known responses are:

- An increase in the concentration of circulating haemoglobin [Hb]—within days of ascending to altitude fluid shifts trigger an increase in [Hb]. Later, this is supplemented by an increase in red cell production.
- An increase in arterial oxygen saturation (SaO_2)—over the course of several hours the depth and frequency of breathing increases. This elevates the partial pressure of oxygen in the lungs and enhances movement of the gas across the alveolar capillary membrane.

Acclimatization may take several weeks to occur. While the speed at which acclimatization takes place varies between individuals, above 3000 m most can tolerate an ascent rate of 500 m per day provided rest days are taken every 3–4 days.

Inadequate acclimatization may lead to high-altitude illnesses such as AMS, HAPE, and HACE.

Those who spend many years at high altitude may develop pathological features (➔ Chronic mountain sickness, p 706–707).

Table 21.2 Atmospheric characteristics at high altitude

Altitude (m)	Pressure (kPa)	Temperature (°C)	Inspired oxygen tension (kPa)
Sea level	101.3	0	21.3
2500	76	−13.75	16
5000	56	−27.5	11.7
7500	40.3	−41.25	8.5

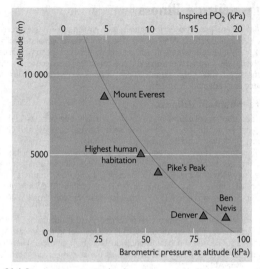

Fig. 21.4 Barometric pressure at altitude.

High-altitude illness

A rapid ascent predisposes individuals to high-altitude illnesses such as AMS, HAPE, and HACE. AMS is by far the commonest high-altitude illness and typically affects between one-third and two-thirds of those who ascend to high altitude. Overlap between all three conditions can occur and should be considered when a high-altitude illness presents. Acclimatization is a slow but necessary adaptation process.

Acute mountain sickness

AMS describes a collection of symptoms typically beginning 6–12 h following arrival at altitude, including headache, fatigue, dizziness and GI disturbance (including anorexia, nausea, and vomiting).

AMS symptoms evolve gradually and are often worse at night. The throbbing headache seen in AMS tends to be diffuse and constant, worsening with straining, lifting, or coughing. Lying down tends to bring some relief. Unlike a common migraine, it resolves after 10–15 min of supplementary oxygen therapy (2 L/min). Most resolve with simple analgesic treatment and adequate hydration.

Clinical and routine laboratory tests do not reveal abnormalities in AMS. While arterial oxygen saturation (SaO_2) is often lower in those with AMS, this may also be seen in healthy individuals at high altitude. Therefore, SaO_2 measurements should not be used as the sole means of predicting or diagnosing AMS.

From a practical point of view, if someone has a headache and feels unwell at high altitude, without another obvious cause, AMS is the most likely diagnosis.

AMS often precedes HAPE and HACE. Always consider these life-threatening conditions when managing those with AMS. The main predictors of AMS are:

- Rapid rate of ascent above 2500 m.
- Altitude attained (>4500 m).
- Previous history of high-altitude illness.
- Low altitude residence.

Minor risk factors include chronic lung disease, obesity, and a history of migraine.

There is no single clinical feature or laboratory test for AMS. However, the Lake Louise Acute Mountain Sickness Score (LLAMSS) (updated in 2018) may be used to monitor symptoms (Table 21.3). Nevertheless, it should be noted that this was originally devised as a tool for investigators studying AMS and not intended for use in the diagnosis or management of the disease. Nevertheless, it does have significant value in the field as an educational tool and is a valuable starting point in raising awareness in those who are new to high altitude. Measurement of the LLAMSS should take place 6 h after arriving at a new altitude.

AMS is defined as the presence of a headache and a score of 3 or more.

HACE can sometimes be mistaken for AMS. HACE can be rapidly fatal if not treated appropriately. All those who are suspected of having AMS should also be assessed for HACE. This should be done by assessing mental status and testing for ataxia (➡ High-altitude cerebral oedema, p. 698–701). If any abnormalities are present, the victim should be assumed to have HACE and treated as a medical emergency.

The LLAMSS is sensitive but not specific. Other illnesses may present in a similar way (Box 21.1).

Table 21.3 Lake Louise Acute Mountain Sickness Score 2018

Headache	
0	None at all
1	A mild headache
2	Moderate headache
3	Severe headache, incapacitating

Gastrointestinal symptoms	
0	Good appetite
1	Poor appetite or nausea
2	Moderate nausea or vomiting
3	Severe nausea and vomiting, incapacitating

Fatigue and/or weakness	
0	Not tired or weak
1	Mild fatigue/weakness
2	Moderate fatigue/weakness
3	Severe fatigue/weakness, incapacitating

Dizziness/light-headedness	
0	No dizziness/light-headedness
1	Mild dizziness/light-headedness
2	Moderate dizziness/light-headedness
3	Severe dizziness/light-headedness, incapacitating

AMS Clinical Functional Score	
Overall, if you had AMS symptoms, how did they affect your activities?	
0	Not at all
1	Symptoms present, but did not force any change in activity or itinerary
2	My symptoms forced me to stop the ascent or to go down on my own power
3	Had to be evacuated to a lower altitude

www.liebertpub.com/doi/pdf/10.1089/ham.2017.0164

> **Box 21.1 Differential diagnoses of acute mountain sickness**
> - Anaphylaxis.
> - Asthma.
> - Cardiac arrhythmia.
> - Chest trauma.
> - High-altitude pulmonary oedema.
> - MI.
> - Panic attack.
> - Poor acclimatization.
> - PE.
> - Respiratory tract infection.
> - Sepsis.

Aetiology

High-altitude illnesses are triggered by hypoxia. Individuals with AMS tend to be more hypoxic than those who adapt well to the high-altitude environment. This may be due to an increase in oxygen consumption (e.g. moving fast or carrying heavy loads) or inadequate delivery (e.g. a low hypoxic ventilatory response or the presence of subclinical pulmonary oedema).

However, the link between hypoxia and the headache of AMS is poorly understood and multiple factors are likely to be responsible. Pain receptors in the brain are concentrated in the meninges and large blood vessels. Headache may therefore be triggered by pressure and distension of the meninges and/or distension of the vasculature. MRI studies have shown that a small increase in brain volume (<10 mL) occurs in those who are exposed to hypoxia. A clear correlation between increase in brain volume and LLAMS score has not been identified. While resting intracranial pressure (ICP) measurements are normal in hypoxia, those with AMS experience a greater increase during exercise. This may represent a loss of autoregulation and result in the sensitization of pain receptors.

Changes in cerebral blood flow—both arterial and venous—have also been proposed as triggers for AMS. However clear correlations between flow and AMS symptoms have not yet been demonstrated. Emerging population studies are slowly revealing a complex interplay between different genetic factors that may in the future help shed light on the underlying pathophysiology of AMS in the future.

Risk factors
- Rapid ascent to 2500 m.
- Altitude above 4500 m.
- Previous history of high-altitude illnesses.
- Long-term residence at low altitude.
- Physical exertion at altitude.
- Pre-existing lung diseases.
- Limited awareness of high-altitude illnesses.

Symptoms
- Headache.
- Anorexia.
- Nausea and vomiting.

- Fatigue.
- Dizziness.

Symptoms typically evolve gradually and are worse at night. Headache is typically throbbing in nature, and aggravated either by bending down and/or by Valsalva's manoeuvre.

Signs

While there are no absolute diagnostic clinical findings, signs may include peripheral oedema, tachycardia, and scattered crackles on auscultation. Those with AMS are often pale, unduly fatigued and sometimes having lower peripheral saturations than other more acclimatized individuals.

Management

- *Stop:* do not ascend further if symptoms are present.
- *Rest:* try lying with head and shoulders elevated on a comfortable surface.
- *Treat:* simple analgesia (the combination of paracetamol 1 g and ibuprofen 400 mg every 6 h is highly effective) and an antiemetic (e.g. ondansetron 4–8 mg 6 h) if required. Encourage sufferer to drink slowly: 500–1000 mL of water, tea, or soup over the course of 1 h. Avoid alcoholic drinks.
- *Descend:* in cases that do not improve it is advisable to *descend* 500 m or further, to an altitude where the individual was well. To aid descent consider using:
  - Dexamethasone: 4 mg PO, IM, or IV four times a day.
  - Supplemental oxygen: 1–5 L/min. Aim for SaO_2 >95%.
  - Hyperbaric chamber: 1–2 h spent in a portable hyperbaric chamber often improves symptoms. Although these effects may only last for a few hours, the use of a chamber may allow those with AMS to descend quicker and more safely.

Prevention of AMS

- Adequate acclimatization—as a guide, consider when above an altitude of 3000 m, sleeping elevation should not increase by >500 m/day, resting every 3 or 4 days.
- Avoid hard physical exertion for 2–3 days after arrival at altitude.
- Acetazolamide 125 mg twice daily starting 1 day before ascent. Although dexamethasone up to 4 mg four times a day has been used and may offer some protection, the use of steroids prophylactically is highly questionable and sudden cessation may trigger AMS and other high-altitude illnesses.
- For further details, see Wilderness Medical Society clinical practice guidelines for the prevention and treatment of acute altitude illness: 2019 update.[3]

High-altitude pulmonary oedema

HAPE is a potentially fatal high-altitude illness in which there is movement of fluid from the capillaries into the alveoli of the lungs. The accumulation of oedema creates a mechanical barrier which impairs gas exchange. The commonest symptoms are poor exercise tolerance, tiredness, cough, and shortness of breath. Breathlessness is first seen during exercise but rapidly develops at rest. HAPE resolves quickly on descent.

3 ⌁ https://www.wemjournal.org/article/S1080-6032(19)30090-0/fulltext

HAPE typically occurs within 2–4 days of arriving at altitude (>2500 m). AMS is frequently, but not always, seen first. There is a strong correlation with altitude attained—6% at 4500 m and 15% at 5500 m. HAPE may be commoner in those who undertake heavy physical exercise and therefore porters from lowland areas may be at particular risk.

Aetiology

The condition is incompletely understood. However, the formation of oedema is likely to be due to an imbalance between fluid entering and exiting the alveolus:

An increase in the build-up of alveolar fluid—this results from the breakdown of the membrane separating the alveoli and capillaries. When blood vessels in the lungs are exposed to hypoxia they respond by contracting (hypoxic pulmonary vasoconstriction). In HAPE this response is patchy, with some blood vessels contracting more than others. There is a resulting stress failure of the alveolar–capillary membrane that results in a leak of fluid and cells into the alveoli. In those with a pre-existing inflammatory condition (i.e. URTI) the risk of developing HAPE is believed to be significantly greater.

A decrease in the reabsorption of alveolar fluid—even at low altitude small quantities of fluid accumulate in the alveoli. This is normally removed by the lymphatic system and relies upon Na^+/K^+-ATPase pump activity in alveolar epithelial cells. In those susceptible to HAPE, drugs such as salmeterol can increase Na^+/K^+-ATPase activity and prevent the condition from developing.

Risk factors and susceptibility

In addition to those risk factors that predispose to AMS, HAPE is also associated with:

- A history of recent AMS or HACE.
- Male sex.
- Cold ambient temperatures.
- Fast ascent (including fast re-ascent in a pre-acclimatized individual).
- Recent respiratory or systemic infection.
- A previous episode of HAPE.
- Blunted hypoxic ventilatory response.
- Diseases that predispose individuals to pulmonary hypertension (including structural cardiac defects such as absent right pulmonary artery and respiratory disorders such as COPD).
- Genes responsible for transcribing substances which regulate changes in pulmonary artery pressure (endothelin, angiotensin II, and nitric oxide) and alveolar fluid removal (surfactant, Na^+/K^+-ATPase) have been found in those with HAPE. However, their contribution to the condition's development is not yet clear.[4]

Symptoms

- Fatigue.
- Shortness of breath.
- Cough, initially dry, becoming wet.
- Haemoptysis.
- Chest pain.
- Symptoms of AMS and HACE can also commonly occur.

4 Scherrer U, Rexhaj E, Jayet PY, et al. New insights in the pathogenesis of high-altitude pulmonary edema. *Prog Cardiovasc Dis.* 2010;52(6):485–492. https://doi.org/10.1016/j.pcad.2010.02.004

Signs

- *Grade 1: mild.* Minor symptoms with heavy exertion. Mild tachycardia and increased respiratory rate at rest. No limitations to normal activities.
- *Grade 2: moderate.* Patient is ambulatory, but normal activities are reduced. Tachycardia and tachypnoea are present. Weakness, dyspnoea, and cough are evident to others. Crackles may be present.
- *Grade 3: serious.* Symptoms are present at rest. The patient may be unable to walk and prefers to rest. Simple tasks may be impossible. Senses may be dulled. Confusion and disorientation may be present. Tachycardia and tachypnoea are present. Crackles are easily heard.
- *Grade 4: severe.* Patient is unconscious and cannot be roused. Exhibits noisy breathing with sounds of fluid in the airways. Breathing and pulse are both rapid.

Investigations (when available)

- Pulse oximetry: most HAPE sufferers will have a low arterial oxygen saturation when compared to healthy, well-acclimatized individuals who have shared the same ascent profile.
- Radiology: changes can be highly variable. However, those with HAPE eventually develop asymmetric areas of 'cotton wool' infiltrates in the mid and lower zones of the lung fields. These often begin in the right mid zone and eventually spread across to the left. The apices and costophrenic angles are usually spared. Signs of cardiogenic pulmonary oedema are usually absent. X-ray and CT changes resolve quickly following recovery.
- Electrocardiography: typically shows a sinus tachycardia and changes compatible with acute pulmonary hypertension including right axis deviation and bundle branch block; peaked P waves in leads II, III, and aVF; and an increase in the depth of precordial S waves.
- Cardiac catheter studies have shown elevated pulmonary artery pressure.
- Chest ultrasound: the presence of pulmonary oedema can result in the formation of 'comet-tail artefacts' on ultrasound scanning. These can provide an objective assessment of pulmonary oedema and can be used to monitor the course of the disease.
- Blood tests: most laboratory investigations are normal in HAPE; however, a mild neutrophil leucocytosis is sometimes seen.

Management

Descent is the main treatment for HAPE. A descent of just a few hundred metres can often prove beneficial. In severe cases the subject should not be self-ambulatory and should ideally be carried by pack animal, porter, or mechanized transport. When descent is not possible (weather, terrain night-fall, etc.) the following approach may help prevent further deterioration:

- Sit patient up and keep warm.
- Supplemental oxygen by face mask (titrate to SaO_2 >95%—up to 10 L/min) and/or hyperbaric chamber.
- Nifedipine 30 mg PO twice a day or 20 mg PO three times a day slow-release preparation.
- Dexamethasone 8 mg initially then 4 mg PO/IM/IV four times a day.

Prevention
- Slow ascent: above 3000 m, ascend at a rate of 500 m/day and include a rest day every 3–4 days. Avoid strenuous exertion while acclimatizing.
- Manage AMS: in the event of AMS symptoms developing follow the 'Stop, Rest, Treat and Descend' approach.
- Modify behaviour: avoid heavy physical exertion for 2–3 days after arriving at a new altitude and descend quickly if HAPE symptoms arise.

In those with a prior history of HAPE, the following have been shown to reduce the incidence and severity of a relapse:
- Nifedipine 30 mg PO twice a day or 20 mg PO three times a day. Slow-release preparation is 'gold standard' prophylactic treatment for those with a previous history of HAPE.
- Salmeterol 125-microgram inhaler twice a day—limited clinical evidence. It is thought to act by improving clearance of lung fluid. Many experts recommend its use only in combination with nifedipine.
- Tadalafil 10 mg twice a day—limited clinical evidence. Along with other phosphodiesterase inhibitors, tadalafil reduces pulmonary artery pressure in those with a history of HAPE.

Khumbu cough is a dry persistent cough that is sometimes seen in lowland residents who spend several days or weeks above 4000 m. While the condition is not life-threatening, it is very uncomfortable and can lead to muscle injury and rib fractures in the most severe cases. Facemasks have been used with limited success to help prevent the inspiration of cold, dry air. The cough quickly resolves on descent.

High-altitude cerebral oedema

HACE is a rare but potentially fatal condition that can occur at altitudes above 2500 m. Approximately 0.5–1% of those travelling above 5000 m will develop the condition. Up to 20% of those who present with HAPE will also have signs of HACE, while up to 50% of those who die from HAPE also have evidence of HACE on autopsy. A low threshold to treat both conditions is needed.

In most cases those who develop HACE will first have symptoms of AMS. However, at very high altitudes (>6000 m) HACE can occasionally develop without symptoms of AMS.

Aetiology
Hypoxia is the underlying trigger of HACE. However, like AMS, it is unclear what distinguishes those who develop the condition from others who remain healthy. It is widely believed that AMS and HACE are on the same pathophysiological spectrum.

A lack of a CSF volume buffering occurs in individuals who are thought to be susceptible to high-altitude illness. There appears to be a predisposition to an earlier rise in ICP when there is oedema formation or increased blood volume. As HACE develops, victims develop an increase in intracerebral pressure. This stems from a disruption of the blood–brain barrier that leads to an influx of water (vasogenic cerebral oedema). As homeostatic mechanisms start to fail, further swelling takes place within the cells (cytotoxic cerebral oedema).

A number of different processes, both mechanical and molecular, have been implicated in the disruption of the blood–brain barrier. In particular, several animal studies have pointed towards vascular endothelial growth factor (VEGF) as playing a significant part in the development of this condition. Expression of this protein is blocked by dexamethasone.

For more information, see Wilson et al.[5]

Risk factors

These are similar to AMS and HAPE. Gradual acclimatization and correct treatment of AMS reduce the risk of brain oedema during the early stages of ascent to high altitudes. Little can be done to prevent sudden brain oedema at extreme altitudes—it is vital to recognize the condition promptly and act swiftly.

A previous history of HACE is widely believed to be a risk factor for developing the condition.

Symptoms

HACE sufferers are often unaware of any changes in their condition. Colleagues may report recent symptoms of other high-altitude illnesses such as AMS and HAPE.
* Headache.
* Nausea.
* Hallucination.
* Disorientation.
* Confusion.

Signs

HACE is distinguished from AMS by the presence of neurological signs. In those with AMS, the appearance of new neurological signs should necessitate urgent evacuation and treatment for HACE.
* *Ataxia:* commonest sign identified in those with HACE. Identified by observing a short distance of heel-to-toe walking interrupted by a 180° turn. A positive Romberg test is often seen. Ask the patient to stand upright with feet together and eyes closed. In severe cases victims may be unable to stand. Differences in tone, power, and reflexes can also occur.
* *Behavioural changes:* victims may appear unusually tired, irritable, confused, forgetful, elated, or prone to bouts of irrational behaviour. Memory and orientation are often impaired. Hallucinations are occasionally seen.
* *Plantar reflexes:* are abnormal in a third of HACE sufferers.
* *Cranial nerve palsies:* although rare, palsies to cranial nerves III, IV, VI, and XII are seen.
* *Urinary signs:* urinary incontinence or retention is reported in about half of those with HACE.
* *Visual:* papilloedema can be seen on fundoscopy.

5 Wilson MH, Newman S, Imray CH. The cerebral effects of ascent to high altitudes. *Lancet Neurol.* 2009;8(2);175–191. https://doi.org/10.1016/S1474-4422(09)70014-6

Investigations

HACE is a clinical diagnosis. Anyone exhibiting these symptoms and signs following a recent ascent to altitude should be assumed to have HACE and evacuated as soon as possible.

In hospital the following tests are useful:
- *CT scan*: an increase in ICP reveals compression of the ventricles and changes to the gyri and sulci on the surface of the cerebral hemispheres.
- *MRI scan*: shows formation of oedema in the white matter. This is often concentrated in the splenium of the corpus callosum. Grey matter is largely unaffected by HACE.

Changes seen on CT and MRI scanning may take weeks or even months to resolve after clinical recovery.

Management

Like HAPE, descent is the main treatment for HACE. When this is prevented by significant compromise or poor conditions, other treatments may help prevent further deterioration:
- Supplemental oxygen by mask (aim for SaO_2 >95%).
- Dexamethasone 8 mg (IV or IM) initially, followed by 4 mg every 4 h.
- If coexistent HAPE is suspected, nifedipine 30 mg PO twice daily or 20 mg PO three times daily slow-release.
- Use of a hyperbaric recompression bag.

Prevention

- Adequate acclimatization.
- Above an altitude of 3000 m, sleeping elevation should not increase by >500 m a day, resting every 3–4 days.
- Avoid hard physical exertion for 2–3 days after arrival at altitude (anecdotal evidence).
- Early descent on any appearance of symptoms (rapidly reversed in early stages).

Portable hyperbaric chambers

Now carried by many high-altitude expeditions, these are capsules constructed from lightweight airtight materials into which a person can be zipped (Fig. 21.5). The chamber is then inflated with a foot or hand pump. This results in a rapid increase in barometric pressure within the chamber and a simulated descent. Manual pumping, with hand or foot pump, must continue intermittently, even after inflation, to allow carbon dioxide clearance.

Single-person portable devices weigh ~5 kg and can be bought or hired in popular mountain regions. Portable hyperbaric chambers have been shown to treat all forms of altitude illness effectively; however, the effect does not persist for long after removal from the chamber and should not replace descent as the primary treatment. Such bags must be used with care:
- Prior to setting out on an expedition the chamber needs to be checked that it is complete (including piping and foot pump) and airtight and the supervisor is familiar with its operation.
- Ensure the subject can clear their ears (to avoid barotrauma).
- Ensure a constant clean air supply to the casualty.

- Position so that casualty lies in head-up position.
- The chamber should be placed in a flat, sheltered area that is set away from any potential dangers.
- Monitor the casualty's condition continuously to ensure that they remain breathing and do not vomit (it is dangerous to put a patient who cannot protect their airway into the bag).

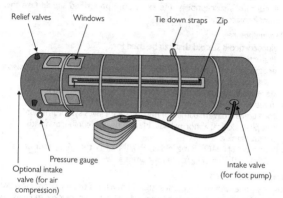

Relief valves   Windows   Tie down straps   Zip

Pressure gauge
Optional intake
valve (for air
compression)

Intake valve
(for foot pump)

Fig. 21.5 Gamow bag.

High-altitude retinal haemorrhage

(See ➲ Colour plate 3.)

Retinal haemorrhages (in the nerve fibre layer) are common above 5000 m and are not necessarily related to AMS. They do not predispose to cerebral oedema and rarely interfere with vision unless they occur over the macula. No treatment is usually necessary but if vision becomes blurred or fails, descent is advisable. Permanent visual loss is exceptional. Haemorrhages that do not affect vision are not known to have any clinical significance. Descent is not necessary in these cases.

Drugs in altitude illness

Acetazolamide

Acetazolamide is a carbonic anhydrase inhibitor which increases bicarbonate excretion from the kidneys and produces a metabolic acidosis that increases respiratory drive. This can be used for:

- *AMS prophylaxis:* drug of choice in at-risk individuals. Recommended dose: 125 mg twice a day, beginning 1 day before ascent to altitude; child 2.5 mg/kg twice a day. Acetazolamide 125 mg twice a day has been shown to improve sleep disturbance at altitude. Smaller doses may also be effective.
- *AMS treatment:* there is only one study supporting acetazolamide in treatment of AMS. 250 mg three times a day; child 2.5 mg/kg three times a day (maximum 250 mg/dose).

Common side effects

Nausea and vomiting, anorexia, dizziness, tingling in hands, and an odd taste in the mouth. While most people tolerate acetazolamide well, others experience significant side effects and it is recommended that people try it before using it as prophylaxis at altitude. It has been argued that since the risk of AMS depends upon the ascent rate, the absolute altitude attained, and the individual's susceptibility, the exact dose prescribed should take these factors into account.

Dexamethasone

A glucocorticoid steroid that can be used for:

- *Prevention and treatment of AMS* (in individuals intolerant to acetazolamide): unknown action. Unlike acetazolamide, dexamethasone does not aid acclimatization. If stopped suddenly, AMS can quickly develop. 8 mg/day in divided doses (e.g. 4 mg twice a day).
- *Treatment of AMS:* 4 mg four times a day; child 0.15 mg/kg/dose four times a day (maximum 4 mg/dose). Relieves symptoms but not physiological abnormalities. May be used in conjunction with acetazolamide.
- *Treatment of HACE:* 8 mg initially PO, IM, or IV then 4 mg four times a day; child 0.15 mg/kg/dose four times a day.

Common side effects

Usually none with short courses; steroid psychosis occurs rarely. However, if used for more than a few days side effects can quickly multiply. An 'Addisonian crisis' has been reported on Mount Everest after 4 weeks' usage. It was further complicated by GI bleeding and a number of other side effects.

Nifedipine

A calcium channel blocker that inhibits hypoxic pulmonary vasoconstriction at altitude and therefore causes pulmonary artery pressure to fall. It can be used for:

- *Prevention of HAPE* in susceptible individuals: has been shown to reduce the incidence significantly in people of known susceptibility. 30 mg twice daily.
- *Treatment of HAPE:* drug treatment is secondary to descent and/or supplementary oxygen which address the primary cause. 20 mg PO slow-release preparation four times a day. Child 0.5 mg/kg/dose PO three times a day—ideally slow-release preparation (maximum 20 mg/dose).

Common side effects

Headache, dizziness, and postural hypotension. The latter, which is serious as it may hamper descent, is less likely with a slow-release preparation.

Phosphodiesterase-5 inhibitors

These drugs lower pulmonary artery pressures with a lesser effect on systemic arterial BP.

Tadalafil 10 mg twice daily can be used for HAPE prophylaxis, and could be used if nifedipine was unavailable or, not tolerated.

Children at altitude

Improved access and the growth of adventure tourism mean that increasing numbers of lowland children are travelling to high altitude. Here they are exposed to the same risks as those described for adults, including environmental and meteorological hazards, and altitude illness, for which the parent, guardian, school, or guide must recognize responsibility. While a carefully planned adventure in high-altitude areas with older children can be beneficial, taking young children to high altitude in remote regions may not be in their best interests.

Altitude illness in lowland children ascending to height

- Although there are few studies that have considered altitude illness in children, the majority found that AMS and HAPE probably occur at about the same rate as in adults.
- Intercurrent illness may increase the risk of altitude illness in children.
- Symptoms of altitude illness are especially difficult to recognize in preverbal children and the classic symptoms of AMS are not reported by children <5 years of age.
- In preverbal children, irritability, fussiness, food refusal, lethargy, decreased playfulness, difficulty sleeping, and excessive crying may be the symptoms noted, but these are difficult to distinguish from symptoms related to other causes including intercurrent illness and even just a change of normal routine.
- The risk of late recognition of altitude illness in children can be reduced by vigilance and an assumption that any non-specific symptoms may indicate the onset of AMS or early HAPE/HACE.
- AMS, HAPE, and HACE in children should be managed in the same way as described previously for adults (paediatric doses of drugs for prophylaxis and treatment are given elsewhere; see ⊃ Drugs in altitude illness, p. 701–702).
- Following treatment for HAPE children should be investigated for underlying congenital cardiorespiratory abnormalities.
- As with adults, AMS may be prevented by slow graded ascent: above an altitude of 3000 m, sleeping elevation should not increase by >500 m a day, resting every 3–4 days.
- Where a rapid ascent with a child is unavoidable, the use of drug therapy for prophylaxis is reasonable, as for adults.

Infants residing at altitude

There is evidence that infants (<1 year of age) who are exposed to high-altitude environments for prolonged periods may develop symptomatic complications as a result of maladaptation:

- Newborns at altitude have low oxygen saturations at birth which may interfere with normal adaptation of the circulation to *ex utero* life. Persistence of a patent ductus arteriosus is more common at altitude and all infants should receive supplementary oxygen after delivery to encourage ductal closure.
- Both infants born at altitude and infants travelling to altitude during the first year of life may develop symptomatic high-altitude pulmonary hypertension (SHAPH) in response to altitude hypoxia.

- The length of exposure necessary for SHAPH is unknown and it is recommended that infants residing at high altitude are monitored by a cardiologist.
- SHAPH is associated with muscularization of peripheral pulmonary arterioles and right ventricular hypertrophy, which may lead to heart failure.
- Treatment of SHAPH includes oxygen therapy and descent.

Environmental factors

As a result of their high surface area to volume ratio, children are especially susceptible to the cold (including wind chill), particularly if they are being carried and are therefore not generating heat through exercise.

- Minimize risk of hypothermia and cold injury by paying attention to thermal balance.
- Ensure they wear adequate windproof, waterproof, insulating clothing.
- Children being carried in packs or slings are at risk of hypothermia and/or frostbite of the extremities.
- Goggles should be worn to avoid snow blindness.
- Sun protection should be provided using clothing and sunblock creams.

Chronic mountain sickness

Some of those who live for many years at high altitude are prone to the development of a high haemoglobin concentration that may subsequently trigger pulmonary hypertension and cardiac failure. This condition is commonly referred to as chronic mountain sickness (CMS or Monge's disease). It is most commonly found in South America. Ethnic Tibetans are rarely affected. However, lowland Chinese immigrants settling on the Tibetan plateau are particularly prone to the disease.

Definition

CMS is a clinical syndrome that occurs in natives or long-term residents above 2500 m. It is characterized by:
- Erythrocytosis—a high haemoglobin concentration of >190 g/L in females and >210 g/L in males.
- Pulmonary hypertension that can develop into cor pulmonale and congestive cardiac failure.
- Typically, clinical features of CMS gradually disappear with descent and return following re-ascent.

Prevalence

CMS increases with altitude of residence—ranging from 1.1% (<3000 m) to 11.9% (>4000 m). CMS is more commonly found in men, elderly, smokers, those exposed to environmental pollution, and individuals with respiratory disease. Conditions associated with hypoventilation (e.g. kyphoscoliosis, obstructive sleep apnoea, and obesity) are also associated with CMS.

CMS is rarer in those populations who have resided at high altitude for many generations. On the Tibetan plateau, CMS occurs in 5.6% of Han Chinese compared to just 1.2% of Tibetan natives.

Pathophysiology

It has been widely believed that hypoventilation leads to an exaggerated erythrocytosis in those with CMS that leads to pulmonary hypertension and cardiac failure. However, it is now clear that many of those with CMS do not hypoventilate. This would suggest that CMS is a far more complex disease than was once thought and a range of different factors play a part.

Clinical picture

- *Symptoms*: decreased exercise tolerance, disturbed sleep, confusion, dizziness, headache, paraesthesia, tinnitus, joint and muscle pain.
- *Signs*: clubbing, deep purplish colour of nail beds, ears, gums and lips, watery eyes. In severe cases there are signs of congestive cardiac failure.
- *Investigations*: chest X-ray reveals cardiac enlargement and prominent pulmonary blood vessels. Evidence of pulmonary hypertension can be seen on ECG and echocardiography.

Treatment

- *Acute*: rapid descent. Supplemental oxygen (SaO_2 >95%).
- *Chronic*: the long-term 'gold standard' treatment is permanent residence at low altitude. Erythrocytosis settles within weeks of descent, however cardiovascular changes may take months or even years to resolve. For those who choose to remain at altitude medical therapies are available. Acetazolamide (250 mg/day) has been shown to be among the safest and most effective treatments.

Chapter 22

Inland and coastal waters

Chapter editor
Chris Johnson

Contributors
Paddy Morgan
Andy Watt

Aquatic environments

Drowning is the third leading cause of accidental death worldwide (after road traffic injuries and falls) and results in ~320,000 deaths a year; 90% of these deaths occur in low- and middle-income countries, where young children are particularly at risk of drowning in ditches and ponds. Worldwide, there is a strong association between alcohol and young adults drowning in lakes and rivers.[1] Serious medical problems such as seizures, ischaemic heart disease, and strokes may cause a person to collapse into water and then drown as a secondary event. A riverside fall into cold water may result in 'cold shock' and drowning (➔ p. 652).

In 2019, the Royal National Lifeboat Institution in the UK and Republic of Ireland assisted 9379 people at sea with a further 29,334 aided by beach lifeguards. Of those rescued, 1835 required casualty care. The service saved 374 lives during the year—but such sophisticated rescue services are not universally available.

Aquatic environments, whether oceans, rivers, or lakes, are very complex, being affected by the flows of water, their interaction with surrounding land, and the interplay with other physical forces such as the wind. Expeditions using rivers or lakes as routes of communication also have to contend with the nature of the surrounding terrain and the local weather conditions.

Inshore boating expeditions may involve kayaking, canoeing, or rafting. Stand-up paddleboarding (SUP) and coasteering (navigation along the intertidal shoreline using a combination of walking, rock climbing, and swimming) are increasing in popularity.

All expedition risk assessments should consider aquatic hazards. In many locations, coastlines and rivers may be polluted by industrial, agricultural, or pathogen containing effluent, especially soon after heavy rains that overwhelm sewage systems. The possibility of water-borne disease must always be considered (➔ p. 719).

Water's edge

Most deaths from drowning occur close to shore. Effective risk assessment requires an understanding of the nature of the coastal terrain or river hydrology.

Gradient

- *Cliffs:* may prevent landing by sea kayak and small boats and may generate strong downdrafts or erratic wave patterns.
- *Vertical or steep edges:* increase the risk of a slip into water of unknown depth, the edges may be unstable (e.g. decaying canal banks), and make it difficult to self-rescue, or retrieve someone in the water. Unfenced river or harbour-side walls are a particular risk.
- *Steeply sloping beaches:* create dumping waves and are prone to fast run-offs that can knock people off their feet.
- *Shallow beaches:* often have long tidal ranges with rapid flows that can strand people on sandbanks.

---

1 World Health Organization. *Global Report on Drowning: Preventing a Leading Killer.* Geneva: World Health Organization; 2014.

- *Rapids:* are formed by gradient, volume of water, or constriction, encouraging white-water activities, but fast currents increase risk for anyone in the water.

Construction

- *Shale/coral:* painful to walk on, sharp pieces can penetrate the skin and cause infections. Sea urchins (→ p. 296, 600) may be present. Formal surgical exploration may be required to remove an infective focus.
- *Sand:* difficult to see animals such as rays (→ p. 597, 598) that may be trodden on. May produce inshore holes, sandbanks, and rip currents.
- *Rock type:* softer limestone and sandstone riverbeds erode into 'holes' that can trap or damage feet and equipment.
- *Boat launching areas:* should avoid coral, urchins, dangerous currents, and other water users. The most significant hazard is wet slippery rock that can led to falls or lower limb injuries.

Landscape

- *Piers and coastal outcrops:* can create rip currents. May be surrounded by sharp barnacles, submerged objects, and waste.
- *Sandbanks:* may falsely reassure about water depth; an incoming tide may produce a deep inshore zone between bather and the shore.
- *Inshore holes:* troughs that run parallel to the shore may be unexpectedly deep, up to 50 m wide, and several hundred metres long. Rip currents develop as waves break over an offshore sandbar and then run out to sea via the inshore hole.
- *Submerged objects:* rocks, tree roots, beach groynes, and outlet pipes may be difficult to recognize. In calm areas look for unexpected waves breaking over an obstruction. Glass, oil, and other discarded objects are common at locations close to civilization. Obstructions can form 'strainers' in a river system, trapping swimmers against them.
- *Flora:* falling coconuts can cause severe head injuries. The Manchineel tree (*Hippomane mancinella*), found in countries bordering the Caribbean, has caustic sap and highly toxic fruits and leaves; don't shelter under these trees. In some countries they are marked by a red cross or band on their trunk, elsewhere you need to be wary.
- *Fallen trees* lying above or in the current of small fast-flowing rivers are very hazardous to small craft, which may become jammed underneath. Push the obstacle away but don't grab onto it as this could lead to capsize.

Water

Offshore

- *Tides, currents, and weather* can vary unpredictably. Assess regularly during the day to evaluate changes and whenever possible, seek local knowledge. Incoming tides can isolate people on sandbanks, and at the midpoint of 'flooding' can raise the level of the sea very quickly. Outgoing tides can pull people and boats offshore. Both flows can be exacerbated by strong winds or storms.
- *Waves* may 'dump', 'spill', or 'surge' depending on their height and the gradient of the beach. Swimmers may be tumbled by the waves, incurring the risk of spinal injury, while those on the beach may be dragged into deeper water. Often the most hazardous part of a sea-kayak trip is landing in surf.

- *Inshore drift*: a current lateral to shore. Can displace water users into more dangerous areas.
- *Rip current*: a body of water moving in a direction other than the general flow. If it is trapped behind a sandbank, as the tide retreats water will flow quickly through deep channels. Rip currents can vary from a couple of metres wide to >50 m, and on rare occasions flow hundreds of metres offshore. The flow will vary with the tides. Identifying features include:
  - Discoloration of the water from disturbance of silt or sand.
  - Darker water surrounding the main current flow.
  - Floating debris or foam on the surface.
  - Surface changes such as rippled water while the surrounding area is calm.
  - Waves breaking on either side of the rip.

If caught in a rip current: float, attract attention, and wait. Some rip currents will re-circulate you to the shore, sandbank, or out to sea. If you are a competent swimmer, you can consider swimming out of the rip aiming parallel to the shore and towards the breaking waves.

Rivers
Risks vary markedly according to their gradient, depth, and flow and will vary by season and time of day. Drop a stick in the river—if it moves faster than walking pace, the energy of the system is enough to knock you off your feet.

- *Fast-flowing rivers* are likely to have stony bottoms, with sudden variations in depth; slow-flowing rivers have muddy bottoms, often with weeds. The outer side of a river bend will have the faster flow.
- *Rapids* may change from year to year, affected by alterations to the riverbed and the volume of water flowing. Define the extent and complexity of portage if craft need to be transported around waterfalls and rapids. Turbulent, aerated water has a reduced density therefore reduced buoyancy for objects (victims) attempting to float in it.
- *Gorges* may contain multiple hazards, such as trees and unscoutable rapids; once entered, escape may be very difficult.
- *Marshes and mud* may make access and egress difficult.
- *Artificial weirs* on managed rivers result in fast currents and steep drops.
- *River confluences* produce eddy currents and chaotic waves.
- *Riverside paths* may be narrow, muddy, or wet, increasing the risk that a slip will result in an injury or fall into water, especially during portages.
- *Tidal river bores* are predictable phenomena that sweep up estuarine rivers. Surfing them is increasingly popular, but significant skill is required.
- *Standing* waves, seen on rivers, maintain their position relative to the current. They can trap craft and people wearing buoyancy aids.
- *'Stoppers'* are the big hazard on rivers. They recirculate vertically upstream, creating a wave that can trap boats in a pounding maelstrom that has a high risk of retention and capsize.
- *Plants and reeds* can easily entrap swimmers or waders; use small gentle strokes to escape. Dense vegetation may hide snakes, crocodiles, etc.
- *Communications*: away from centres of population and tourist destinations, communities at the water's edge are often small, remote, and poor, possibly with limited road access to the outside world. Deep gorges will reduce or block mobile phone and radio signals. Turbulent

water is incredibly noisy. Whistles can be useful provided they do not contain a 'pea' that obstructs when wet.

Tsunami, jøkulhlaup, and flash floods

Although rare, these natural phenomena can be catastrophic—devastating everything in their path and leaving infrastructure wrecked. Many coastal countries have tsunami warning systems; expeditions must be aware of local alarms, the escape routes to higher ground, and designated muster points. In mountainous areas, the overflow or breaching of glacial outflow lakes occasionally leads to catastrophic flooding, heralded by a sound like the roaring of an approaching train. Upstream hydroelectric dams may suddenly release water.

Many landscapes in Iceland have been formed as a result of massive floods secondary to volcanic activity under the ice-caps—jøkulhlaup.

The immediate priority is to get as high above the water as you can:

* If you have time: exit buildings and run to high ground.
* If the water level is already rising, or high ground is too far away, go to the top of a well-constructed building near an exit and wait for the initial surge to pass.
* If time allows, put passport and communications (PLB, satellite phone) into a waterproof bag and fix firmly to yourself.
* If buoyancy aids are available, put them on as soon as possible.
* If on a boat, head offshore as the wave height will be less.
* Post disaster: identify all party members and contact the local embassy or consulate to inform them of your situation.
* Secondary floods, landslides, and building collapse are common.
* Water will be contaminated; purification of drinking water is essential. Typhoid and other illnesses are common post disaster.
* You may feel morally obliged to assist with disaster relief. Balance your involvement with the risk to yourself and your group of exposure to pathogens, depletion of expedition equipment, and the inevitable difficulties in finding clean food and safe water (➲ Chapter 4).

Weather

Always be aware of prevailing and forecasted conditions, adjusting your plans accordingly.

* *Wind* affects wave strength and formation, cools the skin, masks sunburn, and increases the risk of hypothermia. Down drafts near cliffs can be fierce.
* *Rain* reduces visibility, increases the risk of hypothermia, and steep catchment areas can result in rapid changes in river levels. For kayakers and canoeists, cold, wet weather reduces safe time on the water and schedules should be adjusted accordingly.
* *Ultraviolet light* from the sun reflects off the surface of the water, increasing exposure to radiation. Tropical climates encourage scanty clothing. Splash water washes off protective sun block creams. Reflected glare may affect the underside of chin, nose, eyebrows, and eyes. Minimize hazards by appropriate behaviour, clothing, UV protection, and sunglasses.

Rescue

However stressful the situation, never add to the death toll; maintain your own and others' safety. Have a realistic view of your own abilities and, unless highly skilled, avoid direct contact with a panicking casualty. Local rescue services may be basic or non-existent.

Preventing accidents

Risk management

All expeditions working on or near water must consider the possibility of immersion and plan rescue procedures. Many incidents can be avoided with good risk assessment and education of team members.

- Drowning often occurs very quickly and unexpectedly.
- A personal flotation device dramatically improves the chance of surviving an immersion—but only if it is both appropriately sized, and worn. If you are not already wearing it, you may not have enough time to put it on.
- Accidents often happen out of reach of other party members. Use a buddy system to keep in touch with other team members.

Rivers

- Shouted commands are unreliable above the roar of moving water. If possible, agree hand, whistle, or paddle signals between rescuers before starting the rescue. Personal radios, if available, can be a great help provided that the signal is not blocked by the landscape.
- At rapids: identify hazards, agree run, and decide running order.
- In difficult areas, 'set safety' by distributing team members with appropriate rescue equipment in advance of the boats in case rescue is required.
- Remember 'reach, throw, wade, tow'; recognizing the hazards with each technique. Learn and practise proper use of throw-bags.
- Wading risks foot entrapment and is best done with a paddle for support; or better as a pair or threesome, supporting the upstream wader using a wide leg stance in a triangle 'tripod' formation and with safety set downstream. See Fig. 22.1.
- Ropes and karabiners may assist during rescues but add to the hazard if people are not properly trained in their use. The key principles being 'no-knots' and that any system is 'quick release' to a clean line.

Around coasts

- Groups travelling offshore should be able to contact help. There are many options for communication around coasts. Mobile or satellite phones and VHF radios enable surface-to-shore communications. Equipment should ideally allow communication with both rescue centres and rescue craft on a variety of frequencies. These should be researched in the expedition planning phase.
- PLBs (⊃ p. 179–180, 644) can provide a backup if other means of communications are lost or damaged.
- Other vessels may be involved in rescue, so read relevant textbooks on managing such a rescue and also understand actions to take during helicopter rescue (⊃ Helicopter evacuation, p. 169–170, 756).

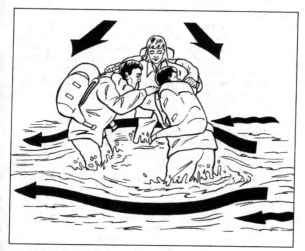

Fig. 22.1 River crossing 'tripod'.

Rescue techniques
See Table 22.1.

Table 22.1 Rescue techniques

Choice	Intervention	Suitability and risk
1st	Signal and shout	Effective for disorientated, weak, or injured swimmer. Low risk to rescuer
2nd	Reach	Casualties that are within physical reach, or in reach with pole/stick, etc. Potential to be pulled into water
3rd	Throw	Floatable aids or rope effective for weak/injured swimmers. Rope throwing requires practise
4th	Boat or dinghy	Limited by availability, operator skill, time to set up, and water conditions
5th	Swim with an aid	Swimming with floatable aid, can allow a small distance to be kept from casualty or assist tow
6th	Swim and tow	High risk owing to physical contact with panicking casualty. Energy sapping procedure. Avoid obstructing victim's airway with towing technique

Unconscious casualty

Approach swiftly; turn the casualty into a supine position. Prompt expired air ventilation (EAV) increases survival if the casualty is not breathing properly. Balance difficulties of administering rescue breaths against the time taken to exit the water, and rescuer's capability to perform the skill. If there is only a short distance to safety—exit and then resuscitate; if a longer swim is involved, and you have the skill and strength, attempt in-water EAV (ideally with the casualty on a flotation aid). Casualties often vomit—be prepared.

Post-immersion collapse syndrome

Prolonged immersion creates dehydration as intravascular fluids are redistributed, with BP supported by hydrostatic pressure of water on limbs. Decreasing water temperature and longer duration of immersion increase the risk. Rescue in horizontal position if practical. Vertical extraction carries the risk of cardiovascular collapse and death. Be aware of the possibility of hypothermia and its associated unstable cardiac rhythms.

Injuries

Certain aquatic accidents predispose to life-threatening injuries. These include fractures and head injuries from high-velocity impacts such as fast watercraft, cliff diving, or anybody in heavy surf. Surfers and those diving into shallow water are at high risk of cervical spine injuries, which are otherwise relatively uncommon.

Mass rescue

If more than one casualty is present, rescue must be prioritized (Table 22.2).

Table 22.2 Priority of rescue

1st	Non-swimmer	Head going under water and unable to maintain a direction
2nd	Weak swimmer	Able to hold position and direction of sight but not move
3rd	Injured swimmer	Holds position, swims slowly, communicates injury
4th	Unconscious	Usually face down. If the casualty is seen to go unconscious, they are first priority to minimize period of hypoxaemia. But if period of hypoxia is unknown, victim may be dead and extraction of body from water will prevent rescue of other casualties

Humans in aquatic environments

- *Non-swimmers* are obviously at greater hazard and require close supervision when near water.
- *Buoyancy aids* (also called personal flotation devices (PFDs)) should always be worn when close to or on the water. Attach a pea-less whistle for attracting attention. Buoyancy aids vary in cut, distribution of buoyancy, availability of pockets, and rescue fittings. Beware of excess loops hanging from PFDs, which can snag on other objects, especially after a capsize.
- Besides being flotation devices they:
  - Provide insulation in cool conditions.
  - Pad the body if in a collision.
  - Can be used as splints for fractured limbs.
  - Act as emergency insulation if resting or sleeping on the ground.
- *Clothing*: appropriate waterproofs, wet or dry suits, and helmets and may be required.
- *Body temperature*: humans are aware of peripheral rather than core temperature. Wet suits, which maintain peripheral temperatures, may disguise insidious drops in core temperature. Regular wave splashes in rough water can lead to insidious loss of heat and serious impairment of judgement. Hypothermia may occur even in relatively warm water if exposure is prolonged (➲ Hypothermia, p. 654–657). Both wet and dry suits are effective at reducing cold shock following sudden immersion in icy water and may save lives under these circumstances (➲ p. 652).
- *Diving and jumping into water*: risks spinal, neck, and head injuries, depending on depth of water and submerged objects.
- *Surfing*: because surf is best in shallow waters, this sport is associated with an increased risk of head or spinal injuries and lacerations from submerged objects.
- *Kite surfing/windsurfing*: carry similar risks to surfing but with the added risk of joint dislocations and back injuries. Injuries secondary to line entanglement are a particular hazard for kite surfers.
- *Kayaking*: occasionally craft can be caught between rock and current, or continuous battering by surf prevents 'righting'.
- *Swimming*: swimmers, surfers, and small craft risk being caught in currents and pulled into areas of water they do not want to be in. People often overestimate their ability in open water, risking cramps, hypothermia, and fatigue.
- *Time of day*: fatigue at the end of a long day, together with fading light increase the risk of accidents at dusk.
- *Trekking groups*: a slip, fall, path subsidence, or surging wave may unexpectedly lead to a member of a trekking group getting into difficulties in the water. Consider how to deal with this eventuality.
- *Relaxing and socializing*: there is a strong correlation between alcohol and drowning; tragedies have occurred when a group has been relaxing at a beach resort following a successful expedition.

Water quality

- Sea, rivers, and lakes are recipients of sewage, chemical pollutants, and, in urban areas, street run-off with oils and both animal and human faeces. In rural areas, flow dilutes pollutants, so a brief immersion or splashes are less likely to result in an infection risk.
- Lakes and coastal seas may develop harmful algae blooms containing toxic or otherwise harmful phytoplankton such as dinoflagellates of the genera *Alexandrium* and *Karenia*, or diatoms of the genus *Pseudonitzschia*. Such blooms often take on a red or brown hue and are known colloquially as 'red tides'.
- Hepatitis A (→ Hepatitis A, p. 486–487).
- Weil's disease (leptospirosis)—bacterial disease transmitted in the urine of rats and found in stagnant or polluted water. Urban canoeists are particularly at risk (→ Leptospirosis, p. 503).
- Cholera—at greatest risk in urban environments (→ Cholera, p. 422–424).
- Onchocerciasis: filarial worm spread by flies, causing 'river blindness' in the tropics (→ Onchocerciasis (river blindness), p. 526–527).
- Schistosomiasis ('bilharzia')—the animal vector is aquatic snails, often found in the tropics in still water or reeds (→ Schistosomiasis (bilharzia), p. 530–531).
- Biting insects may breed in water and transmit diseases such as malaria (→ Malaria, p. 512–520) and dengue.
- Other causes of GI upset. Common causes of diarrhoea include *Shigella*, *Salmonella*, and *Campylobacter* (→ Diarrhoea and vomiting, p. 67, 420–424).

Hazardous wildlife

(Also see → Chapter 17.)
- Fish: lionfish, stonefish, weaver fish, candiru, sting ray, and sharks.
- Mammals: hippopotamus, polar bears, and seals.
- Reptiles: alligators and crocodiles.
- Coral.
- Jellyfish.
- Anemones.
- Birds.
- Snakes.

Resource

Beachsafe (contains well-illustrated information and advice on beach safety, dealing with aquatic hazards such as rip currents, together with advice on marine creatures and marine stingers): ℘ http://beachsafe.org.au

Immersion and drowning

Definitions (World Health Organization)

- *Drowning* is the process of experiencing respiratory impairment from submersion or immersion in a liquid medium such that normal breathing is prevented. The outcomes of drowning may be death, morbidity, or recovery. Non-fatal drownings can be further categorized based on the severity of respiratory impairment immediately after the drowning process has been halted.
- *Immersion* implies that at least the airway and face are under the water, though the rest of the body may be floating.
- *Submersion* requires that the whole body be below the surface of the fluid.
- *Aspiration* is the process of solids or fluids entering the lungs.

Whether the casualty survives or not, they have been involved in a drowning incident. No significant physiological difference exists between salt water and freshwater aspiration. The terms 'wet drowning', 'dry drowning', 'near drowning', and 'secondary drowning' are no longer used.

Hazards of being in the water

- *Cardiac arrhythmias* may occur as a result of a fall into cold water. The elderly and anyone with a history of hypertension or ischaemic heart disease are particularly at risk. The concept of 'autonomic conflict' has been proposed as a cause of sudden cardiac death in water at any age. This involves simultaneous sympathetic (fear/anxiety upon sudden immersion, cold shock response to peripheries) and parasympathetic (dive reflex from cool water on the face) discharge converging on the myocardium and precipitating arrhythmias.[2]
- *Swim failure*: very cold water can cause violent shivering, muscular in-coordination, and gasping, which combine to prevent effective swimming and reduce ability to keep the head above water. Wet suits, dry suits, or habituation to cold water reduce this response. Despite these mitigations swim failure will eventually occur once peripheral limbs cool to the extent they can't function.
- *Hypothermia* develops during prolonged immersion and is a common cause of death following shipwreck if victims survive the initial cold shock responses and maintain flotation on the surface. Survival time in cold water will depend upon the temperature of the water, the build of the swimmer and their habituation to cold water. Unprotected survival times are given in Table 22.3. Survival can be extended to hours by use of an immersion suit and buoyancy aid and days in a covered life raft.
- *Wave splash*: those close to the surface can aspirate water following the slap of a wave on the face. Turn your face away from waves; some survival jackets include face splashguards.
- *Accidental immersion*: being able to swim does not protect you from drowning if you are fully clothed and carrying a heavy rucksack. During river or rope-bridge crossings, balance the risk of loose straps and a wobbly rucksack against the need to escape from the pack if you fall

2 Shattock MJ, Tipton MJ. 'Autonomic conflict': a different way to die during cold water immersion? *J Physiol*. 2012;590(14):3219–30. https://doi.org/10.1113/jphysiol.2012.229864

or are swept away. Training in the ability to float following accidental immersion increases survival.[3]

- *Aerated water*, which may be created by heavy surf, white-water rapids, or waterfalls is less dense and therefore less supportive of people or objects than still water. Combined with the likelihood of churning currents these environments are very hazardous, even for strong swimmers.

Table 22.3 Expected survival times in cold water

Water temperature	Exhaustion or unconsciousness in	Expected survival time
21–27°C	3–12 h	3 h–indefinitely
16–21°C	2–7 h	2–40 h
10–16°C	1–2 h	1–6 h
4–10°C	30–60 min	1–3 h
0–4°C	15–30 min	30–90 min
<0°C	<15 min	<15–45 min

Source: https://www.ussartf.org/cold_water_survival.htm

Immersion

There are four phases following immersion into water below the thermoneutral temperature of 30°C (Fig. 22.2):

- Initial response.
- Short-term response.
- Long-term response.
- Post-immersion response.

The colder the water, the more dramatic the response. Consider whether a sudden illness such as epileptic seizure, hypoglycaemia, or MI may have caused the casualty to fall into the water.

Basic resuscitation

Follow international guidelines such as the European Resuscitation Council guidelines but, as the likely cause is primary respiratory failure, complete five initial breaths and 1 min of CPR before going for help. Victims in respiratory arrest only have a good chance of full neurological recovery if early resuscitation (oxygenation) occurs. Approximately two-thirds of drowning victims will vomit—try to keep the airway clear by turning the head to face downhill. This will allow any fluid or vomit to drain away. Overall, only 0.5% of drowning victims will have associated spinal injuries so care of the spinal cord is of secondary importance unless there is a high index of suspicion: head injury or mechanism (e.g. dive into shallow water). If suspected, and enough rescuers are present, extract the casualty horizontally from the

3 Royal National Lifeboat Institution. How to float: would you know what to do if you were in trouble in the water? https://www.youtube.com/watch?v=iPsJPbjEETE

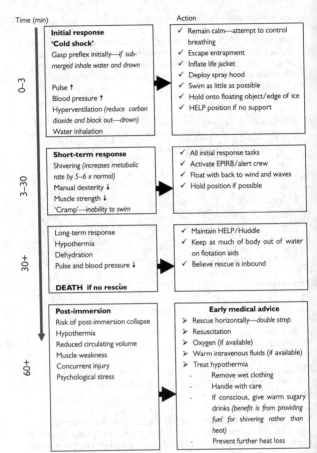

Fig. 22.2 Responses to immersion.

water with cervical spine control and log-roll to clear the airway if required. Hypothermia and shock are common, even in tropical climates.

Advanced techniques

- All post-drowning victims are hypothermic until proven otherwise. Shivering is a good prognostic sign. Warm appropriately (➲ Field management, p. 655).

- Administer high-flow oxygen (if available) during resuscitation and recovery, ideally titrated to pulse oximetry (if available).
- Dehydration and acidosis can develop from hypoxia and physiological effects of prolonged immersion. Consider warm cautious IV fluid boluses if available, monitor urine output and respiratory rate.
- Nasogastric drainage in the acute phase will reduce diaphragmatic splinting, aspiration risk, and cooling effect of ingested water.
- Non-invasive ventilation/assisted ventilations can be considered in hypoxic, conscious patients to bridge to definitive care.
- Acute respiratory distress syndrome (ARDS) can develop up to 72 h post immersion. It presents as a non-cardiogenic pulmonary oedema caused by the irritation of water in the lungs and requires hospitalization and ventilatory support.[4] If there is likely to be a delay in getting the patient to hospital and the casualty develops wheeze, consider regular IV hydrocortisone together with salbutamol inhalers/nebulizers, and furosemide.[5]

Aspiration pneumonia can develop later. Antibiotics are usually not required, but prophylactic antibiotics may be appropriate in remote areas, or if the casualty shows signs of fever or sepsis (➔ p. 250). Consider other fungal or parasitic pathogens if aspirated water was potentially dirty, e.g. ditches, sewers, or frequented by rodents (➔ Leptospirosis p. 503).

> All survivors of an immersion incident who may have inhaled water should be triaged to ascertain whether they require admission to a hospital capable of offering advanced respiratory support.
> A cough post immersion is not a criterion for admission.
> Immediate (as is practicable) admission is required if a cough is present *plus* one of productive sputum or 'foam', fever, respiratory distress, or cardiac compromise.

Discontinuing resuscitation and rescue attempts

Good-quality survival following prolonged immersion can occur, particularly if water is very cold. Attempt basic resuscitation wherever practical and, if possible, evacuate to a hospital capable of advanced rewarming techniques such as cardiopulmonary bypass. After prolonged hypothermia or cardiac arrest, the core temperature should be re-stabilized at 33°C for 24 h before returning to normothermia.

Survival is extremely unlikely if the victim has been submerged (head under) for >30 min in water warmer than 6°C, and >90 min in water <6°C. Expeditions in remote areas should attempt to resuscitate and rewarm a casualty but will have to adopt a pragmatic approach to ceasing resuscitation attempts (see also ➔ Hypothermia, p. 654–659).

Resources

Surf Life Saving GB: ✍ http://www.surflifesaving.org.uk
Transport Canada. Marine safety: ✍ http://www.tc.gc.ca/MarineSafety

4 Tipton MJ, Golden FS. A proposed decision-making guide for the search, rescue and resuscitation of submersion (head under) victims based on expert opinion. *Resuscitation*. 2011;82(7):819–24. https://doi.org/10.1016/j.resuscitation.2011.02.021

5 Van Berkel M, Bierens J, Lie R, et al. Pulmonary oedema, pneumonia and mortality in submersion victims; a retrospective study in 125 patients. *Intensive Care Med*. 1996;22(2):101–7. https://doi.org/10.1007/BF01720715

Canoeing and kayaking

Canoes are open boats manoeuvred by sitting or kneeling using single-blade paddles, but the term is often used generically to include kayaks, which are enclosed craft, paddled sitting using a double-blade paddle. Kayaks are more manoeuvrable and manage waves and white water better. Sea kayaks can carry reasonable loads and manage longer trips; river kayaks have limited space for gear and food. Canoes are more suitable for lakes or slow rivers and can carry heavy loads. These craft may be used to explore remote areas, for other recreations such as fishing, or for the challenge of white-water trips. Lightweight, inflatable 'packrafts' allow access to water after hiking into remote areas but lack directional stability and are more influenced by wind than conventional craft. SUPs are increasingly used for multi-day trips. They are portable but more susceptible to wind and waves.

Preparation

- Fitness appropriate to the challenge is vital, especially for multiday trips, which are more tiring than day trips.
- Good paddling technique reduces the risk of shoulder and back injury. If suffering pain, review your exercises.
- Learn to lift weights like loaded boats safely and efficiently.
- Know the accessibility of start and end points together with escape routes and any 'bad' headlands or rapids that could require scouting or portage.
- Team working is vital for a successful expedition. Disputes about goals are a major cause of conflict. Before departure establish whether the trip is to be a challenging paddle, a holiday, or something in between.
- Arrange appropriate immunizations, prophylactic drugs for endemic diseases, and treatment for dental problems.
- Do a trial pack of your gear to ensure it will fit in your craft and the contents will remain dry.
- Consider taking a course covering sea safety or white-water safety and rescue.

Accommodation and campcraft

- Camp sites are the commonest site for accidents, especially if alcohol is involved.
- Acceptable sites can be infrequent and may have limited space for camping. Keep gear, especially boats, above the high-water mark.
- Lightweight tents take up space in boats. If weather is warm and biting insects not an issue, save weight with a lightweight tarpaulin for the group, propped up with paddles and throwlines, and/or bivi bags. Down sleeping bags pack small but are unreliable if damp. Double bag them or choose the bulkier artificial fibre bags that retain insulation even if damp.

Heat, light, and fuel

- Driftwood makes good fires but may not be available.
- Gas canisters are light, but always check local availability as they cannot be taken on aircraft.
- Kerosene or petrol will probably be available locally, but quality may vary and soot may clog stove nozzles: take several prickers. Fuel bottles

must have perfect seals to prevent smelly contamination and damage of other gear and food.

Water supplies

(See also Water quality, p. 719, and ◆ Water purification, p. 108–114.)

- At sea on coastal trips, it is vital to know the next source of fresh water. If location is unknown prior to departure, take adequate water. Water bladders with pipe to mouth are useful for daytime paddling.
- Water filters are usually too bulky for river kayaks, although they may be carried in canoes, rafts, and sea kayaks. Chlorine dioxide or other water purification tablets are an alternative.

Nutrition

Have enough food and water supplies available during the day to counteract fatigue. In remote locations it may be difficult to buy food; expedition rations may then be restricted to less palatable freeze-dried or tinned alternatives. Keep food and water cool by storing low in the boat's hull, with heavy items central to maintain balance.

Sanitation

At sea, some carry a marked pee bottle, but its use can be difficult in rough water, and groups may need to raft up. More difficult for women, although some use a 'slipper' type bottle or Shewee®.

Faecal matter degrades slowly in toilet pits on beaches. Small or popular beaches can get overloaded unless a management plan is in place. In many North American National Parks, you are required to carry out your toilet waste.

Clothing

Wind and water combine to chill the body, so effective protective gear is necessary, but overheating can also be an issue with hard exercise and impermeable fabrics.

Wetsuits tend not to be used in kayaking expeditions—if you're expecting to get wet, then a dry cagoule is better at keeping you dry and warm, although damaged and leaking dry cagoules are hard to repair effectively. If you are only expecting exposure to spray, then wear a comfortable paddling top cuffed at neck and wrists over a synthetic or merino wool vest. Dry suits can cause overheating, chafing, become punctured, and may be uncomfortable. Following coastal trips, wash all kit in fresh water each evening to minimize damage and chafing. Effective UV protection of exposed skin is necessary in sunny places.

Footwear should cope with carrying loaded boats on rough, slippery ground but with soles flexible enough to fit in a cramped cockpit.

Spectacles should be tied firmly with thin yachting cord; proprietary cords with quick-fit rubber ends don't hold them well in turbulent water.

Safety

- Get used to wearing buoyancy aids whenever close to water.
- Experienced paddlers may choose to do trips alone, or with only one buddy, but the risks are greatly increased if you run into trouble. A safe motto is 'Less than three should not be'.
- Use a buddy system; in bigger groups appoint front and rear paddlers. Split large groups into smaller units.

- Work as a team and know where everyone is. Communication within the group is vital; even small, experienced groups make a point of having a daily briefing on the day past and the day to come. With sea trips, and when the weather is poor, the morning briefing should include a 'Go/No Go' decision.
- Sea kayakers often carry VHF radios for both inter-group and outside contact.
- Agree hand signals and methods of communication that will work despite wind or water noise.
- When scouting rapids, agree routes and running order with safety crafts or throw lines positioned below rapids.
- Helmets, paddles, and cagoules should be brightly coloured, perhaps even using fluorescent tape on dark-coloured gear.
- If travelling with a guiding company using their equipment, check the experience, qualifications, and first-aid training of the guides, together with the age and serviceability of the vessels.
- Self-rescue is important; kayakers should be able to self-right after a roll even in heavy water, and practise other rescue techniques such as towing. If defensive swimming on your back down a river, point your feet downstream, angle your body by pointing your hand and head towards the direction you wish to travel to 'ferry-glide' to a safe area to exit.

White-water rafting

White-water rafting is an exhilarating active sport usually led by professional guides, who can safely guide novices through reasonably hard rapids. Multiday trips are true river journeys, offering unique access to wilderness areas.

Although white-water rafting may appear dangerous, accident rates are low if basic safety rules are followed.

Evaluating the raft company

Good companies should run well-organized trips, but local competition can reduce prices to the detriment of safety. Check:
- The experience of the guides and their qualifications.
- How often they have run the river.
- Age and serviceability of the rafts.
- Buoyancy aids and helmets provided.
- Appropriateness of safety briefing.
- Whether another safety craft will accompany your raft.

Preparations

- You need to be reasonably fit, capable of manoeuvring in the water to float, swim several metres in open water wearing protective equipment, and have respect for the water without fearing it.
- Consider hepatitis A vaccination in endemic areas.
- Clothing should include a peaked sun cap, and good river sandals with either buckles or Velcro® fastening.
- Take a small personal medical kit including paracetamol, plasters, sun screen, iodine for grazes and cuts, and emergency water sterilization.

On the water

- Use sun-protection, which may require regular reapplication.
- Drink plenty of clean water to prevent dehydration.
- Wear a buoyancy aid whenever close to flowing water.
- Consider sunglasses with the appropriate level of protection.

At camps

- Sterilize water effectively and follow local sanitation rules.
- Careful hand hygiene using soap and water or alcohol gel.
- Beware of twists and sprains on rocks especially at night.
- Beware of the campfire.

Stand-up paddleboards

With the rise in SUP use, more people are making multi-day trips, usually with longer boards, and sometimes with coast support. SUPs are very portable, and can carry a small load, strapped to the board, usually forward of the paddling stance. They are more influenced by waves or wind than other craft.

Windspeed and wave forecasts are available in some areas as smartphone apps. Windspeed >10 mph makes head on or beam paddling difficult. The upright stance of the paddler means more exposure to the cooling effects of the wind.

A good leash is essential, perhaps strapped to the knee rather than ankle, with quick-release shackles at one or two points. It is useful to have a grab handle fitted somewhere on deck, as the smooth board edges are difficult to grab in an emergency. Fins can snag in shallow water.

Medical problems in small craft

Serious medical issues

Immersion and drowning

(See also ➲ Immersion and drowning, p. 720–723, and ➲ Cold shock, p. 652.)

Sudden immersion in very cold water, especially in those less habituated to it, activates the cold shock response—'gasp and hyperventilate'—which reduces the time available to attempt a roll and can increase the risk of drowning. Above rapids, experienced paddlers may douse their faces in cold water to reduce the reflex.

Non-freezing cold injury

(See also ➲ Non-freezing cold injury, p. 666–667.)

Also known as trench foot, or in its localized type, pernio or chilblains, cold injury can develop if feet are immersed in cold water for prolonged periods. May occur during spring rafting especially in high latitudes and at altitude in areas such as Nepal. Recognized by pain and discoloration of the foot; it can result in prolonged disability. Prevention is thus vital, and feet should be fully dried and warmed for at least 8 h in any 24 h.

Hypothermia

(See also ➲ Hypothermia, p. 654–657.)

Clearly a risk with prolonged exposure to water and spray, not necessarily very cold. More likely at end of the day, if people are less experienced, have rolled, or have inadequate clothing. Look out for non-specific, poorer functioning, often in a less experienced team mate, who likely won't recognize it, and therefore you will have to take decisions on their behalf. Cut the day short as other group members are also likely to be close to hypothermia. Head for the nearest shelter, camp, rewarm, drink hot fluids, and feed.

Shoulder dislocation

(For relocation see ➲ Shoulder and upper arm injuries, p. 444–445.)

A particular risk for less experienced paddlers unfamiliar with the power of, and the reaction times needed, on big water. Once injured, the risk of a recurrent dislocation is high (up to 50% in first-time dislocations), while a weakened vulnerable shoulder will reduce future capability to deal with difficult waters. Older paddlers with a dislocation tend to injure the rotator cuff muscles surrounding the shoulder joint. Dislocation is common when the paddle arm is lifted high and forcibly abducted: as when bracing against a wave, or during an imminent capsize. Proper paddling technique involves keeping the hands low and not reaching too far to the side: 'Keep hand in a box in front'.

Common medical problems

Seasickness

(See also ➲ Seasickness, p. 750–751.)

May be debilitating and hazardous during rough water paddling. Risk factors include fatigue, cold, fear, and watching compass regularly. Sea-sickness is exhausting; sufferers may require rest, food, fluids, and understanding from the team.

Dehydration

An easily overlooked problem particularly common when rafting in the heat, but risk is high even in the Arctic where humidity can be very low. Early signs are vague symptoms such as headache, light headiness, and lethargy and are difficult to recognize unless you are on the lookout for them. Some people avoid drinking much during the day to reduce toilet trips, but then rehydrate during the evening; a risky strategy unless you are very aware of your fluid status.

Back, neck, and muscle problems

Stiff and knotted muscles, especially in neck and between shoulder blades, are common in paddlers. Stretching exercises after paddling and firm massages of 'knots' or 'trigger points' at the end of the day can help. If non-specific shoulder pain affects your paddling, try keeping the elbow low while paddling.

Sea paddlers can get leg strain through constant sitting in the same position. Take the weight off the leg muscles especially in the groin by placing a filled drybag under the knees.

Low back trouble is common in kayakers. The kayaking posture flexes the lower lumbar spine against its natural lordosis.

- Fit a good backrest with effective lumbar or pelvic support.
- Review your flexibility exercises before departure.
- Use proper lifting techniques and aids such as straps and trolleys.
- Back, pelvis, and thigh strains are a risk in contemporary tightly strapped play boats. On the flatter river sections, you should be able to release your legs easily.

Tenosynovitis

(See also ➔ Wrist injuries, p. 450.)

Tenosynovitis of wrist is a repetitive strain injury due to flexion and extension of the wrist while using a feathered paddle. Pain can be severe and crepitus dramatic. Point tenderness distinguishes this from a non-specific sprain.

Treatment requires complete rest, but on a long journey the paddler may be unable or unwilling to comply. Prescribe an NSAID painkiller such as ibuprofen or diclofenac, or a simple analgesic if NSAIDs are contraindicated (➔ Painkillers, p. 618–625). A wrist splint or neoprene support, together with cooling and elevation in a sling, may assist recovery.

Alterations to paddling technique may help:

- A common cause is gripping the paddle too tightly ('overgrip'). Try a looser grip when the injured wrist is on upper part of stroke.
- Try a larger diameter paddle shaft, cranked shaft, change the feather angle, or use a Greenland paddle.
- Change from right to left paddle feather, or vice versa.

Blisters

(See also ➔ Blisters, p. 295.)

Water softens the skin. Blisters are fairly common on multi-day trips, even among experienced paddlers. Strap tape or Moleskin® over 'hot spots' or early blisters and change the way you grip the paddle. If blisters burst, treat as a simple cut.

Burns
(See also ➔ Burns, p. 300–302.)

Common when wood fires are used. Immediate action to cool the burn is vital—usually best achieved by immersing the affected area in water for a period. If the burn is severe enough to require a burns dressing, then the challenge on the water is keeping that dressing dry: on hands or feet use plastic bags sealed with duct tape.

Piles
(See also ➔ Haemorrhoids (piles), p. 419.)

Common in kayakers, they may be precipitated by diarrhoea, or by constipation associated with dehydrated foods. Sufferers should consider treatment before departure.

Ear problems
A common complaint of kayakers is a sensation of 'water in the ear' with deafness. One cause is extensive wet wax in the ear canal, which can be difficult to remove in the wilderness. May also be caused by a blocked Eustachian tube due to an upper respiratory tract infection or excessive immersion while kayak rolling. Try to unblock the Eustachian tube:
• By inhaling steam.
• Using a decongestant such as Actifed® (for a maximum of 5 days).
• Using a Valsalva manoeuvre—but avoid this technique if the paddler has an active nasal infection with a blocked nose, as it can lead to middle ear infection.

You are unlikely to persuade an enthusiastic kayaker to avoid rolling, so the symptom is unlikely to clear up until after the trip ends. Flying, especially during descent, can be painful if Eustachian tubes are blocked and occasionally leads to tympanic rupture.

Bony exostoses of the ear canal ('surfer's ear') are associated with frequent cold-water impact during years of kayak rolling. When ear canal obstruction exceeds 50%, the risk of infection increases, and hearing is impaired. Some paddlers have >80% obstruction. Operations to excise the exostoses don't always give symptom-free recovery. Prevent with a neoprene hood and custom earplugs with an inbuilt narrow hole to mitigate hearing loss from the plug. Prevention is especially important for athletic youngsters who capsize their playboats frequently.

Otitis externa is infection of the external ear canal, can be itchy or painful, and is common in tropical humid zones. Treatment requires good aural toilet, helped by acetic acid (or vinegar) and alcohol. Use an ear plug of cotton wool with an ointment such as Vaseline® or aluminium acetate. Persistent or severe infections may require antibiotic drops.

Cuts, grazes, and skin problems
(See also ➔ Wound types and management, p. 290–296.)

Cuts and grazes should be cleaned with filtered or sterilized water to eliminate risk of contaminating wound with sand or pathogens. Cuts on the water have a significant risk of infection. Clean and close them as soon as possible with sutures or glue, although glue often wears off after a couple of days. Most adhesive skin closure don't work in the wet. Leukosan SkinLink® reinforced adhesive strips may be helpful. Uninfected wounds become waterproof after 24 h, but until initial healing has taken place try to keep the cut dry.

Fungal skin infections are common in hot climates, while sun and wind can lead to chapped lips.

Jellyfish stings

(See also ➜ Venomous marine animals, p. 596–602.)

- Don't rub the skin as pressure increases discharge from sting.
- Scrape skin with stiff plastic like an old credit card.
- Rinse area well with sea water (fresh water is hypotonic to nematocyst stinging cells and they will discharge in its presence—exacerbating the irritation).
- Use hot water as for fish stings and elevate the affected area.
- Use an antihistamine cream or spray.

Burn out and stress

Rushed itineraries lead to chronic mild exhaustion. On challenging sea trips, safe landings can be hours away, but all team members have to be able to the face consequent fatigue and fear. Don't push weaker members into challenging coastlines or attempting rapids above their skill level. On week-long trips, the nadir of physical fatigue and emotions can come around day 4, then improves. Recognition of variation in moods is important to prevent over-reaction to apparent 'difficult behaviour'.

Limited medical kit items for small craft

(See also ➜ Chapter 28.)

Often lack of space restricts choice of supplies. Pack in several small zipper plastic storage bags or waterproof container/dry bags, leaving air in the bag or barrel so it may float if displaced in a capsize.

- One large bandage (cut to size required).
- Suitable painkillers (➜ Table 28.1, p. 856).
- Multitool with knife and/or scissors (in main repair kit).
- Antibiotic ear drops (e.g. Betnesol-N®), cotton wool, and petroleum gel.
- Hand cream, lip salve.
- Seasickness tablets.
- Tape—duct tape sticks best but doesn't stretch.
- Sub-tropical trips—cotton wool, petroleum gel, and consider aloe vera for sunburn.
- Personal medications (e.g. inhalers, antacids, migraine relief).

Resources

American Whitewater. Safety code: ℘ http://www.americanwhitewater.org/content/Wiki/safety:start

Brown G. *Sea Kayak.* Bangor: Pesda Press; 2006. Available as DVD and ℘ http://www.seakayakwithgordonbrown.com

Ferrero F. *Whitewater Safety and Rescue,* 2nd ed. Bangor: Pesda Press; 2006. ℘ http://www.pesdapress.com

Joliffe B, Shannon S. White water safety and rescue videos: ℘ https://www.youtube.com/c/WhiteWaterSafety

Offshore

Chapter editor
Chris Johnson

Contributors
Spike Briggs
Campbell Mackenzie (1st and 2nd editions)

The offshore environment

Physical characteristics

- *Isolation* from assistance is a major factor when assessing the physical and emotional fitness of crew, planning medical kits, and arranging medical shore support.
- *Extreme weather conditions*—high winds, wave impact, motion, salt water, humidity, heat, cold, and frequent immersion—should be expected, and prepared for.
- *Trauma, illness, and physical danger* are medical and emotional challenges, and are common; pre-existing medical conditions may relapse.
- *Seasickness* is a frequent and often disabling condition. It can usually be treated effectively, but vomiting may prevent absorption of other important oral medications such as antiepileptics, immunosuppressive drugs, and diabetic medications.
- *Living conditions* are enclosed, cramped, and often difficult to keep clean, leading to the risk of community infection. Well-planned watch-keeping schedules are essential to minimize fatigue.
- *Nutrition and hydration* are essential factors in maintaining team health and performance.
- *Team dynamics* are central to every facet of boat performance; a happy and healthy crew performs well.

Weather

Weather forecasts are increasingly accurate and can be accessed anywhere. GRIB (GRIdded Binary) files are readily available from a variety of websites[1] via satellite phone, or single side band radio (SSB), giving high definition of weather conditions local to a yacht's position, but a forecast is only helpful if accessed in good time and interpreted correctly. Think ahead, get information, and plan accordingly.

Be prepared for anything. Bad weather takes a toll on crew and boat; both must be in the best condition possible, and both require regular maintenance. Hot, humid tropical weather in the tropics can lead to exhaustion, dehydration, infections, and sunburn. Prolonged cold conditions make it hard to dry anything and can lead to insidious development of hypothermia (→ Hypothermia, p. 654–657).

Trauma and deterioration of medical conditions are most likely during poor weather. Plan accordingly: where is the best place for the medical kit to be accessed when the boat is falling off 10 m waves, and where is the best place to put a casualty so they do not come to further harm, and can be examined and treated?

Navigation

You should always know where you are and where you are heading. Keep in contact with a shore-based facility; if disaster strikes, rescuers need to know where to look for you.

- *Global positioning system (GPS)*: over the past 30 years, universal access to GPS has made navigation far more accurate and less dependent

---

1 For example: ℰ www.predictwind.com

upon weather conditions. Always have at least one backup system, and another system that gives latitude and longitude that can be plotted on a paper chart.

- *Electricity*: all technical systems require electricity, which also requires multiple backups. Solar panels or a wind turbine can provide an alternative power source to the ship's generator. Electrical power for several days must be available in a life raft as well.
- *Paper charts* (Standard Nautical Charts) and Pilots (Sailing Directions) covering all sail areas and ports of call are still essential items.
- *Astronavigation* is the ultimate backup plan but requires detailed training and frequent practice to be reasonably accurate.

Risk assessment

Both yacht racing and cruising involve significant risk.[2] The hazards depend upon boat activity and crew type.

- Requiring treatment: ~1:10,000 crew miles or 50 crew days at sea.
- Requiring external advice: ~1:100,000 crew miles or 500 crew days at sea.
- Evacuation: ~1:1,000,000 crew miles, or 5000 crew days at sea.
- Life threatening injury: ~1:10,000,000 crew miles or 50,000 crew days at sea.

Specific risk factors

- Crew composition and fitness.
- Proposed route:
  - Distance from land (within or beyond maximum rescue helicopter range of 200 miles).
  - Distance from frequented shipping routes.
  - Special obstacles (e.g. ice, fog, other shipping).
  - Piracy is a risk in some regions.[3]
- Length of time at sea.
- On-board medical skill.
- Shore support.
- Medical kit contents.
- Communication availability.

Search and rescue

Ocean sailing can put a yacht crew >2 weeks from useful medical help. Crews might have to cope with serious medical problems during this time, and must have a realistic expectation of what is possible if someone is seriously injured or falls ill. Communication must be reliable, and may be via:

- Mobile phone when within range of shore.
- VHF radio to shore or other vessels if within range.
- SSB radio from long range offshore.
- Satellite telephones (email or voice).
- Inmarsat-C (data such as emails).

Telemedicine advice services are increasingly common but require video or image transmission and reception, together with the medical expertise to interpret those images. Shore support for medical emergencies is possible via international maritime rescue coordination centres such as MRCC Falmouth (a Maritime and Coastguard Agency service). There are various other organizations that provide support for expeditions to remote places, such as Medical Support Offshore Ltd, based in Southampton, UK, and the British Antarctic Survey Medical Unit (BASMU), based at Derriford Hospital, Plymouth, UK. Larger expeditions may organize their own shore medical support team that can then be tailored to the crew's specific requirements.

Helicopters can fly about 200 nautical miles from the nearest base, and expeditions beyond this range should be planned more rigorously.

2 Nathanson A. Sailing Injuries, A review of the Literature. http://www.rimed.org/rimedicaljournal/2019/02/2019-02-23-wilderness-nathanson.pdf

3 🔖 https://www.gov.uk/sea-river-and-piracy-safety

Environmental impact of sailors

- Sailing takes place in some of the most pristine environments on the planet. Respect this.
- Plastic and other non-perishable detritus already despoil every ocean—do not add to this; take all rubbish to land.
- Do not release oil or other hydrocarbons at sea—oil slicks can have a profound impact on sea life and birds.
- Do not release sewage if it could make landfall within 24 h.
- Consider where you drop the anchor and the effect of the chain when the boat swings on its mooring.
- Do not closely pursue marine animals such as cetaceans and sharks, and do not stray close to seabird nesting colonies.
- Make full use of solar and wind generators, and minimize use of the ship's engines and generators.
- Think about the type of anti-foulant used—this can have serious detrimental effects on local wildlife in crowded moorings.
- Music can add to the atmosphere on board, but not in a quiet anchorage. It will annoy local wildlife and those anchored nearby.

Humans on long voyages

Sailing in remote areas is no longer the preserve of the young and fit.

Journeys—rigorous, remoter, longer, colder, or tropical routes require fitter crew and better medical training for skipper and medic.

Crew should be physically fit prior to the expedition, with particular attention paid to cardiopulmonary fitness and lower limb strength, which will decline when confined on board a yacht for several weeks. Short-handed crew work harder, become more exhausted, and consequently incur more injuries and illnesses.

Personal space is limited, but will be ameliorated by having ownership of at least some space, no matter how small.

Weather—cold, hot, or rough conditions can be exhausting. With no escape crew have to cope, whatever the weather. Storms don't blow forever, although at the time they may feel as if they do.

Eating at sea is a communal activity. Personal choice is reduced with less opportunity for 'grazing' or indulgences. Food supplies must take into account personal dietary restrictions. Occasional treats may prevent mutiny.

Patience and tolerance are essential if the crew are to remain happy and efficient. When in close proximity, noises and smells must be tolerated by the observer, and minimized by the emitter.

Boredom may sometimes beset crew; youngsters are particularly at risk. Usually they can be distracted by a never-ending list of maintenance tasks, but reading, schooling, a structure for the day, and pastimes such as musical instruments may alleviate occasional tedium.

Fear and danger are real concerns offshore. Rough weather, accidents, other emergencies, and even possibly the catastrophic experience of having to take to a life raft after a vessel sinks bring out both the worst and the best in crew. They may react by becoming aggressive or withdrawn and depressed. Mutual watchfulness and support, with honesty about one's own emotions, will result in a strong team more likely to remain cohesive, and survive.

Accommodation

Typically, about half of all injuries happen below-decks. Think what below-decks would be like should the boat turn on its side, or even upside down. Consider how you would escape if the boat remained upside down (a problem with yachts if they lose their keel), and how you would do this in the dark.

Formal standards for accommodation at sea only apply to commercial vessels. Other vessels come in all shapes and sizes, accommodation varies from air-conditioned state rooms with en-suite facilities on superyachts, to hot-bunking cots on racing boats.

Racing boats are stripped out, with no soft coatings on surfaces, which are unforgiving as a result. Crew sleep in sleeping bags on 'cots': fabric slung between two longitudinal poles with a 'lee cloth' to prevent unscheduled exits in rough weather. Commonly members of the off-watch climb into the bunk just vacated by the on-watch, a process known as 'hot-bunking'. Sleeping weight is kept on the windward side, or towards the stern when sailing downwind.

Cruising boats tend to be heavier, but better equipped than racing boats. They may have recognizable bunks, but still with lee cloths to prevent falls. *Dampness* due to the saltwater environment and humidity is ever-present. Take any opportunity when it rains to wash clothing in fresh water coming off the boom, (let the rain wash the salt off the mainsail first). Damp bedding has reduced insulation and is less pleasant to sleep in, so take any opportunity to dry it out.

Heat, light, and fuel

Fuel is invariably diesel—used to run the main boat engine, power a generator for recharging the boat's batteries, and possibly a desalinator for producing freshwater from seawater.

Heat can be supplied by solid fuel stoves, gas heaters, or diesel drip-feed heaters, either on a demand basis or as a 'central heating' system. Each type of system has advantages and disadvantages in terms of cost, responsiveness, ease of use, and service requirements.

Electricity is usually supplied from a 12 V or 24 V DC system battery bank, with inverters to create a 240 V AC supply. The battery bank can be charged by a diesel generator, possibly supplemented by solar panels, wind turbine, or water turbine. A boat without fuel or electricity will have no outside communication (apart from emergency systems), no meteorological information or external navigational aids, and perhaps only a limited supply of water. During pre-voyage planning it is essential to anticipate fuel usage and add a generous safety margin. Fuel consumption should be monitored regularly to ensure the lights and computers stay on.

Water supplies

Fresh water consumption on boats varies enormously, but generally ranges from 5 to 30 L/day per person on a well-run cruising yacht.

Fresh water tanks

Boats are usually equipped with several freshwater tanks, to ensure that the entire freshwater supply is not lost if one tank is breached or contaminated. These tanks are situated low in the boat to keep the centre of gravity low, and also distributed symmetrically to minimize effect on boat trim. When re-filling tanks from a shore supply, test for taste and clarity. Discovery of contaminated water in the tanks when at sea may terminate a voyage prematurely.

Desalinators

At sea a desalinator is commonly used to replenish supplies. Water is pumped under pressure through a fine filter, removing sodium chloride, other electrolytes, larger particles, and bacteria by a process known as 'reverse osmosis'. Desalinators may be powered by electricity, or can be manually powered—a process very tiring for the crew. Apart from collecting rainwater, manual desalination is the only available means of producing fresh water in a life raft.

Rainwater

Rainwater can provide sporadic supplies of freshwater, but collection systems must initially be thoroughly flushed to prevent salt contamination of existing supplies.

Nutrition

Energy expenditure varies enormously offshore but may reach 6000 calories/day, depending on weather conditions, ambient temperature, and body size. Plan accordingly for the number of crew and anticipated length of voyage, then add a generous safety margin.

- Think about where you may be able to re-provision—local ports and local foods.
- It is common sense not to run out of provisions, but it does happen on racing boats when weight is pared to a bare minimum with little margin for error.
- Arranging provisions by day and week is a sensible way to make sure food is used at a sustainable rate.
- Airtight containers are mandatory for dry provisions.
- Tins, jars, and other pre-prepared meals are heavy so food in bags is more efficient in terms of weight and storage space. It is a good idea to remove paper labels from tins and jars and write the contents on the tin with an indelible marker pen.
- Dried provisions are often used, including freeze-dried food. It is critically important that this is rehydrated properly prior to eating, as partially hydrated food may cause catastrophic constipation.
- Frozen foods require a freezer and perishable foods require a fridge, both run by electricity or gas. Make a plan in case fridge or freezer fails, and don't depend on the foodstuffs kept in them.
- Fresh foods are a boon, but after a week at sea, there won't be much left. Plan a balanced diet once the fresh food has run out.
- Convenience foods and the occasional treat will keep the crew going during an extended period of rough weather, and may prevent discord.

Cleanliness

It is mandatory to keep the boat and crew clean at all times. This must be built into the ethos of the crew, and a rota for cleaning below decks helps. Personal cleanliness is personal, but excessive body odour affects others, and does nothing for team dynamics. Main routes of infection are faecal–oral, skin to skin, and skin to infected surfaces to skin. Skin infections such as impetigo can run through a crew in a very short period of time, as can gut infections.

Develop a culture in which hand washing is mandatory:

- After using the toilet.
- Before any form of food handling or preparation.
- Antiseptic wipes or alcohol gel dispensers are convenient and effective on any sort of boat.

Waste water

(See ♒ http://www.rya.org.uk for additional advice.)

Toilets

Toilets on boats may range from one that looks like the one in your home, to a bucket for chucking. In between, most boat toilets (or 'heads') have small-diameter outlet drainpipes and a hand-operated pump, using seawater to flush the toilet. They block easily and are difficult to unblock, so it is forbidden to put sanitary products or other items down them. Toilet paper is usually acceptable. Provide a bin with plastic bag liner for waste that cannot be put down the toilet. This will need to be stored until disposed of ashore.

Sewage

- Empty holding tanks >12 nautical miles offshore, in the open sea, where waste will be quickly diluted and dispersed by wave actions and currents. Preferably where sewage will take >24 h to reach land.
- In marinas, use shore facilities and brief your crew to do likewise. Use holding tanks or a portable toilet if you regularly sail in areas of poor flushing such as estuaries, inland waterways, and inlets, and when visiting crowded anchorages.
- Chemical toilets use toxic substances and must be emptied ashore into the regular sewage system. Plan ahead as they can be difficult to carry and few pump out (sanitation) facilities will accept chemical toilet waste.
- When visiting new sites, give consideration to the environmental sensitivity of the area before using your sea toilet.

Grey water

- Choose environmentally sensitive products—avoiding chlorine and bleach that can be toxic to flora and fauna, and phosphates that encourage algal growth.
- Keep oils and other food waste onboard and dispose of with non-recyclable rubbish.
- Minimize use of soaps and detergents in onboard sinks, showers, and washing machines. The sink on your boat needs to be treated differently to those in your home—it will block more easily.
- If using a washing machine on board, switch to a detergent-free washball, or use less ecologically damaging washing powders—a must in inland waterways.
- Consider re-plumbing your wastewater system so that all sewage, and grey and black water, including that from dishwashers and washing machines, is diverted to a holding tank, especially if you keep your boat in enclosed waters such as inland waterways and marinas.

Preparations for voyage

Numerous tasks demand attention prior to departure, such as:

- Fitting out.
- Planning for safety.
- Victualling.
- Examining charts, pilot books, and weather information.

Thought must be given to the crew's health and welfare, an area at worst neglected, at best given low priority in the work schedule. Such time is well spent and may dictate the success or failure of the trip.

Crew selection

- Crew should be generally physically fit prior to the expedition, with particular attention paid to cardiopulmonary fitness.
- There is greater risk when taking crew on a voyage who are dependent on oral medication for life-threatening conditions, such as organ transplant, epilepsy, or severe heart disease. Seasickness may prevent absorption of the medication. Conditions such as type 1 diabetes mellitus and severe asthma also carry greater risk offshore.
- More stringent exclusion criteria should be applied to expeditions beyond helicopter range, possibly excluding sailors with those conditions mentioned here.
- The Maritime and Coastguard Agency (MCA) guidelines[4] provide a structure for assessing potential crew with pre-existing medical conditions.

Medical screening

- Mostly, there is little choice in who makes up the crew, and often their medical problems will be well known. However, it is worth taking a step back and formally assessing the risk.
- Medical screening may take the form of a self-declaration questionnaire, with or without confirmation by the family doctor who is aware of the medical history, or it may be formal physical examination and testing.
- Such screening will appear onerous but will avoid potentially serious complications that may endanger the whole boat.
- All crew should have a dental check-up and appropriate treatment before departure.
- Crew should have current immunizations for tetanus, diphtheria, meningitis ACWY, hepatitis A and B, and typhoid. Other immunizations (e.g. for yellow fever) and chemoprophylaxis (e.g. for malaria) may be required depending on the ports of call.

Crew medic

Crew will understandably expect that, should they be struck down, treatment on board will be the best available in the circumstances. Ideally, a suitable crew member, preferably with some form of medical or paramedical background such as paramedic, nurse, fire-fighter, or police officer, should be designated to provide medical care on-board. In the absence of

4 Maritime and Coastguard Agency. *Medical Examination System: Appointment of Approved Doctors and Medical and Eyesight Standards. Merchant Shipping Notice 1886(M+F).* Southampton: Maritime and Coastguard Agency; 2018.

someone with professional qualifications, the most important factors are motivation and knowledge. Whether or not medics have a qualification, appropriate training for working in remote and difficult conditions, together with early involvement, gives ownership of the process and will improve outcomes. Both the medic and the skipper should receive appropriate training. There should be clear mechanisms of support including medical manuals on board, and guidance on how to seek shore advice and help.

Medical support

In all medical emergencies, the universal advice is to seek medical advice early. This requires some form of communication system that works reliably in all locations, and the sources of advice must be known beforehand. Medical support may be arranged with a specific provider or, in an emergency, shore support is possible through the system of Maritime Rescue Coordination Centres.[5]

Ports of call

It is worthwhile investigating facilities at all ports of call, both scheduled and ones identified for use in an emergency. Local rescue facilities and hospital services may be limited, so prior knowledge may affect planning a suitable response in an emergency.

Restocking medical supplies may be a problem in areas where the local language is not English. However, most drugs are available in most places, although names and packaging will vary. Ensure the local port customs office knows you have a medical kit on board, so it is properly cleared in and out of port. This is particularly important with scheduled drugs and may save time and red faces if the kit comes to light as part of a search of the vessel.

Insurance

Medical insurance is advisable for all crew. It should provide cover for:
• Rescue from remote locations.
• Emergency treatment in local hospitals.
• Repatriation.
• Cost of medicines.

The medic and skipper may require additional insurance to cover them to treat fellow crew members in territorial waters or in ports of call. Adequate insurance is particularly important if a crew member might be landed in the US and associated territories, as medical costs there can be extremely high.

Clothing

Clothing is the barrier between the crew and the elements. It has to be right for each crew, and no one solution is suitable for all. A triple-layer system is most commonly used:
• *Base layer*—close fitting, usually made from merino wool, silk, or other synthetic material, but always a material with good wicking properties that can be worn for extended periods of weeks or more. Long sleeves and long legs are usual.
• *Mid layer*—reasonably close fitting, made from a fleece-type material, its main function being thermal insulation. The mid-layer may range from a

5 ⌁ https://www.inmarsat.com/services/safety/maritime-rescue-co-ordination-centres/

relatively thin, micro-fleece one-piece suit, to a waterproof, breathable jacket and salopettes combination. The shell layer may have a degree of water and wind resistance.

- *Outer layer* is the main barrier against the elements, and typically comprises a jacket or smock top, with trousers that reach up to chest level. The jacket will usually have a high collar, incorporating a hood that can be zipped up to protect the majority of the face. The outer layer invariably has reflective patches on the shoulders to aid locating crew in the event of a man overboard at night. A safety harness may sometimes be built into the structure of the jacket.
- *Seaboots* must be properly fitted before departure. Loose boots are hazardous and may cause a trip and fall, whereas excessively tight boots may restrict blood supply to the feet, causing uncomfortably cold feet, and possibly other complications such as 'cockpit foot'—a non-freezing cold injury (⊙ Non-freezing cold injury, p. 666–667). Boots should allow adequate space for a pair of reasonably thick socks.
- *Gloves and hats*—essential in cold climes. Take spares. Sun hats are also essential in virtually all areas of the oceans.
- *Sunglasses*—although strictly not clothing, these are essential due to the increased glare from the water (similar to the effect on snow) and may cause photokeratitis after a relatively short period of exposure. Wrap-around glasses are the most effective type.

Offshore medical kits

(See also Chapter 28.)

Contents and quantities

The contents and quantities of the medical kit are similar for any expedition to a remote location, and must take into account:

- Duration of expedition.
- Number of crew.
- Type of voyage—racing is inherently more dangerous than cruising.
- Proposed route and distance from definitive help.
- Medical expertise on-board.
- Medical history of the crew members.
- Opportunities for re-supply in ports of call: generally English-speaking countries are easier for replenishment—drug availability, dosages, and names vary widely in other countries.

The MCA have formulated a recommended kit list[6] for various classes of commercial vessel, with proposed quantities of medications.

Other kit lists have been proposed for non-commercial vessels, such as different types of yacht,[7] taking in to account the specific requirements of boats that are racing, or those venturing to isolated and stormy areas of the world's oceans, and for smaller yachts with less storage space.

Organization

Kits need to be *clearly planned and organized*:

- By body system into separate transparent bags or boxes.
- Additional separate bags should contain:
  - Emergency/resuscitation drugs.
  - Hardware.
  - IV/IM drugs, needles, syringes.
  - IV fluid (if carried).
- Controlled drugs (e.g. morphine) must be kept secure and usage fully documented.
- First-aid books, medical reference manuals, and the *BNF* (or similar pharmacopoeia) should be included, both as hardcopy and electronically if possible.
- Oxygen cylinders and concentrators, and marine defibrillators are also possible additions to the medical kit, but involve regular update training, servicing, and are only one link in a chain of survival.

Grab bag

A specific medical kit to be taken to the life raft if abandoning ship that may also double as emergency treatment bag should contain:

- Emergency analgesics (oral and IM).

6 Maritime and Coastguard Agency. *Ships' Medical Stores. Merchant Shipping Notice1905 (M&F) Amendment 1. Application of the ships medical stores regulations 1995.*Maritime and Coastguard Agency; 2022. https://www.gov.uk/government/publications/msn-1905-mf-application-of-ships-medical-stores-regulations-1995

7 Briggs S, Mackenzie C. *Skipper's Medical Emergency Handbook*, 2nd ed. pp. 205–207. London: Adlard Coles Nautical; 2018.

- Seasickness medications (a large stock and including drugs that can be absorbed by routes other than oral).
- Antibiotics.
- Rehydration salts.
- Suturing kit.
- Immobilization splints, strapping, bandages.

Always restock from the main kit if an item is used.

Offshore medical problems

Seasickness

- The three stages of mal de mer:
  - 'I feel sick.'
  - 'I think I'm going to die.'
  - 'I'm worried I'm not going to die.'
- A common and disabling condition; untreatable in <10%.
- Symptoms include nausea, sweating, vomiting, fatigue, loss of appetite, reduction in bowel action, and dry mouth.
- Prevention is better than a cure; commencing medication 24 h before leaving port is likely to be most effective.
- Behavioural adaptations may lessen the effects of motion: staying on deck, focusing on the horizon, helming, avoiding chart work down below, avoiding unpleasant smells, and eating small meals regularly.
- Drug therapy may be effective in >90% of sufferers (Table 23.1); however, each individual varies in their response and it is worth finding the best drug or combination of drugs for each person.
- There is a wealth of evidence for and against most common remedies which include cinnarizine (Stugeron®), hyoscine hydrobromide (Scopoderm®), domperidone (Motilium®), prochlorperazine (Stemetil®), and ondansetron (Zofran®).
- Drug delivery may be cutaneous, buccal, PO, PR, IM, or IV.
- Some remedies have side effects such as dry mouth, blurred vision, drowsiness, and urinary hesitancy.
- Dehydration and hypothermia may occur more readily in severe seasickness, requiring active treatment.
- Seasickness susceptibility in females is linked to the menstrual cycle, and women may suffer more at these times.
- Sickness usually improves after 48 h but may return if rough weather follows a period of relative calm.
- Remember that if a sufferer is dependent on oral medication (antiepileptics, treatments for heart conditions, oral contraceptive pill, etc.) they may well not absorb the medication, and be at considerable risk of untoward medical deterioration. In these circumstances, there should be increased emphasis on treating seasickness. Pre-planning is essential.
- Being sick over the side carries the real risk of following the vomit. Use a bucket.

Table 23.1 Seasickness drugs

Medication	Route	Dose	Way it works	Notes
Cinnarizine	Oral	30mg 6-12 hours before departure, then 15mg every 8 hours	Antihistamine	Although an antihistamine, usually has little sedative effect
Cyclizine	Oral	50mg every 8h	Antihistamine	Slight sedation only
	IM	50mg every 8h		Painful injection
Domperidone	Oral	10-20mg every 6h	Peripheral antidopamine	Well tolerated, non-sedating. Convert from suppositories once vomiting stops
	Suppository	30mg every 6h		
Hyoscine hydrobromide	Patch behind ear	Replace patch every 72h, on the opposite side	Anticholinergic	Sedative effects, dry mouth; rarely, difficulty passing urine. Take care with patch as contamination will dilate pupil and blur vision. Wash hands after use
	Oral	0.3 mg every 8h		
Ondansetron	Oral	4-8mg every 8h	Antiserotonin	Non-sedating, occasional constipation
	Under tongue	4-8mg every 8h		
Prochlorperazine	Oral	10mg every 6h	Central antidopamine	Some sedative properties, dry mouth, rarely causes abnormal movements, tremor, and restlessness.
	Under tongue	3mg every 6h		
	IM injection	12.5mg, then oral therapy 6h later		
Promethazine	Oral	25mg every 6-8hr	Antihistamine	Significant sedation, which may be an advantage. Dry mouth; rarely difficulty passing urine

Trauma

All types of sport and impact injuries may be encountered. Half of all injuries occur below decks.[8] The susceptibility to injury does not seem to be related to age of crew, but may be affected by work pattern on-board.

Injuries may be life-threatening and include:

- Head injuries (➲ Head injury, p. 320–337).
- Long bone fractures (➲ Fractures, p. 438–472).
- Blunt chest and abdominal trauma (➲ Chapter 7).
- Pelvic fractures (➲ Pelvic fractures, p. 458).
- Therapeutic manoeuvres that may be required include:
  - Chest drains.
  - Limb splints and cervical spine immobilizers.
  - Reduction of fractures and dislocations.
  - Simple LA nerve blocks.
  - IV access and fluid resuscitation.
  - Nasogastric tubes and urinary catheters.
  - Skin suturing or stapling (Steri-Strips™ and tissue glue are of limited use in the marine environment).

Skin

Sun, salt water, heat, cold, damp, and friction have a deleterious effect on the skin. Common complaints include:

- Salt water boils (➲ Other infective skin lesions, p. 313).
- Gunwale bum (sitting for long periods, in clothing damp with salt water).
- Prickly heat (➲ p. 810).
- Cockpit foot (non-freezing cold injury; ➲ Non-freezing cold injury, p. 666–667).
- Rope friction burns.
- Sunburn.

Skin infections (such as impetigo and fungal infections of groin and foot) in the confined yacht environment are also common. Personal hygiene is essential, and regular below-decks cleaning should occur. Skin and wound infections should be treated with antibiotics which include activity against the bacterium *Staphylococcus aureus*. Hypertrophy of the skin leads to the development of 'sausage fingers' and a dangerous reduction in dexterity. A barrier cream such as Sudocrem®, moisturizers, and protective clothing such as gloves may reduce this process. Skin and lips must be protected against the sun.

Dehydration

A serious and potentially life-threatening condition, which can have many causes, including:

- Seasickness.
- Hot weather.
- Hard physical work in heavy clothing.
- Inadequately rehydrated freeze-dried food.

8 Price CJS, Spalding TJW, McKenzie C. Patterns of illness and injury encountered in amateur ocean yacht racing: an analysis of the British Telecom Round the World Yacht Race 1996–1997. *Br J Sports Med*. 2002;36:457–462.

- Distraction from the process of regular rehydration.
- Unwillingness to undress to urinate regularly, so intentional limitation of fluid intake.

Rehydration may be undertaken orally (with balanced oral rehydration fluids (such as Dioralyte®)), PR, or IV, which requires special medical training.
Proper personal hydration must be part of the team ethos.

Immersion and drowning

(See also **⊃** Immersion and drowning, p. 239, 721–723.)
- Prevention is better than cure.
- The man-overboard drill should be clearly understood and practised by all on board, to facilitate rapid recovery.
- The routine use of harnesses, life jackets with spray hoods, immersion-activated lights, and personal EPIRBs (emergency radio beacons) should be part of the ethos of the boat.
- Concurrent injury is common in the process of being swept over the side.
- Immersion in cold water causes uncontrolled rapid breathing and tachycardia.
- Initial action in the water should be to stay still, trying to minimize seawater aspiration during initial gasps, then limit physical exertion, and heat loss by facing away from the weather. Adopt HELP position if practicable (Fig. 23.1 and Fig. 23.2). In calm waters these positions help to conserve heat, but they are less effective and safe in rough seas, where individuals could be thrown against each other, risking injury.
- Recovery should be in the horizontal position as far as possible to prevent circulatory collapse.
- Victims may require full resuscitation, rewarming, and supportive therapy for a prolonged period following recovery.

See **⊃** Field management, p. 721–723, for more details.

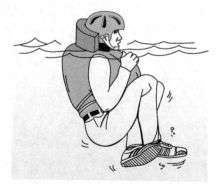

Fig. 23.1 HELP (heat escape lessening posture) survival position. If alone in the water, assume this position to minimize heat loss from head, neck, sides of body, and groin region.

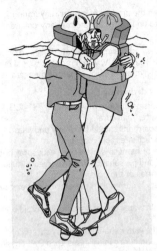

Fig. 23.2 HELP survival position. If two or more people are in water together, form a huddle so that sides of body are close together.

Emergency procedures

Helicopter evacuation

- A very costly resource to be used wisely. Not without risk to boat and helicopter crew. Training exercises are invaluable.
- Good communication with shore and helicopter crew is essential to ensure coordination and convey medical information regarding the victim.
- The normal range for helicopter rescue is within 200 nautical miles, occasionally using a fixed-wing plane to locate the boat initially.

Method

- Brief your crew beforehand—it will be too noisy later.
- Communicate with the helicopter on VHF.
- The boat should steer a straight course close hauled on port, with the helicopter hovering off to port (avoids downdraft hitting yacht).
- Rescue will take place from the starboard door of the helicopter and the port side of the boat.
- Be prepared:
  - Clear the deck of loose objects.
  - Do as the helicopter crew tell you; they are the experts!
  - Use gloves.
  - The victim should be dressed and ready, with medical record attached.
  - All crew should be clipped to the boat.
- Initially, a weighted 'hi-line' is dropped from the helicopter. Do not touch until it has earthed in water or on the boat.
- Do not attach the line to the boat and avoid it getting snagged. For safety, coil it into a bucket.
- A diver descends on the main lifting wire; pull him in to the boat.
- Follow his directions.
- A single or double strop or stretcher may be used.
- In rough weather, recovery may be from a life raft trailed astern, or directly from the water.

Life raft evacuation

- Only abandon a boat if it is sinking under your feet.
- Anticipate the possibility and be prepared. Life rafts must be serviced regularly. Each crewman should have a pre-assigned abandonment task.
- All crew get very seasick in a life raft; take medications beforehand.
- Take the grab bag (→ Grab bag, p. 748–749, 862).
- Water (as much as possible) and portable water maker if carried.
- Weatherproof clothing and life jackets (put on before entering raft).
- VHF radio. Satellite/mobile phones (the latter if inshore).
- Flares and EPIRB(s).
- Polythene or waterproof bags for vomit, faeces, urine.
- Toilet paper.
- Torches.
- Handheld GPS.
- Food.
- Crew get very sick, dehydrated, may be injured, and mentally traumatized by losing their boat.

Man overboard (MOB)

See Fig. 23.3.

- A frightening experience for all on-board, particularly for the one in the water.
- Staying on-board is obviously the best plan. Do this by adopting the following strategies:
  - Use safe techniques on deck and avoid overt risk-taking behaviour.
  - One hand for the boat and one for yourself.
  - Embed the use of harnesses, lifelines, jackstays, and life jackets in the ethos of the boat.
  - Consider all crew carry a personal EPIRB, mini-flares, waterproof torch, proximity- or water-activated alarm.
- Practise regularly, particularly recovery from the water. Decide the best route for recovery—over the sides, from the stern, etc. Plan practices thoroughly, so they don't themselves become an emergency.

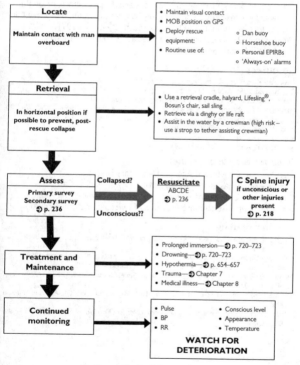

Fig. 23.3 Man overboard algorithm.

- Specific actions in the event of MOB:
  - A loud shout to alert all on-deck.
  - One crew keeps pointing and tracking the crew in the water.
  - Press the MOB button on the boat GPS to record position of event.
  - Deploy all MOB equipment—Dan buoy, horseshoe buoy.
  - Adopt a sailing pattern to return to the crew in the water (e.g. crash stop, reach–turn–reach).
  - If using the engine, approach alongside the crew in the water in neutral or engine stopped.
  - Recover in the horizontal position if the crew member has been in the water for an extended period. If this isn't possible, do not delay recovery, but place in horizontal position when on deck, and reassess.
  - It may be necessary, in the event the crew in the water is unconscious, to put a suitably clothed crew into the water on a line, to assist with recovery.
  - Remember—the crew may have sustained injury before, or on the way over the side, so once recovered from the water, perform a full assessment using the ABCDE approach (➔ p. 236–237).
  - If the MOB is not recovered immediately, consider making a MAYDAY call for assistance.

Resources

Adventure Medical Kits: ℔ http://adventuremedicalkits.com
Cruising Association: ℔ http://www.cruising.org.uk
Maritime and Coastguard Agency: ℔ http://www.mcga.gov.uk
Maritime and Coastguard Agency. *Ships Captain's Medical Guide*, 23rd ed. London: HMSO; 2019. ℔
    https://www.gov.uk/government/publications/the-ship-captains-medical-guide
Medical Support Offshore: ℔ http://msos.org.uk
Royal Ocean Racing Club: ℔ http://www.rorc.org
Royal Yachting Association: ℔ http://www.rya.org.uk

Maritime medical training courses

Maritime and Coastguard Agency: Elementary First Aid.
Maritime and Coastguard Agency: Proficiency in Medical Care.
Maritime and Coastguard Agency: Proficiency in Medical First Aid.
Royal Yachting Association: Sea Survival Course, Elementary First Aid.

Further reading

Briggs S, Mackenzie C. *Skipper's Medical Emergency Handbook*, 2nd ed. London: Adlard Coles Nautical; 2018.
Cold Water Casualty Video. British Defence Library A3788. Institute of Naval Medicine; 1990.
Golden F, Tipton M. *Essentials of Sea Survival*. Leeds: Human Kinetics; 2002.
Howarth F, Howarth M. *The Grab Bag—Your Ultimate Guide to Liferaft Survival*. London: Adlard Coles Nautical; 2002.
Weiss EA, Jacobs M. *A Comprehensive Guide to Marine Medicine*. Oakland, CA: Adventure Medical Kits; 2012.
World Health Organization. *International Medical Guide for Ships*, 3rd ed. Geneva: World Health Organization; 2007.

Chapter 24

Underwater

Chapter editor
James Moore

Contributors
Robert Conway
Craig Holdstock
Lesley F. Thomson
Andy Pitkin (1st edition)

Reviewer
Rose Buckley

The underwater environment

Increased ease of travel and the rise in adventure tourism has enabled many more people to explore the underwater world. A range of specialist breathing equipment has been developed to extend the duration and range of underwater exploration. However, prolonged immersion under pressure can lead to a variety of medical problems.

Medical personnel on diving expeditions should not only understand the medical problems associated with underwater work but also broader medical conditions common to all expeditions. Appropriate medical equipment and casualty evacuation plans should be in place prior to the start of the expedition. Underwater activities on expeditions include:

- Marine biology and conservation work.
- Underwater archaeology including wreck diving.
- Cave diving.
- Marine salvage.
- Fishing—shellfish collection or spear gun.

Commercial activities within the oil or mining industries, governed by stringent commercial diving regulations and medical examinations, are not covered in this chapter.

Contrary to popular belief, shark attacks and the bends are rare on diving expeditions. Common medical problems include:

- GI upsets.
- Minor trauma.
- Ear problems secondary to repetitive diving.
- Soft tissue injuries.
- Secondary infections.

Both decompression illness (DCI; encompassing decompression sickness (DCS) and barotrauma) and immersion pulmonary oedema (IPO) are rare but may be life-threatening and require immediate intervention either at site or in a specialist centre for recompression and hyperbaric oxygen (O_2) treatment.

Physical characteristics of the underwater environment

Environmental conditions expose divers to risks of seasickness, hypothermia, drowning, and marine envenomation. Waves and swell may lead to trauma during water entry or exit from boat or shore; strong currents, tides, or poor visibility may cause a diver to become separated and lost, along with risks of physical exhaustion. Intensely hot or cold climates also expose equipment and divers to physical and physiological stresses.

Weather

Climatic conditions at depth may be both different and more constant than those on the surface, but atmospheric conditions govern the ease with which the transition between land and water is made. Both currents and squalls may make it difficult to return to boat or beach.

Travel

Diving equipment is bulky and transport may be logistically difficult. Cabin pressures in commercial airliners are equivalent to a journey to altitude (about 2500 m/8000 feet) and may precipitate DCS. There are recommendations for the limits to diving for a time period before flying, and these should be strictly imposed for safety. Divers should not fly within 12 h of a single, non-decompression dive or within 24 h after repetitive, multiple day, or decompression diving.

Types of underwater activity

The simplest methods to explore underwater include snorkelling or breath-hold diving (free-diving). Most expeditions use self-contained underwater breathing apparatus (SCUBA), using cylinders filled with compressed air. Nitrox (higher O_2 concentration than air) can be used to reduce the risks of DCS or to increase the duration of safe diving. Technical divers tend to use more complicated equipment configurations to extend the depth and/or duration of the dive. This may involve multiple cylinders with different mixtures of O_2, nitrogen (N_2), and helium. It may also involve rebreathing apparatus, diver propulsion vehicles, heated suits, long periods of decompression and solo-diving.

Snorkelling and breath-hold ('free') diving

A snorkel enables a diver to breathe at the surface while still visualizing objects beneath. Many swimmers use snorkels for short breath-hold dives without training in free-diving.

Free-diving is both a recreational activity and a competitive sport where breath is held throughout a period underwater. The term may include activities such as underwater hockey or synchronized swimming, but at the more extreme end competitive free-diving involves apnoea during swims for maximum distance or depth, or static breath-hold duration. Athletes train to endure high carbon dioxide (CO_2) levels, low O_2 levels, and lactic acidosis. Movement in swimming is relaxed and energy efficient. Competitors winning depth records often have unique morphology and an unusual amount of blood fills the space left in the chest by compressed lung tissue as depth increases. Specific risks include aspiration, drowning, otitis externa, ear barotrauma during descent or ascent, lung squeeze causing pulmonary haemorrhage and haemoptysis, and shallow or deep water blackout.

SCUBA

SCUBA divers breathe compressed air or nitrox from cylinders. Dive depth and duration is calculated from decompression tables or dive computers. These utilize mathematical algorithms to guide dive time according to the maximum depth reached during the dive. The dive should be planned with maximum depth established prior to diving, and calculations to ensure the cylinders contain sufficient gas for the whole dive including any safety or decompression stops. Divers usually dive in buddy pairs for safety and enjoyment. This chapter mainly concentrates on the medical problems associated with SCUBA diving.

Technical diving

A breathing mixture of O_2, N_2, and helium can be used with specific equipment to expand the depth and duration of diving (e.g. cave or wreck penetration). Technical diving in remote locations may require extensive logistical planning. Dives are usually significantly longer and deeper than recreational SCUBA diving, with lengthy decompression schedules of several hours, restricting when the diver can surface. Technical diving requires advanced training and use of either open (produces bubbles like SCUBA) or closed rebreathing circuits.[1] Treatment of DCS is the same for SCUBA; however, if injury occurs during the dive it may prove fatal, with mortality quoted up to 1:100 divers.[2]

1 Mitchell SJ, Doolette DJ. Recreational technical diving part 1: an introduction to diving and technical diving methods and activities. *Diving Hyperb Med*. 2013;43(2):86–93.

2 Fock AW. Analysis of recreational closed-circuit rebreather deaths 1998–2010. *Diving Hyperb Med*. 43(2):78–85.

Risk assessment for diving expeditions

General risk assessments should be made as for all expeditions (➔ Risk assessment, Risk management, p. 70–75). Diving practice and safety can often be improved by running introductory talks on diving-related illness and treatment including first aid, not least because the non-diving expedition members will form the main team helping to treat a sick diver.

Store O_2 cylinders carefully; keep them cool and away from sources of fire. Check where they can be refilled locally and when they were last serviced, as scheduled maintenance may not be possible on expedition. Keep the generator for refilling air cylinders away from vehicle fumes or personnel smoking; both of which could lead to carbon monoxide (CO) entering the breathing gas, which is dangerous at pressure.

Be aware of specific points of danger—the entry and exit from water to shore or boat; and managing boat handling during the pick-up. Have and practise a search protocol to use if a diver is lost underwater or on the surface. Surface marker buoys help to locate divers on surfacing, and there are several electronic diver-locating systems on the market.

Search and rescue

Dive profiles should be planned (and checked) using tables or dive computer algorithms. Divers should have adequate equipment to signal boats. These include whistles, surface marker buoys, and torches or strobes at night. If a boat crew loses a dive team then they should begin the search at the point of last contact, taking into account prevailing currents. Searching should take the form of a systematic approach using linear, sweeping, or circular search patterns. If after initial searching dive teams are still missing, emergency services should be contacted, if available, in order to broaden search patterns.

Environmental impact

Look but do not touch. Training, good buoyancy control, and diving within one's limits are key to protecting the marine environment. Never remove or disturb the underwater environment. In particular, be aware of damaging fragile coral structures with fins and only collect marine animals if warranted, and correct permissions have been sought prior to diving. Respect wreck diving policies on war graves and do not disturb remains.

Preparations before travel

Clothing

Be familiar with diving equipment. Buoyancy is greater in new wet- or dry-suits leading to unexpected rapid ascent. Over-weighted divers may sink. Longer and repetitive exposure may lead to the necessity for a thicker wet-suit in any given water temperature so consider extra thickness. Seek expert advice if unsure.

Specific equipment

Many diving accidents involve the use of new, unfamiliar, or faulty equipment. Induced panic is common. Appropriate experience is more important than paper qualifications. Train and practise in a safe environment. Medics should work closely with expedition leaders to ensure divers are familiar with their equipment and safety procedures, and that initial 'check' dives are in shallow water with good visibility.

Pre-departure medical preparations

A medic with SCUBA diving qualifications is often better placed to understand and influence the diving practice on an expedition and its implications on potential illness or injury. Familiarization with practical issues, equipment, safe use of decompression tables, and dive computers is vital. Diving medicine courses are widely available, and a diving expedition doctor should possess appropriate knowledge.

Medical kits

Diving expeditions should consider including the following additional items to their general medical kit (➲ Chapter 28):

- O_2 supplies with an appropriate delivery system. The filling system in the host country will need to be compatible with the equipment taken, and appropriate volumes for evacuation must be calculated. Rebreathing systems are available; by using lower gas flows these provide longer duration of supply.
- IV fluids and cannulae.
- Seasickness prophylaxis.
- Urinary catheter for neurological bends.
- Antibiotic ± steroid eardrops.
- Liquid decongestant.
- Alcohol ear drops.
- Auriscope and tendon hammer.
- Chest drain/underwater seal drain or Heimlich valve.
- Diuretic (e.g. furosemide).
- Vaseline® for wetsuit sores.

Fitness to dive

Fitness to dive requirements vary between international training organizations. Ultimately, some general standards apply, modified according to the remoteness of the expedition and physical diving activity. Decisions regarding fitness to dive should be made prior to the expedition departure; if necessary, seek advice from experienced diving physicians. The basic principle is that any condition that may unexpectedly impair a diver's ability to exert themselves physically or that may cause a sudden alteration in conscious level will usually mean that the candidate is unfit to dive. Potential medical conditions and acceptability for diving are shown in Table 24.1.

Table 24.1 Potential medical conditions

System	Condition	Acceptability for diving
Cardiac	Hypertension	Normally compatible providing BP control is adequate and no evidence of end-organ damage
	Dysrhythmias	Normally absolute contraindication
	Ischaemia	Strict criteria must be met to dive
	Septal defect/PFO	Shunt dependent, closure currently often advised. Obtain specialist cardiology input
Respiratory	Obstructive airway disease	COPD/emphysema, asthma. Asthma requires acceptable lung function on their normal medication, which can be optimized to achieve this
	Acute URTI	No diving until fully resolved
Neurological	Epilepsy	Contraindicated unless convulsion free and off medication for 5 years
	Severe head injury	May return to diving after review by diving physician
Metabolic	Type 1 diabetes	Allowed if no hypoglycaemic unawareness or end-organ damage and review by diving physician
ENT	Tympanic membrane barotrauma	Perforation 4 weeks, otherwise 24–48 h
	Sinusitis	Acutely is a contraindication; avoid decongestants
Psychiatric	Depression/anxiety	Requiring medication requires discussion with diving physician
Other	Lack of physical fitness	BMI >30 kg/m²
	DCI	Review by diving physician
	Poor dental work	May result in dental pain, review dental work pre-departure (➲ Chapter 11)
	Pregnancy	No research on effects on fetus, therefore diving should be avoided
	Age	There is no maximum age limit

Diving medicine

Safe practice when diving

For medical concerns, see Table 24.2.

Table 24.2 Medical concerns on diving expeditions

Environment	Trauma	Heat illness/ hypothermia
	Sunburn	Marine envenomation
	Dehydration	Near drowning
	Motion sickness	Waterborne disease
Diving	Barotrauma	DCI
	IPO	
Breathing gas	N_2 narcosis	CO poisoning
	Hypercapnia	O_2 toxicity (e.g. nitrox)
Other	Local diseases, e.g. tropical	Otitis externa
	GI upset	Psychological problems/ panic

Dive conservatively and well within limits, guided by tables or computer algorithms. Minimize the number of dives each day (preferably a maximum of two or three depending on depth) with rest days (no diving) every 3–4 days. Safety stops at 3–6 m for 3–5 min significantly reduce intravascular bubbles. Beware of psychological pressure to push diving limits if a project is behind schedule. Occasionally, diving may take place at higher altitudes. In this instance, dive computers or tables will need to be configured to account for the lower ambient partial pressure.

Casualty evacuation (medevac) plan

Introduce yourself to the local recompression chamber at the start of the expedition. This can help to establish the facilities available and make the chamber facility aware of the diving expedition. Local staff will have knowledge of diving conditions or venomous marine life. It may be useful to visit the local hospital(s) to ascertain appropriateness of other medical facilities.

A casualty evacuation plan should include:
- Recompression chamber—emergency phone number, staff contact numbers.
- Transport—type (e.g. boat, road vehicle, aircraft); how many patients fit into vehicle (buddy may also need treatment).
- Distance/time to and from recompression facility.
- Aeromedical transfer (pressurized or fly close to sea level).
- Calculation of O_2 requirement for two people (plus contingency). Is O_2 supplied on transport?
- Are medical personnel available with the transport. Should the expedition medic go with them (and if so, how will they return)?

Always remember to take passport, insurance details, patient family contact details, credit card, and mobile phone.

Medevac letter

In addition to the information supplied in the previous medevac section, a letter with the following details should accompany the affected diver and their buddy:

1. Diver—name, date of birth.
2. Maximum depth, duration, and any mandatory decompression stops. Include the diver's computer if possible.
3. Gases used (e.g. air/nitrox/trimix) and equipment used (e.g. open/closed circuit).
4. Details of precipitating factor (e.g. rapid ascent).
5. Time of surfacing.
6. Time of onset of symptoms.
7. Description of symptoms.
8. Symptom progression (improving/worsening).
9. Treatment given—any improvement?
10. Previous dives (maximum depth, duration, surface intervals) including preceding days.
11. Past medical history, including previous DCS.
12. Prescription medicines/use of recreational drugs or alcohol.
13. Any allergies.

Diving physics

Most diving expeditions will use SCUBA with cylinders containing breathing gas, typically compressed air at 200 bar (atmospheres). A regulator valve reduces this high pressure so the diver breathes at a pressure equal to that of the surrounding water. For every 10 m/33 ft depth, water pressure increases by one atmosphere. The density of breathed air increases with depth; at 10 m it is twice the density of surface air, so more N_2 molecules are inhaled and absorbed with each breath. The N_2 dissolves in blood and tissues and can result in DCS during or after ascent.

Air may be enriched with O_2 to make 'nitrox'. Reducing the inhaled N_2 concentration enables longer dive durations and reduces the risk of DCS. However, it increases the risk of acute O_2 toxicity and the permitted maximum diving depth must take this into account. See Table 24.3.

Table 24.3 Diving physics

Depth (m)	Relative volume of balloon	Density	Partial pressure of oxygen (PO_2)	Partial pressure of nitrogen (PN_2)
Surface	1	×1	0.21	0.79
10	½	×2	0.42	1.58
20	⅓	×3	0.63	2.37
30	¼	×4	0.84	3.16
40	⅕	×5	1.05	3.95

The risk of DCS and circulatory microbubbles following a single dive has been well researched; tables and computer algorithms give consistent analysis of the risks. However, multiple dives, particularly on consecutive days, may lead to accumulation of N_2 in the tissues and very few repetitive dive profiles have been fully researched. Any mathematical error in the DCS tables or physiological variation between divers could increase the risk of DCS.

Effects of high-pressure gases

Nitrogen narcosis

High partial pressures of N_2 cause anaesthetic-like effects. The pioneering diver Jacques Cousteau lost friends to this condition and described it as 'rapture of the deep'. Euphoric effects develop between 10 m and 30 m, below 50 m the effects can be life-threatening. Individual susceptibility varies; divers are usually unaware of being affected and, without appropriate training, oblivious to its danger. They may react inappropriately and put themselves at risk.

Typical symptoms (with increasing depth):
- Tunnel vision, euphoria, apprehension.
- Inability to manage complex tasks.
- Tinnitus.
- Drowsiness.
- Loss of consciousness.

The condition may be exacerbated by hypercapnia, exertion, cold water, and darkness. Symptoms resolve rapidly on ascent. Buddy divers need to take charge of an affected diver.

Hypercapnia (CO_2 retention)

The increased density of gas at depth affects resistance to breathing, and so with increased depth the compressed air 'feels thicker'. Alongside this, diving equipment can increase work of breathing and dead-space. Exertion, such as swimming against a current, will magnify these effects leading to build up of CO_2 and 'air hunger'.

Risk factors include:
- Resistance to breathing in regulator.
- Excessive exertion, over-weighted diver.
- High gas density (excessive depth for gas mixture used, e.g. gas densities >5.2–6.2 g/L (29–39 m depth on air)).[3]
- Exhaustion of CO_2 scrubber in divers using re-breathing system.
- Poor dive practice (e.g. some divers may exhibit 'skip-breathing', deliberately hypoventilating in order to conserve air!).

Symptoms include:
- Headache.
- Strong feelings of panic.
- Flushing.
- Palpitations.
- Breathlessness.
- Eventual loss of consciousness.

Once recognized, try to rest and reassure the affected diver. Ascend at normal rate to minimize risk of barotrauma or DCS. Assistance may be required if diver is over-weighted or panicking.

---

3 Anthony G, Mitchell S. Respiratory physiology of rebreather diving. In: Pollock NW, Sellers SH, Godfrey JM, eds. *Rebreathers and Scientific Diving. Proceedings of NPS/NOAA/DAN/AAUS June 16–19, 2015, Workshop.* Durham, NC; 2016: 66–79.

Carbon monoxide poisoning

Carbon monoxide (CO) is colourless, odourless, and hazardous as it binds to haemoglobin to prevent O_2 transport in the bloodstream. SCUBA cylinder supplies may be contaminated if the breathing gas compressor intake is sited downwind of a source of combustion. Even a small amount of CO may cause symptoms as the partial pressure of CO will increase with depth, increasing the likelihood/severity of symptoms, which include:

- Headache.
- General malaise.
- Nausea.
- Poor coordination.
- Weakness.
- Unconsciousness leading to death.

Management

- 100% O_2 reduces the half-life ($t_{1/2}$) of CO from around 4 h to 1 h.
- In severe cases, hyperbaric O_2 therapy (at 3 atm—if available) can reduce the $t_{1/2}$ to <30 min.
- Check compressor, servicing schedules, tanks, and semi-closed circuits.

Acute (CNS) oxygen toxicity

O_2 breathed at partial pressures of PO_2 >1.6 bar (160 kPa) can be harmful. The risk of toxicity increases with PO_2, duration of exposure, degree of exertion, and associated hypercapnia.

Symptoms include:

- Facial (especially lip), diaphragmatic, and other muscle twitching.
- Visual disturbances (e.g. central and peripheral visual field defects).
- Nausea, vertigo, tinnitus.
- Dysphoria ('sensation of impending doom').
- Convulsions (may be the first manifestation).

Management

- Reduce PO_2 immediately (e.g. ascend, switch gas mix).
- Convulsions occurring under water are potentially fatal:
- Maintain diver's depth during initial tonic phase of the seizure, to prevent barotraumas caused by uncontrolled ascent.
- Attempt to keep mouthpiece in casualty's mouth if possible.
- Recover to the surface and treat any secondary illness e.g. barotrauma.
- The seizure will resolve immediately once PO_2 is reduced and will not require further treatment or restriction of diving. O_2 toxicity is a risk in recompression chambers when breathing 100% O_2.

Decompression illness

DCI describes a group of illnesses that result from a reduction in ambient pressure surrounding the diver. The two conditions that fall into this DCI group are DCS and arterial gas embolism (AGE). See Table 24.4.

Table 24.4 Symptoms of decompression illness

System	Symptoms
Musculoskeletal	Limb pain
Neurological	Paraesthesia (often with limb pain)
	Epigastric/girdle/back pain
	Limb weakness (most commonly legs)
	Loss of balance/coordination
	General malaise or fatigue
	Cognitive dysfunction
	Urinary retention
	Visual disturbance (often 'wavy lines')
Temporary	Petechial rash (may indicate high inert gas load)
	Marbled rash (rare)
	Lymphatic obstruction (rare)
Cardiorespiratory	Cough, frothy bloodstained sputum—'the chokes'
	Dyspnoea
	Chest pain
	Collapse

Decompression sickness

DCS, or 'the bends', is caused by gas that has dissolved within body tissues under pressure during a dive, re-emerging as bubbles when pressure reduces during or after ascent. It is therefore sometimes termed an 'evolved gas disease'. The bubbles (usually N_2) may be intravascular, extravascular, or both depending on gas load, and cause clinical syndromes depending on their location. Small bubbles merge into larger ones leading to bubble growth. Intravascular bubbles cause emboli leading to hypoxic damage. Secondary clotting and inflammatory cascades are activated at bubble/blood interfaces. Rapid recompression and O_2 administration compress gases back into solution, provide a concentration gradient for N_2 elimination and supply O_2 to hypoxic tissues.

Arterial gas embolism

AGE is caused by barotrauma. Gas enters the vascular system leading to intravascular bubbles that cause emboli and hypoxic damage. It is therefore termed an 'escaped gas disease'. It is often associated with rapid ascent, breath holding on ascent, and pneumothorax. Like DCS this can lead to clotting and inflammatory activation. See → p. 779 for cerebral arterial gas embolism (CAGE).

Symptoms of decompression illness

It is often difficult to determine if severe symptoms are due to AGE or DCS. Onset of symptoms varies from several minutes to hours after a dive. Early symptoms may point to AGE (minutes), while later symptoms may indicate DCS (minutes to hours). DCI may be precipitated by ascent to altitude even days after diving or occur following a single dive within decompression limits.

There is an increased risk of DCI following:
- Rapid ascent.
- Missed decompression stops.
- Repetitive diving over several days.
- Physical exercise soon after diving.
- Ascent to altitude (flights, mountain passes).
- Coincidental illness (particularly if dehydrated: fever or hungover).

Field treatment

DCI is often hard to recognize. Concealment and denial are common among divers because of the perceived stigma attached to DCI, as well as possible cognitive dysfunction and lethargy in the patient. Encouragement and awareness should be addressed prior to expedition departure.

Initial management

- Resuscitation: ABC.
- Administer 100% O_2 via rebreather mask or demand regulator.
- Lie flat if there is any concern for CAGE.
- Give fluids: oral if the diver is alert, otherwise IV.
- Early neurological examination, repeated regularly (Box 24.1).
- Seek expert advice (via available communications system).
- Do not forget the buddy.
- Consider early evacuation to recompression facility.

NB: symptoms may resolve during treatment with O_2, but (especially with neurological presentations) relapse is common without hyperbaric therapy. Do not stop transfer to medical facility even if symptoms appear to have resolved.

Box 24.1 Five-minute neurology exam for divers

Work through the following examination, marking abnormal findings.

Orientation:

a. *Person:* diver can tell you their name and date of birth.
b. *Place:* diver states where they are.
c. *Time:* to the nearest hour.

Eyes:

a. *Eye movements:* have the diver hold head still. Ask the diver to follow your hand (~18 inches (45 cm) from diver's face) while you draw an 'H' shape with your finger. Note any nystagmus.

(Continued)

Box 24.1 (Contd.)

b. *Vision*: diver can count fingers. Test each eye in turn.
c. *Pupils*: check they are equal and response to light.

Ears:

a. *Hearing*: close their eyes. Rub your thumb and finger together 10 cm from the diver's ear, check each side.

Face:

a. *Sensation*: check skin.
b. *Movements*: get diver to do the following in turn:
   • Raise eyebrows.
   • Screw up eyes tightly.
   • Show teeth.

Mouth:

a. *Movements*: get diver to:
   • Stick out tongue (tongue should be central).

Arms:

a. *Sensation*: test several points on both arms and shoulders.
b. *Movements*: get diver to do the following:
   • Shrug shoulders against resistance.
   • Straighten and bend the elbows against resistance.
   • Squeeze fingers.

Legs:

a. *Sensation*: test several points on both legs.
b. *Movements*: get diver to do the following:
   • Raise and lower the entire leg against resistance.
   • Straighten and bend the knee against resistance.

Coordination/balance:

If no symptoms since the dive and normal examination so far, ask diver to:
a. Walk normally.
b. Walk heel to toe.
   If any abnormalities are present, assume that you have a diving accident.

Evacuation

• Recompression becomes less effective as each hour passes. Most benefit is obtained within 6 h of onset, but some cases respond even after several days.
• First aid (O_2, fluids) should continue during transport.
• Keep dive computers/record of previous dives with the casualty.
• Unpressurized aircraft should be flown at the lowest safe altitude.
• Recompression treatment (and evacuation) is very expensive and divers should be appropriately insured.

Recompression treatment

Recompression protocols typically start with compression to 2.8 atmospheres (18 m/60 feet) on 100% O_2, with subsequent treatment based on clinical response. Most cases are treated using US Navy Table 6 (RN Table 62) with extensions if necessary. In remote areas, hyperbaric facilities may be limited and unable to sustain a treatment longer than this, even if it is required. Further hyperbaric O_2 sessions may then be given to improve any residual manifestations.

In water recompression

A controversial technique. It has been used when a diver is in an extremely remote location with no means of evacuation to dedicated facility or awaiting retrieval. If conscious level is reduced use a full face mask and have an attendant in the water. Hypothermia, seizures, and aspiration are significant risks. No high-level evidence currently supports its use.[4]

Intracardiac shunts

A patent foramen ovale (PFO) is a common opening in the heart between the left and right atria, which normally closes after birth. PFOs that are around 0.5–1 cm in size can cause bubbles to pass directly from venous to arterial circulation, bypassing the usual filtering of bubbles by the lungs, leading to emboli which causes damage to tissues.

Rapid onset of neurological, cardiovascular, and skin DCS (occurring within 30 min of surfacing) has been linked with the presence of a large PFO. The risk of DCS increases with the size of the shunt, and divers are often advised to be screened for a PFO using bubble contrast echocardiography after developing DCS. Options for a confirmed PFO include stopping diving, diving more conservatively (no-decompression dives, <15 m depth, one dive per day, nitrox with air planning) or PFO closure.[5]

4 Lippmann J, Mitchell S. *Deeper into Diving*, 2nd ed. Victoria: JL Publications; 2005.

5 Smart D, Mitchell S, Wilmshurst P, et al. Joint position statement on persistent foramen ovale (PFO). and diving. *Diving Hyperb Med*. 2015;45(2):129–131.

Barotrauma

Barotrauma is tissue damage due to a change in pressure altering the volume within gas-filled spaces such as sinuses, middle ear, facemask, teeth, gut, and lungs. Pressure must be equalized to avoid 'squeeze' during descent or 'overpressure' during ascent from a dive. The volume of an enclosed gas-filled space varies inversely with pressure (Boyle's law). Gas volume changes are greatest closest to the surface and most problems occur within 10 m (33 feet) of the surface.

Middle ear (tympanic membrane) barotrauma

- Common.
- Pressure/pain on ascent or descent.
- 'Muffled' hearing post dive owing to middle ear effusion.
- Transient vertigo.
- Sudden-onset relief of pain with or without vertigo.
- Tympanic membrane may appear inflamed and retracted.
- Return to diving: 24–48 h if no perforation has occurred. If perforation is present, diving should be avoided for at least 28 days and full otolaryngological review should be sought.

Inner ear barotrauma

- Rare.
- Rupture of the round window caused by pressure differential between inner and middle ear, usually because of excessive Valsalva manoeuvres.
- Severe persistent vertigo, distinguishable from transient vertigo on ascent and caloric vertigo from tympanic membrane perforation. Associated with a sensorineural hearing loss.
- Difficult to differentiate from DCI affecting the inner ear which may also cause severe vertigo; diagnosis may rest on the response to hyperbaric O_2 therapy.

Pulmonary barotrauma

Rapid expansion of alveolar gas during a fast ascent must be vented through the transmitting airways. If this cannot occur, owing to the diver forgetting to exhale, a closed glottis, or obstruction, it may rupture into surrounding structures or pulmonary blood vessels. *Always* consider life-threatening CAGE (see following section) following rapid ascent. Air expansion may cause the following:

Pneumothorax

- Air escapes into the pleural cavity.
- Symptoms include chest pain, breathlessness, and cardiovascular collapse.
- ABC approach, standard needle decompression using large-bore cannula plus chest drain.

Pneumomediastinum

- Air enters the mediastinum.
- Symptoms include central chest pain, voice change, neck swelling, subcutaneous emphysema, and cardiovascular collapse.
- ABC, O_2 (may be required for several hours) and evacuation to a specialist centre.

Cerebral arterial gas embolism

- Air enters pulmonary capillaries and is carried to the cerebral circulation.
- CAGE is difficult to distinguish from DCS, but rapid time of onset (often within minutes of surfacing) may influence the likely diagnosis.
- Symptoms include loss of consciousness, convulsions, and/or neurological deficits such as hemiparesis, weakness, or dysphasia.
- Treat as for DCS. ABC, 100% O_2, and hyperbaric recompression.
- Examine for other signs of barotrauma.

Immersion pulmonary oedema

IPO is a life-threatening condition that affects surface swimmers, including snorkellers and divers.

IPO is poorly understood and the relative risk is unknown. In IPO there is accumulation of fluid in the alveoli causing dyspnoea, cough, and frothy or blood-stained sputum. Progression leads to hypoxia and unconsciousness can occur. During diving, hypoxia may be exacerbated during ascent due to decreasing partial pressure of O_2. Divers often report that their equipment was not working properly, although tests confirm that it was working fine. The precise incidence is unknown.

Risk factors

- Hypertension and pre-existing cardiac disease.
- Cold water immersion.
- Exercise and stress.
- Excessive hydration.
- Inspiring against negative pressure while diving.
- Previous IPO.

Treatment

- Terminate dive, ascend safely, and exit water.
- ABC approach including O_2.
- Sit upright if conscious.
- Keep warm.
- May require hospitalization for further O_2 therapy, non-invasive ventilation, and diuresis.
- Avoidance of further diving until specialist opinion sought.

Other problems

Otitis externa

A common problem associated with repetitive diving. Exposure to water and subsequent shifts in pH cause bacterial growth in the external ear canal leading to skin inflammation. Symptoms include:

- Painful ears.
- Inability to equalize pressures.
- Hearing loss if severe.

Treatment

- Meticulous attention to hygiene—ensure ears are dried thoroughly after immersion.
- Some divers recommend alcohol drops to dry out outer ear after diving.
- Breaks in diving schedule may be required.
- Antibiotics are not normally required.
- Steroid plus antibiotic eardrops may help in severe cases.
- Condition increases incidence of tympanic membrane perforation.

Hypoxia

Altered consciousness as a result of reduced inspired O_2 concentrations is rare but should be excluded as a cause if a diving using a semi- or closed-circuit rebreathing apparatus develops an impaired cognitive state during a dive.

Other conditions

- Trauma—⮕ Chapter 7.
- Sunburn—⮕ p. 284–285.
- Dehydration—⮕ p. 67, 258, 420, 648, 687, 716, 731, 752, 800, 804.
- Motion sickness—⮕ p. 750–751.
- Heat illness—⮕ p. Hot, dry environments, Chapter 25.
- Hypothermia—⮕ p. 654–657.
- Marine envenomation including coral cuts—⮕ p. 314–315.
- Near drowning—⮕ p. 721–723.
- Water-borne disease—⮕ p. 710–713.

Expert advice

Relevant bodies include

- UK water: at sea call the Marine Coastguard Agency on VHF Channel 16, DSC Channel 70, or call 999 and ask for the Coastguard.
- British Hyperbaric Associations National Diving Helpline (England and Northern Ireland): Tel. +44 7831 151523.
- Scotland: Tel. +44 345 408 6008 (Aberdeen).
- Europe: Tel. +39 6 4211 8685 (Divers Alert Network).
- Africa: Tel. +27 828 106010 or 0800 020111 in South Africa (Divers Alert Network).
- Asia: Tel. +10 4500 9113 (Korea); Tel. +81 3 3812 4999 (Japan).
- Australasia and the Pacific: Tel. +61 8 8212 9242 (Australia); Tel. +64 9 445 8454 (New Zealand).
- In the USA/Caribbean: +1 919 684 8111 (Divers Alert Network).

Resources

Divers Alert Network: ℘ www.diversalertnetwork.org
UK Sports Diving Committee: ℘ http://ukdmc.co.uk/

Further reading

British Thoracic Society Fitness to Dive Group, Subgroup of the British Thoracic Society Standards of Care Committee. British Thoracic Society guidelines on respiratory aspects of fitness for diving. *Thorax*. 2003;58(1):3–13. https://doi.org/10.1136/thorax.58.1.3

Doolette D, Mitchell S. In-water recompression. *Diving Hyperb Med*. 2018;48(2):84–95.

Edmonds C, Bennett M, Lippmann J, et al. *Diving and Subaquatic Medicine*, 5th ed. Boca Raton, FL: CRC Press; 2015.

Chapter 25

Hot, dry environments: deserts

Chapter editor
Shane Winser

Contributors
Jon Dallimore
Tom Mallinson
Shane Winser
Sundeep Dhillon (1st and 2nd editions)

Reviewer
Harvey Pynn

The desert environment

Two of the most popular expedition destinations, deserts and tropical forests, seem very different. Deserts appear barren, arid, and have a very limited range of highly adapted plants and animals, while in contrast the hot and humid tropical forests (❍ Chapter 26) offer the world's richest land ecosystem.

Both environments require humans to live and work in high temperatures, but the high humidity in tropical forests places additional stresses on body physiology. Those living in temperate climates such as Northern Europe only occasionally experience heat waves and may be physically and mentally unprepared for heat stress. Heat illness is an important cause of death among travellers, including previously fit young adults. Endurance athletes and the military are especially at risk as they deliberately push their bodies even when environmental conditions are hazardous. An occasional short spell of heat in an otherwise temperate zone is especially hazardous to endurance competitors as they will have little physiological acclimatization to the conditions.

Deserts

A desert is a region with little vegetation and much exposed bare soil, where average annual rainfall is <20% of the amount needed to support optimum plant growth, and where plants and animals show clear adaptations for survival during long droughts. Covering almost 20% of the earth's landmass, deserts are mainly found between 25° and 35° north and south of the equator and are home to >1 billion people.

Some deserts consist of the sand dunes of popular imagination, but others are rocky wastelands or semi-arid grasslands. Diurnal and seasonal temperature ranges can be considerable, with the landscape sculpted by freeze/thaw cycles and by powerful winds driving sand, soil, or snow.

Clothing and footwear

Wear light-coloured, loose-fitting clothes made of natural materials that allow air to circulate and sweat to evaporate. Protect the head with a hat, scarf, or keffiyeh (shemagh). Shorts and T-shirts are also convenient and usually perfectly adequate but be conscious that such dress may cause offence in some countries. Where possible, check the UV protection factor offered by clothing—some materials are more effective at preventing sunburn than others. Exposed skin must be properly protected by sunblock, while in some conditions sunglasses or goggles may be essential.

Footwear needs to be light, comfortable, and tough; boots, shoes, and trainers all have disadvantages. Enclosed feet become sweaty, smelly, soft, and prone to fungal infections. On the other hand, bare feet or light shoes expose the feet to heat from the ground, injury by rock or thorns, and bites from snakes or scorpions. In sand and gravel deserts, walking sandals, trainers, or desert boots suffice; heavier footwear is required in stony or volcanic areas.

Bases and campsites

It is possible to travel for months in deserts without the need for formal shelter. A camp bed off the ground is protection against snakes and scorpions (but remember to shake your shoes and clothing out in the morning) and a tent, or impregnated mosquito net, will protect against insects. In many areas, the location will also need to be guarded against human or large animal invasion. Beware of making camps in dry riverbeds or wadis, which can be susceptible to flash flooding from rainfall many miles away.

Travel

Most desert expeditions use vehicles. These must be well maintained and have adequate tyres, tool kits, and spares to cope with the stresses of travel. Fuel consumption will be high. Ensure the party knows how to extricate a bogged vehicle, and do not lose the vehicle keys.

Travellers relying on more traditional travel methods will usually enlist the assistance of local stockmen or guides. If not, they will require suitable skills in animal husbandry, to keep pack animals healthy, content, and safely tethered at night.

Navigation

Journey times are often very long. Maps may be unreliable and roads little more than parallel tracks on the ground, invisible if the wind is blowing. GPS devices are invaluable but ensure suitable back-ups are available.

Risk management

Difficult travel

Considerable reserves of water, fuel, and food are essential to ensure safety in the event of bad weather, mechanical failure, navigational problems, or other unforeseen circumstances.

Dust storms

Dust storms can develop with little warning in any arid or semi-arid environment. These take the form of an advancing wall of dust and debris that may be kilometres long and over a thousand metres high; they can appear from any direction though generally follow the prevailing winds. Most storms pass within an hour, but some persist for several hours. High winds can destroy tents and strip campsites bare. Health risks include suffocation and silicosis from dust inhalation, and extremely low visibility both on roads and in the air leading to disorientation and the possibility of serious accident.

Survival strategies in a dust storm

- Don't panic!
- Avoid travelling in dust storms if possible.
- If caught in a dust storm while driving, get off the road. Turn off driving lights and turn on emergency flashers.
- If out in the open with a dust storm coming your way, sit down with your back to the wind, and cover your head with your clothes to keep dust out of your eyes, nose, mouth, and ears (a dry shemagh or bandana is ideal—wet clothing will quickly become clogged up). Goggles or other protective eyewear will provide much-needed protection when available.

Flora and fauna

Snakes and scorpions (➲ Chapter 17) live in deserts and may enter discarded footwear, clothing, or containers; both pose a significant danger to travellers and a fatal dose of toxin can be delivered by snakes such as the Nubian cobra (*Naja nubiae*) and side-winder adders (*Bitis peringueyi*), or potentially through the sting of scorpions such as the deathstalker (*Leiurus quinquestriatus*). Plants in arid areas can have thorns, tough spiny surfaces, or serrated leaves.

Heat-related illnesses

In hot weather, a major environmental risk is that of developing some form of heat-related illness (HRI). Humans originated in tropical regions and most people can adapt well to heat, but only after a period of acclimatization. Individuals vary considerably in their tolerance to heat stress, and the underlying mechanisms are not fully understood. Many people successfully complete endurance races such as the Marathon des Sables and Amazon Marathon in hot environments without incident, yet others may die while exercising on a hot day in temperate latitudes. Ultimately, if the duration and intensity is sufficiently challenging, everyone is vulnerable. Prolonged heat adds to the physiological stress and the risk of serious HRI is greatest following several days' exposure to hot and humid conditions.

Epidemiology

Classical HRI affects humans trapped in hot, unventilated environments; e.g. workers in mines, stowaways in freight containers, or children left in cars during heat waves. Individuals with impaired thermoregulation such as infants, the elderly, people with underlying medical conditions, or those taking drugs known to interfere with thermoregulation are at greater risk Problematic classes of drugs include: thiazide diuretics, Beta blockers, anti-histamines, anti-cholinergics prescribed for bladder disorders, stimulant medications for ADHD and some psychiatric medications. Increasing summer temperatures in normally temperate areas (exacerbated by urban environments where buildings can store heat and so raise night-time temperatures by 5°C) are increasingly producing urban heat waves and deaths among the frail and elderly. Heat waves have caused tens of thousands of premature deaths in Europe since 2000. It is predicted that heat waves will increase in the future.

The constant heat of jungles and urban environments constitutes a greater physiological stress than that found in deserts, where the nights are often cool.

Exertional HRI occurs as a result of physical exercise, and cases may develop even in otherwise temperate conditions if someone becomes dehydrated or overexerts themselves, sometimes in inappropriate clothing. It typically occurs during military exercises or during endurance sporting events. Exertional HRI is much more likely on expeditions than classical HRI.

Hyperthermia is also associated with some prescription drugs (such as suxamethonium or methoxyflurane) and recreational drugs such as cocaine, ecstasy, or amphetamines.

Heat exhaustion

Heat exhaustion is the most commonly encountered form of HRI. It occurs when the cardiac output is insufficient to meet the demands of increased blood flow to the skin, working muscles and vital organs. The effects are compounded by a decreased effective plasma volume (redistribution of blood), dehydration, and salt loss due to sweating. Heat exhaustion does not result in any organ damage and some individuals may be fit to resume normal activities after 24–48 h.

Exertional heat stroke

Exertional heat stroke (EHS) is defined as a core body temperature of >40°C caused by strenuous exercise and/or environmental heat exposure which is associated with CNS dysfunction and multiple-system organ failure (usually cardiovascular collapse). Heat shock proteins and cytokines contribute to a systemic inflammatory response syndrome (SIRS) similar to that seen in other critical illnesses.

EHS is most often associated with pale, sweaty skin, as opposed to the hot, dry, flushed skin of classical HRI. As tissue temperatures rise, cell membranes and enzyme-dependent energy systems are disrupted leading to cell and organ dysfunction and death. The extent of injury relates both to the duration of exposure and the severity of the rise in core temperature, but the seriousness of the condition cannot be predicted from these two parameters alone and requires laboratory confirmation.

Unfortunately, the symptoms of EHS are non-specific. Anyone looking unwell, or behaving abnormally in a hot or humid environment, or during vigorous exercise in a temperate climate, should be managed as a victim of heat illness until proven otherwise. Typically, sufferers from EHS will have more than two-thirds of the symptoms in Box 25.1, while someone who has a febrile illness instead of a HRI will show one-third or less. Box 25.1 may be used as a prompt and all symptoms and signs should be sought.

> **Box 25.1 Exertional heat stroke may present with the following features**
>
> - Anxiety.
> - Collapse.
> - Coma.
> - Confusion.
> - Convulsions.
> - Diarrhoea.
> - Delirium.
> - Dizziness.
> - Fatigue.
> - Headache.
> - Hyperventilation.
> - Impaired judgement.
> - Irrational behaviour.
> - Lethargy.
> - Loss of consciousness.
> - Muscle cramps.
> - Nausea.
> - Seizures.
> - Staggering.
> - Vomiting.
> - Weakness.

Incidence

EHS is not always recognized and may be diagnosed as exercise-associated collapse. The incidence appears to be on the rise as more people take up long-distance and endurance sporting events.[1]

Differential diagnosis of EHS in a previously fit person

- Acute-onset fever (especially malaria).
- Cerebrovascular event (stroke).
- Drug toxicity (including alcohol).
- Epilepsy.

1 Vicedo-Cabrera AM, Scovronick N, Sera F, et al. The burden of heat-related mortality attributable to recent human-induced climate change. *Nat. Clim. Chang.* 2021;11:492–500. https://doi.org/10.1038/s41558-021-01058-x

- Head injury.
- Hypoglycaemia (especially if diabetic).
- Hyponatraemia (excess rehydration with plain water).
- Ischaemic heart disease.
- Exertion collapse associated with sickle cell trait (ECAST).
- Arrhythmia.
- Inability to reduce core temperature to <39°C with evaporative cooling suggests that a febrile comorbid condition may be present.

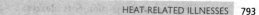

Pathophysiology of heat-related illnesses

Core temperature is the temperature of the vital organs such as brain, heart, liver, and kidneys. Normally it should remain relatively constant regardless of environmental conditions and at rest should be between 35.5°C and 37°C, with a measurement >37.5°C being abnormal. However, during vigorous and prolonged exercise, such as long-distance running on a hot day, core temperature rises and measurements up to 41°C have been recorded without apparent harm to the subject. Temperatures >41°C are almost always abnormal and harmful.

The human body is constantly working to maintain a stable core temperature. One way of doing this is to regulate the transmission of heat from the body core to the skin and extremities. Such transmission can be varied through modalities such as altering peripheral blood flow and sweat production.

The most critical factor in predicting the severity of injury in HRI is the duration of heat exposure following collapse. An elevated core temperature of 42–43°C can be tolerated for short periods (5–10 min) with little damage. For example, EHS during military training usually involves short exposures and rapid treatment, so while there may be large numbers of casualties, the mortality rate is often relatively low.

If core body temperature remains persistently elevated, metabolism becomes deranged and enzymes denature. The destructive processes are listed in Box 25.2.

Box 25.2 Pathophysiology of exertional heat stroke

- Cellular oxidative phosphorylation becomes uncoupled at temperatures >42°C.
- Cellular damage is directly proportional to the temperature and exposure time.
- Compensatory mechanisms for heat dissipation fail.
- Dehydration increases the sodium/potassium pump activity and increases metabolic rate.
- Complications may arise in multiple organ systems:
  - *CNS*: oedema and petechial haemorrhages cause focal and generalized damage.
  - *Muscle*: skeletal muscles show widespread degeneration of fibres. Rhabdomyolysis releases myoglobin, potassium, creatinine phosphokinase, and purines (which are metabolized into uric acid) into the circulation.
  - *Lungs*: non-cardiogenic pulmonary oedema.
  - *Kidneys*: oliguric acute kidney injury due to renal ischaemia, muscle breakdown products, DIC, hyperuricaemia, and hypovolaemia. Renal failure occurs in up to 35%.
  - *Blood*: DIC (poor prognosis), thrombocytopenia, leucocytosis. Thermal injury to endothelium releases thromboplastins which result in intravascular thrombosis and secondary fibrinolysis.
  - *Metabolic*: metabolic acidosis, respiratory alkalosis, hypoglycaemia, hyper- or hypokalaemia.

Physics of heat transfer

Heat transfer and hence changes in body temperature take place as a result of radiation, conduction, convection, and evaporation.

- *Radiation*: the direct transfer of heat between the body surface and all other sources of radiant energy. The main source of radiant energy in hot climates is the sun. Under clear daytime desert skies the sun can cause great heat stress, but at night heat radiates away from warm bodies.
- *Conduction*: the direct transfer of heat between the body and any solid or liquid in contact with it, particularly the ground. Conduction ceases when the two materials in contact reach thermal equilibrium.
- *Convection*: the removal of heat through the flow of one substance over another. Convection augments conductive heat transfer and prevents thermal equilibrium developing by constantly replacing one of the materials so heat transfer can continue.

The rate of heat transfer by conduction, convection, and radiation is dependent on the difference in temperature between the body surface and the materials, or radiating surfaces, in the environment. If the body surface is warmer than the environment, the body will lose energy to the environment. However, very warm air or surfaces will transfer heat to the body by conduction/convection, and sunlit surfaces or sky will transfer heat to the body by radiation.

- *Evaporation*: heat can be lost indirectly by evaporation of sweat. Each litre of sweat evaporated from the body surface at 30°C removes ~580 kcal of heat energy. If sweat drips off the body, it has not been allowed to evaporate, and therefore no heat is lost. Sweating (and therefore evaporative heat loss) occurs when internal heat production exceeds the capacity of direct routes of heat transfer to dissipate it. Importantly, when the environment is sufficiently hot to cause heat gain by the direct transfer routes, evaporative cooling is the only thermoregulatory mechanism available to control body temperature.

Biology of heat transfer

Approximately 80% of metabolic energy is produced as heat in muscles—by normal metabolism, during exercise, and through shivering—and is conducted to the skin, where it is lost to the environment. The circulation of the blood augments and regulates this heat transfer by varying superficial blood flow. Clothing further modifies heat loss by acting either as a conductor or an insulator. At rest with an ambient temperature of 20°C, conduction and convection account for only ~10% of our heat loss, the majority occurring by radiation.

Once environmental temperature rises to >35°C it is impossible to lose significant heat through conduction, convection, or radiation. Our ability to survive and function in higher temperatures depends upon the ability to sweat.

Sweating allows the body to lose heat at any environmental temperature through evaporation, but evaporative heat loss can only occur if the air is not saturated with water vapour. So, sweating is most efficient in hot, dry deserts and is less effective in hot, humid rainforests. Therefore, humidity has a greater effect on the ability to lose heat than the absolute temperature.[2] See Table 25.1.

---

2 Morimoto T. Heat loss mechanisms. In: Blatteis CM (ed) *Physiology and Pathophysiology of Temperature Regulation*. Singapore: World Scientific Publishing; 1998: 80–90.

Table 25.1 Heat transfer

Mode of heat transfer	Contribution		
	25°C	30°C	35°C
Radiation	67%	41%	4%
Conduction and convection	10%	33%	6%
Evaporation	23%	26%	90%

The body's response to thermal stress

Changes in temperature are detected by both sensory nerve endings in the skin and by direct sensing of blood temperature in the hypothalamus of the brain. At rest, the skin receives ~9% of the total circulating blood flow. A rise in core temperature of as little as 0.1°C will increase skin blood flow to dissipate the heat, and under high heat stress skin blood flow can increase fourfold. Heat energy is then lost directly to the environment by a combination of radiation, conduction, convection, and by evaporation of sweat. High environmental temperatures also lead to behavioural changes such as reduced activity, seeking shade, and drinking more.

During physical work, blood flow is directed to the working muscles and away from the intestines. This limits the ability of the gut to absorb water to around 1200 mL/h. If the rate of fluid lost in sweat exceeds this amount, then dehydration will occur. Anyone working in these conditions must be allowed adequate rest periods with fluid replacement. If blood flow is further distributed to the skin to allow evaporative heat loss, then the effective circulating volume is further decreased. An adequate blood volume is therefore required to ensure that thermoregulatory blood flow can occur.

Measurement of core temperature

Measuring body temperature accurately is difficult and medics need to be aware of the limitations of the various techniques. In hospital the best ways to measure core temperature are by the use of central venous or oesophageal sensors but neither is practical on most expeditions.

Rectal temperature can be measured using simple portable equipment, but there may be poor correlation between the rectal temperature and the severity of symptoms; fatalities have been reported with rectal temperatures of 39.5°C, while victims have survived core temperatures of 47°C. During active cooling, there may be rapid changes in temperature of the blood as demonstrated by the sudden onset of shivering, but there is a significant lag before this body temperature change is seen rectally.

A systemic review of febrile critically ill patients concluded that rectal temperatures were overestimated and inaccurate, but oral and tympanic temperatures more accurately reflected core (pulmonary artery catheter) temperature.[3]

---

3 Jefferies SS, Weatherall MM, Young PP, et al. A systematic review of the accuracy of peripheral thermometry in estimating core temperatures among febrile critically ill patients. *Crit Care Resusc.* 2011;13(3):194–199.

Oral temperature measurement requires a conscious and cooperative patient to allow accurate placement of the bulb underneath the tongue for sufficient time to ensure thermal equilibrium. Furthermore, the patient should not breathe through the mouth during temperature measurement.

The tympanic membrane shares its blood supply with the hypothalamus (the body's thermostat) and changes in body temperature are measurable sooner at the tympanic membrane than at other external sites. Tympanic measurements can, however, be inaccurate if localized cooling to the face or head has occurred. Ear temperature probably offers the best compromise between the lag associated with rectal temperature measurement and the impracticalities and inaccuracies of oral temperature measurement, particularly in a semi-conscious patient.

However, for ease of use, most infrared ear thermometers are calibrated to read the mid-canal temperature, rather than the temperature of the tympanic membrane. Some thermometers (e.g. Braun Thermoscan® models) correct for the site of measurement, but false readings may occur for a variety of reasons. Proper technique is important; a clean probe cover should be used each time, the ear must be free of wax and water, and the ear canal should be straightened (pull the ear up and back). If in doubt, treat the clinical signs rather than be reassured by a single measurement of temperature.

Acclimatization to heat

Full acclimatization to heat develops at different rates in different individuals; typically, 10–14 days are required for all the physiological changes to develop. The rate of acclimatization depends upon several factors, including body shape, the severity of the heat stress, and pre-existing physical fitness.

Benefits of acclimatization
- Reduced resting HR.
- Increased blood volume.
- Reduced core and skin temperature.
- Decreased salt loss in sweat (may drop from 60 mmol/L to 5 mmol/L).
- Increased sweat production (at lower core temperatures).
- Increased blood flow to skin.
- Improved renal sodium and water retention (aldosterone mediated).
- Increased plasma proteins maintain extracellular fluid volume and reduce tachycardias.
- Decreased glycogen consumption.
- Improved ability to exercise (➲ Fig. 25.1, p. 803).

Physiological acclimatization enhances evaporative heat loss while reducing cardiovascular strain. Exercise becomes easier and exercise syncope, common on day 1, rapidly declines to zero by day 5. The increased sweat rate (0.5 L/h to 2 L/h), coupled with the increased blood flow, can increase heat loss by a factor of 20, but requires a significant increase in water consumption before, during, and after activity.

Some degree of acclimatization can be obtained in temperate climates before departure. Hot baths twice a day, saunas, and exercising while wearing more clothing than normal may be effective. In a hot, dry climate, rapid acclimatization requires about 2 h of exercise per day sufficient to raise HR to around two-thirds of maximum, which should be conducted during the cooler hours of the morning or evening. Acclimatization may be delayed if substantial portions of the day are spent in air-conditioned environments. In comparison to dry heat, acclimatizing to hot, humid climates, especially if the heat is unremitting, is much harder, and initial exercise tolerance will be substantially lower.

Sweating can only remove heat if there is sufficient fluid to spare. Sweat production rates can reach 2 L an hour for short periods and can be up to 15 L a day. In low-humidity environments such as deserts where evaporation is rapid, the daily cooling capacity of the sweating mechanism is adequate to maintain body temperature even during vigorous work, but in humid environments such as tropical forest, evaporation is ineffective and slow, so exercise must be limited to avoid overheating.

Sweat is a hypotonic (dilute) solution of sodium chloride. The concentration of sodium chloride in sweat depends on the sweat rate and the degree of acclimatization. Higher sweating rates reduce the opportunity to conserve salt, and the sweat salt concentration rises, but acclimatized sweat glands conserve salt more effectively by producing more hypotonic sweat. In addition to conserving salt in sweat, humans acclimatized to heat start sweating at lower body temperatures and their kidneys conserve salt more effectively. As a consequence, an acclimatized person in a hot environment requires no more salt than an unacclimatized individual in temperate conditions and can maintain lower body temperatures for any degree of heat stress.

Jungle acclimatization readily transfers to desert climates (hot and dry) but the reverse journey requires further acclimatization to humidity. The benefits of acclimatization are lost over 20–40 days after returning to a temperate environment.

Prevention of heat illnesses

Heat stress is the product of the interaction between:
- The individual.
- The environment: temperature, wind, sun, and humidity.
- The workload of the task being undertaken.

Assessment of risk must consider each of these factors.

> **Prevention of heat illness**
> - Identify individuals at risk.
> - Monitor environmental heat stress (ideally the wet bulb globe temperature (WBGT) index; see **→** Evaluating environmental heat stress, p. 801–802).
> - Adjust the daily expedition activities accordingly.
> - Educate everyone about the nature of heat illness: prevention, early recognition, and treatment.
> - Provide adequate clean drinking water, shade, and latrines (inadequate toilet facilities may discourage drinking).
> - Ensure that a robust medical evacuation system is in place.

The individual

An individual is best able to cope with heat stress when:
- Fully hydrated.
- Physically fit.
- Acclimatized.
- Well nourished.
- Well rested.

Dehydration reduces both blood flow and sweating, so that a dehydrated person has reduced ability to maintain a constant body temperature in the heat. Acclimatization and physical fitness enable high temperatures to be better tolerated, but do not reduce water requirements; indeed, a fit acclimatized person will usually drink more than a new arrival to a hot environment.

Thermoregulation can be impaired by:
- Lack of sleep.
- Missed meals.
- Fever or recent pyrexial illness.
- Sunburn in the previous 3 weeks increases the risk of heat illness.
- Recent air travel.
- Use of therapeutic medications (Box 25.3).
- Other causes of relative dehydration such as diarrhoea.

People with any of these conditions should be watched closely for signs of heat distress and should avoid excessive exertion. If one member of a party develops symptoms of heat stress, then leaders and medics should assume that everyone else in that group who has been exposed to similar heat stress is a potential heat casualty.

A few individuals appear to have a genetic predisposition to developing heat illness. Previous heat illness should alert one to a recurrence. However, the data are variable and victims of previous EHS may cope perfectly well with subsequent heat stress.

Box 25.3 Medications that increase risk of heat illness
- ACE inhibitors.
- Alcohol.
- Amphetamines.
- Anticholinergics.
- Antihistamines.
- Beta-blockers.
- Calcium channel blockers.
- Cocaine.
- Desmopressin.
- Diuretics.
- Laxatives.
- Major tranquillizers.
- Phenothiazines.
- SSRI antidepressants.
- Theophylline.
- Tricyclic antidepressants.

Evaluating environmental heat stress

Four environmental characteristics influence heat stress:
- Air temperature.
- Solar (or radiant heat) load.
- Absolute humidity.
- Wind speed.

Environmental heat stress can vary greatly and unpredictably over short periods of time and space. On a calm, sunny day, an open field may present a greater heat stress than an adjacent forest, but on a windy, cloudy day the forest may present the greater heat stress.

Three of these four factors are combined into an internationally accepted measure of heat stress, the WBGT index, developed by the US military in the 1950s.
- Wet bulb (Tw)—measures absolute humidity.
- Black globe (Tg)—measures solar load.
- Dry bulb (Tamb)—measures ambient air temperature in the shade.

$$\text{WBGT} = 0.7\text{Tw} + 0.2\text{Tg} + 0.1\text{Tamb}$$

Several manufacturers now produce relatively cheap devices capable of measuring and calculating WGBT; suppliers can be readily accessed online. In some states in the US, measurement of WGBT is mandatory before sports are played in hot weather, with risk management procedures dependent upon the heat stress. Elsewhere, organizers of sporting events and expedition leaders should consider planning activities around the value of WGBT. Further details of this and other temperature indices, are available through the websites listed at the end of the chapter (➔ Resources, p. 811).

If you do not have access to equipment for measuring WBGT, consider evaluating heat stress using the workload calculations described in the following section and Table 25.2.

Table 25.2 Recommended maximum workloads in various conditions

	Workload			Work-rest cycle (per hour)
	Light	Medium	Heavy	
WGBT	30.0	26.7	25.0	Continuous work
	30.6	28.0	25.9	45 min work/15 min rest
	31.4	29.4	27.9	30 min work/30 min rest
	32.2	31.1	30.0	15 min work/45 min rest

The wet bulb temperature is the most important component of the WBGT index, which reflects the thermoregulatory importance of evaporation in hot (especially humid) environments, but the index does not include wind speed, another important environmental modifier, within its calculation. Air movement increases convective heat transfer and will assist evaporation; cool winds reduce heat stress, but hot winds increase it. The American College of Sports Medicine provides guidelines for exercise in hot environments and recommends cancelling sporting events if the WBGT is >28°C.

Workload calculations

For expeditions lacking meteorological facilities, an alternative method of judging a safe workload pattern has been suggested[4]:
- Each individual should work out their maximum HR (220 minus their age in years) (e.g. a 40-year-old will have a maximum HR of 220 − 40 = 180 beats/min). Many people will have a smart watch or similar HR-measuring device which can be very valuable.
- Multiply the age-adjusted maximum HR by 0.75 (e.g. 75% age-adjusted maximum = 180 × 0.75=135 beats/min).
- The group should all work to the lowest figure obtained.
- The group should undertake the proposed activity for one work period (e.g. 30 min) under close supervision.
- Immediately after this initial work period everyone should recheck their HR.
- If anyone's HR exceeds the 75% age-adjusted maximum, the next working period should be reduced by one-third (e.g. to 20 min with 40 min rest).
- The group should rest in the shade and rehydrate for the remainder of the hour.
- Repeat the process until the 75% age-adjusted maximum is not exceeded.
- Unless they are lean, athletic, and very fit, women tend to tolerate heat less well than men, and their exercise rates should be adjusted accordingly.
- Fig. 25.1 indicates the rapid improvements in exercise tolerance that develop with acclimatization.

4 https://doi.org/10.1152/ajpregu.1999.276.6.R1798

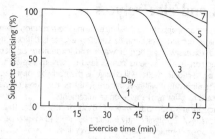

Fig. 25.1 Improved exercise duration with acclimatization during a standard exercise regime in hot conditions. Reproduced from Piantadosi CA (2003). *The Biology of Human Survival.* Oxford University Press.

Fluids and electrolytes

Maintaining an appropriate fluid balance during the transition from a cool to a hot climate, or during endurance sporting events is difficult. Inadequate fluid intake, excessive ingestion of water, and inadequate or inappropriate use of electrolyte supplements can all lead to serious health issues. Fluid and electrolyte requirements will change as the body becomes acclimatized to heat. Each individual will have different needs at different times and this makes it hard to offer firm advice on requirements.

A reduction in total body water (TBW) of 1% affects thermoregulation and losses of 2% significantly impair physical and mental performance. Thirst is a poor stimulus to drink and TBW losses of 5–10% have been tolerated in experiments. Fluid must be consumed before, during, and after physical activity to maintain normal hydration (euhydration). This is most easily assessed by dipstick measurement of the specific gravity of the first urine of the day (a specific gravity of ≤1.020 can be considered as euhydrated), along with changes in daily body weight performed at the same time (and before and after activity). Weight loss is common on expeditions and caused not only by dehydration, but also by increased work-load, GI upset, and decreased appetite due to heat and unfamiliar food.

Even when a person is significantly dehydrated, urine is still produced and the volume of fluid required to return to full hydration must be at least 1.5 times that lost in sweat (assuming the individual was fully hydrated before the onset of activity). Women have a lower proportion of water in their bodies and may be at greater risk of dehydration than men.

Dehydration

If an individual drinks only enough to satisfy their thirst they may become chronically dehydrated, particularly if they drink substantial amounts of caffeine-containing drinks, which act as diuretics. It is essential that personnel working hard in any environment are made aware of the need to drink water despite not feeling thirsty. Expedition leaders must enforce work/rest cycles, and provide adequate shade. If toilet facilities are unpleasant or lack privacy, travellers may seek to avoid visits by drinking less. Clean and screened facilities will encourage proper drinking habits—especially if the party consists of easily embarrassed youngsters.

Thirsty = dehydrated. Dehydrated *does not* = thirsty.

Hydration can be monitored by the colour and quantity of urine along with how often one needs to pass urine. Dark yellow urine is a sure indicator that the individual is dehydrated, as is the need to urinate less than twice a day. Lying and standing BPs may be useful when assessing heat casualties; a difference of >15 mmHg in the systolic pressure suggests dehydration.

People with diabetes need to maintain good glucose control as blood glucose >10 mmol/L will result in glucose in the urine and consequent osmotic diuresis producing lighter coloured urine. This could be mistaken as indicating adequate hydration whereas in reality it would be masking, and at the same time worsening, dehydration.

Water supplies

In hot environments, water losses can reach 15 L/day per person. Complete replacement requires realistic estimates of potable water requirements, adequate water logistics, and individuals who understand and act on their water requirement. Water for hygiene and cooking will be needed in addition to water for drinking.

Where water supplies are unsafe, expedition leaders must ensure that adequate provision exists to purify sufficient water for the group's requirements. This may be flavoured to increase palatability. If chlorine or iodine is used, there should be a method of removing the unpleasant taste at the point of use (→ Water purification, p. 108–114). Locally purchased bottled water may not be a safe alternative, as such supplies may be recycled plastic bottles which have been refilled from a local, and possibly contaminated, water source.

As it is harder to tamper with, carbonated water may be a preferred alternative. However, as carbonated water and fizzy soft drinks may fill the stomach with carbon dioxide before sufficient water has been ingested to combat dehydration, they should not be relied upon as the only source of fluid.

Choice of replacement fluid

New arrivals in a hot climate will lose more salt in their sweat than normal and should supplement their salt intake until they become acclimatized. Salt tablets are best avoided as they contain an unknown amount of sodium and may irritate the stomach. Salt tablets may also cause an osmotic gradient and retain water in the gut. Table salt should be made readily available at meal times, and this can also be added to fluids in sensible amounts (around half a teaspoon of salt in 1 L of water with sugar added to improve palatability). Soups are an excellent source of both fluid and salt.

The oral rehydration solution recommended by the WHO has a sodium content of 60–90 mmol/L, but this high sodium content significantly reduces palatability, with resultant reduced consumption. Therefore, while this recipe is life-saving in cases of diarrhoeal illnesses, its use cannot be recommended for fluid replacement in healthy people operating in the heat.

Sports drinks manufacturers have heavily promoted their products as the ideal way for active adults to replace the water and salt lost in sweat. Their value is controversial, with some athletes believing that they increase endurance and reduce the risk of heat cramps, while others doubt their value. Some sports drinks are sold as powders. Dissolving excessive amounts of powder in the hope of increasing absorbed energy produces hypertonic fluids that do not quench thirst and enhance the effects of dehydration. Always mix such powders according to instructions.

A 2012 *BMJ* review concluded that water remains the best replacement fluid, but that overhydration is a bigger risk than dehydration during running events up to marathon length.[5] However this advice may not apply when prolonged heat exposure leads to substantial additional salt losses.

5 Cohen DD. The truth about sports drinks. *BMJ*. 2012;345:e4737–e4737. https://doi.org/10.1136/bmj.e4737

Fluid-induced hyponatraemia

In the absence of serious HRI or renal failure, dehydration by itself does not cause unconsciousness. Competitors participating in endurance races can develop symptomatic hyponatraemia if they drink excessive amounts of plain water or hypotonic fluids. Stomach bloating, weakness, and collapse may be followed by unconsciousness. The risk increases with endurance activities >4 h in length.

* Hospitalization is necessary.
* Cerebral oedema can develop.
* Avoid giving further water.
* The bladder should be catheterized and urine output monitored.
* Salt-containing foods may be given during recovery.
* Extreme hyponatraemia results in coma, collapse, or decreased GCS score.
* Hypertonic saline (150 mL of 3% saline) can be given IV over 20 min. This can be repeated until serum sodium has risen 5 mmol/L or to >125 mmol/L.

Without laboratory facilities it will probably be impossible to distinguish between collapse from symptomatic hyponatraemia and collapse because of a HRI. Both are life-threatening conditions and require urgent medical support.

The use of desmopressin (DDAVP) for the treatment of nocturnal enuresis has been linked to the death of a young traveller on an expedition (➔ Nocturnal enuresis, p. 554).

Treatment of heat illnesses

The goal of treatment is to return the casualty's core body temperature to within the normal range as rapidly as possible in the prevailing situation.

Remove the casualty from sources of heat and place them in the shade. Lying down maximizes heat loss through conduction, but only if the ground or mattress is no warmer than the surrounding environment. A string hammock is ideal for encouraging heat loss as it enables air to circulate over the whole body.

The most rapid cooling (with lowest morbidity and mortality) is achieved by immersing a casualty in a bath or pool of iced-water (2–15°C). Therefore, a children's paddling pool may be a suitable piece of first-aid equipment for expeditions or event organizers to provide. Cold water immersion does hold certain risks, most notably airway compromise if the patient subsequently falls unconscious or has a seizure. Aggressive cooling using ice-water-soaked towels or ice packs achieves reasonable cooling. If using ice-cold water, immerse only to the level of the umbilicus as there is a risk of vagal response with slowing of the HR and drop in BP. Evaporative cooling using wet towels and fanning is less effective, especially in humid conditions, but is probably the mainstay of treatment on expeditions. The casualty should be continuously sprayed with cold water and fanned to encourage evaporation. Alternatively, a wet sheet may be wrapped around the casualty and kept constantly moist with cold water.

In some countries, a simple solution to heat exhaustion is to lie the victim in a tepid running stream, but beware that they could become unconscious, that the stream could be polluted, or that aggressive animals may be encountered.

Oral or IV fluids may be given, the latter being more effective in serious cases. At the Hajj pilgrimage, cold IV infusions of up to 1 L of normal saline or glucose saline at 5°C for heatstroke and 12°C for heat exhaustion have been used successfully. Frequently casualties also suffer from hypoglycaemia, and glucose could be administered orally or IV when a capillary blood glucose monitor is not available. No more than 2 L of IV fluids are normally required.

A heat-injured casualty who has not been cooled and yet is shivering is seriously ill. They may complain bitterly of feeling cold. They will not feel hot or thirsty. They will look pale and have cold skin. They will want to be wrapped in warm clothing, which only increases their core temperature further, as does shivering. They must have their core temperature measured to exclude heat illness or a febrile illness such as malaria.

During cooling, the return to a normal temperature is often associated with shivering. It is important to continue to monitor core temperature, as the casualty's thermoregulatory capacity has been damaged and these individuals are at continued risk of either hyperthermia or hypothermia.

Some of the effects of heatstroke, such as renal or hepatic failure, only develop after 24–72 h. As it is impossible to distinguish accurately between heat exhaustion and heatstroke, all casualties with neurological signs or symptoms (particularly confusion) should be evacuated to a hospital with intensive care facilities.

Management of heat stroke

- Undertake a primary survey using the CABCDE mnemonic.
- Ensure adequate oxygenation and ventilation; consider ventilatory support and supplemental oxygen.

- Remove from heat source where possible.
- Undress the casualty while commencing rapid cooling.
- Start rapid cooling (Table 25.3). Aim to reduce core temperature to <39°C as rapidly as possible.
- Consider administering 1 L of cold 0.9% saline over 10 min (at 5–10°C).
- Seizures should be managed as normal (➜ p. 272–273).
- Monitor urine output.
- Monitor HR and BP.
- Body temperature characteristically remains unstable for several days following a severe acute episode. Aim to avoid further heat stress for several days.
- Make plans for evacuation to an appropriate facility, but do not delay cooling to facilitate transport.

Advanced medical care

- Airway—unconscious patients require support and may need intubation and ventilation.
- Cardiorespiratory collapse—IV fluids and BP monitoring may be required.
- Fitting—may require IV lorazepam, PR diazepam, or buccal midazolam.
- Renal failure—may require catheterization to monitor urine output, careful fluid balance, and possibly dialysis.
- Liver failure—may develop several days after the initial episode.
- Dantrolene—used in the treatment of malignant hyperpyrexia does *not* appear to help in other HRIs.
- Antipyretics—including anti-inflammatories such as NSAIDs and paracetamol (acetaminophen) are valueless and may exacerbate renal and hepatic failure.
- In serious cases of heat stroke, the value of a period of controlled induced hypothermia, similar to that employed following cardiac arrest, should be considered.

Table 25.3 Methods of casualty cooling

Cold water immersion	Water temperature should be between 2°C and 15°C
	Immersion for 15–20 min should lower core temperature by ~3–4°C
Icy wet towels	Immerse towels in ice water. Remove from water and cover the patient's body
	Leave in place for 2–3 min then replace with fresh icy wet towels
Running water	Where ice water is unavailable, place the casualty under a cold shower of water
Wet and fan	Cover casualty with wet sheets and direct fans onto their body. Ensure the sheets are kept cool and wet
Cold IV fluids	1–2 L of cold saline (4°C) over 30 min to 1 h
Ice packs	Apply ice packs to the whole body, being cautious not to cause cold injury

Other heat-related problems

Heat syncope

Fainting on standing in the heat is thought to occur because of blood pooling in the legs and increased blood flow to the skin. When standing, the blood supply to the brain is temporarily reduced, causing loss of consciousness. Although most cases of heat syncope are harmless, the potential for heat illness should be considered, especially following physical work in the heat, or if occurring after the acclimatization period. Treat by allowing the patient to rest in a cool environment and oral fluids, recovery should occur within 20 min. Underlying cardiac disease or medication such as beta-blockers may precipitate heat syncope.

Heat oedema

Mild swelling of the limbs may be experienced during the first few days of exposure to heat, as the plasma volume increases to facilitate increased blood flow to the skin. Cutaneous vasodilatation and pooling of increased interstitial fluid in dependent extremities results in swelling of the hands and feet. It is self-limiting, resolving in a few days; elevating the affected extremities, resting in cool environments, and compression stockings may help. Diuretics should not be used.

Exercise-associated muscle (heat) cramps

Heat cramps are painful skeletal muscle spasms following prolonged exercise, often in the heat. They usually occur in the arms, legs, or abdomen from prolonged exercise and are thought to be due to dilutional hyponatraemia, but also occur in cool conditions (e.g. swimming). Treatment is rest, prolonged stretches of affected muscle groups, and oral sodium replacement, either with isotonic drinks or by adding half a teaspoon of salt to 1 L of water with two tablespoons of sugar. If the individual is otherwise well, there is no association with heat illness, but a raised core temperature should be treated promptly. Prolonged heat cramps not responding to treatment should prompt the measurement of serum sodium and the consideration of other possible causes (e.g. sickle cell crisis, rhabdomyolysis, etc.).

Heat tetany

Hyperventilation, triggered by exposure to a high heat environment, can cause a relative alkalosis. Subsequent increased binding of free calcium to circulating albumin leads to a relative calcium deficit in the blood, resulting in paraesthesia (often in extremities and around the mouth) and spasm of the muscles in the hands and feet. It is less painful than heat cramps, with the large muscle groups not being involved. Treatment is through removing the casualty from the hot environment and coaching their breathing back to a normal rate.

Miliaria rubra ('prickly heat')

Miliaria rubra is an inflammatory skin eruption, which appears in actively sweating skin in humid conditions (or skin covered by clothing in dry environments). Each lesion represents a sweat gland which has become blocked in the dermis or epidermis, usually by keratin and therefore cannot function properly. The risk of heat illness is increased in proportion to the amount of skin surface involved. Sleeplessness due to itching and secondary infection or inflammation of occluded glands (miliaria pustulosa) may further affect thermoregulation. Miliaria is treated by cooling and drying affected skin, avoiding sweating, controlling infection, and relieving itching. Sweat gland function recovers with replacement of the damaged skin, which takes 7–10 days.

Prevent if practicable by wearing loose, airy cotton clothing and taking regular cool showers. Treatment consists of frequent bathing in cool water, gently dabbing skin dry to prevent further damage, and application of calamine lotion. Talcum powder should not be routinely used, as it may block sweat glands. Air conditioning can help if available. Sedative antihistamines such as chlorphenamine (Piriton®) may help to relieve symptoms and promote sleep at night, but sedative drugs should be avoided during the daytime as they may increase risk of accidents (e.g. with machetes, machinery, or when driving). Topical steroids such as hydrocortisone 1% cream may help to relive itching and inflammation.

Sunburn

Sunburn reduces the thermoregulatory capacity of skin and also affects central thermoregulation; aim to prevent sunburn by insisting on the use of adequate sun protection. Sunburnt individuals should be protected from significant heat stress until the burn has healed (see also ➲ p. 65, 284–285).

Skin infections

Wound and skin infections are common in hot conditions and are covered in ➲ Chapter 9.

Resources

American College of Sports Medicine Position Stands:
Exertional Heat Illness during Training and Competition: ℘ http://journals.lww.com/acsm-msse/Fulltext/2007/03000/Exertional_Heat_Illness_during_Training_and.20.aspx
Exercise and Fluid Replacement: ℘ http://journals.lww.com/acsm-msse/Fulltext/2007/02000/Exercise_and_Fluid_Replacement.22.aspx
Australian government: Bureau of Meteorology. Thermal comfort observations and details of temperature calculation and estimation. ℘ http://www.bom.gov.au/info/thermal_stress/
Singapore Army. Evidence-based guidelines for the management of heat illness. ℘ http://www.smj.org.sg/sites/default/files/5110/5110cpg1.pdf

Further reading

Bennett BL, Hew-Butler T, Hoffman MD, et al. Wilderness Medical Society practice guidelines for treatment of exercise-associated hyponatremia: 2014 update. *Wilderness Environ Med.* 2014;25(4):S30–S42.
Lipman GS, Gaudio FG, Eifling KP, et al. Wilderness Medical Society clinical practice guidelines for the prevention and treatment of heat illness: 2019 update. *Wilderness Environ Med.* 2020;30(4S):S33–S46.
O'Brien KK, Leon LR, Kenefick RW, et al. Clinical management of heat-related illnesses. In: Auerbach P, Cushing TA, Harris NS (eds). *Wilderness Medicine*, 7th ed, Mosby; 2017: 267–274.

Chapter 26

Hot, humid environments: tropical forests

Chapter editor
James Moore

Contributors
Jon Dallimore
Larry Goodyer
James Moore
Paul Richards
Shane Winser

Reviewer
Harvey Pynn

NB: this chapter should be read in conjunction with ➲ Chapter 25, particularly the sections on heat illness.

The tropical forest environment

Tropical forests cover a dwindling 5% of the Earth's landmass and are defined by their location (between the tropic of Cancer and the tropic of Capricorn). They can be broadly separated into five types:

- *Lowland equatorial evergreen forests*: archetypical tropical forest such as the Amazon and Congo Basins.
- *Moist deciduous forests*: Central American, Caribbean, Indian, and Indochina.
- *Montane rain forests*: cloud forests found between 1500 and 3000 m, e.g. Bolivian Yungas or Malaysian Cameron Highlands.
- *Flooded forests*.
- *Freshwater swamps*.

Expedition preparations should be tailored to the particular biome visited. Primary (un-logged) tropical forest, where the high tree canopy suppresses ground growth, is more open and easier to travel through than logged forest. Logging removes the tall canopy trees allowing more light to reach the forest floor and creating greater secondary plant growth. Travel becomes restricted to pre-cut trails.

Weather

During the day tropical forests are hot and humid, often with little breeze to give respite, but at night they become much cooler, and travellers in montane forests will require a blanket or lightweight sleeping bag. The forest floor, especially in flooded forests, may be under water for much of the year.

Rainfall varies between biomes and may exceed 2 m annually. Seasonal variations in weather patterns (such as dryer seasons or monsoons) can be expected, depending on the forest type and location. Typically, cumulonimbus storm clouds develop during the day, leading to intense rainfall mid to late afternoon.

Humidity

The combination of high temperatures and high rainfall ensures the humidity remains high for much of the year in most tropical forests, affecting not only the health of individuals, but also the operation of equipment. Everything gets damp, and it is very difficult to dry things out. Silica gel sachets may help to reduce moisture in medical kits, bags, and containers holding sensitive and electronic equipment.

Biting insects

Insects are the most prolific of all creatures in the tropical forest environment and will rapidly invade every part of camp life. Insects can bite, irritate, and infest; they may transmit serious illnesses such as malaria (➲ p. 512–520) and dengue fever (➲ p. 494–495), filarial diseases, and a variety of tick-borne diseases.

They may be attracted by:

Carbon dioxide from respiration or stoves.

- Scented deodorants or antiperspirants.
- Smelly feet and boots.
- Food.
- Poor personal hygiene.

There is a three-tier approach to insect bite avoidance and all three methods should be used. Barrier (e.g. clothing), area (e.g. mosquito coils), and applied repellent methods.

Barrier

During the day, wear appropriate clothing that should include good ankle and leg protection. The hazardous malaria-carrying mosquitoes emerge at dusk and usually bite during the night. During daylight, clothing needs to be appropriate to the task in hand. Once dusk falls, it is sensible to spend as much time as possible wearing appropriately protective clothing, which may include items impregnated with permethrin (➲ p. 516–517), and remaining inside screened accommodation. At night, sleep under permethrin impregnated mosquito nets.

Area

An area method of discouraging mosquitoes involves the use of an insecticide or other irritant released into the atmosphere. A smoky campfire will provide this to some extent, and local people will often burn the remains of disused insect nests. Probably more effective is burning 'mosquito coils' near a seating area in camp. An insecticide spray is useful for clearing a tent of insects before retiring.

Repellents

Repellent products containing the active ingredients shown in Box 26.1 should be used. If applied at the same dose, each of these active ingredients is probably equally efficacious at preventing mosquito bites, though IR3535 may be less effective against malaria-carrying species. Overall, DEET has been the most widely researched and shown to be reliable against a range of species of mosquitoes.

Two key elements should be considered when applying repellents: how much of the active ingredient is applied, and the activities/environmental situation. For the first parameter, use of a product containing 30–50% of active ingredient is recommended. Quite a generous application is required (as with sunscreen). Once applied, the length of protection will be determined by the numbers/biting pressure of mosquitoes, sweating, unintentionally rubbing off repellent, and wet/rainy conditions.

The rule of thumb is to consider reapplying the repellent should the mosquitoes be 'taking an interest' again after previous application. Note that when manufacturers state the product lasts 'up to 12 h', it really means that in many tropical jungle situations, this time could be as little as 1 h.

Box 26.1 Insect protection and repellents[1]
(See also ➲ Box 15.3, p. 516.)

The annoyance and hazard of insects may be reduced by use of:
- *DEET* which can help in the prevention of mass insect invasion. A few squirts on tassels wound around the strings of a hammock, or on the guy ropes of a tent will divert insects elsewhere. Note: DEET in high

---

1 Goodyer LI, Croft AM, Frances SP, et al. Expert review of the evidence base for arthropod bite avoidance. *J Travel Med*. 2010;17(3):182–192. https://doi.org/10.1111/j.1708-8305.2010.00402.x

concentrations will dissolve man-made fibres and plastics. 50% DEET is adequate.
- *20% picaridin*: a modern repellent of comparable efficacy to DEET that does not degrade man-made fibres.
- *P-menthane-3,8-diol (PMD)* is an isolate of the lemon eucalyptus plant and has been shown to have similar efficacy to DEET although much shorter duration of action. It must not be used on children <3 years and can cause irritation to the eyes.
- Smoke from a campfire. Smouldering, vacated insect nests are often used in the Amazon.
- Insecticides such as permethrin.
- Insect repellent coils can help in enclosed spaces, but there must be ventilation.
- Reducing the amount of artificial light used after sunset.

Other repellents such as citronella oil or candles, or Skin So Soft® have *not* been shown to be as efficacious and should be avoided. Remember that the half-life of most repellents applied to skin is reduced in hot, humid conditions, as sweat will remove the agent.

See also ➲ Arthropods, p. 590–591.

Other animals

Tropical forests are home to several species of animals large enough to cause harm to humans (➲ Chapter 17). To minimize the risk of a dangerous encounter:
- Obtain good local knowledge about dangerous animals.
- When siting camp, avoid animal tracks—especially if they lead to a waterhole. Be particularly wary of wild boars, peccaries, hippos, crocodiles, and elephants.
- Store food in appropriate containers, away from sleeping and communal areas.
- Be cautious around rivers and lakes. Large reptiles and animals will attack while humans and animals are near the water's edge.
- Be especially cautious using head torches by the water's edge at night. This may attract animals.

Birds

Generally birds do not pose a threat to humans although large birds such as the cassowary have been known to cause serious injuries if provoked. They may, however, be vectors for transmissible diseases such as salmonella, bird flu, and Japanese encephalitis.

See also ➲ Ectoparasitic infestations, p. 306–310, and ➲ Leeches, p. 310–311.

Plant hazards

(See also ➲ Chapter 18.)

Approximately two-thirds of all plant species grow within tropical forests. Consuming any part of an unidentified plant is hazardous, as is remaining below a rotten tree whose branches could break, or where any species is liable to drop nuts or fruit. Many plants and grasses can cause irritation and or injury.

Plants are a natural source of food for insects and animals and so have developed defence mechanisms. Many contain poisons in their fruit, sap, flesh, or foliage, e.g. *Solanum americanum* (American nightshade) that contains the neurotoxin solanidine, or the highly poisonous *Strychnos nux-vomica*, also known as the strychnine tree. If human skin comes into contact with these plants, it should be irrigated as rapidly as possible; itching and discomfort can be relieved using topical steroids. In more serious cases both parenteral corticosteroids and hydrocortisone cream may be required, and very occasionally these plants may cause an anaphylactic reaction (➲ p. 256–257).

Identification of the toxic plant will be difficult without extensive subject knowledge, but useful for appropriate treatment guidelines. Where possible the use of telemedicine and remote-photographic identification should be considered. Individuals should be made aware of the dangers of eating unidentified plants and fruit found in the tropical forest, or drinking water collected from vines or leaves.

Other plants protect themselves by spines, barbs and needles, e.g. *Acacia cuspidifolia* (wait-a-while), or many of the 600 species of *Calameae*—commonly known as rattan. Foreign bodies left in the skin after contact with spine-bearing plants should be removed rapidly, observed for infection, and treated accordingly.

Finally, some plants use a combination of needles and poisons, such as *Dendrocnide moroides*, or the 'stinging bush' native to northeastern Australia and Indonesia. This species is clothed in hollow silica hairs filled with a potent neurotoxin. On contact, silica hairs penetrate the skin and remain stuck, releasing toxin and causing pain and discomfort for several weeks. The irritant hairs can be removed using adhesive tape or hair-removal waxing strips.

Hazards of tropical forests

Before embarking on a tropical forest expedition, consider how the environment is likely to affect the participants' safety. Important risk factors include:

Topography

- Falls due to steep-sided ravines and cliffs.
- Rivers prone to flash flooding.
- Thick vegetation hindering communications and navigation.
- Camp design and layout.

Climate

- High rainfall.
- High humidity.
- High temperatures.

Forest living and travel

- Deadfall—dead trees and branches supported by the canopy but which can fall down in even light winds.
- Falling branches and debris in recently logged forest.
- Trip hazards—muddy, slippery paths, roots, rattan.
- Lack of ambient light—particularly at dusk when sunset occurs in a matter of minutes.
- Sunburn especially during the middle of the day; in clearings and if travelling in the open or on boats.
- Contact with biting insects and hazardous spine-bearing plants.
- Disorientation and navigation errors. Plan lost-person search procedures (→ p. 154–156).
- Journey times must take account of difficulty of terrain.
- Consider how a non-ambulant casualty could be evacuated.
- Appropriate jungle equipment and clothing.

Health and well-being

- Heat—new arrivals must acclimatize to the environment, heat, and humidity. Physical exertion must be limited until full acclimatization has occurred. Death from heat stroke may occur. Visitors should be aware of the hazards of both dehydration and hyponatraemia (→ p. 804–806).
- Water supplies must take account of high fluid requirements—especially among poorly acclimatized newcomers.
- Insect-borne diseases, especially dengue and malaria (→ Chapter 15).
- Cuts and grazes can quickly become infected and untreated can lead to tropical ulcers (→ p. 312).
- Tropical immersion foot and fungal infections (→ Chapter 9).
- Jungle psychology (→ p. 826–828).

Safe travel in tropical forests

Traditionally, travel through forests has been by foot or waterway, but in recent years roads have been cut through many tropical forests to obtain natural resources. Planning should consider not only normal movement through the forest, but also how supplies can be brought in or a casualty evacuated.

For most non-indigenous groups, the forest micro-topography, high temperatures, and humidity mean that travel by foot will be slow and physically demanding. Waterways provide easier and faster passage, and can provide access to remote areas by canoe, powerboat, float plane, or helicopter, although they have their own hazards including fast currents, waterfalls and cataracts, submerged obstacles and debris, and reptiles, hippopotamuses, and other large animals.

Forest roads may be poorly maintained and hazardous with large vehicles travelling at speed. Avoid driving at night. In the event of a traffic collision, warning signals should be placed by or in the road several hundred metres either side of the accident and it is essential to carefully search the surrounding jungle for casualties thrown clear but hidden by dense foliage.

Navigation

The absence of visible references, such as the sun or landmarks, makes navigation in tropical forests difficult. Without visual references, winding paths and difficult terrain can be very disorientating. Any available maps are likely to be small-scale, making accurate navigation and pacing difficult although large navigable waterways are often well charted.

Steep valleys and high tree canopies restrict the use of satellite navigation and communication equipment. Electronic navigation equipment should not be relied on in tropical regions—as with anything electronic, they are prone to failure.

The most accurate and safest method of navigation in tropical regions is by using reliable local guides and a good compass.

Search and rescue

(See also ➋ p. 154–156).

Locating lost or injured casualties is very difficult in tropical forests. Shouts and cries do not carry far, while visibility is very restricted both on the ground and from above, limiting the use of aids such as heliographs, smoke, or flares. Electronic communications can warn rescue agencies of a problem but amid dense vegetation on steep hillsides it can still be very difficult to locate a party. Even if a helicopter is available, topography, weather conditions, and tall trees can make it impossible to land or winch a casualty, who may have to be transported some distance to a clearing and then nursed for an extended period until medevac becomes possible. No member should leave camp without a personal survival kit (➋ p. 828).

Living safely in tropical forests

Living safely in the jungle requires knowledge and sound fieldcraft, which should be learned and practised before arrival. Managed successfully, tropical forests can be an immensely satisfying environment in which to live and work.

Campsite management

- Look upwards when setting camp: site shelters away from rotting trees or branches that could crash down ('deadfall').
- Consider the animals and insects likely to be affected by setting up camp. Minimize interference with animals' natural food supplies and carefully assess areas for the presence of insect colonies such as hornet nests.
- Low river banks are access points to and from the water for wild animals. Check potential campsite for animal spoor and droppings.
- Ensure all paths around the camp are well marked and clear from obstacles.
- Provide group areas with some form of shelter.
- Sleep off the ground to avoid snakes, scorpions, etc. A hammock, mosquito net, and basha combination is the best form of accommodation in the jungle. Hammocks are now available with an integrated mosquito net, which reduces complicated sleeping set-ups and the number of guy-ropes needed.
- Expedition medics will benefit from an 'over-sized' basha or tarpaulin, allowing more space should they need to assess and treat patients.
- Leaf litter can hide snakes and scorpions, so this is best cleared from the ground beneath hammocks.
- Abandoned shelters may be structurally unsound and can harbour spiders, ants, rodents, and snakes which feed off them. Even when the fauna have left, they are potential sources of infections such as histoplasmosis (➔ p. 848) and Chagas' disease (➔ p. 524–525).

Fuel

- Fuel is one of the most important components of survival in a tropical forest. Fuel is needed for heating, cooking, sterilizing water, and generating light. The most common source of fuel used in a tropical forest is wood and one should not underestimate quantities required for even modest use. Wood should be collected and stored with care as snakes and scorpions will often use woodpiles as homes or shelters. Keep wood piles well away from the kitchen and living areas.
- Those responsible for collecting and using wood fuel should learn to use it efficiently, reducing the environmental impact.
- Petroleum and diesel should be stored in a well-marked place away from any fires or cooking areas. When siting the fuel dump ensure there is no possibility of accidental spillage reaching water sources.
- Ideally, there should be a method of extinguishing any fire around fuel storage areas, such as buckets of water/sand or fire extinguishers.

Light

- Tropical sunsets are considerably shorter than those in the northern and southern latitudes and it is important that individuals have a torch with them at all times. The jungle canopy dims sunlight during the day and causes an almost complete 'blackout' at night.
- Key areas of camp should be well lit or easily identified at night:
  - Communal area.
  - Latrines.
  - Kitchen.
  - Medic's basha.
- Even with a generator it may be impractical to keep a camp lit at all times for the duration of the expedition. Small LED lights last longer than traditional battery-powered lights, and solar-powered lights may have some benefit although may struggle with charging under a canopy. Teams must learn to conserve light source energy and always have a back-up in case of emergency.
- Glow-sticks are a useful source of emergency light. However, they have a limited light duration.
- Lanterns are commonly used for light on expeditions. These are generally run on liquid fuels (sometimes under pressure) or gas. Not only are these an obvious fire hazard, but they also emit fumes which are poisonous in enclosed spaces.
- Single-cell LED lights are very useful as an emergency light. They are low cost and often have intermittent or flashing settings. Placing one inside a balloon will create a large, glowing sphere.

Water and sanitation in tropical forests

Water

In the tropics daily drinking fluid requirements may rise from 3 L/day to as much as 8 L/day, depending on work load and humidity. By their very nature, tropical forests have an abundance of water; however, it is not always easily accessible.

Water can be collected from streams, wells, rivers, and lakes but must be treated appropriately. If a ground water source is unavailable, consider the use of tarpaulins or bashas to collect and funnel rainwater. It is wise to filter and treat rainwater to remove particles collected from the canopy. See ➔ Water purification, p. 108–114.

Each member of the team should carry at least 2 L of water with them at all times.

Sanitation

Careful disposal of human waste in the jungle is important as it can quickly find its way into water sources or the animal food chain.

Jungle latrines

In tropical forests the top 15 cm is where most bacterial activity takes place, so only a shallow scrape or latrine trench is required. Latrines should be sited downstream of any local water source to minimize risk of contamination.

'Long-drop latrines' are not appropriate in most jungle environments. Unless professionally designed and sited, they do not allow for the natural decomposition process to occur.

Toilet paper and sanitary items

If storing toilet paper and sanitary items at the latrine, make sure they are kept in a container suitable for the conditions present, preferably animal- and waterproof.

Toilet paper and sanitary items should be burnt. This can be on an individual basis, or stored and collected as part of the latrine rota, then burnt at the end of the day with other rubbish.

Latrine rota

Where possible, a latrine rota should be established. Tasks include:
- Digging new trenches.
- Re-siting urinals.
- The marking of new/old latrines.
- Ensuring an adequate supply of toilet paper is available.
- Ensuring that there is sufficient alcohol gel for hand cleaning.
- Ensuring there is soap/detergent by the water.
- Burning toilet paper and sanitary items.

See also ➔ Sanitation and latrines, p. 115–116.

Humans in the tropics

Humans in heat and high humidity

In hot climates, the human body becomes increasingly dependent upon sweating to maintain normal body temperature. In tropical forests, high humidity and lack of breeze limit evaporation rates. At ~80% relative humidity, perspiration fails to evaporate, drastically reducing its cooling effect. Evaporation of sweat is only an effective cooling mechanism if the moisture evaporates on or close to the skin surface, but in hot, humid conditions sweat frequently runs off ineffectively, continuing to dehydrate the individual. Until acclimatized, this fluid loss will be associated with salt depletion.

Expedition leaders must be very aware of the debilitating and potentially hazardous combination of heat and humidity experienced by new arrivals in the tropics. Heat illness and evaluation of heat stress are discussed in ➲ Chapter 25.

- Weather conditions in the tropics are usually consistent which should permit analysis of likely heat stresses before departure. However, heat waves or unusually high humidity on arrival may require plans for activity to be further modified.
- Pressures of an expedition may make it hard to limit exercise in certain circumstances, but youngsters in particular should not be required to trek long distances in high levels of heat and humidity.
- Until team members have acclimatized, maximum work intensity and duration must be adjusted according to the ambient heat and humidity levels (➲ Table 25.2, p. 802).
- It is important to get both fluid balance and salt intake correct. Both dehydration and excessive intake of water can be hazardous (➲ p. 804–805). Fluid loss through sweat alone in humid environments can exceed 2 L/h, therefore fluid and electrolyte replacement is vital. Ensure adequate fluid, salt, and carbohydrate intake throughout the day. Add salt to food rather than relying on salt tablets. Oral rehydration sachets are useful for electrolyte replacement but ideally should only be used in the presence of illness. Excessive fluid intake can lead to hyponatraemia (➲ p. 806).

Clothing and equipment

The tropical forest environment is unforgiving in its treatment of clothing and equipment. Without proper care both will degrade rapidly, as a result of environmental conditions and effects from flora and fauna. Clothing should be manufactured from tough, snag-proof man-made fibres. Natural fibres rapidly become waterlogged with sweat and rain. Clothing should cover arms and legs to prevent scratches and reduce the effect of insect, animal, and reptile bites. In some areas of the tropics, local people will wear 'snake-gaiters' or 'leech protectors'—canvas or cloth over-socks up to the knees.

- Waterproof clothing will keep rainwater out, but increase the wearer's body temperature, thus leading to counterproductive sweating inside the clothing. Consider a waterproof poncho or compact umbrella as an alternative.

- Accept daytime wetness. Rinse kit in camp and re-wear wet next day. Keep a set of clothing in a dry bag, as well as your sleeping system for evening and bedtime use to preserve comfort and skin.
- Never go barefoot or wear sandals; you risk cuts, insect or snake bites, larva migrans, jiggers, etc.
- Use boots with good tread (Panama soles) that dry quickly. De-roofed blisters could develop into ulcers, so ensure that boots are properly worn-in before entering the jungle.
- Waterproof socks, such as Sealskinz™ (or even plastic bags) are useful should one need to get up at night and keep feet dry.
- Cover up—long sleeves and trousers protect you from irritant plants and insect bites.
- Lycra shorts will help to prevent leeches and other insects from reaching the more intimate body parts.
- Gloves protect against sawgrass cuts, especially when using a machete.
- Hats with a brim protect against sun, rain, and barbed leaves.

Personal skills

- In camp, personal sleeping space should be kept clean and tidy. When not in use, kit should be kept packed away and bags fastened shut to prevent infestation by insects, snakes, or other small animals. Mosquito nets should be tied up and off the ground.
- At night, ensure boots are kept off the ground, upside-down on sticks, or with the boot-neck fastened shut or blocked. Open boots can attract scorpions, snakes, and spiders. Check every time you put your boots back on!
- Minimize risk of insect bites (➲ p. 305, and ➲ Box 15.3, p. 516).
- Be wary of snakes (➲ p. 580–590) and scorpions (➲ p. 594–595).
- Avoid trauma. Learn correct use of machete—sheathed when carried and not in use.
- Practise crossing rivers safely but avoid whenever possible.
- On log bridges, balance is aided by fixing eyes ahead and use of a walking pole.
- Beware water contamination with heavy metals such as mercury from gold mining in the Amazon. This will not be removed by boiling, but filters using activated carbon should reduce the risk (➲ p. 108–114).
- Learn to navigate using map and compass. GPS is useful but may require wide clearings as the canopy impedes the signal. Use trails, walk in file keeping team members in sight, use guides, and place a designated person at the back of the group as tail marker.
- Rise at dawn and make a camp an hour before nightfall.
- Cicadas singing indicate ~30 min of daylight remaining. Ensure you have a torch handy and get a fire lit before the arrival of the tropical night.
- Respect local customs, including those of dress (➲ p. 122–124).
- Theft—many expeditions are supplied with food, equipment, and clothing costing more than the local village's annual income. Overt displays of wealth should be avoided.
- Avoid ingesting local hallucinogenic plants or drugs (➲ Chapter 18).

Useful equipment

- *Machete:* a key piece of tropical forest kit is the machete or parang. It should be made of a tool-grade steel or similar and come with a file or sharpening steel to maintain a sharp edge. Before using a machete ensure the area is safe and free from others. Only the first person in the column should have an open machete. A wrist loop is useful. Ensure the knife has a full tang (the blade metal extends into the handle as one continuous piece) Cut using small movements and stand leading with the dominant leg and hand, i.e. if you hold the machete in your right hand, have your right leg forward. Ensure inexperienced group members are given sufficient training in the use of machetes.
- *Dry bags:* very helpful to keep your kit dry in camp, during rain, or while crossing rivers.
- *Slings and karabiners:* useful for keeping kit off the ground.
- *Paracord and 'gaffa' tape* will fix most things in the jungle.
- *An umbrella:* ideal for walking around camp in a downpour.
- *Personal survival kit:* many seasoned tropical forest veterans will recommend keeping an army-style 'belt kit'. This holds, within a few belt pouches, enough equipment to survive a night or two in the jungle alone. Among other things it would contain:
  - A sturdy pocketknife.
  - A whistle.
  - A compass.
  - A torch.
  - A fire lighting kit:
    - Lighter.
    - Tinder/accelerant.
    - Flint and steel.
  - Water purification tablets.
  - Paracord.
  - An energy bar or other snack.

The most important thing about any piece of equipment is to know how to use it before it is required. This is especially true in the tropics.

Tropical-related illnesses

Heat illnesses—see ➲ Heat-related illnesses, p. 790–792.
Acclimatization to heat—see ➲ Acclimatization to heat, p. 798–799.
Treatment of heat illnesses—see ➲ Treatment of heat illnesses, p. 808–809.

Psychological stress

Unfamiliar sounds, smells, fear of animals, disease, the intense darkness of night, or the isolation of sleeping exposed in a hammock in a strange place may contribute to anxiety. Encourage team members to learn about the environment, listen to the local guides, and become informed. Fear arises from unfamiliarity and uncertainty; knowledge helps you to find the forest accommodating rather than intimidating.

Prolonged exposure to wet discomfort saps morale, so regular return to a comfortable environment such as a well-constructed base camp is important. 'Social time', particularly for sharing the evening meal and general relaxed chat, is important for team integrity and morale. All expedition members should be briefed on:

- Bite prevention and malaria chemoprophylaxis.
- Safety, lost person, and SAR plan.
- Hammocks/machete/clothing.
- Dangers of the heat and humidity.
- Ensuring an appropriate water intake.
- Deadfall (dead timber in the canopy that may fall in high winds).
- Animal hazards.
- First-aid treatment of snakebite and other bites/stings (➲ Chapter 17).
- Water hazards.

Stress that some diseases such as malaria will not manifest themselves until after return, and that in the event of an illness doctors must be informed of the recent overseas trip. GPs in a temperate country may be unfamiliar with the signs and symptoms of tropical illness and it may be appropriate to seek referral to a specialist infectious or tropical disease unit.

Finally, it is important that team members are sufficiently fit for jungle life. Poor physical fitness makes it harder to cope with the cardiovascular effects of heat stress and acclimatization takes longer. Overweight individuals are at increased risk from HRIs, both because excess body fat acts as insulation and because they have to use extra energy to move around arduous and demanding terrain.

Tropical ulcers

See ➲ p. 312.

Tropical immersion foot

Tropical immersion foot is a dermatological condition resulting from the skin being in contact with warm water for >48 h. The skin becomes hyperhydrated, ulcerates, and breaks down. Although difficult, prevention is far better than cure:

- Allow time every night for foot care.
- In the evenings, ensure feet are clean and dry.
- Use a light dusting of medicated foot powder.
- When possible and where appropriate, use flip-flops or sandals around camp to give feet 'air-time'.

Other fungal infections

See ⊃ Chapter 9.

Tropical infections

See ⊃ Chapter 15:

Yellow fever (⊃ p. 38–40) occurs in South America and Africa with 90% of cases reported from Africa.

African trypanosomiasis (sleeping sickness) occurs in a number of small areas scattered throughout West, Central, East, and southern Africa (⊃ p. 523).

Lassa fever and other viral haemorrhagic fevers (⊃ p. 495).

Leishmaniasis (⊃ p. 522–523).

Marburg and Ebola viruses which have caused epidemics of highly fatal haemorrhagic fever in Equatorial Africa, Congo DR, Sierra Leone, and Uganda (⊃ p. 496).

Elephantiasis (lymphatic filariasis) (⊃ p. 526).

Melioidosis, a dangerous infection caused by soil-dwelling bacteria in South East Asia, Northern Australia, and the tropical Americas (⊃ p. 504–505).

Tropical medical kits

Medical kits for tropical forest expeditions should be robust and designed to keep water out. The rugged and humid nature of the jungle will quickly cause medicine labels to degrade, metal components to rust, and kit bags to fail.

The medical kit should be kept in a dry, well-ventilated area and be sealed sufficiently to prevent insect invasion. Consider the use of silica gel sachets to keep the contents dry.

For discussion of medical kit contents, see ⊃ Chapter 28.

Chapter 27

Caving

Chapter editor
Jon Dallimore

Contributors
Paul Cooper
Simon Flower
Craig Holdstock

The environment underground

Caving, cave diving, and mine exploration are dangerous sports carrying certain specific risks. Any significant trip underground demands a good degree of 'cave fitness', along with specific skills, judgement, and psychological composure, generally acquired through years of practice. Non-caving medics are therefore unlikely to find themselves on cave rescue teams or caving expeditions, where they risk becoming a liability.

While accidents underground are uncommon among experienced cavers, they have significant consequences for the casualty, with extended pre-hospital times and a difficult and often hazardous extrication process. Whether on expedition or not, casualty management will be hindered by limited equipment, a suboptimal and often dangerous working environment, and poor lines of communication. The best qualified medics (such as trauma or pre-hospital specialists), will often be unable or unwilling to assist. Collectively, this puts a unique spin on standard pre-hospital care; a pragmatic approach is often required.

Abroad, cave rescue services may be limited or non-existent (especially in those countries with unexplored caves), and expeditions may not have the means to deal with significant mishap. Thought also needs to be given to the potential for cave-related diseases. Fortunately, most issues on expedition tend to be minor, or at least surface related.

An understanding of the potential risks underground is essential in planning for their eventuality.

Medical problems underground

Hypothermia

(See also ➋ p. 654–657.)

Although modern caving clothing helps protect against hypothermia, the risk remains, particularly in alpine caves—where temperatures hover only a few degrees above freezing; in wet caves outside warm climates; and among injured, dehydrated, and exhausted cavers. A small survival bag and a thin balaclava, carried in a pocket or helmet, provide effective first aid, and all cavers should be encouraged to carry them.

Useful equipment for an underground 'hypothermia' bag include:

- Food (simple carbohydrates) and fluids.
- Group shelter ± candle/solid fuel stove.
- Roll mat.
- Additional insulation (including balaclava/hat).
- Vapour barrier. This will be more convenient than changing into dry clothes, especially for stretcher cases.
- Chemical heat pads, for application to axillae and chest.

A Blizzard® bag or blanket (🖰 www.blizzardsurvival.com) is recommended. They pack up small, and perform as a space blanket, insulation, and vapour barrier, and with optional heat pads are a source of heat. Airways warming devices, traditionally used by cave rescue teams, are unlikely to do much more than prevent further heat loss via the respiratory route.

Casualties with stage 2 hypothermia (non-shivering and/or impaired consciousness), require urgent evacuation to the surface. Dry clothing and vapour barriers will only slow down the rate of heat loss. The casualty must be carefully supervised throughout evacuation and sudden posture changes avoided as they could induce arrhythmias.

If a casualty is unconscious or apparently dead (stage 3 or 4 hypothermia) provide oxygen (O_2) if available, and *carefully* package and evacuate the casualty to the surface. Even if there are no signs of life, it is usually better to wait until out of the cave to start CPR unless a mechanical device is available. Rough handling (including heavy-handed insertion of airway adjuncts, changing into dry clothes, and CPR) can precipitate ventricular fibrillation. Once in ventricular fibrillation, it will be impossible to reverse underground. Even intermittent CPR (5 min on, 5 min off) will be impractical in most cave rescue situations and will slow evacuation to an unacceptable degree.

Trauma

While any type of trauma may occur, dislocations of the patella and shoulder are disproportionately common underground, as are ankle injuries. Consider in advance how to manage these underground (➋ p. 842–843).

Cold casualties and ubiquitous mud mean that IV analgesia/sedation should be avoided if possible. Consider using medications that can be given via inhalation, intranasal, or buccal/sublingual routes (e.g. methoxyflurane, ketamine, fentanyl, buprenorphine), balancing the narcotic and sedative effects against the ideal of keeping the casualty mobile and so avoiding a stretcher rescue. Prolonged and often rough rescues mean that nerve blocks (particularly a fascia iliaca block) should also be considered (➔ p. 630–631).

See discussion of cervical spinal injuries (➔ p. 218–221).

Crush injury

(See Fig. 27.1.)

In caves, crush injury typically occurs following a rockfall, but can result from smaller forces applied over longer periods, such as when a caver slips into a tapering rift.

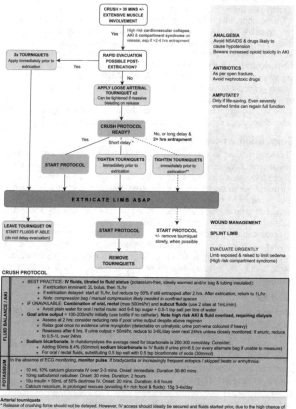

Fig. 27.1 Crush injury algorithm.

Aside from the immediate injury to the limb, there is a significant risk of cardiovascular collapse, acute kidney injury, and compartment syndrome on release ('crush syndrome'). The severity of this reaction will depend upon both the muscle mass involved, and the magnitude and duration of the crushing force. The crushing force should therefore be released as soon as possible. However, IV access should ideally be obtained prior to this, with fluids started and the heart monitored for signs of hyperkalaemia. Underground, these resources will either be unavailable, or take a considerable time to assemble. Although still debated, consideration should be given to the application of a temporary tourniquet, which will allow the crushing force to be released and the evacuation process begun while keeping the casualty safe from reperfusion injury.

If evacuation time will be short, the tourniquet can be kept on until more definitive care is reached. However, if the evacuation will be prolonged, and resources fail to materialize or cannot be improvised (e.g. oral, rectal, and SC fluids), this decision will be more difficult; extended tourniquet times are themselves associated with local tissue damage, loss of limb, and a more pronounced reperfusion injury on release. While up to 2 h of ischaemic time is generally considered 'safe', nerve injury can occur beyond this and, by 6 h, many casualties will need amputation. It may therefore be best to reserve tourniquets in these circumstances for those in whom reperfusion injury will present a significant risk to life (e.g. large muscle mass, >2 h crush).

Suspension syncope ('harness hang')

Pooling of blood in motionless, gravitationally dependent legs leads to presyncopal symptoms even in healthy individuals. Ultimately, it causes loss of consciousness and, if not addressed, death within a few minutes. It is a particular risk to cavers who are rendered unconscious while suspended in a sit harness (which further impedes venous return) or tilted upright for a period of time during a stretcher rescue (when shock or dehydration can exacerbate the effect—see ⊃ p. 716).

Presyncopal symptoms can be improved by movement, raising the legs, or, ideally, standing in a foot loop. An unconscious casualty on rope is a medical emergency. They should be urgently lowered to a horizontal surface, raising the legs to the level of the core as a temporary measure. Familiarity with mid-rope rescue techniques is paramount in achieving this.

Bad air

Bad air can be encountered in both natural caves and mines, but the latter are particularly hazardous (Table 27.1): high concentrations of carbon dioxide (CO_2), hydrogen sulphide (H_2S), carbon monoxide (CO), or methane (C_2H_4) can displace O_2, poison someone outright, or create an explosion. Coal mines are especially prone to containing these gases. It is important to seek out local knowledge before entering disused mines and, where appropriate, employ gas analysers.

Carbon dioxide

The most important underground gas hazard. Levels are usually elevated in caves, and easily approach 1% (vs atmospheric levels of 0.04%). However, they can be much higher because of poor ventilation, traffic build-up in small passages, rotting vegetation (especially in tropical areas), or nearby geothermal activity. Naturally occurring levels of up to 7% have been recorded.

Hyperventilation is the first sign (often mistaken for lack of fitness or nerves). Respiration rates and fatigue increase in proportion to rising levels, along with headaches and nausea with prolonged or higher exposures. The exact physiological response depends on the O_2 concentration (itself variable, depending on the cause of CO_2 build-up), and varies widely between

Table 27.1 Types of bad air in caves and mines

CO_2	*Found in caves and mines (see main text)*
	1% increased respiration (barely perceptible)
	2% headache after several hours
	3% ×2 respiratory rate, slight headache
	4% ×3 respiratory rate, bad headache, nausea, flushed
	7–10% violent respiratory distress and loss of consciousness after a few minutes
O_2	*Low O_2 rare in natural caves unless associated with rotting organic matter (when CO_2 will be elevated)*
	<17% laboured breathing ± impaired judgement
	<16% flame extinguished
	<10% risk loss consciousness
H_2S	*Found mainly in mines (especially coal). Rare in natural caves, unless nearby geothermal activity*
	0.003 ppm: odour detectable (rotten eggs)*
	250 ppm: unconscious
	1000 ppm: death
	Safe working limits: 8 h = 5 ppm, 15min = 10 ppm
	* Prolonged exposure and higher concentrations nullify the senses, leading to false reassurance that the gas has gone. If smelt, retreat, as highly toxic
C_2H_4	*Found mainly in mines (especially coal). Rare in natural caves unless copious rotting organic matter*
	Odourless, highly explosive >50 000 ppm
	May asphyxiate in higher concentrations
CO	*Found in mines (a by-product of combustion)*
	400 ppm: headache, collapse after 2 h rest/45 min work
	2000 ppm: loss of consciousness after 30 min rest/10 min work
	Safe working limits: 8 h = 30 ppm, 15 min = 200 ppm
NO_2	*Produced by explosives*
	Effects depend on concentration and duration of exposure:
	0.12–0.5 ppm: odour detectable (pungent, acrid, ammonia-like)
	13–25 ppm: eye, nose, throat irritation (though may occur at 4 ppm if exposed for 1 h)
	When suspected, use a gas analyser. Do not rely on your senses alone for detection, as higher concentrations and prolonged exposure can cause severe/fatal respiratory effects (may take 3–30 h to develop). Safe working limits: 8 h = 0.5 ppm, 15 min = 1 ppm

individuals. Some deteriorate and collapse when levels reach 3–6%, while others may tolerate effects for several hours. There is ordinarily one 'canary' on a team who will serve as a warning to others that levels are elevated.

Consider taking a CO_2 monitor if caving in areas where CO_2 is known to be a problem, particularly if abseiling. The effects of CO_2 poisoning may not be recognized until well committed when dropping into a CO_2-rich pit, by which time the changeover and prusik out may prove extremely difficult. A flame test can be useful but relies on low O_2, which may not be sufficiently depleted to extinguish the flame. While evacuating from affected areas, life-line even simple climbs as judgement can be affected and even minor exertion will be difficult. Symptoms resolve rapidly on removal from the contaminated atmosphere but, after significant exposure, headaches and nausea can persist for many hours.

Fumes from explosives

Explosives (usually used to progress exploration or widen passages for rescue) are generally safe in trained hands. However, their fumes are a highly toxic mix of gases including CO_2, CO, and nitrous oxides (especially NO_2), all of which can linger for some hours after an explosion—a hazard therefore to cavers too close to, or returning too soon after, the site of a 'bang'. The use of small diameter detonating cord has greatly reduced this risk, although its plastic covering can release other harmful gases such as cyanide. It is generally advised to delay returning to the explosion site until the following day, although fumes may still persist if airflow is sluggish.

Radon

Radon is a radioactive gas that can cause lung cancer. While certain caving regions and caves have elevated levels of radon, mine explorers are at particular risk. In the UK, concentrations are particularly high in granite. The gas is heavier than air and will concentrate in pockets just above the floor or water level, particularly when ventilation is poor or the atmospheric pressure is low. While probably not a great risk to the recreational caver, it makes sense to avoid frequent visits to higher-risk places. Choose mines with more than one entrance and try to avoid blind headings and shafts where the air is stale (themselves a risk for other noxious gases). Individuals who spend hundreds of hours per year underground (e.g. cave guides) should consider carrying a dosemeter to limit annual exposure to below 1×10^6 Bq/m³/h.

Decompression illness

(See → p. 774–777.)

Cave divers are at risk from decompression sickness, particularly after prolonged trips in cold water.

Follow the advice in → Chapter 24, with the following caveats:

- Do not allow casualty to exert/self-extricate without input from a specialist dive doctor, due to the risk of gas embolism.
- Give analgesia only under the advice of a specialist dive doctor. Entonox, widely used by cave rescue teams, is contraindicated within 24 h of diving, whether or not the diver shows signs of decompression illness. Methoxyflurane (Penthrox®) is safe.

- There will be a lower threshold for 'in-water recompression', although it remains a last resort due to the many risks involved (➲ p. 777).

Acute coronary syndrome

(See ➲ p. 393.)

Given the energetic nature of the sport, acute coronary syndrome is not that uncommon. Casualties should be stretcher evacuated if possible. If this is impossible, consider beta-blockers to limit HR, together with the usual pre-hospital treatment.

Cardiopulmonary resuscitation and recognition of life extinct (ROLE) underground

CPR will be futile in almost all underground situations. Nevertheless, the default should be to attempt it:
- *Start resuscitation.* Unless:
  - Any injuries incompatible with life.
  - Cardiac arrest >15 min with no bystander CPR.
  - Apparent death due to hypothermia (➲ p. 654–657).
  - Not possible, unsafe, or unable to maintain.
  - Submersion >30 min (60 min for very cold water—a further 30 min if young or small).
- *Stop after 20 min.* Unless:
  - The resources to deal with potential causes (e.g. O$_2$, fluids, defibrillator, needle thoracotomy, adrenaline, etc), beyond those currently on-scene, are imminently forthcoming.
- *Do not attempt extrication during resuscitation.* Unless:
  - Effective CPR can be maintained (unlikely, unless mechanical device available), *and/or*
  - Exit will be quick, *and*
  - Exit will significantly speed access to the above resources (unlikely on expedition).

If death is uncertain, the casualty should be evacuated promptly as if alive, with regular reassessment. If death is later confirmed during evacuation, the rescue can then be handled as a body recovery.

Medical considerations during a rescue

Medics treating casualties underground will inevitably be involved with the rescue process. While it is beyond the scope of this chapter to discuss rescue techniques, appreciation of the impact of the rescue process on casualty care, and vice versa, is important.

Considerations for the medical team

- Being wet and moving slowly, with little chance of reprieve, you will likely get cold and hungry. Take food and consider additional dry clothing.
- Accept that with limited resources ± skills and support, there may be little you can do. Very sick casualties may die.
- Consider scene safety. Casualties at the base of pitches will be at risk of rocks dislodged by members of the rescue team rigging haul lines above. Move casualties free of danger or set up a tarp.
- Establish communications with the surface early, where possible.

Casualty management at the scene of the incident

- Assume all casualties are cold (➔ Hypothermia, p. 654–657), hungry, and dehydrated, and physically and emotionally exhausted.
- Think ahead regarding resources that may need to be replenished, as it will take time to deliver them. The demand for O_2, especially if used on high flow, may put an unacceptable strain on the rescue effort (a portable 2 L bottle will only last 30–45 min). There is little role for it outside of formal rescue teams and diving expeditions.
- While a period of in-cave 'hospitalization' to stabilize the casualty may be possible, for most sick casualties the best management is to extricate urgently.

Packaging the casualty into a stretcher

- Use a vapour barrier if clothes are wet. Place heat packs inside (if using) and layer additional insulation on top. A Blizzard® bag will perform all these roles.
- Plan for the casualty's need to micturate—consider a portable urine bottle or incontinence pad.
- Provide protective goggles.
- Caving helmets with rear-mounted battery packs will cause the neck to flex forward, potentially creating airway issues. Replace with a lower profile alternative or, if using a SLIX stretcher (which wraps up around the head), remove it altogether.

The extrication process

The route and mode of extrication should be agreed with both the rigging team leader and those in overall command of the rescue. If the cave needs widening to allow for safe extrication, this needs to be communicated as soon as possible.

Self- or assisted extrication is greatly preferred over a stretcher rescue, due to the difficulty and labour intensive nature of the latter. Both methods present potential risks to the casualty, particularly if rescue needs to be expedited (e.g. if time-critical injuries or flood risk).

Considerations for self-extrication

- May exacerbate the casualty's condition (e.g. acute coronary syndrome, hypothermia, injury).
- May precipitate further injury (e.g. if unstable on feet or altered consciousness from head injury or analgesia/sedation). Keep the casualty under very close supervision.

Considerations for a stretcher extrication

- *Monitoring issues:* a well-packaged casualty may deteriorate unnoticed in a busy rescue scenario. Keep them talking, if/when formal observations are impractical. Ensure the stretcher is chaperoned during hauls.
- *Thromboprophylaxis:* consider this if the casualty is immobilized for >12 h.
- *Risks to the casualty in the prone position:*
  - Motion sickness and increased aspiration risk; consider a prophylactic antiemetic and, if reduced consciousness, an airway adjunct.
  - Exacerbation of any breathing difficulties, e.g. due to chest injury.
  - A head-down tilt will increase intracranial pressure. Avoid in casualties with severe head injuries (ideally they should be tilted 20–30° head up).
- *Risks to the casualty when hauling in the vertical position:*
  - Orthostatic effects, with risk of suspension syncope (⏵ p. 838). This is more likely in stretchers without in-built foot stirrups or end plates, and in shocked or unconscious casualties. Use for brief periods, only where the cave dimensions dictate or where it would speed extrication for a time-critical casualty. Employ rigging that is easy to release in case of mishap.
  - Helmets straps can strangle the casualty: if using, undo chin strap.
  - Airway may be compromised if airway unprotected and head allowed to slump forward.
  - Pressure is applied to legs, pelvis, abdomen, or chest, potentially exacerbating injury or restricting breathing.
  - Cervical spine issues (see following section).

Cervical spine injuries

(See ⏵ p. 218–221.)

If a cervical spine cannot be cleared via NEXUS rules, a degree of motion restriction is usually indicated, owing to the rough nature of cave rescues. Even so, the evidence for such measures is weak. Given they will likely increase the complexity and duration of extrication, their use must be balanced against any time-critical injuries (more likely in those with a significant cervical spine injury) and the safety of the rescue team.

- Tape and head blocks, or a vacuum mattress, are the most suitable methods, though the latter are heavy and vulnerable to destruction underground.
- Semi-rigid collars are less appropriate. Cave rescues are prolonged and rough, the casualty often unmonitored, and the collar often poorly applied, amplifying their risks: discomfort, worsening spinal cord injury, aspiration risk, raised intracranial pressure, and even strangulation.
- A semi-rigid collar could be used as a temporary extrication device for manoeuvring casualties through awkward spaces (although manual

in-line stabilization (MILS), if practical, will suffice), then loosened afterwards.
- A softer collar (e.g. foam roll mat, SAM® splint, vacuum limb splint) will protect against big neck movements during extrication (such as 'head bobbing' on vertical hauls if/when head tape migrates) and may help the casualty achieve a position of comfort.
- A degree of neck movement may be inevitable, or even necessary. Fortunately, physiological movements post injury are generally thought to be insufficient to cause further cord damage. Also, conscious casualties will protect their own neck through muscle spasm and (as with any broken bone) a natural reluctance to move out of a position of comfort.
- A mobile, fully conscious casualty could self-extricate, if under close supervision and the risk of further injury (fall, slip, etc.) is low.

Minor ailments on caving expeditions

Common preventable issues that impact the productivity of expeditions.

Gastroenteritis

(See ➔ Caring for people in the field, Chapter 3.)

A dirty environment, limited toilet facilities, close proximity to others, and scarce surface water for cleaning body parts and cooking equipment means that gastroenteritis is a distinct possibility on caving expeditions. Close attention to hygiene is paramount.

Skin problems

Less clothing tends to be worn on expeditions to tropical areas. Cuts and abrasions are therefore common (especially on hands) and, for the reasons explained above, prone to infection. Broken skin also provides a port of entry for cave diseases (➔ p. 848–849).

Foot issues

Painful sores and blisters are common, resulting from prolonged activity in wet, suboptimal footwear. Continually wet feet may become macerated and blanched, with wrinkling of the soles, rendering them yet more susceptible to the effects of friction. Progression to more serious forms of 'immersion foot' is rare (➔ p. 666–667), but it makes sense to take a break from caving if feet don't respond to standard foot care (frequent exposure to air ± cleaning).

Wetsuit issues

Prolonged wetsuit use, particularly when much of the trip is spent in dry passages, can lead to chafed and macerated skin. Vaseline®, or a water-repellent barrier cream, can be applied pre-emptively. Avoid urinating in the wetsuit!

Zoonoses, bites, and stings

American trypanosomiasis (Chagas'disease)

(See ➔ p. 524–525.)

Triatomine bugs have been found residing in caves of Latin America, where the primary hosts are bats and other cave-dwelling mammals.

Escherichia coli 0157/STEC (Shiga toxin-producing *E. coli*)

Found in the faeces of many animals (especially cattle, sheep, and goats), and transmitted faeco-orally, this is a rare but potential risk worldwide in wet caves downhill from farms. Symptoms vary from mild diarrhoea to haemorrhagic colitis. There is a 5% risk of developing life-threatening haemolytic uraemic syndrome (15% risk in children <10 years). Treatment is supportive.

Histoplasmosis ('Spelunker's lung')

A fungal infection causing respiratory illness, inhaled from bats' droppings. It is endemic to various regions worldwide. Visiting cavers from non-endemic regions are at particular risk. It is not readily diagnosable in the field. Most are clinically silent, or mild, and do not require treatment, but those with symptoms of pneumonia not responding to antibiotics would merit evacuation to hospital for assessment. Treatment, if merited, would be with antifungal medication. Avoid disturbing bat guano in endemic countries and be wary of confined passages where bat guano is present.

Leishmaniasis

(See ➔ p. 522–523.)

Transmitted by sandflies, sometimes present in the near reaches of caves (especially if home to rodents or other mammals).

Leptospirosis

(See ➔ p. 503.)

Notorious among cavers, leptospirosis is a potential risk in wet caves downhill from farms and is especially prevalent in tropical and subtropical areas after flooding/rains. It is a particular risk to cavers in the latter regions owing to an inclination to wear less protective clothing. Early infection in these areas will be difficult to distinguish from other tropical illnesses such as malaria, dengue, typhoid, and viral hepatitis. Elsewhere, it seems cavers are much less at risk. In the UK for example, no indigenously acquired caving-related cases have been reported since the mid-1990s. However, underdiagnosis ± under-reporting is likely. The advice in at-risk caves is to wear suitable protective clothing and cover cuts, scratches, and sores with a waterproof plaster. Avoid drinking the water and minimize immersion/submersion. Wash promptly after caving and thoroughly clean any cuts or abrasions received. If infection is suspected, treat promptly due the risk of progression to more severe illness (Weil's disease).

Marburg virus disease

(See ➔ p. 496.)

A frequently fatal infection transmitted by Egyptian fruit bats in central Africa. Outbreaks are usually associated with visits to caves and mines in which large colonies reside, although exact mode of transmission remains unclear. One possibility is via urine and faeces, typically released on or shortly after takeoff when the bats are disturbed; wear protective clothing, including gloves, masks, and eye wear.

Melioidosis

(See ➔ p. 504–505.)

While sporadic cases can occur in a number of (mainly developing) regions worldwide, it is endemic in SE Asia and northern Australia, and is especially prevalent in NE Thailand. Take precautions in water bearing caves, and caves that are currently dry but are prone to flood events, especially if digging (the bacteria can survive in the soil for up to 16 years).

Rabies

(See ➔ p. 490–492.)

Although rabies is often transmitted by bats, cavers do not seem to be at particular risk of bat bites; of the ~30 possible bat-related cases in the US between 1997 and 2017, only one was attributed to bat contact underground (although no bite or scratch was reported, and rabies virus and antigen were undetectable). An exception would be if caving (and especially camping) in the caves of central and northern South America, where vampire bats reside. Immunize as per usual travel recommendations but treat *all* bat bites (often felt rather than seen) as potential rabies exposure, regardless of country. Seek immediate medical attention.

Tick-borne relapsing fever

Caused by several *Borrelia* spirochaete and transmitted by different *Ornithodoros* (soft-bodied) ticks. Cave dwelling species are prevalent in the southwestern US states, as well as in the sweep of drier terrain spreading east from the eastern Mediterranean coast into central Asia. In Israel, where it is known as 'cave disease', it is estimated that 30–60% of caves are infested. The ticks feed at night, and a red bite mark may be the only evidence you've been bitten. Symptoms (after a ~7-day incubation period) include an intermittent fever (~3-day duration, every ~7 days) associated with headaches and myalgia ± GI upset, arthralgia, and confusion. Hepatosplenomegaly and jaundice are possible, but the disease is rarely fatal and complications are rare. Treatment is with tetracyclines, but in >50% of individuals precipitates the temporary but severe 'Jarisch–Herxheimer' reaction, with worsening of symptoms and possible hypotension and seizures.

Bites and stings

(See ➔ Chapter 17.)

Caves often play host to a number of animal species that can deliver nasty, or even deadly, bites and stings depending on the region visited. Be wary of spiders, scorpions, bees, wasps, and snakes in the entrances and entrance passages of caves, noting that on expeditions to warmer climes, less protective clothing tends to be worn.

Further reading

Ecole Francaise de Speleologie. *Caving Technical Guide* [English Edition]. Paris: Editions Gap; 2013.

French Federation of Speleology. *Cave Rescuer's Manual* [English Edition]. Lyon: French Federation of Speleology; 2005.

Merchant D. *Life on a Line*, 2nd ed. London: Lulu Enterprises; 2007. [Specialist cave rescue manual.] ℜ https://www.lifeonaline.com

National Cave Rescue School of CNSAS. *Cave Rescue Techniques* [English Edition]. 2015. Available as a free download: ℜ http://caverescue.eu/cave-rescue-techniques

Medical kits

Chapter editor
Jon Dallimore

Contributors
Alistair Cobb
Jon Dallimore
Robert Conway
Penelope B. Granger
Burjor K. Langdana
Daniel S. Morris

NB: this chapter suggests the type of drug supplies and equipment that would be suitable for a medium-sized climbing expedition spending 6 weeks in a remote area. The kit is compatible with the advice given within individual chapters of this book.

However, this list should not be regarded as definitive, nor do we endorse any individual manufacturer's products. Factors such as the nature of the expedition, the skills of the medics, and the ease of access to high-quality medical facilities, together with cost and weight will all affect the extent of medical kit.

Medical kits and supplies

It is never possible to deal with every conceivable injury or illness—even with a large amount of medical equipment. Items from medical kits are used most frequently for blisters, headaches, minor cuts and sprains, sunburn, diarrhoea, and insect bites. Similar illnesses and accidents occur on all expeditions, but clearly extra drugs and equipment may be needed to deal with problems in particular environments.

It is often difficult to judge how much medical equipment to take and this will depend on:

• The size of the party and how remote.
• The duration of the trip.
• The number of any outlying camps.
• Local medical facilities.
• The medical knowledge of the team members/medic.
• Communications with other camps.
• Ability to access remote medical help.

Obtaining supplies

Buying medical supplies from a retailer can be costly, and acquiring, packing, and labelling a medical kit can be time-consuming. GPs should not give NHS prescriptions for illnesses which may be acquired outside the UK, but will issue a private prescription in some circumstances.

In some parts of the world, prescription drugs are available over the counter but they may be counterfeit and the quality cannot be guaranteed.

Drug export

Expeditions carrying reasonable quantities of drugs are unlikely to encounter problems at customs when entering a country. However, it may be useful to have a doctor's letter stating that the drugs are for the personal use of the expedition team members and are not the subject of any commercial transaction.

Controlled drugs

Wherever possible, avoid taking 'controlled' drugs. A Home Office licence is required and must be returned within 28 days of return to the UK. (For more details see: ℅ www.gov.uk/controlled-drugs-licences-fees-and-returns.) Any controlled drugs dispensed should be recorded in a controlled drugs register.

Be aware that drugs that are freely available in one country may be controlled or prescribed in another.

Storage and transport

• Where possible, avoid liquid medicines because of bulk and weight.
• Obtain tablets in blister packs—loose-packed tablets can disintegrate during the rigours of an expedition.
• Avoid splitting the medical kit between several team members—it is better to keep the first-aid and medical supplies together.

- Wrap the whole kit in waterproof/dustproof packaging (e.g. re-sealable polythene bags or in plastic boxes) (➲ Colour plate 24).
- Try to pack items which are used together in the same box, e.g. cotton buds, fluorescein strips, tetracaine, and chloramphenicol ointment for eye problems.
- Label each box with a laminated, waterproof list of its contents on the lid. If the kit is marked with a large red cross it may attract attention and be a target for thieves—medical supplies are very valuable in many parts of the world.
- Detailed instructions should be provided with each medical kit.
- A small personal medical kit should be carried by each expedition member at all times.

Personal medical kit

Each team member should carry a small supply of first-aid equipment for their own personal use. This should be kept in a compact waterproof and re-sealable container or bag.

- Paracetamol or preferred painkiller.
- Adhesive plasters.
- Antiseptic wipes.
- Blister kit.
- A non-sedating antihistamine.
- Insect repellent.
- Sunblock cream.
- Water purification tablets.
- Rehydration sachets.

In addition, team members should carry sufficient personal medication for the duration of the trip, including antimalarials.

Team medical kit

Table 28.1 indicates the types of drugs and equipment that a group of 20 people on a 6-week high-altitude mountaineering expedition might wish to assemble. However, this list should only be regarded as indicative of the sort of kit required which may vary according to the exact nature of the work, the logistics available, and the skills of the medics.

In this text, our treatment recommendations have been restricted to a relatively limited range of drugs and equipment that we feel most medics could use with reasonable safety. It is likely that a specialist in a particular area of medicine would want to take additional materials and more specialist kit (➲ p. 862–863).

Table 28.1 Drugs and equipment list

	Amounts
Antimicrobials	
Azithromycin 500 mg	20 tablets
Ceftriaxone for injection 2 g	5 ampoules
Chloramphenicol (eye) ointment 1%	3 × 4 g
Clarithromycin 250 mg	40 tablets
Co-amoxiclav 250/125	84 tablets
Doxycycline 100 mg	56 capsules
Fluconazole 150 mg	4 tablets
Gentamicin with hydrocortisone (ear drops)	10 mL × 4
Mebendazole 100 mg	20 tablets
Metronidazole 400 mg	96 tablets
Metronidazole suppositories 1 g	10
Valaciclovir 500 mg	10 tablets
Riamet® malaria treatment pack	2
Rabies vaccine 1 mL (lyophilized)	2
Painkillers, local anaesthetics/sedatives	
Aspirin 300 mg	32 tablets
Bupivacaine 0.5% injection	10 mL ×5
Co-codamol 30/500	56 tablets
Diclofenac 50 mg	56 tablets
Diclofenac 100 mg suppositories	5
Ibuprofen 400 mg	84 tablets
GTN spray	1
Ketamine for injection (50 mg/mL)	2 vials
Lidocaine 1% for injection	5 mL × 10

Table 28.1 (Contd.)

	Amounts
Lidocaine 5% gel	2 tubes
Lorazepam for injection 2 mg	5 ampoules
Midazolam for injection (10 mg/5 mL)	5 ampoules
Paracetamol 500 mg	100 tablets
Penthrox® inhaler (methoxyflurane)	2
Tetracaine (amethocaine) eye drops	6 minims
Gastrointestinal	
Antacid tablets	100 tablets
Bisacodyl 5 mg	60 tablets
GlucoGel® 75 g	4 ampoules
Loperamide 2 mg	50 capsules
Prochlorperazine 3 mg buccal tablets	16 tablets
Prochlorperazine 5 mg	56 tablets
Omeprazole 20 mg	56 tablets
Ondansetron 4 mg	10 tablets
Oral rehydration solution sachets	40 sachets
Prochlorperazine injection 12.5 mg	5 ampoules
Prochlorperazine suppositories 25 mg	10
Cardiovascular	
Atropine for injection 600 micrograms	5 ampoules
Bisoprolol 5 mg	20 tablets
Furosemide 40 mg	28 tablets
Respiratory/allergy	
Adrenaline (epinephrine) 1:1000	5 × 1 mL
Beclometasone inhaler 100 micrograms	2
Chlorphenamine 4 mg	40 tablets
Chlorphenamine injection 10 mg	5 ampoules
Emerade® adrenaline auto-injector 500 micrograms	2
Hydrocortisone injection 100 mg	10 ampoules
Prednisolone 5 mg	112 tablets
Salbutamol CFC free inhaler 100 micrograms/actuation	2
Sodium cromoglicate eye drops 20 mg/mL 10 mL	2
Spacer device	1

(Continued)

Table 28.1 (*Contd.*)

	Amounts
Altitude	
Acetazolamide 250 mg	100 tablets
Dexamethasone 2 mg	40 tablets
Dexamethasone for injection 3.3 mg/mL, 1 mL ampoules	5
Nifedipine MR caps 10 mg	20 capsules
EmOx® (chemical oxygen)	1 set
Portable altitude chamber	1
Creams and ointments	
Aciclovir cream	2g × 6
Aqueous cream	50 tube
Clotrimazole cream	20 × 6
Haemorrhoid cream	1
Hydrocortisone cream 1%	30 × 4
Mupirocin cream	15 × 6
Silver nitrate cautery sticks	5
Terbinafine 1% cream	30g × 4
Topical steroid/antibiotic ear drops	10mL × 4
Tropicamide 1%	5 minims
Airway care—for appropriately trained individuals	
Oropharyngeal airways, sizes 2, 3, 4	2 of each
Nasopharyngeal airway, sizes 5, 6	2
Bag-valve mask apparatus	1
Insertion bougie for endotracheal tubes	1
Endotracheal tube 6 mm for tracheostomy	1
Endotracheal tubes 7, 8 mm	2 of each
i-gel™ sizes 3, 4, 5	2 of each
Catheter mounts for above	2
Handheld suction unit	1
Laryngoscope	1
Oxygen cylinder	1
Oxygen tubing	1
Pulse oximeter	1
Major trauma	
Bladder syringe 50 mL	2
Blizzard® blanket	1
Catheter bag and tubing	2

Table 28.1 (Contd.)

	Amounts
Chest drain 32 F	2
Combat application tourniquet	2
Disposable scalpels	2
Heimlich valve	2
Kendrick traction device	1
Nasogastric tube 12 F	2
Needle holder	1
Haemostatic gauze/sponges	Pack of 5
Safety pins	12
Sam splint (R)	2
Scissors for dressings	1
Skin staples and remover	1
Sutures:	4
2/0 silk straight	5
4/0 non-absorbable suture	5
5/0 non-absorbable suture	
Tissue glue	1
Toothed forceps	1
Tranexamic acid 100 mg/mL, 5 mL ampoules	5
Tuff Cut® scissors	1
Urinary catheter 14 F	2
Examination / other	
Alcohol gel	250 mL
Automatic sphygmomanometer	1
Blood glucose monitoring equipment	1
Dental first aid kit (➲ p. 864–865)	1
Facemasks	1 box
Fluorescein eye test strips	10
Gloves sterile (medium)	10 pairs
Clinical gloves (non-sterile)	100
Head torch, pen torch	1
Malaria immunochromatographic test	1
Sterile saline sachets	20
Stethoscope	1
Thermometer (digital)	1
Thermometer (low reading)	1

(Continued)

Table 28.1 (Contd.)

	Amounts
Tick remover	2
Tongue depressors	1 box
Urine pregnancy kit	2
Waterproof paper and pencils	1
Dressings	
Adhesive plasters	50 assorted
Alcohol swabs	100 × 2
Burn dressings 10 × 10cm	5
Crepe bandages 5 cm	5
Gauze swabs 5 cm²	100
Non-adherent dressing 5 cm²	5
Non-adherent dressing 10 cm²	5
Hypoallergenic tape 2.5 cm	2 rolls
Steri-Strips™, assorted	4 packets
Triangular bandages	8
Tubigrip (knee/ankle)	10 of each
Paraffin gauze 10 cm²	10
Cling wrap	1 roll
Zinc oxide tape	2 rolls
Injection equipment and intravenous fluids	
2 mL, 5 mL, 10 mL syringes	20 of each
1 mL insulin syringes (for rabies intradermal injection)	5
Blue, green, orange needles	20 of each
IV cannulae 14 G, 18 G	10 of each
Giving sets	5
Glucose 5%	500 mL × 4
Hartmann's solution 1 L	1000 mL × 3
Normal saline 1 L	1000 mL × 3
Sharps box	1

Reference texts

This handbook is available in a digital as well as a printed version. An up-to-date *BNF* or other pharmacopoeia should be carried at all times—to check drug doses, side effects, and contraindications. Digital drug guides such as the *BNF* app or *Epocrates* app can reduce the need for a relatively heavy book—although rely upon a charged and functioning phone or tablet. Also see: ℛ http://www.bnf.org/bnf/index.htm

Specialist equipment

The use of these items requires special training and so will depend on the medical skills in the group:

- Stethoscope.
- Anaeroid sphygmomanometer.
- Auriscope/ophthalmoscope.
- Oropharyngeal/nasopharyngeal airways.
- i-gel™ supraglottic airways.
- Endotracheal tubes.
- Portable capnograph.
- Nasogastric tube.
- Urinary catheter.
- Portable ultrasound.
- Chest drains and Heimlich valves for pneumothorax.
- Suturing equipment.
- Dental forceps, if skilled.
- Snake (or other) antivenom.

Extra drugs and equipment for special environments

Malaria medication

(See ➔ p. 64, 517–520.) Take spare prophylactic antimalarials if the expedition is going to a region where malaria is endemic—someone always loses their tablets! Also take a different and appropriate drug for standby (prospective) treatment of a fever that could be malaria (e.g. Riamet® (coartemether) or Malarone® (atovaquone–proguanil)). Rapid diagnostic tests for malaria can be very useful (➔ p. 514). Mosquito nets should be retreated with permethrin every 3–6 months (depending on the amount of rain and UV exposure); always carry spare permethrin together with protective gloves.

Sailing, boating, or canoeing

(See ➔ Chapters 22 and 23.) Participants develop chapped hands, salt water boils, and sunburn. Lanolin-based hand cream is useful and cinnarizine is recommended for seasickness.

Grab bag

A specific medical kit to be taken to the life raft if abandoning ship that may also double as an emergency treatment bag should contain:

- Emergency analgesics (oral and IM).
- Seasickness medications (a large stock and including drugs that can be absorbed by routes other than oral).
- Broad-spectrum antibiotics.
- Rehydration salts.
- Suturing kit.
- Immobilization splints, strapping, bandages.

Tropical areas

(See ➔ Chapter 26.) Wound infections are common, and small individual iodine tincture bottles are recommended to clean wounds plus additional topical antibiotics. Antivenoms for snakes, scorpions, etc. may be considered for high-risk areas and occupations plus several long 10 cm-wide crepe bandages for pressure pad immobilization (➔ p. 584–585).

Diving expeditions

(See ➔ Chapter 24.) Otitis externa (diver's ear) is common; take extra antibacterial eardrops (e.g. gentamicin with hydrocortisone) and consider aluminium acetate or distilled water after each dive. Oxygen, chest drains, and ventilation equipment may be needed. Find out where decompression facilities exist before you need them! Consider additional antibiotics for marine wound infections.

Mountain expeditions

(See ➔ Chapter 21.) Oxygen is bulky and heavy but is essential for any trip above 6000 m. EmOx® is used by some groups—chemical oxygen from the reaction of percarbonate, manganese dioxide, and water. Acetazolamide, nifedipine, and dexamethasone should certainly be carried. Consider a femoral traction device for thigh fractures as these can be life-saving in remote areas—they are lightweight (~500 g) and are very popular with mountain rescue teams. Pelvic binders can be improvised but specialized equipment such as the Sam Sling® are relatively cheap and effective.

Desert environments

(See ⊋ Chapter 25.) Dehydration and heat-related illnesses are of major concern. Strongly consider IV fluids and plenty of cannulae and giving sets. Total block sun cream and goggles to keep sand out of eyes are recommended.

Extra materials for those with special skills

Ocular first-aid kit

The first-aid kit listed here is lightweight and will fit into a small pouch.

Equipment
- Pentorch and blue filter.
- Pocket ophthalmoscope.
- Magnifying loupe.
- Eye pads.
- Eye shield.
- Surgical tape.
- pH paper.
- Minor operations kit.
- Single use drops ('Minims'™):
  - Tetracaine (amethocaine)/benoxinate (topical anaesthetic).
  - Fluorescein 1% (use only after topical anaesthetic for corneal staining).
  - Cyclopentolate 1% (pupil dilation and pain relief).
  - Artificial tears (dry eyes and snow blindness).
  - Tropicamide 1% (for pupil dilation).
  - Pilocarpine 2% (for reversal of pupil dilation by tropicamide).

Other topical medication:
- Antibiotic ointment and drops, e.g. chloramphenicol (conjunctivitis, any minor infection, or snow blindness).
- Ofloxacin (reserve for more serious corneal infection and all contact lens-related infection).
- Sodium cromoglicate (allergic conjunctivitis).
- Fluorometholone (mild steroid; use cautiously in snow blindness).
- These drops are given four times daily except ofloxacin, which can be given hourly for serious corneal infection.
- Remember: oral analgesia is required for a painful eye.

Useful equipment and drugs for ENT problems

- Head torch.
- Forceps.
- Nasal tampons such as Rapid Rhino®.
- Gentamicin with hydrocortisone drops.
- Amoxicillin.
- Silver nitrate sticks for nasal cautery.

Remote dentistry kit list

Suppliers: The Dental Directory, 6 Perry Way, Witham, Essex, CM8 3SX, UK. Tel: 01376 391 100; 0800 585 586. ℅ www.dental-directory.co.uk

Some items may well be duplicated within your standard medical kit.

Instruments (sterile disposable kits available which come with their own tray):

- Two dental mirrors (size 3) (a bent spoon serves as an excellent intraoral retractor).
- One flat-plastic (a stainless steel instrument for placing dental filling material onto tooth).
- College tweezers.
- Spoon excavator (medium)—for scraping out soft caries.
- Spencer Wells suturing forceps.
- Fine curved surgical scissors.
- One double-ended stainless steel cement mixing spatula.
- One glazed mixing paper pad for mixing and moulding temporary filling materials.
- Disposable scalpel (number 15 blade).
- Cold sterilization tablets.

Medicaments

- Temporary filling materials—glass ionomer powder + liquid and either intermediate restorative material or Cavit™ or Coltosol™.
- Chlorhexidine 0.2% mouthwash or 1% Corsodyl® gel.
- Duraphat® (high-fluoride varnish).
- Ledermix® paste.
- Antibiotics—co-amoxiclav 500/125 mg, metronidazole 400 mg, and clindamycin 150 mg.
- Painkillers—ibuprofen, paracetamol, codeine-phosphate.
- Dental LA cartridges—2% lidocaine with 1:80,000 adrenaline (epinephrine) or articaine 4% with 1:100,000 adrenaline.
- Eugenol (oil of cloves) topical analgesic.

Others

- Sterile gloves.
- Cotton wool rolls.
- 3/0 black silk or Vicryl® suture on fine semilunar needle.
- Stainless steel wire for eyelet wiring (24 G for eyelets, 26 G for ligatures) or electrical cord for harvesting copper wire.
- Dental cartridge syringe—27 G long (can be used in upper and lower jaw).
- 5 mL syringe with blunt needles (for irrigation and flushing out debris below operculum).
- Nasal clip from face masks (five)—can be used as dental splints.
- Head torch + spare batteries.
- Gas aerosol suitable for camera cleaning—ideal for drying teeth and cavities.

Optional equipment (if gained experienced in their use)

- Upper single root extraction forceps.
- Upper molar extraction forceps left and right.
- Lower molar extraction forceps.
- Lower single root extraction forceps.
- Medium Luxator® or elevator—Coupland's chisel size 2.

Index

For the benefit of digital users, indexed terms that span two pages (e.g., 52–53) may, on occasion, appear on only one of those pages.

Tables, figures, and boxes are indicated by *t*, *f*, and *b* following the page number